ADVANCES IN PROSTAGLANDIN, THROMBOXANE,
AND LEUKOTRIENE RESEARCH
VOLUME 23

Prostaglandins and Related Compounds
Ninth International Conference
Florence, Italy

Advances in Prostaglandin, Thromboxane, and Leukotriene Research

Series Editors: Bengt Samuelsson and Rodolfo Paoletti

Volumes not listed are out of print.

Advances in Prostaglandin, Thromboxane,
and Leukotriene Research
Volume 23

Prostaglandins and Related Compounds
Ninth International Conference
Florence, Italy

Editors

Bengt Samuelsson, M.D.
*Department of Medical Biochemistry
and Biophysics (MBB)
Division of Physiological Chemistry
Karolinska Institute
Stockholm, Sweden*

Peter W. Ramwell, Ph.D.
*Department of Physiology and
Biophysics
Georgetown University Medical Center
Washington, D.C., U.S.A.*

Rodolfo Paoletti, M.D.
*Institute of Pharmacological Sciences
University of Milan
Milan, Italy*

Giancarlo Folco, Ph.D.
*Institute of Pharmacological Sciences
University of Milan
Milan, Italy*

Elisabeth Granström, M.D.
*Department of Woman and Child
Health
Division of Reproductive
Endocrinology
Karolinska Hospital
Stockholm, Sweden*

Simonetta Nicosia, Ph.D.
*Institute of Pharmacological Sciences
University of Milan
Milan, Italy*

Raven Press **New York**

Raven Press, 1185 Avenue of the Americas, New York, New York 10036

Made in the United States of America

International Standard Book Number 0–7817–0238–0
Library of Congress Catalog Card Number 83—645438

9 8 7 6 5 4 3 2 1

Preface

The Ninth International Conference on Prostaglandins and Related Compounds was held at Palazzo dei Congressi in Florence, Italy on June 6–10, 1994. This volume contains most of the papers presented orally during the conference.

The eicosanoid field is still developing rapidly. Significant progress is being made in both basic and applied areas. Studies of the molecular biology of the enzymes involved in the formation of various oxygenated products of arachidonic acid and other polyunsaturated fatty acids have generated new knowledge that can be applied in many different areas. It serves as a basis for understanding the regulation of eicosanoid formation and the role of the various derivatives of arachidonic acid in both normal physiology and disease processes. The new knowledge about the enzymes also plays a key role in the development of drugs. This is particularly noteworthy with respect to the new inducible cyclooxygenase-2.

Considerable progress was also reported in the area of eicosanoid receptors during the conference and a special session on receptor nomenclature was held. There was considerable coverage of areas such as cardiovascular and renal systems, inflammation, immunology, and the respiratory system. Other sessions dealt with blood cells and vascular wall, cell differentiation and proliferation, isoprostanes, PAF, nitric oxide, and cytochrome P450.

A special session was devoted to development of drugs where the use of leukotriene antagonists and biosynthesis inhibitors in the treatment of human bronchial asthma and other human diseases was discussed. In addition, this session included work on the development of specific cyclooxygenase-2 inhibitors and the use of prostaglandins in fertility control and as ocular hypotensive agents.

The Editors

Acknowledgments

We express our gratitude to Dr. Emanuela Folco and her associates of the Fondazione Giovanni Lorenzini for their important work in connection with the conference. We are also grateful to the local organizing committee, the international program committee, and the international advisory committee for their valuable contributions. It is a pleasure to acknowledge the generous financial support of a number of pharmaceutical companies.

We also thank the authors for their prompt submission of the papers which has made the rapid publication of this volume possible.

Contents

Phospholipases

Cyclooxygenase Pathways

Lipoxygenase Pathways

Cytochrome P450 and Other Oxygenase Products

Isoprostanes

Receptors

Immunology

Inflammation

Respiratory System

Cardiovascular and Renal System

Blood Cells and Vascular Wall

Cell Differentiation and Proliferation

Platelet Activating Factor

Nitric Oxide

Round Table on Advances in Ocular Prostaglandin Research

Round Table on Use of PGE_1 in Erectile Dysfunction

Contributors

ADVANCES IN PROSTAGLANDIN, THROMBOXANE,
AND LEUKOTRIENE RESEARCH
VOLUME 23

Prostaglandins and Related Compounds
Ninth International Conference
Florence, Italy

Advances in Prostaglandin, Thromboxane, and Leukotriene Research, Vol. 23,
edited by B. Samuelsson et al.
Raven Press, Ltd., New York © 1995

5-Lipoxygenase: structure and stability of recombinant enzyme, regulation in Mono Mac 6 cells.

Olof Rådmark+, Ying-Yi Zhang+, Tove Hammarberg+, Birger Lind#, Mats Hamberg+, Martina Brungs*, Dieter Steinhilber*, and Bengt Samuelsson+

+*Dept. of Medical Biophysics and Biochemistry, and* #*Institute of Environmental Medicine, Karolinska Institutet, Stockholm, Sweden.* *Department of Pharmaceutical Chemistry, University of Tübingen, Auf der Morgenstelle 8, D-72076 Tübingen, F.R.G.*

Human 5-lipoxygenase (5LO) catalyzes the first two reactions in the conversion of arachidonic acid to leukotrienes (1), compounds with biological functions related to inflammation and hypersensitivity reactions. Iron is a cofactor necessary for activity of 5LO (2), and we have recently studied the amino acids functioning as ligands to iron in 5LO, by site directed mutagenesis of recombinant enzyme expressed in E. coli (3, 4). In conjunction with these studies, a method for stabilization of purified 5LO was developed (5). Regarding regulation of 5LO in leukocytes, transforming growth factor ß (TGFß) was found to increase 5LO activity in differentiating HL-60 cells (6). More recently, when the monocytic cell line Mono Mac 6 was treated with TGFß and vitamin D3 (VD3), profound effects on 5LO activity, and also on expression of 5LO protein, were obtained (7). This paper gives a summary of these studies.

LIGANDS TO IRON IN 5-LIPOXYGENASE

Soybean lipoxygenase was first shown to contain iron, and subsequently this was also demonstrated for mammalian lipoxygenases. The role for iron in the generally accepted scheme for the lipoxygenase reaction (the radical reaction mechanism), is to act as electron acceptor and donor, during hydrogen abstraction and peroxide formation. In this reaction mechanism, the lipoxygenase is first converted from the resting ferrous state to the ferric form. It then cycles between the ferric form and the substrate reduced ferrous form (8).

1

Heme or iron-sulfur clusters were not found in soybean lipoxygenase, and it was suggested that the iron should be bound directly to functional groups in the protein (9). Extended X-ray absorption fine structure analysis of soybean lipoxygenase indicated that the iron was bound by 4 ± 1 nitrogen ligands (imidazole) and 2 ± 1 oxygen ligands (10). The iron center is thought to be similar among the lipoxygenases, and six histidines are conserved in all cloned lipoxygenases. The involvement of histidine residues as iron ligands in lipoxygenase was thus strongly inferred, and the six conserved His were the initial targets in our mutagenesis studies of 5LO. There are also nine conserved Asp/Glu among the lipoxygenases, the functional importance of these residues in 5LO was also tested by mutagenesis. During this work, crystal structures for soybean lipoxygenase I were presented (11, 12), confirming the function of three of the conserved His as ligands. Those studies also gave additional suggestions regarding possible iron ligands in 5LO, the C-terminal Ile and Asn 554.

Site directed mutagenesis was followed by expression in E. coli, purification by ATP-agarose affinity chromatography, and analyses of iron content (graphite furnace atomic absorption spectrophotometry) and enzyme activity. For detailed methods, see (3, 4).

Table 1 summarizes the results. The mutated residues are divided in three groups. The first contains two of the conserved histidines, and the C-terminal isoleucine. When these amino acids were mutated, both iron and enzyme activity were lost. Thus, these residues are regarded as permanent ligands, existing in all forms of the enzyme that appear during the 5LO reaction cycle (see above). Each of them is

Table 1. Putative iron ligands in 5LO.

	Fe-content mol/mol	Enz. act. µmol/mg	
Nonmutated control	0.9	23	
Mutation			**Ligand status**
His 372 Gln	0	0	Yes
His 550 Gln	0	0	Yes
Ile 673 deleted	0	0	Yes
His 367 Gln/Asn/Ser	0.5/0.2/0.5	0/0/0	?
Glu 376 Gln	0.7	0	?
Asn 554 Gln/Asp	0.7/1	0/0.3	?
His 362 Gln	0.9	2	No
His 390 Gln	0.8	13	No
His 399 Gln	0.9	12	No

required to keep the iron in place.

The second group contains one of the conserved histidines (His 367), Glu 376 (one of the conserved acidic residues), and Asn 554. Mutations of these residues led to partial iron contents, but activity was lost. These results exclude that any of these residues should be a permanent ligand, but any of them could be a replacable ligand. Such a ligand should be temporarily replaced, for example by a reaction intermediate, during catalysis. It seems reasonable that a replacable ligand would not be obligatory to retain iron, but that it would be necessary for proper catalysis. In this group, His 367 seems most interesting. Thus, by EXAFS it was found that one of the His-ligands in the resting FeII form of soybean lipoxygenase was replaced by an oxygen ligand in the FeIII form (8). Other spectroscopic studies supported this concept (13). Two findings pointed out His367 as the replacable His. First, the corresponding His ligand in soybean lipoxygenase has a stereochemistry which is different from that of the other two His ligands (11). Second, His367 is the only conserved His in 5LO that was found not to be necessary for iron association, while it was necessary for enzyme activity (4, 14).

Regarding Asn554, an alternative function was suggested for the corresponding Asn in soybean lipoxygenase, where this residue is part of a network that stabilizes the iron centre by hydrogen bonds (11). It seems that our data are compatible with such a function for Asn554 in 5LO. Exchange of Asn to Gln may lead to a shift of the iron from its correct position, thus preventing catalysis.

The third group contains three of the conserved histidines. Mutants of these residues retained both iron and enzyme activity. Thus, none of these histidines appear to function as a ligand, permanent or replacable. However, these His appear important for proper folding or maintenance of stability (4).

Mutations regarding eight of the nine conserved Asp/Glu, gave mutants which retained partial activity. Therefore, these residues should not function as permanent ligands, and the mutants of these acidic residues (D166, D176, D229, D358, D473, D496, D502, and E504) were not subjected to purification and iron analysis.

In summary, our mutagenesis data, and the comparison to spectroscopic data and crystal structures of soybean lipoxygenase, together indicate four iron ligands in 5LO. These are His 372, His 550 and the C-terminal Ile as permanent ligands, and His 367 as a possible replacable ligand.

STABILIZATION OF PURIFIED 5-LIPOXYGENASE

A major obstacle encountered during studies of 5LO is the instability of the purified enzyme, which has hampered further structural and mechanistic studies. For stability tests, freshly purified 5LO (0.25-0.45 mg/ml) was mixed with various reagents. The activity of a sample at various time points was measured in aliquots, which were diluted 200-400 fold in the enzyme assay.

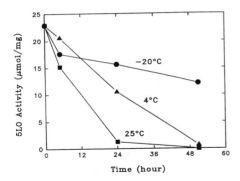

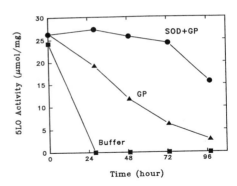

FIG. 1. Stability of 5LO at different temperatures.

FIG. 2. Stability of 5LO at 37°C in presence of GP, or GP plus SOD.

Protective effect of glutathione peroxidase and superoxide dismutase

Time courses of inactivation of purified 5LO are shown in Fig. 1. The enzyme lost 50% of its activity within 10 h at 25°C, and 24 hrs at 4°C. Loss of activity at -20°C was in part due to freezing and thawing, which caused 10 - 20% inactivation.

GP (150 ng/ml) extended the half inactivation time of 5LO to 36 hrs, activity still remained after 96 h (Fig 2). With higher concentration of GP (1.5 µg/ml), stabilization of 5LO was the same (Fig. 3). Even higher concentrations of GP gave an apparent lower protection, probably due to the interference of GP with the 5LO activity assay (15). Experiments in which GP was inactivated by heat treatment or inhibitors, clearly indicated that GP itself, and not a contaminant, protected 5LO.

Reductions catalyzed by GP require a hydrogen donor. In most experiments, 10 mM BME (present in the purified 5LO) was the hydrogen donor. The protective efficiencies of GP, in presence of BME, GSH, and DTT were compared. As shown in Fig. 4, the best protection was obtained with 1 mM BME. GSH was about half as efficient, and with DTT 5LO activity was lower than for the control (3.6 µmol/mg without addition of reducing agent).

The possibility that the declining protection by GP (Fig. 2) was due to GP itself being inactivated was considered. Glutathione peroxidase, in its active reduced form, can be inhibited by superoxide anion, and the inhibition can be prevented by SOD (16). Therefore, a combination of SOD and GP was investigated (Fig. 2). SOD alone did not protect 5LO, but SOD (1 µg/ml) together with GP (0.15 µg/ml) gave a persistent effect, the 5LO activity was almost constant for 3 days at 37°C.

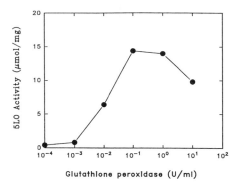

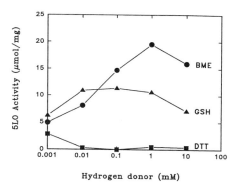

FIG. 3. 5LO protection by GP at various concentrations (1U= 1.5μg). At 37°C for 25h.

FIG. 4. 5LO protection by GP with different hydrogen donors. At 37°C for 25h.

Mechanism for inactivation and protection

The stabilizing effect of GP suggested that a hydroperoxide caused the inactivation of 5LO. However, no hydroxy fatty acids could be detected in a 5LO extract, and no polyunsaturated fatty acids were found in the E. coli cells from which recombinant 5LO was purified. Thus, inactivation of 5LO during storage was not caused by lipid hydroperoxide. Hydrogen peroxide is known to inactivate soybean lipoxygenase (17). Recently, also 5LO was found to be susceptible to hydrogen peroxide, and catalase protected purified 5LO against inactivation (18). Small amounts of hydrogen peroxide are probably sufficient for gradual inactivation of 5LO during storage. A two step reaction sequence could lead to formation of hydrogen peroxide in the 5LO solution. This would involve the initial reduction of molecular oxygen to superoxide by the reducing reagent added to the buffer, in presence of trace amounts of metal ions (19). Some of the superoxide anion could undergo slow spontaneous dismutation, to give hydrogen peroxide. It thus appears reasonable that the protective effect of GP was due to removal of hydrogen peroxide.

It has been suggested that the susceptibility of metalloproteins to hydrogen peroxide is due to generation of hydroxyl radical, at the site of the prosthetic metal ion, via a Fenton type reaction. The very reactive hydroxyl radical thus formed would immediately react with closely located amino acid residues, causing inactivation if the metal binding site coincides with the catalytic site.

REGULATION OF 5-LIPOXYGENASE IN MONO MAC 6 CELLS

Leukotrienes are produced by granulocytes, mast cells, monocytes and macrophages after stimulation, and the capacity for leukotriene biosynthesis of these cells is supposedly acquired during cell maturation. Transforming growth factor ß (TGFß) was found to upregulate 5LO in DMSO differentiated HL-60 cells (6), the most prominent effect was observed regarding the 5LO activity of intact cells.

Human monocytes and macrophages express 5LO mRNA and protein, while Mono Mac 6 cells, which have characteristics of mature monocytes, did not express detectable amounts of 5LO mRNA (20). To identify factors which induce 5LO activity during monocytic differentiation, we studied effects of TGFß and other differentiation promoters on the human monocytic cell line Mono Mac 6. A profound upregulation 5LO activity, and also of 5LO protein and mRNA, was obtained in cells treated with a combination of TGFß and vitamin D3 (VD3). Detailed descriptions of experiments are provided in ref 7.

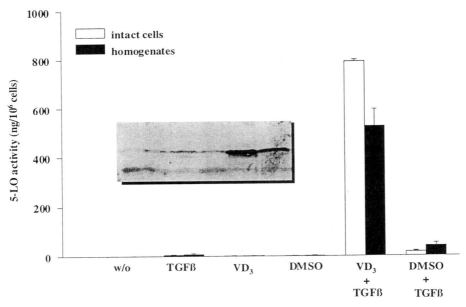

FIG. 5. Effects of TGFß, VD3 and DMSO on 5-LO activity and protein of Mono Mac 6 cells. Cells were grown without additives (lane 1), with TGFß (1 ng/ml), VD3 (50 nM), DMSO (1.2%), TGFß plus VD3, or TGFß plus DMSO. After 4 days, intact cells and homogenates were assayed for 5-LO activity. Mean + SE of three experiments. Aliquots of the same samples (corresponding to 4×10^5 cells) were analyzed for 5-LO protein by Western blot (insert, same order of samples).

Effects on 5LO activity

Mono Mac 6 cells were grown in the presence of TGFß (1 ng/ml), VD3 (50 nM), DMSO (1.2%) or combinations of these compounds. After 4 days, TGFß, VD3 or DMSO induced only low 5LO activities in intact cells and cell homogenates (fig. 5). For example, after culture with TGFß the activity in homogenate was 7 ng /10^6 cells. Combination of TGFß and VD3 strongly upregulated 5LO activity in intact cells and cell homogenates (791±7 and 524±70 ng /10^6 cells, n=3). Thus, increase of 5LO activity required presence of both VD3 and TGFß, either of these agents alone was almost ineffective. Also the combination of TGFß and DMSO gave a modest increase of 5LO activity, of both intact cells and homogenates (17±4 ng and 40±12 ng, n=3).

Effects on 5LO mRNA and protein

Total RNA was isolated, reverse transcribed and analyzed by PCR. 5LO mRNA was nearly undetectable in undifferentiated cells (fig. 6 left panel, lane 1), while clear bands were observed in samples from cells treated with TGFß, VD3 or DMSO (lanes 2-4). Combination of TGFß with VD3 lead to apparent induction of 5LO mRNA (lane 5), but also treatment with TGFß and DMSO lead to a stronger signal (lane 6) as compared to TGFß or DMSO alone.

The differences in 5LO mRNA expression were determined with competitive PCR. Samples from undifferentiated cells (fig. 6 right), from cells differentiated for 4 days with TGFß, or VD3 and TGFß, were analyzed. For undifferentiated cells, PCR products of similar intensities were obtained when cDNA corresponding to 100 ng of RNA was multiplied for 32 cycles together with 12 x 10^{-21} mole of internal standard. Assuming that the reverse transcriptions were equally efficient for the different samples, TGFß gave 8-fold increase of 5LO mRNA as compared to undifferentiated cells, while TGFß plus VD3 gave a 64-fold induction.

5LO protein expression was analyzed by Western Blot. No 5LO was detected in samples from untreated Mono Mac 6 cells, while small amounts were found in cells cultured with TGFß, VD3 or DMSO (fig 5 insert). As expected from 5LO activity determinations, combination of VD3 and TGFß gave a strong induction of 5LO protein. A prominent 5LO band was also observed in samples from cells differentiated with TGFß and DMSO.

Discrepancies between 5LO activity, mRNA and protein

The combination of TGFß and VD3 resulted in upregulation of 5LO activity, mRNA and protein. The effect on activity was most prominent, a 72-fold increase

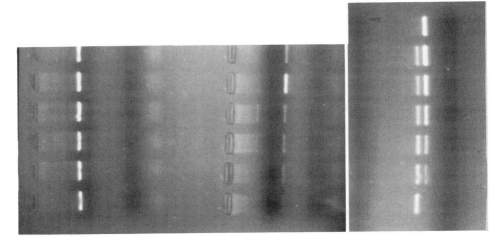

FIG. 6. Left. Mono Mac 6 cells were treated as in fig. 5. Total RNAs were subjected to reverse transcription-PCR for analysis of 5-LO mRNA. ß-Actin mRNA served as control. Bottom lane, without additives. Right. Competitive PCR analysis of 5-LO mRNA of undifferentiated Mono Mac 6 cells. Total RNA was extracted and transcribed into cDNA. Competitive PCR was performed (32 cycles) with defined amounts of internal standard pEMBL 5BS XL2. Lane 1 (bottom), standard only, 49×10^{-21} mole, Mono Mac cDNA (100 ng) plus 49, 24, 12, 6, 3 x 10^{-21} mole of standard, (lanes 2-6, respectively), cDNA only, 100 ng (lane 7, top).

in cells treated with TGFß plus VD3, as compared to cells which only received TGFß. At the same time, 5LO mRNA increased 8-fold, and 5LO protein 13-fold Comparisons indicate that TGFß and VD3 induces 5LO expression, and in addition leads to either a modification of the 5LO protein which increases its specific activity, or induces or modifies other cellular components of importance for 5LO activity.

Synergistic effects of TGFß and VD3 on leukemic cell lines have been described previously (21, 22). A number of differentiation related parameters were affected, and it was concluded that TGFß plus VD3 together stimulate the terminal differentiation of monocytic cells. It appears reasonable that the effects on 5LO are part of such a differentiation process.

We previously found that TGFß had an upregulatory effect, primarily on 5LO activity, when given to HL-60 cells together with DMSO. The combination of TGFß plus VD3 gave a more prominent upregulation of the activity in HL-60 cells, and also induced 5LO mRNA and protein, as shown in a paper by Steinhilber et al in this volume (23).

ACKNOWLEDGEMENTS

These studies were supported by the Swedish Medical Research Council (03X-217, 03X-5710, and 03X-7464), and from Konung Gustaf V:s 80-års fond.

REFERENCES

1. Samuelsson, B., Dahlén, S-E., Lindgren, J.A., Rouzer, C.A., Serhan, C.N. (1987) *Science* 237, 1171-1176.
2. Percival, M.D. (1991) *J. Biol. Chem.* 266, 10058-10061.
3. Zhang, Y., Rådmark, O. and Samuelsson, B. (1992) *Proc. Natl. Acad. Sci. USA* 89, 485-489.
4. Zhang, Y., Lind, B., Rådmark, O. and Samuelsson, B. (1993) *J. Biol. Chem.* 268, 2535-2541.
5. Zhang, Y., Hamberg, M., Rådmark, O. and Samuelsson, B. (1994) *Anal. Biochem.*, accepted for publication.
6. Steinhilber, D., Rådmark, O. and Samuelsson, B.(1993) *Proc. Natl. Acad. Sci. USA* 90, 5984-5988.
7. Brungs, M., Rådmark, O., Samuelsson, B and Steinhilber, D., in preparation.
8. Van der Heijdt, L., Feiters, M., Navaratnam, S., Nolting, H.-F., Hermes, C., Veldink, G.A., Vliegenthart, J.F.G. (1992) *Eur. J. Biochem.* 207, 793-802.
9. Veldink, G.A. and Vliegenthart, J.F.G. (1984) *Advances in Inorganic Biochemistry* vol VI, 139-162.
10. Navaratnam, S., Feiters, M.C., Al-Hakim, M., Allen, J.C., Veldink, G.A. and Vliegenthart, J.F.G. (1988) *Biochim. Biophys. Acta* 956, 70 - 76.
11. Boyington, J., Gaffney, B., and Amzel, L. (1993) *Science* 260, 1482-1486.
12. Minor, W., Steczko, J., Bolin, J.T., Otwinowski, Z., and Axelrod, B. (1993) *Biochemistry* 32, 6320-6323.
13. Zhang, Y., Gebhard, M.S., and Solomon, E.I. (1991) *J. Am. Chem. Soc.* 113, 5162-5175.
14. Percival, M.D. and Ouellet, M. (1992) *Biochem. Biophys. Res. Commun.* 186, 1265-1270.
15. Haurand, M. and Flohé, L. (1988) *Biol. Chem. Hoppe-Seyler* 369, 133-142.
16. Blum, J. and Fridovich, I. (1985) *Arch. Biochem. Biophys.* 240, 500-508.
17. Aoshima, H., Kajiwara, T., Hatanaka, A., Nakatani, H. and Hiromi, K. (1977) *Int. J. Peptide Protein Res.* 10, 219-225.
18. Percival, M.D., Denis, D., Riendeau, D. and Gresser, M.J. (1992) *Eur. J. Biochem.* 210, 109 - 117.
19. Misra, H.P. (1974) *J. Biol. Chem.* 249, 2151 - 2155.
20. Claesson, H.-E., Jakobsson, P.-J., Steinhilber, D., Odlander, B. and Samuelsson, B. (1993) *J. Lipid. Mediators* 6, 15-22.
21. Morikawa, M., Harada, N., Soma, G. and Yoshida, T (1990) *In Vitro Cell. dev. Biol.* 26, 682-690.
22. Testa, U., Masciulli, R., Tritarelli, E., Pustorini, R., Mariani, G., Martucci, R., Barberi, T., Camagna, A., Valtieri, M. and Peschle, C. (1993) *J. Immunol.* 150, 2418-2430.
23. Steinhilber, D., Brungs, M., Rådmark, O., Samuelsson, B , this volume.

Advances in Prostaglandin, Thromboxane,
and Leukotriene Research, Vol. 23,
edited by B. Samuelsson et al.
Raven Press, Ltd., New York © 1995

LIPOXYGENASE STRUCTURE AND MECHANISM

B.J. Gaffney*, J.C. Boyington†, L.M. Amzel†, K.S. Doctor‡, S.T. Prigge††, & S.M. Yuan††

Chemistry Department, ‡ Biophysics Department, and ††IBRMA, Johns Hopkins University Baltimore, MD 21218 and †Department of Biophysics and Biophysical Chemistry, Johns Hopkins University School of Medicine, Baltimore, MD 21205 .

Characterizing the structure and mechanism of lipoxygenases has presented many challenges over a number of years: what kind of non-heme iron center is consistent with redox cycling during turnover, how does the iron remain stable in the ferrous form in the presence of air, how are positional and stereochemical specificity achieved in the enzymatic reaction, what is the significance of conserved residues and why are plant and animal enzymes of different size are among these questions. New insights on these questions from studies by x-ray crystallography, electron paramagnetic resonance (EPR) spectroscopy and differential scanning calorimetry are the subjects of this chapter. The effort to give a structural basis to the lipoxygenase mechanism has only begun: at present, the x-ray structure is being refined and a survey is being made of crystals containing inhibitor and substrate analogs. Our present understanding of the relation of structure to mechanism of lipoxygenases will be described. References to positions in the lipoxygenase sequence refer to the sequence of soybean lipoxygenase-1.

RELATION OF LIPOXYGENASE STRUCTURE AND MECHANISM

Overall Structure of Soybean Lipoxygenase-1

Several lipoxygenases have now been crystallized [1-4] and two structures of the L-1 isozyme of soybean have been presented[1,2]. X-ray analysis to 2.6 Å resolution reveals a structure of two domains for soybean lipoxygenase L-1 (a 15-, arachidonic acid lipoxygenase)[1]. The first 146 amino-terminal amino acids form domain I, an eight-stranded β-barrel. Most of this region is missing from the sequences of animal lipoxygenases. The first α-helix is closely associated with this β-barrel, so that domain-I may actually extend as far as the first ~200 amino acids. Domain-II includes the rest of the sequence and is made up of 22 helices (or 23, if helix-1 is included) and 8 β-sheets. These secondary structure elements include 55-60% of the amino acids in domain-II. A striking feature of domain-II is a long helix (43 amino acids) that spans the entire domain. The catalytic iron atom is buried nearly in the center of domain-II and two of the histidine ligands to iron are on the long helix. A second long helix (30 amino acids) crosses the first at the point where the third histidine iron ligand lies. The carboxy terminal region of the chain makes a long loop on the surface until the last 8 residues where it turns toward the center of the molecule, ending with a carboxyl oxygen of the C-terminal isoleucine as the fourth ligand to iron.

Histidine-rich Region

When sequences of soybean lipoxygenase isozymes were first compared[5], Axelrod and coworkers pointed out that there were six conserved histidines in a stretch of about 40 amino acids. They also suggested that this region might contribute to the binding site for iron. This proposal gained support from numerous mutagenesis studies of the five histidines conserved[6-9] in all but one[10] of lipoxygenases from plant and animal sources. Substitutions at the second and third His-residues in this region gave mostly inactive proteins, while other substitutions gave partial, or even enhanced, activity. In the x-ray structure, this highly conserved region of lipoxygenase is found in the long, central helix (helix 9) and the loop and short helix 10. The amino-end of helix 9 also contains the five-amino acid sequence (WLLAK), conserved in all lipoxygenase sequences.

The spacing of the two essential histidines in helix 9 is i and i+5, inconsistent with an α-helical arrangement if both are bound to iron. In fact, the helix expands in the middle so that the two histidine ligands are on the same side of the helix. Most of the carbonyls of the peptide backbone in this region have the same orientation as in an α-helix, but the hydrogen bonding scheme is from i to i+5, instead of i to i+4. This is the spacing of a π−helix; the π-helical region extends from Tyr493 to Ala506.

The Iron Center

The x-ray structure reveals that His690 and the carboxy terminus are ligands to iron, in addition to the two histidines on helix-9. The His-ε-nitrogens are the iron ligands in each case. A hydrogen-bonding network includes the His-δ-nitrogens and, at least, Gln495, Asn539, Asn694, Gln697 and Leu754 (main chain carbonyl). In our structure[1], the closest approach of iron to Asn694 is 3.3Å. Another group gives Asn694 as a fifth ligand to iron[2]. The differences between these structures probably is due more to placements of iron than to crystallization conditions.

The symmetry of ligands around iron is intermediate between tetrahedral and octahedral. Viewed as a distorted octahedron with two empty sites, the empty sites are *cis* to each other. The structure is consistent with the possibility of transient addition of ligands to iron during the catalytic cycle.

Cavities

There are only two paths by which substrates could approach iron in the structure. One is a conical cavity that is wide at the protein surface and narrow as it approaches the position on iron opposite His504. The other cavity follows a 40Å-long, winding path from the surface to the interior, passing the unoccupied site on iron that is opposite His690. Mutations of human 15-lipoxygenase[11] and human platelet 12-lipoxygenase[12] at sites that correspond to residues lining this cavity in the L-1 structure lead to altered positional specificity. These results, together with the cavity shape, support assignment of this cavity as the fatty acid binding site. Figure 1 has the side chains of the residues that line these two cavities highlighted with space-filling representations. The entrance at the surface to cavity II is located between helix 6 and the long helix 9 and is blocked by the side chains of Leu480 and Met341. The structural elements contributing side chains to the walls of the two cavities include nine helices and three strands of β-sheet. It is evident that a large portion of the protein structure is involved in forming the cavities that approach iron.

Location of Sulfhydryls

The side chains of the four sulfhydryls in L-1 are also highlighted in Figure 1. Some insight into the chemical reactivity of these side chains results from preparation of heavy atom derivatives for calculating initial phases in the structure determination[1]. The reagents used were $Hg(CN)_2$, $KAu(CN)_2$ and mersalyl (sodium(o-[3-hydroxymercuri-2-methoxypropyl)carbamoyl]phenoxyacetate). Cys357 in L-1 reacts with all three reagents when crystals at pH 7.0 are soaked for two days with the reagents at 0.8-1.0 mM. Cys127 reacts with the two mercury reagents, but not with the gold reagent, under the same conditions. Cys492 reacts with a single reagent after prolonged (71 days) incubation with mercury dicyanide. The fourth cysteine, Cys679, is completely unreactive.

Several authors have demonstrated that one or two sulfhydryls in L-1 may be labeled with mercury reagents with little loss of activity[13]. These sites probably correspond to the ones that are most reactive in the crystal. Cys357 is in cavity-I leading to iron and Cys127 is in the β-barrel domain that is missing from animals lipoxygenases; both of these residues are easily accessible from solvent. Although Cys492 is sequentially close to two histidine ligands to iron, it falls nearly on the opposite side of helix 9 from the iron ligands. It is close to cavity II leading to iron, so that its modification might alter access of fatty acid substrates to the active site. Although Cys127, 492 and 679 are conserved in most plant sequences, they are not in animal ones. It is probably coincidental that 15-LO from rabbit can also react[13] with up to two mercury reagents before losing activity.

EPR EVIDENCE FOR MULTIPLE IRON SITE GEOMETRIES

EPR spectroscopy has provided key insights about the mechanism of lipoxygenases. We have examined the ferric form of the enzyme under a variety of conditions in an effort find evidence for changes in ligation at iron[14]. It has long been known that there are at least two components to the EPR spectra and our goal has been to find conditions that lead to a preponderance of the component with

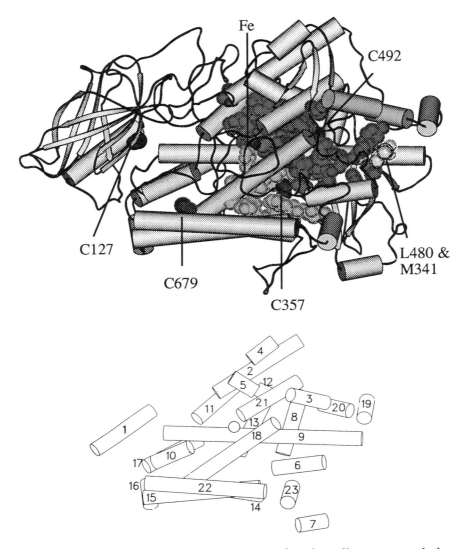

FIG. 1 This diagram (upper) of the structure of soybean lipoxygenase-1 shows regions of α-helix as cylinders and regions of β-sheet as arrows. Shades of grey are used to highlight important amino acid side chains. The side chains are given in space-filling representations without hydrogen atoms. Side chains lining cavity I are the light grey ones in the lower center, those lining cavity II are the dark grey ones in the upper right regions of the structure except for the two (L480 and M341) that block the entrance, which have light shading. The darkest grey side chains are the sulfhydryls. The lower figure gives the sequential numbering of α-helices. The diagrams were constructed using the program SETOR, courtesy of S. Evans[17].

more rhombic symmetry. This component is favored by some anionic buffers and gradually changes to the more axial species in hours after initial activation of lipoxygenase. Although we have made a point of HPLC purifying samples before and after activation to the ferric state (to remove hydroperoxide decomposition products in the latter case), it should be pointed out that the same variations in EPR spectra can be obtained by activating partially pure, commercial lipoxygenase samples. Other experimental conditions that favor formation of the species that changes with time are low protein concentration (<10 mg/ml) and high oxygen concentration when hydroperoxide is added to ferrous enzyme. The origin of the time-dependent changes in EPR signals is not elucidated, but they may reflect some readjustment of the structure when the charge on iron is increased. To examine the apparent involvement of oxygen, we have used a sensitive, thin-layer microcalorimeter[15], but have been unable to detect any heat of oxygen binding to the ferrous enzyme. Apparently the influence of oxygen on EPR spectra of the ferric enzyme is secondary to an initial interaction of the protein with fatty acid hydroperoxide. We also have shown by EPR that the ferrous to ferric conversion can be achieved by soaking crystalline L-1 in solutions containing linoleic hydroperoxide. Interestingly, the reported purple color[5] is not observed in this reaction of crystalline enzyme with hydroperoxide.

THERMAL STABILITY OF LIPOXYGENASES

We have examined the thermal stability of soybean and rabbit reticulocyte lipoxygenases by differential scanning calorimetry[16]. The enzymes exhibit a single, asymmetric transition in the range ~60-75°C and the transitions are modeled as a two-step process: a reversible unfolding followed by an irreversible, kinetically-limited denaturation. The unfolding transitions occur at lower temperatures with higher values of pH. Since thermal stability is often used to characterize lipoxygenase mutants, and incubation temperatures are in the range where we observe calorimetric transitions, we recommend that thermal characterization include several temperatures and information about pH.

ACKNOWLEDGMENTS

This work is supported by The US National Institutes of Health grants GM36232 (BJG) and GM49231 (LMA).

REFERENCES

1.   Boyington JC., Gaffney BJ. and Amzel LM. The Three-Dimensional Structure of an Arachidonic Acid 15-Lipoxygenase. *Science* 1993;260:1482-1486.
2.   Minor W., Steczko J., Bolin JT., Otwinowski Z. and Axelrod B. Crystallographic Determination of the Active Site Iron and Its Ligands in Soybean Lipoxygenase L-1. *Biochem* 1993;32:6320-6323.
3.   Stallings C.; Kroa BA., Carroll RT., Metzger AL. and Funk MO. Crystallization and Preliminary X-ray Characterization of a Soybean Seed Lipoxygenase. *J Mol Biol* 1990;211:685-687.

4.   Sloane DL., Browner MF., Dauter Z., Wilson K., Fletterick RJ. and Sigal E. Purification and Crystallization of 15-Lipoxygenase from Rabbit Reticulocytes. *Biochem Biophy Res Comm* 1990;173:507-513.

5.   Shibata D., Steczko J., Dixon JE., Andrews PC., Hermodson M. and Axelrod B. Primary Structure of Soybean Lipoxygenase L-2. *J Biol Chem* 1988;263:6816-6821.

6.   Nguyen T., Falgueyret J-P., Abramovitz M. and Riendeau D. Evaluation of the Role of Conserved His and Met Residues among Lipoxygenases by Site-directed Mutagenesis of Recombinant Human 5-Lipoxygenase. *J Biol Chem* 1991;266:22057-22062.

7.   Zhang YY., Rådmark O. and Samuelsson B. Mutagenesis of some conserved residues in human 5-lipoxygenase: Effects on enzyme activity. *Proc Natl Acad Sci US* 1992;89:485-489.

8.   Steczko J., Donoho GP., Clemens JC., Dixon JE. and Axelrod B. Conserved Histidine Residues in Soybean Lipoxygenase: Functional Consequences of Their Replacement. *Biochem* 1992;31:4053-4057.

9.   Suzuki H., Kishimoto K., Yoshimoto T. et al. Site-directed mutagenesis on the iron-binding domain and the determinant for the substrate oxygenation site of porcine leukocyte arachidonate 12-lipoxygenase. *Biochim Biophys Acta* 1994;1210:308-316.

10.   Chen X-S., Kurre U., Jenkins NA., Copeland NG. and Funk CD. cDNA Cloning, Expression, Mutagenesis of C-terminal Isoleucine, Genomic Structure, and Chromosomal Localizations of Murine 12-Lipoxygenase. *J Biol Chem* 1994;269:13979-13987.

11.   Sloane DL., Leung R., Craik CS. and Sigal E. A Primary Determinant for Lipoxygenase Positional Specificity. *Nature* 1991;354:149-152.

12.   Chen XS. and Funk CD. Structure-Function properties of human platelet 12-Lipoxygenase: chimeric enzyme and in vitro mutagenesis studies. *The FASEB J* 1993;7:694-701.

13.   Höhne WE., Kojima N., Thiele B. and Rapoport SM. Lipoxygenases from soybeans and rabbit reticulocytes:Inactivation and iron release. *Biomed Biochim Acta* 1991;50:125-138,*and references therein.*

14.   Gaffney BJ., Mavrophilipos DV. and Doctor KS. Access of Ligands to the Ferric Center in Lipoxygenase-1. *Biophys J* 1993;64:773-783.

15.   Johnson CR., Gill SJ. and Peters KS. Thin-layer Microcalorimetric Studies of Oxygen and Carbon Monoxide Binding to Hemoglobin and Myoglobin. *Biophys. Chem.* 1992;45:7-15.

16.   Gaffney BJ., Sturtevant JM., Yuan SM., Lang DM. and Dagdigian E. What Thermal Stability of Lipoxygenases Reveals About Catalytic Activity. *Biophys J* 1994;66:A178.

17.   Evans SV. SETOR: Hardware-lighted 3-Dimensional Solid Model Representations of Macromolecules. *J. Mol. Graphics* 1993;11:134-138.

Advances in Prostaglandin, Thromboxane, and Leukotriene Research, Vol. 23, edited by B. Samuelsson et al. Raven Press, Ltd., New York © 1995

Structures, Properties and Distributions of Prostanoid Receptors.

Shuh Narumiya

Department of Pharmacology, Kyoto University Faculty of Medicine,

Sakyo- ku, Kyoto 606, Japan

Prostanoids including prostaglandins (PGs) and thromboxane (TX) exert a variety of actions in the body. Some are unique to each compound, and others appear overlapping among the prostanoids. In some cases, the apparently opposite actions are evoked by the same compound. The question is how such diverse actions are exerted by these compounds. Because prostanoids are released outside of the cells immediately after synthesis and the cell membrane is practically impermeable to these compounds, most of their actions are believed to be mediated via cell surface receptors. These receptors have been characterized pharmacologically by comparing activities and potencies of various prostanoids and their analogues in many bioassay systems. Based on these findings, Coleman and his colleagues presented the pharmacological classification of the prostanoid receptors, in which they proposed that each prostanoid has its own receptor and that there are at least three subtypes, EP1, 2 and 3, of PGE receptor, which are different in their actions and responses to several analogues (1). The prostanoid receptors have been studied also biochemically by examining the ligand binding of radiolabelled prostanoids and analyzing biochemical changes evoked by these compounds in the cell. These studies suggested that they are the G-protein-coupled receptors. However, none of the receptors was isolated and cloned until we first purified the TXA_2 receptor from human blood platelets in 1989 (2) and cloned its cDNA in 1991 (3). These studies revealed that the TXA_2 receptor is indeed a G-protein-coupled rhodopsin-type receptor with seven transmembrane domains. However, its homology to other rhodopsin-type receptors is limited; about 10 to 20% to the adrenergic and muscarinic receptors. These results led us to hypothesize that the TXA_2 receptor belongs to a new subfamily of the rhodopsin-type receptor superfamily and that the prostanoid receptors as a whole constitute this subfamily. Based on this hypothesis, we performed homology screening in mouse cDNA libraries and isolated cDNAs for seven pharmacologically different prostanoid receptors (4-10). We also found that alternative splicing of mRNA of one of the receptors produces several molecular isoforms which are different in their signal transduction (11). Here I summarize our findings on structures, distributions and functions of these receptors.

MOLECULAR STRUCTURES

Receptor Types and Subtypes encoded by Different Genes

Fig. 1 shows the amino acid sequence alignment of the cloned prostanoid receptors of the mouse. They include the TXA$_2$ receptor (TP), three PGE receptors designated as EP1, EP2 and EP3, PGF receptor (FP), PGI receptor (IP) and PGD receptor (DP). All of them contain seven hydrophobic segments corresponding to the putative transmembrane domains. The overall homology among these receptors is not high, and the conserved amino acids are scattered in the entire sequence, suggesting that they derive from the different genes. Indeed, mapping of the mouse genes encoding TP, EP2 and EP3 revealed that they are on different chromosomes, chromosomes 10, 15 and 3, respectively (12). However, strong conservations are found in the particular regions of these receptors, suggesting that these genes have been evolved from the common ancestor. Some of them are conserved in the rhodopsin-type receptors in general (13). For example, the aspartic acid in the second transmembrane domain is conserved in almost all of the receptors and suggested to be involved in transduction process. Two cysteines, one in the first and the other in the second extracellular loop, are conserved in the majority of the receptors and proposed to form a disulfide bond to give an appropriate configuration. On the other hand, two clusters of conservation are specifically observed in the prostanoid receptors. One is in the seventh transmembrane domain, where the consensus sequence of L-X-A-X-R-X-A-S/T-X-N-Q-I-L-D-P-W-V-Y-I-L-R is found. The other is the sequence of G-R-Y-X-X-Q-X-P-G-T/S-W-C-F found in the second extracellular loop. These conserved sequences presumably reflect structural requirements as the prostanoid receptors. In particular, by analogy to the retinal attachment site of the rhodopsin, the arginine in the seventh transmembrane domain was proposed as the binding site of the carboxyl group of prostanoid molecules. Indeed, the mutation of this residue in the human TP significantly affected the ligand binding activity (14). The homology shared by all the receptors is not high. However, more conservation is found when we compare the sequences of the functionally similar groups of the receptors. For example, TP, FP and EP1, the three receptors evoking calcium mobilization and mediating contractile responses, resemble more closely each other; 47-48% identity in their transmembrane domains. Similarly, the receptors mediating cAMP rise and relaxant response are more closely related; 39% homologous in the entire sequence between DP and IP and 32% between DP and EP2. On the other hand, the identity among the three PGE receptors is less. These results together with the finding that only PGE has three different receptors mediating different responses indicate that the prostanoid receptors have evolved from the primitive PGE receptor to the functionally different groups of receptors mentioned above. The gene strucutre of the prostanoid receptor gene was clarified for the human TXA$_2$ receptor and contains 3 exons devided by two introns in the 5'-noncoding region and at the end of the sixth transmembrane domain (15). This exon-intron relationship appears conserved in other types of the prostanoid receptors. In addition, there appear several exons in the C-terminal regions which lead to formation of several alternatively spliced receptor variants as described below.

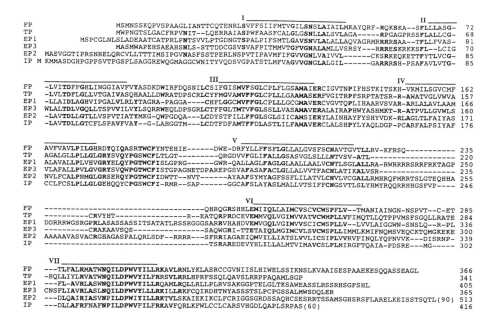

```
              I                                                      II
FP            MSMNSSKQPVSPAAGLIANTTCQTENRLSVFFSIIFMTVGILSNSLAIAILMKAYQRF-RQKSKA--SFLLLASG-  72
TP            MWPNGTSLGACFRPVNIT--LQERRAIASPWFAASFCALGLGSNLLALSVLAGA-----RPGAGPRSSFLALLCG-  68
EP1       MSPCGLNLSLADEAATCATPRLPNTSVVLPTGDNGTSPALPIFSMTLGAVSNVLALALLAQVAGRMRRRRSAA--TFLLFVAS-  81
EP3             MASMWAPEHSAEAHSNLS-STTDDCGSVSVAFPITMMVTGFVGNALAMLLVSRSY---RRRESKRKKSFL--LCIG  70
EP2 MAEVGGTIPRSNRELQRCVLLTTTIMSIPGVNASFSSTPERLNSPVTIPAVMFIFGVVGNLVAIVVL------CKSRKEQKETTFYTLVCG-  85
IP  M KMMASDGHPGPPSVTPGSPLSAGGREWQGMAGGCWNITYVQDSVGPATSTLMFVAGVVGNGLALGIL------GARRRSH-PSAFAVLVTG-  85

                 _____III_____IV
FP            -LVITDFFGHLINGGIAVFVYASDKDWIRFDQSNILCSIFGISMVFSGLCPLFLGSAMAIERCIGVTNPIFHSTKITSKH-VKMILSGVCMF  162
TP            -LVLTDFLGLLVTGAIVASQHAALLDWRATDPSCRLCYFMGVAMVFFGLCPLLLGAAMASERFVGITRPFSRPTATSR-R-AWATVGLVWVA  157
EP1           -LLAIDLAGHVIPGALVLRLYTAGRA-PAGGA----CHFLGGCMVFFGLCPLLLGCGMAVERCVGVTQPLIHAARVSVAR-ARLALAVLAAM  166
EP3           WLALTDLVGQLLTSPVVILVLSQRRWEQLDPSGRLCTFFGLTMTVFGLSSLLVASAMAVERALAIRAPHWYASHMKT-R-ATPVLLGVWLS  160
EP2           -LAVTDLLGTLLVSPVTIATYMKG-QWPGDQA---LCDYSTFILLFFGLSGLSIICAMSIERYLAINHAYFYSHYVDK-RLAGLTLFAIYAS  171
IP            -LAVTDLLGTCFLSPAVFVAY--G-LAHGGTM---LCDTFDFAMTFFDLASTLILFAMAVERCLALSHPYLYAQLDGP-PCARFALPSIYAF  176

                                           V
FP            AVFVAVLPILGHRDYQIQASRTWCFYNTEHIE------DWE-DRFYLLFFSFLGLLALGVSFSCNAVTGVTLLRV-KFRSQ-----------  235
TP            AGALGLLPLLGLGRYSVQYPGSWCFLTLGT---------QRGDVVFGLIFALLGSASVGLSLLLNTVSV-ATL------------------  220
EP1           ALAVALLPLVHVGRYELQYPGTWCFISLGPRG------GWR-QALLAGLFAGLGLAALLAALVCNTLSGLALLRA-RWRRRRSRRFRKTAGP  250
EP3           VLAFALLPVLGVGRYSVQWPGTWCFISTGPAGNETDPAREPGSVAFASAFACLGLLALVVTFACNLATIKALVSR------------------  235
EP2           NVLFCALPNMGLGRSERQYPGTWCFIDWTT---NVT------AYAAFSYMYAGFSSFLIIATVLCNVLVCGALLRMHRQFMRRTSLGTEQHHA  255
IP            CCLFCSLPLLGLGEHQQYCPGSWCFI-RMR---SAP------GGCAFSLAYASLMALLVTSIFFCNGSVTLSLYHMYRQQRRHHGSFVP----  246

                                    VI
FP            ------------------------------------QHRQGRSHHLEMIIQLLAIMCVSCVCWSPFLV--TMANIAINGN-NSPVT--C-ET  285
TP            ----------CRVYHT----------------R--EATQRPRDCEVEMMVQLVGIMVVATVCWMPLLVFIMQTLLQTPPVMSFSGQLLRATE  284
EP1           DDRRRWGSRGPRLASASSASSITSATATLRSSRGGGSARRVHAHDVEMVGQLVGIMVVSCICWSPLLV--LVVLAIGGWN-SNSLQ---R-PL  336
EP3           ----------CRAKAAVSQS----------------SAQWGRI-TTETAIQLMGIMCVLSVCWSPLLIMMLKMIFNQMSVEQCKTQMGKEKE  300
EP2           AAAAAVASVACRGHAGASPALQRLSDF--RRRR---SFRRIAGAEIQMVILLIATSLVVLICSIPLVVRVFINQLYQPNVVK---DISRNP-  339
IP            ------------------------------------TSRAREDEVYHLILLALMTVIMAVCSLPLMIRGFTQAIA-PDSRE---MG------  302

             VII
FP           ---TLFALRMATWNQILDPWVYILLRKAVLRNLYKLASRCCGVNIISLHIWELSSIKNSLKVAAISESPAAEKESQQASSEAGL  366
TP           -HQLLIYLRVATWNQILDPWVYILFRRSVLRRLHPRFSSQLQAVSLRRPPAQAMLSGP  341
EP1          ---FL-AVRLASWNQILDPWVYILLRQAMLRQLLRLLPLRVSAKGGPTELGLTKSAWEASSLRSSRHSGFSHL  405
EP3          CNSFLIAVRLASLNQILDPWVYLLLRKILLRKFCQIRDHTNYASSSTSLPCPGSSALMWSDQLER  365
EP2          ---DLQAIRIASVNPILDPWIYILLRKTVLSKAIEKIKCLFCRIGGSGRDSSAQHCSESRRTSSAMSGHSRSFLARELKEISSTSQTL(90)  513
IP           ---DLLAFRFNAFNPILDPWVFILFRKAVFQRLKFWLCCLCARSVHGDLQAPLSRPAS(60)  416
```

Fig. 1. Amino Acid Sequences of the Cloned Prostanoid Receptors.

The sequences of mouse PGF receptor (FP), TXA$_2$ receptor (TP), three PGE receptors (EP1, EP2 and EP3), and the prostacyclin receptor (IP) are aligned. The putative transmembrane domains are shown by overlines and numbered by Roman numerals.

Isoforms created by Alternative Splicing

In addition to the receptors encoded by different genes, alternative splicing can create several isoforms of the receptors. This is observed in EP3 receptor of mouse, bovine and other species (11, 16-19). Alternative splicing occurs in the C-terminal region and forms the receptor variants which are different only in the carboxyl tails. Because they have the identical structures from the amino terminus to ten amino acids after the seventh transmembrane domain, they show identical ligand binding properties. However, they couple to different G-proteins to induce different signalling (11,16,18). They are also different in their sensitivities to agonist-induced desensitization (17). Whether such splicing variants exist in other prostanoid receptors is a question to be tested in future study.

LIGAND BINDING PROPERTIES AND SIGNAL TRANSDUCTION

Table 1 summarizes the ligand binding properties of the cloned receptors. In general, each receptor binds its own prostanoid ligands with Kd of 1 to 40 nM. The affinities to other prostanoids are more than two orders of magnitudes lower. The binding properties of the three PGE receptors were examined in detail with various synthetic PGE analogues, and found in good agreement with those in the pharmacological experiments (1). For example, EP1 receptor cloned shows about ten times higher affinity to PGE$_2$ and iloprost than PGE$_1$, while the other two

Table 1. Properties of the Cloned Prostanoid Receptors

Type		Kd(nM)	Rank Order of Binding Affinity	Signalling
TP		1.2; [^{3}H]S-145	S-145>ONO-3708>STA$_2$>PGD$_2$ PGE$_2$ PGF$_{2\alpha}$	Gq, Gi PI response cAMP decrease
EP	EP1	21; [^{3}H]PGE$_2$	PGE$_2$>iloprost>PGE$_1$>PGF$_{2\alpha}$>PGD$_2$ 17-Phenyl-PGE$_2$>sulprostone>M&B*>> AH-6809, butaprost	G(?) Ca^{++} rise
	EP2 or EP4	11; '[^{3}H]PGE$_2$	PGE$_2$=PGE$_1$>>PGD$_2$,PGF$_{2\alpha}$, iloprost misoprostol, M&B>>>sulprostone, butaprost=0	Gs cAMP rise
	EP3	3; [^{3}H]PGE$_2$	PGE$_2$=PGE$_1$>>ilosprost>PGD$_2$>PGF$_{2\alpha}$ M&B>>>butaprost, SC-19220=0	Gi cAMP decrease
FP		1.3; [^{3}H]PGF$_{2\alpha}$	PGF$_{2\alpha}$>9,11-PGF$_2$>PGF$_{1\alpha}$>PGD$_2$ > STA$_2$>PGE$_2$>iloprost	Gp PI response
IP		4.5; [^{3}H]iloprost	cicaprost>iloprost>PGE$_1$>cabacyclin> PGD$_2$, PGE$_2$, STA$_2$>PGF$_{2\alpha}$	Gs, Gp cAMP rise PI response
DP		40; [^{3}H]PGD2	PGD$_2$>BW245C>BWA868C>STA$_2$ PGE$_2$>iloprost>PGF$_{2\alpha}$	Gs cAMP rise

*M&B, M&B-28767

receptors bind PGE$_2$ and PGE$_1$ with equal affinities and iloprost with much lower affinty. 17-phenyl-PGE$_2$ shows the highest affinity to EP1, while misoprostol and M&B-28767 are the best ligands to EP2 and EP3, respectively. However, some discrepancies are noted between the cloned and the pharmacologically characterized receptors. One is the failure of butaprost, the well known EP2 agonist, to bind to the cloned EP2 receptor, although the cloned receptor mediates the cAMP increase as suggested for EP2 receptor. The reason for this discrepancy is not known at present. It may imply that the cloned receptor corresponds to a molecular subtype other than EP2. Coleman and his colleagues recently reported another PGE receptor subtype, EP4, which, like EP2, couples positively to adenylate cyclase but is different from it in the ligand binding properties (21).

Table 1 also shows the signal transduction of the cloned receptors. These studies not only confirmed the previous biochemical findings in the crude systems but also revealed several novel characters. For example, the prostacyclin receptor expressed in CHO cells was found to couple to both Gs and Gp and to induce not only cAMP rise but also PI response. It has been reported that prostacyclin induces elevation of free calcium ion concentration in several lines of cultured cells (22,23). Our results thus support the view that these responses are indeed mediated by the prostacyclin receptor and not by cross-reaction on other types of prostanoid receptors. It is also noteworthy that the splicing variants of EP3 receptor described above couple to different siganlling pathways. Thus, bovine EP3A couples to Gi to induce inhibition of adenylate cyclase, EP3B and C couple to Gs to increase cAMP, and EP3D couples to Gp, in addition to Gi and Gs, to evoke pertussis toxin-insensitive PI response (11).

TISSUE DISTRIBUTION

Tissue distribution of the prostanoid receptors was examined by Northern blot analysis of its mRNA expression. As shown in Fig. 2, these analyses together with *in situ* hybridization studies have shown that they are differently distributed in the body. Some of these patterns explain the cellular basis of the known actions of the prostanoid molecules. For example, *in situ* hybridization studies of PGE receptors in kidney (24) revealed that EP3 is mainly expressed by tublar epithels in the medulla, EP1 in the collecting tublus of pappila and EP2 in the glomerulus (21). These distributions appear to correspond to PGE2-mediated regulations in ionic transport, water reabsorption and glomerular filtration rate, respectively. Similar analysis in the nervous system revealed that EP3 receptor is highly expressed in small neurons in dorsal root ganglion (25), suggesting the involvement of this receptor in PGE2-mediated hyperalgesia. The distribution study also reveals novel actions of prostanoid molecules. As shown in the figure, both the TXA2 receptor and the prostacyclin receptor are most highly expressed in the thymus, where little is known on their actions. *In situ* hybridization analysis revealed that both are expressed by thymocytes, but the former is expressed abundantly in the cortex, while the latter exclusively in the medulla. Consistently, we found by the ligand binding study that the TXA2 receptor is expressed in CD4, CD8-double negative and double positive immature thymocytes. We further found that the TXA2 agonist induces apoptosis of these cells via this receptor (26). Thus, this study has revealed the novel immuno-modulatory actions for TXA2, which has been thus far presumed to play an important role only in the cardiovascular and respiratory systems.

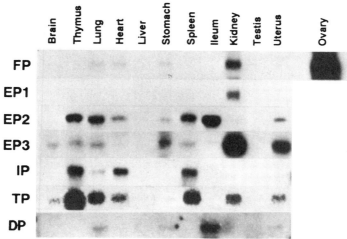

Fig.2. Northern Blot Analysis of the Prostanoid Receptor Expression in Various Mouse Tissues.

ACKNOWLEDGEMENTS.

The author thanks the following people for the studies presented in this review; F. Ushikubi, M. Hirata, Y. Hayashi, T . Namba, H. Oida and A. Kakizuka of Department of Pharmacology, R. Shigemoto and N. Mizuno of Department of Morphological Brain Sciences, Kyoto University Faculty of Medicine, and Y. Sugimoto, M., A. Honda, A. Watabe, A. Irie, M. Negishi and A. Ichikawa of Department of Physiological Chemistry, Kyoto University Faculty of Pharmaceutical Sciences.

REFERENCES

1. Coleman RA., Kennedy I., Humphrey PPA. Bunce K. and Lumley P. In: Emmett, J C.*Comprehensive Medicinal Chemistry vol. 3. Membranes and Receptors* . Oxford:Pergamon Press; 1990: 643-714
2. Ushikubi F., Nakajima M., Hirata M., Okuma M., Fujiwara M. and Narumiya S. *J Biol Chem* 1989;264:16496-16501
3. Hirata M., Hayashi Y., Ushikubi F. et al. Nature 1991;349;617-620
4. Namba T., Sugimoto Y., Hirata M. et al. *Biochem. Biophys. Res. Commun.* 1992;184: 1197-1203
5. Sugimoto Y., Namba T., Honda A. et al. *J Biol.Chem* 1992;267:6463-6466
6. Honda A., Sugimoto Y., Namba T. et al. *J Biol.Chem* 1993;268:7759-7762
7. Watabe A., Sugimoto Y., Honda A. et al. *J Biol Chem* 1993;268:20175-20178
8. Sugimoto, Y., Hasumoto, K., Namba, T. et al. *J Biol Chem* 1994;269:1356-1360
9. Namba, T., Oida, H., Sugimoto, Y. et al. *J Biol Chem* 1994;269:9986-9992
10. Hirata M., Kakizuka A., Aizawa M., Ushikubi F. and Narumiya S. submitted
11. Namba T., Sugimoto Y., Negishi M. et al. *Nature* 1993;365:166-170
12. Taketo M., Rochelle J.M., Sugimoto Y.et al. Genomics 1994;19:585-588
13. Savarese T.M. and Fraser C.M. *Biochem J* 1992;283:1-19
14. Funk, C.D., Furci, L., Moran, N. and Fitzgerald, G.A. *Mol. Pharmacol.* 1993;44:934-939
15. Nüsing R.M., Hirata M., Kakizuka A. et al. *J Biol Chem* 1993;268:25253-25259
16. Sugimoto Y., Negishi M., Hayashi Y. et al. *J Biol Chem* 1993;268:2712-2718
17. Negishi M., Sugimoto Y., Irie A., Narumiya S. and Ichikawa A. *J Biol Chem* 1993;268:9517-9521
18. Irie A., Sugimoto Y., Namba T. et al. *Eur J Biochem* 1993;217:313-318
19. Breyer R.M., Emeson R.B., Tarng J-L., et al. *J Biol Chem* 1994;269:6163-6169
20. Negishi M., Namba T., Sugimoto Y. et al. *J Biol Chem* 1993;268:26067-26070
21. Coleman R.A., Grix S.P., Head S.A. et al. *Prostaglandins* 1994;47:151-168
22. Watanabe T., Yatomi Y., Sunaga S. et al. *Blood* 1991;78:2328-2336
23. Vassaux G., Gaillard D., Ailhaud G. and Negrel R. *J Biol Chem* 1992;267:11092-11097
24. Sugimoto Y., Namba T., Shigemoto R. et al. *Am J Physiol* 1994;266:F823-828
25. Sugimoto Y., Shigemoto R., Namba T. et al. *Neuroscience in press*
26. Ushikubi F., Aiba Y., Nakamura, K. et al. *J Exp Med* 1993;178:1825-1830

Advances in Prostaglandin, Thromboxane,
and Leukotriene Research, Vol. 23,
edited by B. Samuelsson et al.
Raven Press, Ltd., New York © 1995

The Regulation and Role of TIS10 Prostaglandin Synthase-2

Harvey R. Herschman, Rebecca S. Gilbert, Weilin Xie, Steven Luner, and Srinivasa T. Reddy

Department of Biological Chemistry and UCLA-DOE Laboratory of Structural Biology and Molecular Medicine, UCLA Center for the Health Sciences, Los Angeles, CA 90024

We study the molecular and cellular events that occur when non-dividing cells are stimulated by mitogens to leave G_o and re-enter the cell cycle. We isolated mutant Swiss 3T3 cell lines unable to mount proliferative responses to mitogenic stimulation by epidermal growth factor (1) or the tumor promoter and mitogen tetradecanoyl phorbol acetate (TPA, Ref. 2). By identifying mitogenic defects in these mutant cells (3), we can delineate causal steps in the mitogenic pathways. In a second approach, we identified cDNAs for messages whose levels are increased by mitogenic stimulation (4). By screening libraries prepared from cells stimulated with TPA in the presence of cycloheximide, we identified cDNAs for TPA Induced Sequences (TIS genes); "primary response" (5) genes whose message levels are increased by TPA activation of pre-existing, latent transcription factors. Although many mitogen-activated genes encode transcription factors necessary for transcriptional cascades required for commitment to DNA synthesis and cell division, some encode proteins that modulate paracrine communication between mitogen-stimulated cells and their neighbors (5). Sequencing (6), chromosomal mapping (7), and enzyme analysis of transfected cells (8) demonstrated that one TIS gene, TIS10, encodes a second prostaglandin synthase. Other laboratories isolated the TIS10/PGS-2 cDNA as a *v-src*, serum, or platelet derived growth factor induced gene (reviewed in Ref. 9).

THE TIS10/PGS-2 GENE IS INDUCED IN A WIDE VARIETY OF CELLS, BY A NUMBER OF DISTINCT INDUCERS

Although we first identified the TIS10/PGS-2 gene as a TPA-inducible gene in Swiss 3T3 cells (4, 6), we showed in these reports that this gene could also be induced by serum, protein growth factors such as epidermal growth factor (EGF), fibroblast growth factor (FGF), and platelet derived growth factor (PDGF), and by forskolin. Thus inducers that act through protein kinase C (TPA), protein tyrosine kinases (EGF, PDGF), and protein kinase A (forskolin) can all stimulate the accumulation of TIS10/PGS-2 message in 3T3 cells. These data suggested that the regulatory region of the TIS10/PGS-2 gene would be able to respond to transcription factors activated by a number of distinct second messenger pathways. Transient transfection assays with [TIS10/PGS-2 promoter] [luciferase reporter] gene constructs demonstrated this to be the case (8). Subsequent studies from our laboratory and a number of other laboratories have demonstrated that the TIS10/PGS-2 gene can be induced by inflammatory agents such as endotoxin/lipopolysaccharide (LPS) in macrophages and monocytes, by depolarization in central nervous system neurons, by phorbol esters and inflammatory cytokines in epithelial cells, endothelial cells, and muscle cells, by phorbol esters in mast cells, and by pituitary glycoprotein hormones in ovarian granulosa cells. References for these and other studies are not included because of space constraints. These data suggest that expression of the TIS10/PGS-2 gene is likely to be important in a wide variety of biological events in which ligand-stimulated prostaglandin production plays a role.

DEXAMETHASONE INHIBITS TIS10/PROSTAGLANDIN SYNTHASE INDUCTION IN A WIDE VARIETY OF CONTEXTS

Prostaglandin synthesis is one of the hallmarks of inflammation. Nonsteroidal anti-inflammatory drugs such as aspirin inhibit the enzymatic activity of both PGS-1 (EC 1.14.99.1) and TIS10/PGS-2 (10, 11). Glucocorticoid treatment is one of the most common therapeutic approaches to acute and chronic inflammation, and suppresses prostaglandin production in inflamed tissue. We demonstrated that dexamethasone is able to suppress mitogen-induced TIS10/PGS-2 message and protein accumulation at nanomolar concentrations (12, 13). The inhibition of TIS1-/PGS-2 induction by dexamethasone is not general for all mitogen-induced primary response genes; e.g., mitogen induction of the TIS8/egr-1/zif-268/krox 24 transcription factor is not inhibited by dexamethasone concentrations three orders of magnitude greater than that observed to inhibit TIS10/PGS-2 induction (12). Nuclear run-on experiments in our own laboratory (9) and in the laboratory of David DeWitt (14) demonstrate that the inhibition of TIS10/PGS-2 induction by dexamethasone is at the transcriptional level. Induction of TIS10/PGS-2 message and protein accumulation by appropriate stimuli is inhibited by glucocorticoids in fibroblasts, macrophages, monocytes, epithelial cells, endothelial cells, ovarian granulosa cells, muscle cells, and neurons.

TRANSFORMING GROWTH FACTOR BETA MODULATES TIS10/PGS-2 INDUCTION IN A CELL-TYPE SPECIFIC MANNER

Transforming growth factor beta (TGF-beta) is a potent modulator of the immune response. This cytokine is able to suppress expression of a number of responses in LPS-activated monocytes and macrophages. TGF-beta alone has no effect on TIS10/PGS-2 expression in RAW 264.7 cells (a murine macrophage cell line), or in murine peritoneal macrophages. However, TGF-beta, at concentrations as low as 0.1-1.0 ng/ml, is able to *attenuate* TIS10/PGS-2 induction in response to LPS stimulation in both RAW 264.7 cells and in peritoneal macrophages (15).

TGF-beta also modulates gene expression in fibroblasts. This cytokine alone did not induce TIS10/PGS-2 expression in 3T3 cells or in primary murine embryo fibroblast cultures. However, in contrast to the results observed for macrophages, TGF-beta *augments* TIS10/PGS-2 induction by mitogens in 3T3 cells and murine embryo fibroblasts (16). TGF-beta, while not inducing TIS10/PGS-2 expression in macrophages or fibroblasts, suppresses induction of this gene in the former cells and enhances induction in the latter cells. In both cases, the cytokine effect is at the level of transcript accumulation (15, 16). TGF-beta also *augments* TIS10/PGS-2 induction in the IEC-6 intestinal epithelial cell line (in prep).

LIGAND-INDUCED PROSTAGLANDIN SYNTHESIS REQUIRES EXPRESSION OF THE TIS10/PGS-2 GENE IN MURINE FIBROBLASTS AND MACROPHAGES

Swiss 3T3 cells, murine embryo fibroblasts, RAW 264.7 cells, and murine peritoneal macrophages all contain constitutive PGS-1 enzyme, capable of converting exogenously supplied arachidonic acid to prostaglandin. Conventional interpretations of ligand-stimulated synthesis of prostaglandins from endogenous arachidonic acid suggest that the rate limiting step in prostaglandin biosynthesis is the activation of phospholipase following stimulation by growth factors or endotoxin. Prostaglandin synthase activity has been thought to be present in excess; availability of endogenous arachidonic acid, released from membrane stores by the activated phospholipase, has been thought to be rate-limiting in ligand-induced prostaglandin biosynthesis.

We find, however, that the induction of both prostaglandin accumulation and the expression of the TIS10/PGS-2 gene are correlated in a variety of contexts. For example, dexamethasone is able to suppress both mitogen-induced prostaglandin production and TIS10/PGS-2 expression in 3T3 cells (12, 13). TGF-beta augments both mitogen-induced prostaglandin production and TIS10/PGS-2 expression in fibroblasts (16), but attenuates both endotoxin-induced prostaglandin production and TIS10/PGS-2 expression in macrophages (15). Moreover, we find that the induction of prostaglandin accumulation in 3T3 cells in response to mitogenic stimulation, like the mitogen induction of TIS10/PGS-2 antigen accumulation, is inhibited by cycloheximide (12). Our data suggest ligand-induced stimulation of prostaglandin accumulation may *require* expression of the TIS10/PGS-2 gene and production of this isoform of PGS.

To investigate this question more extensively, we utilized antisense oligonucleotides directed against the message of TIS10/PGS-2. When transfected into Swiss 3T3 cells, murine embryo fibroblast (MEF) cultures, RAW 264.7 cells, or murine peritoneal macrophages, TIS10/PGS-2 antisense oligonucleotides (ASO) are able to block mitogen or endotoxin induced TIS10/PGS-2 protein accumulation, without modulating the level of PGS-1 (17). TIS10/PGS-2 sense or random sequence oligonucleotides have no effect on expression of PGS-1 or TIS10/PGS-2 antigen. Cells transfected with TIS10/PGS-2 ASO, when stimulated with either mitogens (for 3T3 cells and MEF cultures) or LPS (for RAW 264.7 cells and peritoneal macrophages) are unable to produce prostaglandins from endogenous arachidonic acid stores. In contrast, these same cells are able to produce prostaglandins from exogenously supplied arachidonic acid, demonstrating the presence of active PGS-1 in these cells.

Although these data suggest that fibroblasts and macrophages are unable to utilize endogenous arachidonic acid for prostaglandin synthesis unless TIS10/PGS-2 enzyme is produced, it is possible that the TIS10/PGS-2 ASO are in some way inhibiting release of arachidonic acid following stimulation. To determine if this is the case, we labelled endogenous arachidonic acid stores with radioactive arachidonic acid, and measured both the production of prostaglandin E_2 and release of free arachidonic acid in 3T3 cells and in RAW 264.7 cells following TPA or LPS stimulation respectively. Once again, ligand-induced prostaglandin production in these cultures was blocked by TIS10/PGS-2 ASO. In contrast, free arachidonic acid levels were increased relative to untreated, sense oligonucleotide, or random oligonucleotide controls. We conclude that endogenous arachidonic acid, released from cells in response to ligand stimulation in macrophages and fibroblasts, is not available to PGS-1. TIS10/PGS-2 protein must be synthesized in response to mitogens or endotoxin, to convert the released arachidonic acid to prostaglandins. We suggest that induced prostaglandin synthesis in a variety of biological contexts --in macrophages, fibroblasts, neurons, epithelial cells, endothelial cells, ovarian granulosa cells, mast cells, and muscle cells-- is likely to *require* induced expression of the TIS10/PGS-2 gene.

ACKNOWLEDGEMENTS

These studies were supported by NIH grant GM24797 and Contract DE FC03 87ER 60615 between the Department of Energy and the Regents of the University of California.

REFERENCES

1.   Pruss, R.M. and Herschman, H.R.   Variants of 3T3 cells lacking mitogenic response to epidermal growth factor. *Proc. Natl. Acad. Sci. USA* 1977;74:3918-21.

2.   Butler-Gralla, E., and Herschman, H.R.   Variants of 3T3 cells lacking mitogenic response to the tumor promoter tetradecanoyl-phorbol-acetate. *J. Cell. Physiol.* 1981;107:59-68.

3.   Herschman, H.R.   Mitogen specific nonproliferative variants of Swiss 3T3 cells.   In:Colburn, N.H., Moses, H.L., Stanbridge, E.J. *Growth Factors, Tumor Promoters, and Cancer Genes, Vol 58.* New York: Alan R. Liss, Inc.; 1988:295-310.

4.   Lim, R.W., Varnum, B.C., and Herschman, H.R.   Cloning of tetradecanoyl phorbol ester induced "primary response" sequences and their expression in density-arrested Swiss 3T3 cells and a TPA nonproliferative variant. *Oncogene* 1987;1:263-70.

5.   Herschman, H.R.   Primary response genes induced by growth factors and tumor promoters. *Ann. Rev. Biochem.* 1991;60:281-319.

6.   Kujubu, D.A., Fletcher, B.S., Varnum, B.C., Lim, R.W., and Herschman, H.R. TIS10, a phorbol ester tumor promoter-inducible mRNA from Swiss 3T3 cells, encodes a novel prostaglandin synthase/cyclooxygenase homologue. *J. Biol. Chem.* 1991;266:12866-72.

7.   Ping, X.W., Warden, C., Fletcher, B.S., Kujubu, D.A., Herschman, H.R., and Lusis, A.L. Chromosomal organization of the inducible

and constitutive prostaglandin synthase/cyclooxygenase genes in mouse. *Genomics* 1993;15:458-60.

8. Fletcher, B.S., Kujubu, D.A., Perrin, D.M., and Herschman, H.R. Structure of the mitogen-inducible TIS10 gene and demonstration that the TIS10 encoded protein is a functional prostaglandin G/H synthase. *J. Biol. Chem.* 1992;267:4338-44.

9. Herschman, H.R., Kujubu, D.A., Fletcher, B.S., Ma, Q., Varnum, B.C., Gilbert, R.S., and Reddy, S.T. The TIS genes, primary response genes induced by growth factors and tumor promoters. In:Cohen, W., and Moldave, K. *Progress in Nucleic Acids Research and Molecular Biology* San Diego, California: Academic Press. 1994;47:113-148.

10. Meade, E.A., Smith, W.L., and DeWitt, D.L. Differential inhibition of prostaglandin endoperoxide synthase (cyclooxygenase) isozymes by aspirin and other non-steroidal anti-inflammatory drugs. *J. Biol. Chem.* 1993;268:6610-14.

11. Mitchell, J.A., Akarasereenont, P., Thiemermann, C., Flower, R.J., and Vane, J.R. Selectivity of nonsteroidal antiinflammatory drugs as inhibitors of constitutive and inducible cyclooxygenase. *Proc. Natl. Acad. Sci. USA* 1993;90:11693-97.

12. Kujubu, D.A., and Herschman, H.R. Dexamethasone inhibits mitogen induction of the TIS10 prostaglandin synthase/cyclooxygenase gene. *J. Biol. Chem.* 1992;267:7991-94.

13. Kujubu, D.A., Reddy, S.T., Fletcher, B.S., and Herschman, H.R. Expression of the protein product of the prostaglandin synthase-2/TIS10 gene in mitogen-stimulated swiss 3T3 cells. *J. Biol. Chem.* 1993;268:5425-31.

14. DeWitt, D.L., and Meade, E.A. Serum and glucocorticoid regulation of gene transcription and expression of the prostaglandin H synthase-1 and prostaglandin H synthase-2 isozymes. *Arch. Biochem. Biophys.* 1993;306:94-102.

15. Reddy, S.T., Gilbert, R.S., Xie, W., Luner, S., and Herschman, H.R. TGF-beta$_1$ inhibits both endotoxin-induced prostaglandin synthesis and expression of the TIS10/prostaglandin synthase 2 gene in murine macrophages. *J. Leukoc. Biol.* 1994;55:192-200.

16. Gilbert, R.S., Reddy, S.T., Kujubu, D.A., Xie, W., Luner, S., and Herschman, H.R. TGF-beta$_1$ augments mitogen-induced prostaglandin synthesis and expression of the TIS10/prostaglandin synthase 2 gene both in Swiss 3T3 cells and in murine embryo fibroblasts. *J. Cell. Physiol.* 1994;159:67-75.

17. Reddy, S.T., and Herschman, H.R. Ligand-induced prostaglandin synthesis requires expression of the TIS10/PGS-2 gene in murine fibroblasts and macrophages. *J. Biol. Chem.*, in press.

Advances in Prostaglandin, Thromboxane,
and Leukotriene Research, Vol. 23,
edited by B. Samuelsson et al.
Raven Press, Ltd., New York © 1995

The Orientation of Prostaglandin Endoperoxide Synthase-1 in the Endoplasmic Reticulum of Transiently Transfected *Cos*-1 Cells

James C. Otto and William L. Smith

Department of Biochemistry, Michigan State University,
East Lansing, Michigan 48824

Both PGH synthases-1 and -2 (PGHS-1 and PGHS-2) are glycoproteins (1,2) associated with the endoplasmic reticulum (ER) and nuclear membranes (3,4). Both isozymes contain signal peptides in their deduced amino acid sequences which are cleaved in the mature proteins (5-8). This indicates that the amino termini of these enzymes are initially inserted into the lumen of the ER. Ovine PGHS-1 is N-glycosylated at three sites: Asn68, Asn144, and Asn410 (2). All known PGHSs-2 have consensus N-glycosylation sites at analogous positions (9-12); in addition, murine PGHS-2 is partially glycosylated at a fourth site, Asn580 (2). Because N-glycosylation occurs in the lumen of the ER (13), each of the N-glycosylated residues in PGHS-1 and PGHS-2 is predicted to reside in the ER lumen. Both purified and microsomal forms of ovine PGHS-1 are cleaved by trypsin at Arg277 (14-16). This has led to the prediction that Arg277 is located on the cytoplasmic side of the ER. Tests of these predictions were conducted by preparing antibodies to the N- and C-termini and the Arg277 trypsin cleavage site of PGHS-1 and then using these antibodies to perform immunocytofluorescent staining following treatments with membrane-selective permeants.

RESULTS

Anti-peptide antibodies reactive with ovine PGHS-1 were prepared against (a) the amino terminus ([25]ADPGAPAVNPC[35]), (b) a domain which includes the tryptic cleavage site at Arg277 (^{272}LMHYPRGIPPQ^{283}C), and (c) a region near the carboxyl terminus of the protein (C^{583}PDPRQEDRPGVE^{594}). Another antibody against an eighteen amino acid cassette located near the carboxyl terminus of murine PGHS-2 and unique to this isozyme was prepared previously (2).

Cos-1 cells were transfected with constructs encoding ovine PGHS-1 (17-19), murine PGHS-2 (20), or β-galactosidase (pSVGAL, Promega). Following fixation, the transfected cells were subjected to immunocytofluorescent staining with various antibodies under different membrane permeabilization conditions. Digitonin (21) and streptolysin O (22) were used for the selective permeabilization of plasma membranes; saponin (0.2%) was used as a general permeant for all cell membranes. The results shown in Fig. 1 are for saponin and digitonin permeabilizations; however, the results obtained with digitonin and streptolysin O were essentially identical. Anti-actin antibodies were used as a control for cytoplasmic staining; in addition, an antibody against β-galactosidase (Promega) was used as a control for the staining of a cytoplasmic protein expressed by transient transfection. The antibody against the carboxyl terminus of murine

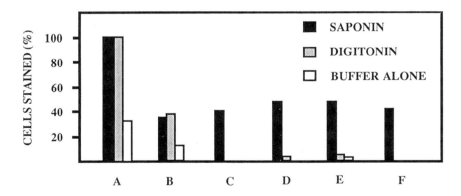

Fig. 1. Determination of the orientation of ovine PGHS-1 in the endoplasmic reticulum by immunocytofluorescence of selectively permeabilized *cos*-1 cells. *Cos*-1 cells were transfected with vectors containing cDNAs encoding either ovine PGHS-1, β-galactosidase, or murine PGHS-2. Cells were fixed in 2% formaldehyde/PBS and permeabilized with either saponin (0.2%) or digitonin (5 μg/ml). Cells were then stained with either (A) a rabbit polyclonal antisera against actin, (B) a purified mouse monoclonal antibody against β-galactosidase, (C) affinity-purified antibody against the carboxyl terminus of murine PGHS-2, and affinity-purified antibodies against the (D) amino terminus, (E) region of the Arg277 trypsin cleavage site, and (F) carboxyl terminus of ovine PGHS-1. Between 100 and 300 individual cells on each coverslip were counted and examined by both phase microscopy and fluorescence microscopy to determine the percentage of cells which exhibited immunofluorescence.

PGHS-2 described above served as a marker for the ER lumen of *cos*-1 cells because this antibody had previously been demonstrated to stain the luminal side of the ER (23). Finally, antibodies against the amino terminus, the Arg277 trypsin cleavage site, and the carboxyl terminus of ovine PGHS-1 were used to examine the orientation of this enzyme in the ER.

Cos-1 cells treated with either digitonin or with streptolysin O to selectively permeabilize plasma membranes were uniformly stained with anti-actin antibodies. The results obtained with saponin and digitonin are shown in Fig. 1. About 30% of the *cos*-1 cells that had been transfected with a pSVGal were stained by anti-β-galactosidase antibodies when the plasma membranes were permeabilized, and this percentage did not increase after permeabilizing the ER with 0.2% saponin; these findings indicate that the staining percentage reflects the efficiency of transfection. When *cos*-1 cells expressing murine PGHS-2 were permeabilized with either digitonin or streptolysin and incubated with antibodies to PGHS-2, no staining occurred (Fig. 1). However, after permeabilization with 0.2% saponin, approximately 40% of these cells became reactive with the anti-PGHS-2 antibody. This pattern of staining observed with anti-PGHS-2 antibodies in *cos*-1 cells treated with different cell permeants is the same as that observed previously in staining murine NIH/3T3 cells, where PGHS-2 is a marker for the lumen of the ER (23).

Cos-1 cells transfected with PGHS-1 were stained with the three different anti-peptide antibodies against this protein following permeabilization of all cellular membranes with 0.2% saponin (Fig. 1), but no staining was seen in cells permeabilized with either digitonin or streptolysin; only about 40% of the transfected cells could be stained because of incomplete transfection. The differential staining for PGHS-1 in the presence of selective permeants parallels that observed for PGHS-2. These results indicate that (a) the amino terminus, (b) the domain containing the unique tryptic cleavage site at Arg277, and (c) a region near the carboxyl terminus of ovine PGHS-1 are all located in the lumen of the ER.

DISCUSSION

PGHSs are integral membrane proteins (2,3) located in the ER and nuclear membranes of prostaglandin-forming cells (3,4). Previous models describing the association of PGHSs with membranes have included one or more transmembrane domains (2,6,15). The arguments for the existence of transmembrane domains have been predicated on the observations that PGHS-1 is N-glycosylated (1,2) and mannose-containing N-glycosyl groups are found exclusively on the luminal side of the ER (13), and that microsomal ovine PGHS-1 is susceptible to cleavage by trypsin which hydrolyzes the enzyme at Arg277 (14-16). To test this model, we prepared antibodies to the domain containing Arg277, as well as to the N- and C-termini, and then performed immunocytofluorescent staining in the presence of detergent treatments which would either expose only the cytoplasmic surface of the ER or both the cytoplasmic and luminal surfaces. The results of these studies have indicated that the domain containing Arg277 and the N- and C-termini of ovine PGHS are only accessible to antibodies following permeabilization of the ER with 0.2% saponin; no staining was observed under conditions found to cause only permeabilization of the plasma membrane. These immunocytochemical results argue that Arg277 is located in the lumen of the ER in cells expressing ovine PGHS-1.

Our work indicates that the N- and C-termini and the Arg277-containing domain of ovine PGHS-1 reside in the lumen of the ER. Combined with the presence of N-glycosylation sites at Asn68, Asn144, and Asn410 in ovine PGHS-1, six regions of the enzyme spaced along the length of the amino acid sequence reside in the ER lumen. The prediction that the amino and carboxyl termini, Arg277, and each of the N-glycosylation sites of ovine PGHS-1 reside on the same side of the ER membrane is in agreement with the recently determined crystal structure of detergent-solubilized ovine PGHS-1 (24). Thus, it appears that the entire enzyme, including both the cyclooxygenase and the peroxidase active sites, reside in the ER.

The luminal orientation of the active sites of PGHS-1 raises questions of how the enzyme acquires free arachidonate for prostaglandin formation and how PGH_2, formed through the action of PGHS-1, is channeled to enzymes downstream in the prostaglandin biosynthetic pathway. Arachidonic acid can diffuse across lipid bilayers, and arachidonate added exogenously to cells expressing PGHS is rapidly converted into prostaglandins, indicating that arachidonate can efficiently pass through cell membranes to reach the ER lumen. One pathway whereby arachidonate is released from cellular phospholipid utilizes a cytosolic phospholipase A_2 ($cPLA_2$), which is activated rapidly in response to hormonal stimuli (25). Upon activation, this enzyme translocates to an intracellular membrane, where it specifically releases arachidonate from phospholipid on the cytoplasmic side of the membrane (25). This intracellular membrane is likely to be the ER membrane, and thus, arachidonate would have to cross a single leaflet of the bilayer to reach PGHS-1. One possibility is that the ω-terminus of arachidonate moves through the center of the helical membrane anchors embedded in the inner bilayer of the ER directly into the hydrophobic channel that forms the core of the cyclooxygenase active site of PGHS (24). Following synthesis of PGH_2 by PGHS-1 in the ER lumen, PGH_2 is converted into active prostanoids by other enzymes. The location of the enzymes which catalyze these conversions may shed light on the mechanism of release of prostanoids from the cell. In the case of PGI_2 synthase, the enzyme is associated with the endoplasmic reticulum. This enzyme has recently been cloned and found to be a P450. The active sites of this family of proteins have been predicted to be located on the cytoplasmic side of the ER (26), suggesting that PGH_2 would need to cross the ER membrane to the cytoplasm for conversion into prostacyclin. PGH_2 added to cells is rapidly converted to PGI_2 (27), suggesting that PGH_2 can move through membranes, and thus, generation of PGH_2 in the ER lumen should pose no difficulty for its subsequent enzymatic isomerization occurring on the cytoplasmic face of the ER.

ACKNOWLEDGEMENTS

This work was supported in part by United States Public Health Service National Institutes of Health Grants DK42509 and DK22042, a National Institutes of Health Predoctoral Training Grant HL07404, and a grant-in-aid from the American Heart Association of Michigan.

REFERENCES

1. Mutsaers JHGM, van Halbeek H, Kamerling JP, and Vliegenthart JFG. Determination of the structure of the carbohydrate chains of prostaglandin endoperoxide synthase from sheep. *Eur J Biochem* 1985;147:569-574.
2. Otto JC, DeWitt DL, and Smith WL. N-glycosylation of prostaglandin endoperoxide synthases-1 and -2 and their orientation in the endoplasmic reticulum. *J Biol Chem* 1993;268:18234-18242.
3. Rollins TE, and Smith WL. (1980) Subcellular localization of the prostaglandin-forming cyclooxygenase in Swiss mouse 3T3 cells by electron microscopic immunocytochemistry. *J Biol Chem* 1980;255:4872-4875.
4. Regier MK, DeWitt DL, Schindler MS, and Smith WL. Subcellular localization of prostaglandin endoperoxide (PGH) synthase-2 in murine 3T3 cells. *Arch Biochem Biophys* 1993;301:439-444.
5. DeWitt DL, and Smith WL. Primary structure of prostaglandin G/H synthase from sheep vesicular gland determined from the complementary DNA sequence. *Proc Natl Acad Sci USA* 1988;85:1412-1416.
6. Merlie JP, Fagan D, Mudd J, and Needleman P. Isolation and characterization of the complementary DNA for sheep seminal vesicle prostaglandin endoperoxide synthase (cyclooxygenase). *J Biol Chem* 1988;263:3550-3553.
7. Yokoyama C, Takai T, and Tanabe R. Primary structure of sheep prostaglandin endoperoxide synthase deduced from cDNA sequence. *FEBS Lett* 1988;231:347-351.
8. Sirios J, and Richards JS. Purification and characterization of a novel, distinct isoform of prostaglandin endoperoxide synthase induced by human chorionic gondadotropin in granulosa cells of rat preovulatory follicles. *J Biol Chem* 1992;267:6382-6388.
9. Kujubu DA, Fletcher BS, Varnum BC, Lim RW, and Herschman HR. TIS10, a phorbol ester tumor promoter inducible mRNA from Swiss 3T3 cells, encodes a novel prostaglandin synthase/cyclooxygenase homologue. *J Biol Chem* 1991;266:12866-12872.
10. Hla T, and Neilson K. Human cyclooxygenase-2 cDNA. *Proc Natl Acad Sci USA*, 1992;89:7384-7388.
11. Jones DA, Carlton DB, McIntyre TM, Zimmerman GA, and Prescott, SM. Molecular cloning of human prostaglandin endoperoxide synthase type II and

demonstration of expression in response to cytokines. *J Biol Chem* 1993; 268:9049-9054.

12. O'Banion MK, Winn VD, and Young DA. cDNA Cloning and functional activity of a glucocorticoid-regulated inflammatory cyclooxygenase. *Proc Natl Acad Sci USA*, 1992;89:4888-4892.

13. Kornfeld R, and Kornfeld S. Assembly of asparagine-linked oligosaccharides. *Ann Rev Biochem* 1985;54:631-664.

14. Chen YP, Bienkowski MJ, and Marnett LJ. Controlled tryptic digestion of prostaglandin H synthase. *J Biol Chem* 1987;262:16892-16899.

15. DeWitt DL, Rollins TE, Day JS, Gauger JA, and Smith WL. Orientation of the active site and antigenic determinants of prostaglandin endoperoxide synthase in the endoplasmic reticulum. *J Biol Chem* 1981;256:10375-10382.

16. Kulmacz RJ, and Wu KK. Topographic studies of microsomal and pure prostaglandin H synthase. *Arch Biochem Biophys* 1989;268:502-515.

17. Shimokawa T, and Smith WL. Essential histidines of prostaglandin endoperoxide synthase: His309 is involved in heme binding. *J Biol Chem* 1991;266:6168-6173.

18. Shimokawa T, Kulmacz RJ, DeWitt DL, and Smith WL. Tyrsoine-385 of prostaglandin endoperoxide synthase is required for cyclooxygenase catalysis. *J Biol Chem* 1990;265:20073-20076.

19. Laneuville O, Breuer DK, DeWitt DL, Hla T, Funk CD, and Smith WL. Differential inhibition of human prostaglandin endoperoxide H synthases-1 and -2 by nonsteroidal anti-inflammatory drugs. *J Pharm Exp Therap* 1994; in press.

20. Meade EA, Smith WL, and DeWitt DL. Expression of the murine prostaglandin (PGH) synthase-1 and PGH synthase-2 isozymes in cos-1 cells. *J Lipid Mediators* 1993;6:119-129.

21. Roitelman J, Olender EH, Shoshana B, Dunn WA Jr, and Simoni RD. Immunological evidence for eight spans in the membrane domain of 3-hydroxy-3-methylglutaryl coenzyme A reductase: implications for enzyme degradation in the endoplasmic reticulum. *J Cell Biol* 1992;117:959-973.

22. Gravotta D, Adesnik M, and Sabatini DD. Transport of influenza HA from the trans-golgi network to the apical surface of MDCK cells permeabilized in their basolateral plasma membranes: energy dependence and involvement of GTP-binding proteins. *J Cell Biol* 1990;111:2893-2908.

23. Otto JC, and Smith WL. The orientation of prostaglandin endoperoxide synthases-1 and -2 in the endoplasmic reticulum. *J Biol Chem* 1994; in press.

24. Picot D, Loll PJ, and Garavito RM. The X-ray crystal structure of the membrane protein prostaglandin H_2 synthase-1. *Nature* 1994;367:243-249.

25. Clark JD, Lin LL, Kriz RW, Ramesha CS, Sultzman LA, Milona N, and Knopf JL. A novel arachidonic acid-selective cytosolic PLA_2 contains a Ca^{2+}-dependent translocation domain with homology to PKC and GAP. *Cell* 1991;65:1043-1051.

26. Ruan KH, Wang LH, Wu KK, and Kulmacz RJ. Amino-terminal topology of thromboxane synthase in the endoplasmic reticulum. *J Biol Chem* 1993;268:19483-19490.

27. Smith WL. Prostaglandin synthesis and its compartmentation in vascular smooth muscle and endothelial cells. *Ann Rev Physiol* 1986;48:251-262.

Advances in Prostaglandin, Thromboxane,
and Leukotriene Research, Vol. 23,
edited by B. Samuelsson et al.
Raven Press, Ltd., New York © 1995

Expression Cloning of Human LTC$_4$ Synthase

Bing K. Lam, John F. Penrose, and K. Frank Austen

Department of Rheumatology and Immunology, Brigham and Women's Hospital and Department of Medicine, Harvard Medical School, Boston, Massachusetts 02115 U.S.A.

The cysteinyl leukotrienes (LTs), LTC$_4$, LTD$_4$ and LTE$_4$, are potent smooth muscle contractile agonists that were once collectively termed slow-reacting substances of anaphylaxis (SRS-A) (1,2). LTC$_4$ synthase catalyzes the conjugation of the unstable epoxide intermediate LTA$_4$ to reduced glutathione (GSH) to form LTC$_4$ (3), the parent compound of the cysteinyl LTs. It is a membrane-bound enzyme whose GSH transferase activity differs from other GSH-S-transferases (GSTs) (4). LTC$_4$ synthase is very substrate specific; it only conjugates LTA$_4$ and does not conjugate xenobiotically with GSH (4).

LTC$_4$ synthase has been recently purified from human myelocytic KG-1 cells (5) and human monocytic THP-1 cells (6) and the respective N-terminal amino acid sequence of each protein determined (6,7). The reduced protein migrates as an 18-kDa protein in SDS-PAGE gel (5,6). The enzyme was proposed to function as a homodimer and its function was attenuated by protein kinase C activation (6). In the expression cloning of LTC$_4$ synthase, we described the utilization of a novel fluorescence-linked immunoassay for the LTC$_4$ produced by cells transfected with the cDNA for human LTC$_4$ synthase derived from a KG-1 expression library (7). The nucleotide sequence and the deduced amino acid sequence of human LTC$_4$ synthase share no significant homology with other GSTs but show significant identity with 5-lipoxygenase activating protein (FLAP) (7,8).

METHODS

Fluorescence-linked Immunoassay for LTC$_4$

Briefly, KG-1 cells were harvested by centrifugation, resuspended in Hanks' balanced salt solution (HBSS) at 10^7 cells/ml, and biotinylated. The biotinylated cells were washed and linked to avidin. The biotin-avidin coupled KG-1 cells were washed and the LTC_2-biotin complex was linked onto the cell surface via the previously bound avidin. After washing, samples of 10^5 cells each were incubated either with 0-200 pg of synthetic LTC_4 or with 5- to 10-μl-portions of the incubation medium from transfected COS cells that contained unknown amounts of released LTC_4. Mouse monoclonal LTC_4 antibodies were added, and the cells were incubated, washed, and incubated with fluorescein isothiocyanate-conjugated goat anti-mouse Fab' antiserum on ice in the dark. The cells were washed, resuspended in 1 ml of HBSA containing 1 mM EDTA, and analyzed by flow cytometry for cell surface fluorescence intensities (7).

Screening of pcDNA3 Library with COS Cell Transfections

A cDNA library was constructed from mRNA of KG-1 cells as described (7). The sequential and stepwise identification of a single clone from the 2.4 x 10^5 clones in 96 pools was described in detail in the original study (7). Briefly, plasmids from the expression library were transfected into COS-7 cells by the DEAE-dextran technique (9). 72 hr later, COS cells were harvested and assayed for LTC_4 synthase activity by adding the substrate, LTA_4. In the first round of screening, 20,000 COS cells were incubated with 20 μM LTA_4 for 30 min on ice

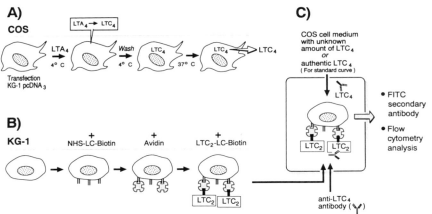

FIG. 1. Fluorescence-linked competitive immunoassay for LTC_4 generated and released from COS cells transfected with cDNA from KG-1 pcDNA mammalian expression library. Schematic presentation of the procedure. **A)** Synthesis and release of LTC_4 from washed, transfected COS cells; **B)** coupling of LTC_2 to KG-1 cell surface; and **C)** competition between released LTC_4 and membrane-bound LTC_2 for anti-LTC_4 as analyzed by decrements in binding of fluorescence-linked secondary antibody by fluorescence flow cytometry.

for the synthesis of intracellular LTC$_4$, washed, and resuspended at 37°C for 10 min for the release of the intracellular LTC$_4$. Supernatants were then assayed for LTC$_4$ level by the fluorescence-linked immunoassay. Once a positive pool was identified, the subsequent rounds of screening were performed with the methyl ester (ME) of LTA$_4$ as substrate and assayed by RP-HPLC for LTC$_4$-ME level as described (7).

RESULTS AND DISCUSSION

A novel fluorescence-linked immunoassay for LTC$_4$ was developed for the primary screening of a mammalian expression library derived from KG-1 cells, as depicted in Figure 1. This immunoassay is capable of detecting as little as 2.5 pg of LTC$_4$ with a linear dose response between 10 and 100 pg of LTC$_4$ (Fig. 2). Using this immunoassay in combination with RP-HPLC, we isolated a clone which contains the human LTC$_4$ synthase cDNA (7). The cDNA insert is 694 bp in length with an open reading frame of 450 bp. It encodes for a 150-amino acid polypeptide with a calculated MW of 16,567 daltons, and a predicted pI of 11.05. The deduced protein contains two putative protein kinase C phosphorylation sites and a glycosylation site.

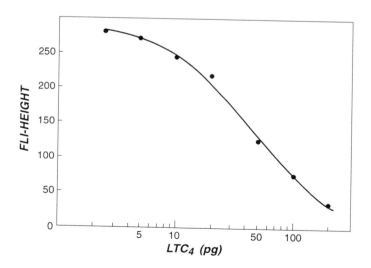

FIG. 2. Standard curve of the fluorescence-linked immunoassay for LTC$_4$.

LTC₄ Synthase   46 F E R V Y R A Q V N C 56
Human FLAP   50 F E R V Y T A N Q N C 60

FIG. 3. Partial sequence comparison of the putative FLAP inhibitor binding site of FLAP (11 of 15 amino acid residues) and human LTC₄ synthase with identical amino acids in bold. Numbers correspond to the amino acid residue position for the respective protein.

The nucleotide and the deduced amino acid sequence of LTC₄ synthase share no significant homology with known GSTs but share 31% overall amino acid identity with FLAP. The amino acid identity at the N-terminal two-thirds of these two proteins is 44% and includes the putative FLAP inhibitor binding site (Fig. 3) (10). Secondary structure analysis of these proteins predicts the presence of three transmembrane domains which almost overlap each other, and intervening hydrophilic loops of similar size which in LTC₄ synthase are arginine rich (7).

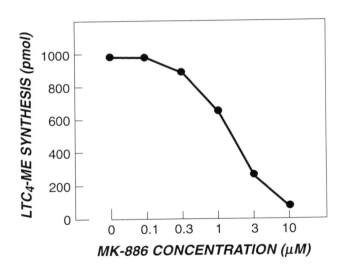

FIG. 4. Dose-dependent inhibition of LTC₄ synthase from transfected COS cell microsome by MK-886.

In agreement with the amino acid identity between LTC_4 synthase and FLAP, the FLAP inhibitor MK-886 inhibits LTC_4 synthase activity in a dose-dependent manner when transfected COS cell microsomes are used as a source of LTC_4 synthase enzyme and LTA-ME as substrate. Similar to the transfected COS cell lysate (7), the IC_{50} of MK-886 is <3 μM (Fig. 4). As LTA_4 and reduced GSH can conjugate spontaneously in a basic environment (4), it may be that the putative binding of LTA_4 to LTC_4 synthase, a protein with a pI of 11.05, allows a favorable microenvironment for the conjugation with bound and/or unbound GSH with only a slight catalytic boost. Regardless of the catalytic mechanism yet to be determined, it is likely that LTC_4 synthase represents a member of a novel gene family in which FLAP is also a member.

REFERENCES

1.   Samuelsson B. *Science* 1983; 220:568-75.
2.   Kellaway CH, Trethewie ER. *Q J Exp Physiol* 1940; 30:121-45.
3.   Yoshimoto T, Soberman RJ, Lewis RA, Austen KF. *Proc Natl Acad Sci USA* 1985; 82: 8399-403.
4.   Yoshimoto T, Soberman RJ, Spur B, Austen KF. *J Clin Invest* 1988; 81:866-71.
5.   Penrose JF, Gagnon L, Goppelt-Struebe M *et al. Proc Natl Acad Sci USA* 1992; 89:11603-6.
6.   Nicholson DW, Ali A, Vaillancourt JP *et al. Proc Natl Acad Sci USA* 1993; 90:2015-9.
7.   Lam BK, Penrose JF, Freeman GJ, Austen KF. *Proc Natl Acad Sci USA* 1994, in press.
8.   Dixon RAF, Diehl RE, Opas E *et al. Nature (London)* 1990; 343:282-4.
9.   Seed B, Aruffo A. *Proc Natl Acad Sci USA* 1987; 84:3365-70.
10.   Vickers PJ, Adam M, Charleson S, Mancini JA. Amino acid residues of human FLAP involved in binding leukotriene synthesis inhibitors. In: *The 8th international Conference on Prostaglandins and Related Compounds.* July 26-31, 1992, Montreal, Canada. Abstract #6, p. 4.

Advances in Prostaglandin, Thromboxane, and Leukotriene Research, Vol. 23,
edited by B. Samuelsson et al.
Raven Press, Ltd., New York © 1995

A BETTER UNDERSTANDING OF ANTI-INFLAMMATORY DRUGS BASED ON ISOFORMS OF CYCLOOXYGENASE (COX-1 AND COX-2).

by J.R. Vane and R.M. Botting

*The William Harvey Research Institute, St Bartholomew's Hospital Medical College,
Charterhouse Square, London EC1M 6BQ, UK*

In 1971 we demonstrated that aspirin inhibits the cyclo-oxygenase enzyme of guinea pig lung homogenates, of human platelets and of dog spleen *in vivo* (1,2,3), thus preventing the synthesis of the then known arachidonic acid metabolites. This inhibition is due to the irreversible acetylation of the cyclo-oxygenase component of prostaglandin endoperoxide synthase, leaving the peroxidase activity of the enzyme unaffected (4). Ser 530 is acetylated (5,6,7), placing a bulky group close to the active site of the enzyme thus hindering access of the substrate to the active site. Ser 530 is not itself part of the active site since its replacement by an alanine residue does not affect cyclo-oxygenase activity. However, the mutant enzyme can no longer be acetylated and inactivated by aspirin (8).

In contrast to the irreversible action of aspirin, other non-steroidal anti-inflammatory drugs such as indomethacin or ibuprofen produce reversible cyclo-oxygenase inhibition by competing with the substrate, arachidonic acid, for the active site of the enzyme (9).

The inhibition of prostaglandin synthesis nicely explains the actions of all aspirin-like drugs. They prevent the overproduction of prostaglandins in inflammatory states (therapeutic effects) and the physiological formation of prostanoids (side effects).

INHIBITION OF PROSTAGLANDIN SYNTHESIS

The inhibition of prostaglandin synthesis by NSAIDs has been demonstrated in a wide variety of cell types and tissues, ranging from whole animals and man to microsomal enzyme preparations. Several classes of inhibitors have been identified (10) and at least 12 major chemical series are known to affect prostaglandin production directly (11).

The release of prostaglandins by inflammatory stimuli is well established. However, the mechanism by which the increased synthesis of prostaglandins is achieved in inflammation has only recently become understood. The other factors which have awaited an explanation have been the difference between the anti-inflammatory action of aspirin and salicylate and the mechanism of action of acetaminophen (paracetamol).

First, salicylate is an order of magnitude less active than aspirin on the crude cyclooxygenase enzyme prepared from lung tissue (1), yet rheumatologists (12) report that salicylate is as potent as aspirin in suppressing arthritis. This observation in patients is supported by the work of Higgs et al. (13) which showed that a crude cyclooxygenase preparation from an inflamed site in the rat had almost the same sensitivity to aspirin as to salicylate.

Second, acetaminophen is antipyretic and analgesic but has little anti-inflammatory activity. Furthermore, it has only weak activity against most cyclooxygygenase preparations but is considerably more active in diminishing prostaglandin synthesis in the brain (14).

SELECTIVE INHIBITION OF COX-2

Four years ago, Needleman and his group reported that bacterial lipopolysaccharide increased the synthesis of prostaglandins in human monocytes *in vitro* (15) and in mouse peritoneal macrophages *in vivo* (16). This increase was inhibited by dexamethasone and associated with de novo synthesis of new cyclooxygenase protein. A year or so later, an inducible synthase was identified as a distinct isoform of cyclooxygenase (COX-2) encoded by a different gene from the constitutive enzyme (COX-1) (17,18,19,20). The amino acid sequence of its cDNA shows only a 60% homology with the sequence of the non-inducible enzyme, with the size of the mRNA for the inducible enzyme approximating 4.5 kb and that of the constitutive enzyme being 2.8 kb. However, both enzymes have a molecular weight of 70 Kd and similar active sites for the attachment of non-steroidal anti-inflammatory drugs.

It should, therefore, be possible to develop new anti-inflammatory drugs which are specific inhibitors of COX-2 but which will not inhibit COX-1 and thus will not harm the stomach. With this in mind, we have developed models to test the activity of non-steroidal anti-inflammatory drugs for inhibitory actions against COX-1 and COX-2. Cultured bovine aortic endothelial cells serve as a source of COX-1 enzyme and J774.2 macrophages (which have little or no COX-1) stimulated with LPS are the means of testing for anti-COX-2 activity. In both instances prostaglandin release from the cells, when incubated with arachidonic acid, is measured. Comparing the activity of the known NSAIDs in these two cell types with their ED_{50} in the original experiment carried out by

Vane (1) on guinea-pig lung homogenates, it becomes clear that in 1971 the drugs were tested for their activity against COX-1. A series of NSAIDs have also been tested for their relative activities against COX-1 and COX-2 and a table of activity ratios constructed with aspirin and indomethacin showing as the inhibitors with the worst COX-1/COX-2 ratios (Table 1). These drugs have strong side effects at antiinflammatory doses. Compounds with decreasing activity ratios should have decreasing side effects and less irritant action on the stomach. BF389 has the best activity ratio for COX-1/COX-2 and also has minimal damaging effects on the gastrointestinal tract (21).

Even though aspirin would not now be the drug of choice for chronic inflammatory conditions such as rheumatism and arthritis because of its potent inhibitory action on COX-1, it will remain the drug of choice in reducing the number of secondary and primary heart attacks and strokes (22) for platelets almost certainly contain COX-1 (23). A low-dose aspirin regimen of 75 mg/day has been recommended while doses of up to 325 mg/day may be administered in acute emergencies.

Interestingly, on COX-2, salicylate (100μg/ml) has a similar IC_{50} to aspirin (50μg/ml), a much better correlation with the clinical effects. Acetaminophen is still a puzzle, unless there is a COX-3.

Table 1. IC_{50} values (μg/ml) of NSAIDs on COX-1 or COX-2 activity in intact cells

NSAID	COX-1	COX-2	Ratio
Aspirin	0.3±0.2	50±10	166
Indomethacin	0.01±0.001	0.6±0.08	60
Tolfenamic acid	0.0003±0.0007	0.005±0.0019	16.7
Ibuprofen	1±0.07	15±5.33	15
Acetaminophen	2.7±2	20±12	7.4
Sodium salicylate	35±11.24	100±16.2	2.8
BW755C	0.65±0.26	1.2±0.78	1.9
Flurbiprofen	0.02±0.01	0.025±0.01	1.3
Carprofen	3±0.41	3±1.72	1
Diclofenac	0.5±0.21	0.35±0.15	0.7
Naproxen	2.2±0.98	1.3±2.2	0.6
BF389	0.15±0.01	0.03±0.01	0.2

The nonsteroidal antiinflammatory drugs (NSAIDs) are arranged in order of ratio of their activities for inhibiting cyclooxygenase-1 (COX-1) and cyclooxygenase-2 (COX-2). The least favourable ratios are at the top of the list.

INTERACTIONS BETWEEN THE CYCLOOXYGENASE AND NITRIC OXIDE SYNTHASE PATHWAYS.

We tested the eicosanoids PGE_1 and its metabolite 13,14-dihydro PGE_1 (PGE_0) on cultured bovine aortic endothelial cells and J774.2 macrophages treated with LPS. Both prostanoids reduced the release of prostaglandins from the cultured cells and inhibited the expression of COX-2 protein measured by Western blot analysis (24).

In the mouse macrophage cell line RAW264.7 treatment for 18 h with LPS causes an increase in the release of nitrite and PGE_2. This is due to increased expression of inducible NOS and of COX-2 in these cells. Lowering the endogenous nitric oxide concentrations with inhibitors of nitric oxide synthase such as N^G-monomethyl-L-arginine reduced the formation of PGE_2 suggesting that nitric oxide was potentiating the activity of COX-2 (25). Conversely, adding nitric oxide donors such as sodium nitroprusside to cultured cells which contained no endogenous nitric oxide increased COX-2 activity and the production of prostanoids (25). However, addition of sodium nitroprusside to LPS-treated cultured macrophages caused dose-related inhibition of prostanoid release (26). Thus, small amounts of nitric oxide (when cells are depleted of endogenous nitric oxide) stimulate COX-2, whereas large amounts of nitric oxide (when NO donors are added to cells which already contain nitric oxide) inhibit the enzyme.

Products of COX-2 and inducible NOS also interact in models of chronic inflammation such as the murine granulomatous air pouch (27,28,29). COX and NOS activities were measured in normal skin and skin samples from the first 24 h after initiation of the air pouch as an index of activities in the acute stage of inflammation. To cover the chronic and resolving stages of the inflammatory process, COX and NOS activities were measured at 3,5,7,14 and 21 days.

In the acute stage, iNOS activity in the skin was raised at 6 h and sustained up to 24 h. In contrast, the increase in COX-2 activity was slower in onset and was maximal at 24 h. These findings support the well-established role for prostaglandins as mediators of the acute inflammatory response (30) and allow a similar interpretation for the role of NO. However, the role of NO in inflammation is not clear as both pro- and anti-inflammatory actions have been reported (31).

In the granulomatous tissue, taken as an indication of chronic inflammation, maximal iNOS activity was between 3 and 7 days, whereas COX-2 expression continued to rise until day 14. This pattern of COX-2 and iNOS induction between 3 and 21 days suggests that there is differential regulation of the enzymes. This may be attributed to the changing profile of cytokines as the inflammatory process progresses. Thus, TGF-β is known to induce COX-2 but inhibit iNOS (32,33) and TGF-β immunoreactivity is greatest on day 14 in this model (28). The rise in COX-2 activity and fall of iNOS activity at 7-14 days may be due to the presence of TGF-β.

The release of large amounts of NO by iNOS can inhibit the induction of COX-2 (34) and suppress the formation of COX metabolites (35,36). In the murine granulomatous tissue, between days 3 and 7 elevated NOS activity was associated with a fall in COX activity. When COX-2 levels were maximal at day 14, NOS activity was depressed. Thus, the modulatory actions of NO on COX-2 activity may also contribute to the dissociation of activities seen in the chronic phase of inflammation.

TARGETS FOR NEW MEDICINES

The path from making a scientific discovery to treating patients with a new drug is a slow one and can take 20 years or more. Prostacyclin was discovered in 1976, but sadly within Wellcome the development of prostacyclin as a therapeutic agent received little support in the early days. The overall lack of vision of the marketing advisers in a pharmaceutical company was once more demonstrated, for they could not analyse effectively the potential market. However, other drug companies, including several in Japan and Schering in Germany, picked up the baton. Schering developed the stable analogue, iloprost, which will be marketed for the treatment of obstructive diseases of the circulation. Orally active compounds are also on their way. Again, the time scale is inordinately protracted with two decades passing between discovery and the marketing of a compound active by mouth. Several companies have produced prostacyclin analogues which display oral activity; indeed, one (beraprost) is on the market in Japan (37,38) and another (cicaprost) is being developed in Germany for its potential anti-cancer activity (39). Oral administration of cicaprost to cholesterol-fed rabbits reduced the proportion of the aortic intimal surface covered by atheromatous lesions from 84% to 63% (40). The availability of a daily tablet which would slow down or even prevent the atherosclerotic process would make a valuable contribution to medicine.

The discovery of COX-2 has stimulated several laboratories to develop selective inhibitors of this enzyme. These potential aspirin-like drugs should have anti-inflammatory activity without the side-effects of damaging the stomach or kidney. Needleman and his group at Searle have made cyclooxygenase inhibitors which are some 1000 fold more potent against COX-2 of inflamed tissues than against COX-1 of the stomach (41). These have been tested on various models of chronic inflammation such as carrageenin-induced oedema of the rat paw, the rat carrageenin-injected air-pouch and rat adjuvant arthritis. However, selective COX-2 inhibitors may not be as potent as steroids, even though the lack of side effects will allow higher dosage. This is because prostaglandins are not the only mediators involved in chronic inflammation. Nevertheless, arthritic patients will surely benefit before the year 2000 from the important discovery of selective COX-2 inhibitors.

ACKNOWLEDGEMENTS
The William Harvey Research Institute is supported by grants from the Ono Pharmaceutical Company, the Parke-Davis Pharmaceutical Division of Warner-Lambert, Schwarz Pharma Limited and the Servier International Research Institute.

REFERENCES

1. Vane JR. Inhibition of prostaglandin synthesis as a mechanism of action for the aspirin-like drugs. Nature 1971; 231: 232-5.

2. Smith JH and Willis AL. Aspirin selectively inhibits prostaglandin production in human platelets. Nature 1971; 231: 235-7.

3. Ferreira SH, Moncada S and Vane JR. Indomethacin and aspirin abolish prostaglandin release from spleen. Nature 1971; 231: 237-9.

4. Van der Ouderaa FJ, Buytenhek M, Nugteren DH, van Dorp DA. Acetylation of prostaglandin endoperoxide synthetase with acetylsalicylic acid. Eur J Biochem. 1980; 109: 1-8.

5. Roth GJ and Majerus PW. The mechanism of the effect of aspirin on human platelets. I. Acetylation of a particulate fraction protein. J Clin Invest 1975; 56: 624-32.

6. Roth GJ, Stanford N and Majerus PW. Acetylation of prostaglandin synthetase by aspirin. Proc Natl Acad Sci USA 1975; 72: 3073-6.

7. Roth GJ and Siok CJ. Acetylation of the NH_2-terminal serine of prostaglandin synthase by aspirin. J Biol Chem 1978; 253: 3782-4.

8. De Witt DL, El-Harith EA, Kraemer SA, Yao EF, Armstrong RL and Smith WL The aspirin and heme-binding sites of ovine and murine prostaglandin endoperoxide synthases. J Biol Chem 1990; 265: 5192-8.

9. Vane JR, Flower RJ and Botting RM. History of aspirin and its mechanism of action. Stroke 1990; 21 (Suppl. IV): 12-23.

10. Flower RJ. Drugs which inhibit prostaglandin biosynthesis. Pharm Rev 1974; 26: 33-67.

11. Shen TY. Prostaglandin synthetase inhibitors. In: Vane JR, Ferreira SH. *Antiinflammatory Drugs*. Berlin: Springer-Verlag; 1979: 305-47.

12. Preston SJ, Arnold MH, Beller EM, Brooks PM and Buchanan WW. Comparative analgesic and anti-inflammatory properties of sodium salicylate and acetylsalicylic acid (aspirin) in rheumatoid arthritis. Br J Clin Pharmacol. 1989; 27: 607-11.

13. Higgs GA, Salmon JA, Henderson B and Vane JR. Pharmacokinetics of aspirin and salicylate in relation to inhibition of arachidonate cyclo-oxygenase and anti-inflammatory activity. Proc Natl Acad Sci USA 1987; 84: 1417-20.

14. Flower RJ and Vane JR. Inhibition of prostaglandin synthetase in brain explains the antipyretic activity of paracetamol (4-acetamidophenol). Nature 1972; 240: 410-1.

15. Fu J-Y, Masferrer JL, Seibert K, Raz A and Needleman P. The induction and suppression of prostaglandin H_2 synthase (cyclooxygenase) in human monocytes. J Biol Chem 1990; 265: 16737-40.
16. Masferrer JL, Zweifel BS, Seibert K and Needleman P. Selective regulation of cellular cyclooxygenase by dexamethasone and endotoxin in mice. J Clin Invest 1990; 86: 1375-9.
17. Xie W, Chipman JG, Robertson DL, Erikson RL and Simmons DL. Expression of a mitogen-responsive gene encoding prostaglandin synthase is regulated by mRNA splicing. Proc Natl Acad Sci USA 1991; 88: 2692-6.
18. O'Banion MK, Sadowski HB, Winn V and Young DA. A serum- and glucocorticoid-regulated 4-kilobase mRNA encodes a cyclooxygenase-related protein. J Biol Chem 1991; 266: 23261-7.
19. Kujubu DA and Herschman HR. Dexamethasone inhibits mitogen induction of the TIS10 prostaglandin synthase/cyclooxygenase gene. J Biol Chem 1992; 267: 7991-4.
20. Sirois J and Richards JS. Purification and characterization of a novel, distinct isoform of prostaglandin endoperoxide synthase induced by human chorionic gonadotropin in granulosa cells of rat preovulatory follicles. J Biol Chem 1992; 267: 6382-8.
21. Mitchell JA, Akarasereenont P, Thiemermann C, Flower RJ and Vane JR. Selectivity of nonsteroidal antiinflammatory drugs as inhibitors of constitutive and inducible cyclooxygenase. Proc Natl Acad Sci USA 1994; 90: 11693-7.
22. Antiplatelet Trialists' Collaboration. Collaborative overview of randomised trials of antiplatelet therapy-I: Prevention of death, myocardial infarction and stroke by prolonged antiplatelet therapy in various categories of patients. Br Med J 1994; 308: 81-106.
23. Funk CD, Funk LB, Kennedy ME, Pong AS and Fitzgerald GA. Human platelet/erythroleukemia cell prostaglandin G/H synthase: cDNA cloning, expression and gene chromosomal assignment. FASEB J 1991; 5: 2304-12.
24. Akarasereenont et al, unpublished.
25. Salvemini D, Misko TP, Masferrer JL, Seibert K, Currie MG and Needleman P. Nitric oxide activates cyclooxygenase enzymes. Proc Natl Acad Sci USA 1993; 90: 7240-4.
26. Swierkosz et al, unpublished.
27. Appleton I, Tomlinson A, Chander CL and Willoughby DA. Effect of endothelin-1 on croton oil-induced granulation tissue in the rat. Lab Invest 1992; 67: 703-10.
28. Appleton I, Tomlinson A, Colville-Nash P and Willoughby DA. Temporal and spatial immunolocalization of cytokines in murine chronic granulomatous tissue. Implications for their role in tissue development and repair processes. Lab Invest 1993; 69: 405-14.

29. Vane JR, Mitchell JA, Appleton I, Tomlinson A, Bishop-Bailey D, Croxtall J and Willoughby DA. Inducible isoforms of cyclooxygenase and nitric oxide synthase in inflammation. Proc Natl Acad Sci USA 1994; 91: 2046-50.

30. Willoughby DA. Human arthritis applied to animal models: towards a better therapy. Herberden Oration 1974. Ann Rheum Dis 1975; 34: 471-8.

31. Gorbunov N and Esposito E. Nitric oxide as a mediator of inflammation. International Journal of Immunopathology and Pharmacology 1993;6:67-75.

32. Bailey JM and Verma M. Analytical procedures for a cryptic messenger RNA that mediates translational control of prostaglandin synthase by glucocorticoids. Anal Biochem 1991; 196: 11-8.

33. Schini BB, Durante W, Elizondo E, Scott-Burden T, Jubquero DC, Schafer AI and Vanhoutte PM. The induction of nitric oxide synthase activity is inhibited by TGF-β_1, PDGF$_{AB}$ and PDGF$_{BB}$ in vascular smooth muscle cells. Eur J Pharmacol 1992; 216: 379-83.

34. Swierkosz TA, Mitchell JA, Tomlinson A, Warner TD, Thiemermann C and Vane JR. Co-release and interactions of nitric oxide and prostanoids in vitro and in vivo following exposure to bacterial lipopolysaccharide. In: Moncada S, Feelisch M, Higgs EA. Biology of Nitric Oxide. London: Portland Press; 1994 (in press).

35. Stadler J, Stefanovic-Racic M, Billiar TR, Curran RD, McIntyre LA, Georgescu HI, Simmons RL and Evans CH. Articular chondrocytes synthesize nitric oxide in response to cytokines and lipopolysaccharide. J Immunol 1991; 147: 3915-20.

36. Stadler J, Harbrecht BG, Di Silvio M, Curran RD, Jordan ML, Simmons RL and Billiar TR. Endogenous nitric oxide inhibits the synthesis of cyclooxygenase products and interleukin-6 by rat Kupffer cells. J Leukocyte Biol 1993; 53: 165-72.

37. Sakaguchi S, Tanabe T, Mishima Y, Shionoya Y, Katsumura T, Kusaba A, Sakuma A. Effect of beraprost sodium (PGI$_2$ derivative) in Rayneaud's Disease or Syndrome. A comparative double blind study with placebo. Clinics and Research 1990; 67: 234-242.

38. Sakaguchi S, Tanabe T, Mishima Y, Shionoya Y, Katsumura T, Kusaba A, Sakuma A. Effect of beraprost sodium (PGI$_2$ derivative) in chronic arterial occlusive disease. A comparative double blind study with Ticlopidine Hydrochloride. Clinics and Research 1990; 67: 575-584.

39. Schirner M and Schneider MR. Antimetastatic potential of the stable prostacyclin analogue Cicaprost. In: Vane J, Rubanyi G. Prostacyclin: New Perspectives in Basic Research and Novel Therapeutic Indications. Amsterdam: Elsevier Sci Publ; 1992: 247-75.

40. Braun M, Hohlfeld T, Kienbaum P, Weber A-A, Sarbia M and Schrör K. Antiatherosclerotic effects of oral cicaprost in experimental hypercholesterolemia in rabbits. Atherosclerosis 1993;103: 93-105.

41. Needleman P. In search of a better NSAID. This meeting.

*Advances in Prostaglandin, Thromboxane,
and Leukotriene Research, Vol. 23,*
edited by B. Samuelsson et al.
Raven Press, Ltd., New York © 1995

DISCOVERY OF A BETTER ASPIRIN

Peter Isakson, Karen Seibert, Jaime Masferrer, Daniela Salvemini,
Len Lee and Philip Needleman.

*Inflammatory Diseases Research
G.D. Searle and Monsanto Corporate Research
700 Chesterfield Village Parkway
St. Louis, Missouri 63198*

Non-steroidal anti-inflammatory drugs (NSAIDs) such as aspirin have been used to treat various ailments for over 100 years. As a class, these drugs possess anti-inflammatory, analgesic and anti-pyretic activity, and are widely used to treat chronic inflammatory states such as arthritis. The available NSAIDs are approximately equivalent in terms of anti-inflammatory efficacy. All of the NSAIDs, however, also cause untoward side effects in a significant fraction of treated patients,and this frequently limits therapy. The most common side effects associated with NSAID therapy are gastrointestinal (GI), with hemorrhage and frank ulceration seen in some patients; these lesions apparently can lead to increased morbidity in long term NSAID users (1). Renal and CNS effects are also observed. Because of these problems, a major goal of the pharmaceutical industry is the development of drugs that possess anti-inflammatory activity but lack the toxic effects associated with current NSAIDS. To date, no NSAIDs with the desired therapeutic profile have been commercially developed.

In the early 1970's NSAIDs were found to prevent the production of prostaglandins (PGs) by inhibiting the enzyme cyclooxygenase (COX), suggesting a biochemical mechanism of action for these drugs (2,3). PGs are produced by most cells and tissues, and have a diverse array of biological functions. Of particular note are the cytoprotective actions of PGs in the gastrointestinal (GI) tract, and the effects of PGs on renal function. In addition to these positive roles in physiology, PGs are associated with inflammatory conditions and can cause many of the signs and symptoms of inflammation including edema, hyperemia and hyperalgesia. For many years it was believed that PGs were formed via the activity of a single enzyme COX, that is present constitutively in most cells (4). Inhibition of COX would lead to decreased production of pro-inflammatory PGs at the site of inflammation while at the same time inhibit the formation of PGs that play a role in sustaining normal cellular or tissue function. A corollary of this view was that the availability of substrate arachidonic acid was the sole means of regulating PG production. This view was challenged by a number of experiments demonstrating that the amount of COX enzyme was regulated in inflammatory conditions. One of the first such observations was in a rabbit model of hydronephrosis, characterized by markedly elevated PG production following ureter obstruction (5). Exaggerated PG production in this model was associated with an influx in inflammatory cells such as macrophages and fibroblasts, and with an increase in the mass of COX enzyme (6,7). *In vitro* experiments then demonstrated that incubation of fibroblasts or monocytes with the inflammatory cytokine IL-1 caused a similar increase in PG synthetic capacity that was associated with elevated amounts of COX enzyme; importantly, increases in PG synthetic capacity and COX enzyme levels were inhibited by the anti-inflammatory glucocorticoid dexamethasone, but the latter drug did not alter basal COX activity observed *in vitro* or *in vivo* (8-11). Based on this data it was hypothesized that there is an inducible form of the COX enzyme that was sensititive to cytokine stimulation and selective inhibition by glucocorticoids. This hypothesis was supported by the isolation of a second COX gene whose expression is induced by a number of inflammatory cytokines, and whose mRNA expression is selectively blocked by dexamethasone (12-21).

The two COX genes are clearly closely related and contain stretches of near identity. Modeling of the active site based on the recently published x-ray structure of sheep seminal vesicle COX (22) suggests that the active sites of the two enzymes are very similar; this close relationship could make it difficult to synthesize compounds that will selectively inhibit one of the enzymes. However, two compounds described in the literature, DuP 697 and NS 398 (23-25) have anti-inflammatory activity without concomitant formation of gastric lesions, a pharmacological profile expected of a selective COX-2 inhibitor. We have cloned and expressed COX-1 and COX-2 and evaluated the activity of these and other NSAIDs on the recombinant enzyme (see Seibert et al, this volume). As shown in Table I, NS398 and DuP 697 were potent inhibitors of COX-2 with much less activity on COX-1. We also evaluated these agents for anti-inflammatory activity and GI toxicity, and confirmed their profile as potentially GI safe NSAIDs.

SC-58125, A SELECTIVE COX-2 INHIBITOR

Based on our observations with DuP 697 and NS 398, we embarked on a program to identify selective COX-2 inhibitors. This led to the discovery of SC-58125, a compound with high selectivity for COX-2 (Table I).

TABLE I

| | IC_{50} (uM) | | ED_{50} (mg/kg) | | |
	COX-1	COX-2	Carrag. edema	Adj. Arthritis	GI ulcers
Indomethacin	0.2	1.2	2	0.1	8
DuP 697	0.8	0.01	5	0.3	>600
NS 398	>10	0.01	3	4.7	>1000
SC-58125	>100	0.09	10	0.4	>600

Role of COX-2 in NSAID-sensitive animal models

The availability of molecular and pharmacological probes specific for COX-2 has allowed us to evaluate the role of this enzyme in inflammation and in the GI tract. We have focused on inflammatory models that have been traditionally used to select NSAIDs such as the carrageenan-induced footpad edema and adjuvant arthritis models.

Carrageenan paw edema. To critically examine the role of COX-2 *in vivo*, the presence and function of COX-2 at the site of inflammation was examined in the carrageenan-induced rat paw edema model. Following injection of carrageenan, paw volume increases markedly over a 3 hr time course, and this edematous response is blunted by NSAIDs such as indomethacin. We found that the increase in paw volume coincided with an increase in tissue TxB_2, and that the latter was completely inhibited by indomethacin. Analysis of tissue expression of COX showed that carrageenan induced marked increases in COX-2 mRNA and protein that coincided with TxB_2 production; COX-1 mRNA levels were unchanged. Importantly, tissue TxB_2 levels were reduced by selective COX-2 inhibitors such as NS-398 and SC-58125 at doses similar to those required to suppress edema formation. These results indicate that COX-2 plays a major role in the rat carrageenan paw edema model, which has been traditionally used to develop NSAIDs.

Adjuvant arthritis The ability of DuP697 and NS-398 to suppress inflammation in adjuvant arthritis suggested that there was a prominent COX-2 component contributing to the pathophysiology of this form of arthritis. This idea has been repeatedly confirmed pharmacologically as we have shown that highly selective COX-2 inhibitors (e.g. SC-58125) are as efficacious as mixed COX-1/COX-2 inhibitors (e.g. indomethacin) in inhibiting edema in this model when administered therapeutically. SC-58125 is anti-inflammtory in this model (i.e. reduces cell influx and synovial hyperplasia) and inhibits the elevated production of PGs in the inflamed paw. We have also examined COX expression in this model with immunological and molecular tools and found that COX-2 mRNA and protein are elevated in arthritic rat paws. Our data suggests that PG production in this model is driven exclusively by COX-2.

Analgesia An important aspect of the clinical activity of NSAIDs is their ability to relieve pain, especially that associated with inflammation. We have evaluated COX-2 selective inhibitors in the Hargreaves model of inflammation induced hyperalgesia and found them to be as efficacious as indomethacin or naproxen. This suggests that COX-2 is involved in some aspect of inflammatory hyperalgesia; whether this is a peripheral or central effect is currently under investigation.

Biochemical efficacy model for COX-2 inhibitors

Carrageenan administration to the subcutaneous rat air pouch induces a rapid inflammatory response characterized by high levels of PGs and leukotrienes in the fluid exudate. We found that COX-2 mRNA and protein were induced by carrageenan over a time course that coincided with the production of PGs in the pouch tissue. COX-2 immunoreactivity was localized to macrophages in the fluid exudate and in cells within the pouch lining (26). Pharmacological analysis was performed using non-selective (COX-1/COX-2) such as indomethacin, and selective (COX-2) inhibitors; PG's were measured in both the pouch and the stomach. Indomethacin blocked PG synthesis in the air pouch and the stomach, and produced gastric lesions. In contrast, selective COX-2 inhibitors such as NS-398 (23,24,26) and SC-58125 completely suppressed pouch PG synthesis without significant effect on gastric PG. These results suggest that PG synthesis in the air pouch model is driven solely by COX-2, and thus provides a useful model for establishing biochemical efficacy of COX-2 inhibitors.

Role of COX-1 in GI toxicity

Our hypothesis is that constitutive COX-1 activity protects the GI tract and inhibition of this activity by current NSAIDs leads to GI toxicity; tissue distribution studies reported elsewhere in this volume (Seibert et al) are consistent with this notion. This hypothesis was examined pharmacologically by comparing the ability of non-selective inhibitors such as indomethacin, and the selective inhibitors NS 398 and SC-58125, to inhibit GI PG production and to cause ulcers. A close correlation between reduction of stomach PG levels by non-selective COX inhibitors and the appearance of GI lesions was observed; in contrast, selective COX-2 inhibitors had no effect on gastric PG production and did not cause lesions even at very high doses (200 mg/kg). Taken together these results provide strong support for the hypothesis that COX-1 is responsible for producing cytoprotective PGs in the GI tract.

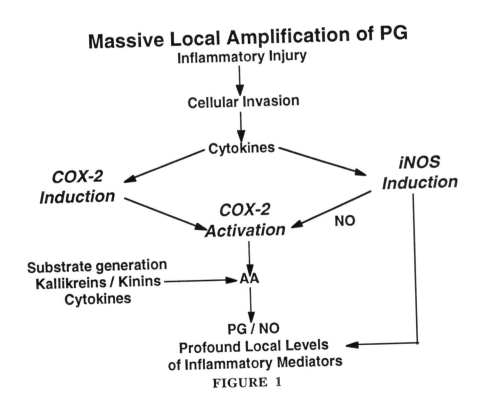

FIGURE 1

INTERACTIONS BETWEEN THE COX AND NO PATHWAYS

Nitric oxide (NO) is another widely distributed molecule that is apparently important in normal physiology and in some disease states. Similar to the COX pathway, NO synthase occurs both constitutively and in an inducible form (27 for review). The inducible NO synthase has been associated with inflammatory states and may directly be responsible for some of the deleterious events of inflammation. Another mechanism by which NO may exert inflammatory effects via increased production of PGs has recently been found (28, 29). Thus, NO synthase inhibitors were found to decrease production of both nitrites and PGs in tissue culture cells and in the intact hydronephrotic kidney; furthermore, NO directly increased PG production by activation of the COX enzyme. This suggests that local production of NO at a site of inflammation could amplify the inflammatory response by augmenting COX-2 activity and subsequent PG production (Figure 1).

In conclusion, we have shown that a highly selective inhibitor of COX-2 is anti-inflammatory *in vivo* without causing gastric lesions, while traditional NSAIDs like indomethacin are both anti-inflammatory and ulcerogenic, consistent with their ability to inhibit COX-1 as well as COX-2. Development of selective inhibitors of COX-2 that spare gastric PG production may represent a significant advance for the treatment of acute and chronic inflammatory disorders.

REFERENCES

1. Allison, M.C., Howatson, A.G., Torrance, C.J., Lee, F.D., and Russell, R. (1992) New England J. Med. 327:749-754.
2. Vane, J.R. (1971) Nature (New Biol.) 231:232-235.
3. Smith, J.B., and Willis, A.L. (1971) Nature (New Biol.) 231:235-239
4. DeWitt, D. (1991) Biochim. Biophys. Acta. 1083: 121-134.
5. Morrison, A.R., Nishikawa, K.A., and Needleman, P. (1977) Nature. 267:259-260.
6. Lefkowith, J.B., Okegawa, T., DeSchryver-Kecskemeti, K., and Needleman, P. (1984) Kid.Intl. 26:10-17
7. Smith, W.L., and Wilkin, G.P. (1977) Prostaglandins 13:873-892.
8. Raz, A., Wyche, A., and Needleman, P. (1989) Proc. Natl. Acad. Sci., USA. 86: 1657-1661.
9. Masferrer, J.L., Seibert, K., Zweifel, B.S., and Needleman, P. (1992) Proc. Natl. Acad. Sci., USA 89: 3917-3921.
10. Masferrer, J.L., Zweifel, B.S., Seibert, K., and Needleman, P. (1990) J. Clin. Invest. 86: 1375-1379.
11. Merlie, J.P., Fagan, D., Mudd,J., and Needleman, P. (1988) J. Biol. Chem 263:3550-3553.
12. DeWitt, D., and Smith, W.L. (1988) Proc. Natl. Acad. Sci. USA 85:1412-1416.
13. Yokoyama, C., Takai, T., and Tanabe, T. (1988) FEBS Lett. 231:347-351.
14. Xie, W., Chipman, J.G., Robertson, D.L., Erikson, R.L., and Simmons, D.L. (1991) Proc. Natl. Acad. Sci. USA 88: 2692-2696.
15. Kujubu, D.A., Fletcher, B.S., Varnum, B.C., Lim, R.W., and Herschman, H.R. (1991) J. Biol. Chem. 266: 12866-12872.
16. O'Banion, M.K., Sadowski, H.B., Winn, V., and Young, D.A. (1991) J. Biol. Chem. 266: 23261-23267.

17. Fletcher, B.S., Kujubu, D.A., Perrin, D.M., and Herschman, H.R. (1992) J. Biol. Chem. 267: 4338:4344.
18. Sirois, J., and Richards, J.S. (1992) J. Biol. Chem. 267: 6382-6388.
19. Kujubu, D.A., and Herschman, H.R. (1992) J. Biol. Chem. 267, 7991-7994.
20. O'Banion, M.K., Winn, V., and Young, D.A. (1992) Proc. Natl. Acad. Scit. USA 89: 4888-4892.
21. Kujubu, D.A., Reddy, S.T., Fletcher, B.S., and Herschman, H. (1993) J. Biol. Chem. 268: 5425-5430.
22. Picot, D., Loll, P.J., and Garavito, R.M. (1994) Nature 367j:243-249.
23. Futaki, N., Arai, I., Hamasaki, S., Takahashi, S., Higuchi, S., and Otomo, S. (1992) J. Pharm. Pharmacol. 45: 753-755.
24. Futaki, N., Yoshikawa, K., Yumiko, H., Arai, I., Higuchi, S., Iizuka, H., and Otomo, S. (1993) Gen. Pharmac. 24: 105-110
25. Gans, K.R., Galbraith, W., Roman, R.J., Haber, S.B., Kerr, J.S., Schmidt, W.K., Smith, C., Hewes, W.E., and Ackerman, N.R. (1989) J. Pharm. Exp. Ther. 254:180-187
26. Masferrer, J., Zweifel, B., Manning, P.T., Hauser, S.D., Leahy, K.M., Smith, W.G., Isakson, P.C., and Seibert, K. (1994). Proc. Natl. Acad. Sci. 26. 91:3228-3232
27. Moncada, S., Palmer, R.M.J., and Higgs, E.A. (1991) Pharm. Rev. 43:109-141.
28. Salvemini, D., Misko, T.P., Masferrer, J., Seibert, K., Currie, M.G., and Needleman, P. (1993) Proc. Natl. Acad. Sci. USA. 90:7240-7244.
29. Salvemini, D., Seibert, K., Masferrer, J., Misko, T.P., Currie, M.G., and Needleman, P. (1994) J. Clin. Inv. 93:1940-1947.

Advances in Prostaglandin, Thromboxane,
and Leukotriene Research, Vol. 23,
edited by B. Samuelsson et al.
Raven Press, Ltd., New York © 1995

THE COMBINED USE OF PROSTAGLANDIN AND ANTIPROGESTIN IN HUMAN FERTILITY CONTROL

E.E. Baulieu

Lab. Hormones, INSERM U 33, Collège de France, 80 rue du Général Leclerc, 94276 Le Kremlin-Bicêtre Cedex

Prostaglandins have been, for a quarter of a century, a very important component of the worldwide biomedical effort to improve human fertility control (1). In the early seventies, in the framework of the Expanded (Special) Programme of Research, Development and Research Training in Human Reproduction of the World Health Organization (WHO), a Research and Training Centre was established in Stockholm, at the Karolinska Institute and Hospital, where most prostaglandin research was performed (2). Prostaglandins have already greatly contributed to modifying the dramatic demographic trend of humanity and to saving the lives of thousands of pregnant women. At present, with ~ 50 10^6 abortions/years, the majority of them under terribly unsafe conditions leading to acute catastrophes and long term sequelae, the situation is still medically and ethically unacceptable, particularly when appropriate technology is now ready for successful application.

The early sixties saw « the pill » (oral hormonal contraception) reaching the market, and besides its efficacy and a number of health benefits, it became a symbol of the progress in the condition of women merging with ongoing science. However, for many reasons, the pill cannot be « the » only method for fertility control. Medically, psychologically and even socially, there is a need for several techniques offered for women's choice (without referring to men here).

Progesterone is the hormone of pregnancy (pro-gestare). It participates in the process of ovulation, is necessary to prepare uterine implantation of the fertilized ovum, and is also indispensable for the continuation of pregnancy. Since the description of the progesterone receptor in the uterus (3), I considered the possibility of decreasing progesterone action in order to have a new way to contraception, and the simplest, and probably the most specific, means seemed to obtain an antihormonal effect at the receptor level (4). Conceiving a particular chemical structure with antihormonal activity, relied on previous physicochemical

(5) and biological (6) work with estrogens and triphenyl-ethylene antiestrogens, such as tamoxifen and derivatives. It was therefore « logical » to suggest that an extra phenyl group grafted perpendicularly to the main plane of the steroidal ring system at its center, might generate antagonistic compounds (Fig. B1.3 in 7). There were also enough similarities between the different steroid hormone receptors, as confirmed by molecular cloning (review in 7), to suggest that they could have similar two and three dimensional features. Therefore, since we had 4-hydroxy tamoxifen with high affinity for the estrogen receptor (9, 10), why should not the addition of an 11β-phenyl group to a steroid also permit high affinity for its cognate receptor? The Roussel-Uclaf chemists and pharmacologists thus obtained compounds of high affinity displaying antiglucocorticosteroid and antiprogesterone activities (11, 12), and we could test the most interesting derivative, RU486 (mifepristone), very rapidly for both voluntary early pregnancy termination and interruption of the luteal phase in non fertile cycles (13).

Already, at that time, an increase of PGF2α was observed in the blood of women having RU486-induced abortion (14), probably reflecting an increase of uterine prostaglandin concentration (the same was observed in the pregnant rat uterus after RU486 administration) (15).

Using RU486 alone in women asking for *early pregnancy termination*, the complete efficacy was rarely > 80% (review in 16). This result established that

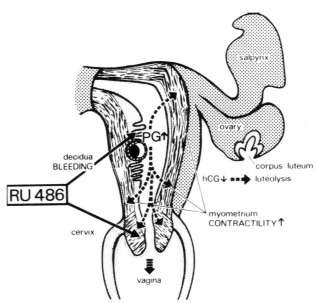

FIG. 1. Physiopharmacological mechanism of action of RU486 on the implanted blastocyst. Temporally, the antiprogesterone effect of RU486 comes first, and then an increase in PG concentration and action, followed by a decrease in hCG-sustained corpus luteum function (7).

we indeed had a second generation of hormonal compounds active for fertility control. The ~ 20% incompletenesses or failures of very early pregnancy interruption are to be compared to the ~ 1/5 miscarriages which necessitate complementary mechanical evacuation.

From current knowledge and available data, the postulated global mechanism (Fig. 1) includes, firstly, the arrest of progesterone support to the decidua, leading to bleeding and (partial) detachment of the product of conception (blastocyst). Thereafter, occurs a second period which involves an increase of locally made prostaglandins, probably due to both the augmentation of synthesis and the decrease of catabolism of prostaglandins PGF2α and PGE2 (17-20). Marc Bygdeman and colleagues (21) indicated the increased sensitivity of the myometrium to small doses of prostaglandin after RU486 treatment. In absence of the antiprogesterone, the prostaglandin was unable to sufficiently increase the frequency and amplitude of contractions, and therefore to be abortifacient (Fig. 2). RU486 softens and opens the cervix, facilitating evacuation of the uterus; prostaglandins may be involved in this response, but no change of prostaglandin metabolism has been found at this level (22).

This potentiation of prostaglandin activity by RU486 in the pregnant uterus, by decreasing progesterone activity, takes about 24-48 h, as would be expected for the « genomic » effects of progesterone via its nuclear receptor. Then RU486

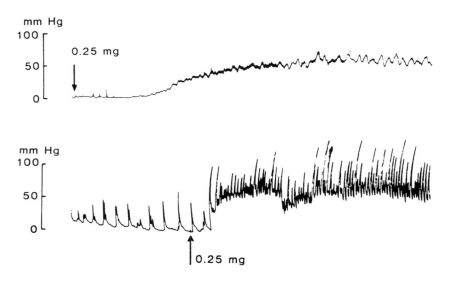

FIG. 2. The figure shows the spontaneous uterine contractility and the effect of an intramuscular injection of 0.25 mg 16-phenoxy-tetranor-PGE2 methyl sulfonylamide in two early pregnant women. The first patient recieved no pretreatment (upper curve), while in the second patient, the recording was performed on the morning of day 4 of treatment with 25 mg RU486 twice daily (lower curve) (21).

transforms the « suppressed » pregnant uterus into an active one, a result which could be predicted from the Csapo studies (23). These results are the basis for the two step regimen currently used: RU486 followed by prostaglandin ~ 48 h afterwards. The efficacy of such a regimen is ≥ 95% as demonstrated in ~ 200,000 women (24, 25). The medical method is applicable and even the most efficient when applied as early as possible after the diagnosis of pregnancy is positive (that is when the chorionic gonadotrophin hCG is detected in the woman by a « pregnancy » test indicating implantation). The current instrumental method, suction, is used later

The prostaglandins available up to now, in conjunction with the standardized dose of 600 mg RU486 taken once ~ 2 days before, are:

1) Sulprostone, a PGE_2 derivative, at the dose of ~ 0.25 mg administered intramuscularly, efficient but responsible for a few severe cardiovascular accidents. It was demonstrated that these accidents were not due to the association with RU486 administration. In France, the distribution of this injectable product has been stopped.

2) Gemeprost, a PGE1 derivative, 0.5-1 mg being given in a vaginal pessary. This prostaglandin administration is safe, very efficient, but relatively painful (cramps), probably by an effect of the high proximal concentration established near to the uterus (however there is also passage into the general circulation).

3) Misoprostol, another PGE1 derivative, orally active at the dose of 400-600 µg taken in one or two ingestions (25, 26).

4) We do not have many reported cases with the 15-methyl PGF2α (1 or 2 injections of 50 µg) which has been used in a few countries (27).

At present, the use of Misoprostol is the preferred one. The product is available, contrary to some other prostaglandins which are also orally active (such as 9-methylene PGE2, 28), is very cheap, easy to store (no refrigeration is necessary), convenient to ingest, very well tolerated (uterine cramps are minimal), safe (hundred of thousands of users have taken the product or other medication without reported accident: this is probably related, at least in part, to the oral way of administration making the distribution in the body slower than after an injection)* Misoprostol use is a turning point in the use of RU486 for two main reasons:

1) The RU486 + Misoprostol regimen is potentially more private, since there is no reason so far for it not to be prescribed and followed by practicing gynecologists, in their office. This may defuse the mandatory use of abortion clinics which are targets for antiabortionists, as seen in the USA.

---

* Misoprostol has been used alone, illegally, for abortion, generally at high dose and in the absence of medical supervision, since it can be obtained relatively easily, being sold in pharmacies, contrary to RU486. In this uncontrolled use, it is taken orally, and sometimes vaginally. It is an abortifacient (29) which in most cases provokes an incomplete result, leading the patient to the hospital for further evacuation and is responsible for a number of hemorrhages and infections, as observed in Brazil (30, 31). Note also that there is a known risk of fetal abnormalities in case of continuation of pregnancy (32).

2) It is possible to envisage a one-step, simplified mode of administration, because of both the safety and convenience of the method. For example, when the women consult for pregnancy termination, the physician[**] could give RU486 and the few pills of Misoprostol to be taken 48 h afterwards. The improvement could be made even better if we had a prostaglandin preparation administered at the same time as RU486 but with delayed release and efficacy (for example, it may be possible to envisage a vaginal delivery system or a skin patch placed at the same time as the ingestion of RU486, but releasing the prostaglandin 36-48 h afterwards).

The association RU486-prostaglandin will continue to be used for a very long time by many women, at least as a back-up for failures of contraceptive methods, whether not used or not efficient. It seems to be the earliest and safest available technique that women could use if necessary.

Of course, much research remains to be done. 1) Synthesis of other antiprogestins (in particular with no antiglucocorticosteroid activity, as displayed by RU486). 2) Definition of appropriate dosages (there is a sort of balance between the necessary amounts of antiprogestin and prostaglandin: a lower dose of RU486 may necessitate more prostaglandin, and conversely, the 600 mg dose of RU486 currently used permits a very small dose of prostaglandin to be efficient. The best balance may not be yet found. 3) A one-step method for the administration of prostaglandin is badly needed, specially in developing countries, and the research on prostaglandin with delayed activity is of importance. It is known that available prostaglandins are not directly luteolytic in human beings (luteolysis takes place secondarily after detachment of the blastocyst when the supply of hCG decreases). A luteolytic prostaglandin would obviously be welcome.

Other uses of prostaglandin associated with RU486 include:

1) *Therapeutic pregnancy interruption, late* in the first trimester and after. Several trials have indicated the possibility of decreasing the amount of administered prostaglandin, and its beneficial effect when the administration is preceded by RU486. There is decreased pain and acceleration of the process (33, 34).

2) The use of RU486 to *induce labor* (which physiologically involves an increase of prostaglandins), when there is abnormally prolonged pregnancy,

---

[**] We insist that RU486 + prostaglandin should be taken after a medical decision and remain under medical supervision. It is unwise to suggest that it can be sold « over the counter », since, for this method as for any other intervention during pregnancy. I believe it is the right of women to have medical assistance in all circumstances related to their reproductive life. Here the risk is not the drug, but the pregnancy itself: for instance the increasing number of ectopic pregnancies, not interrupted by RU486, is a grave danger. However, there is a respectable argument that the overall number of accidents due to medical deficit, in the case of RU486 use, is certainly lower than that due to the current non-use of RU486 in developing countries. More generally, to compensate for the insufficient access to family planning and reproductive health providers, imperfectly distributed RU486 may provide a definitive improvement of the present situation in some countries.

particularly if there is cervical dysfunction. Experiments in animals have indicated that in RU486 induced delivery, several hormonal and metabolic parameters, including prostaglandin increase do not follow the same order as observed in spontaneous delivery (35-37). Administered oxytocin in cases of retarded delivery is potentialized by RU486 in monkeys (38) and human (39). Whether the administration of prostaglandin would be better than that of oxytocin in association with RU486, is yet not known.

3) As a *once-a-month menses inducer*. The use of RU486 at the end of the cycle has been proposed for induction of menses (40, 41). It is not yet an acceptable method of contraception, because of dysregulation of the cycles due at least in part to the high doses which have been used (42). The appropriate combination of RU486 and prostaglandin, with a low dose of RU486 and the use of a convenient form of prostaglandin, may avoid disturbing the regularity of the ovarian cycle, and therefore become a once-a-month inducer. Trials are currently being performed in Paris.

It is remarkable that, *separately*, two of the main *basic research* avenues in the field of cellular communications, into cellular receptors and the arachidonic acid cascade, have led to the creation of *active drugs*, antiprogestins[*] and prostaglandins[**], the « encounter » of which may decrease the suffering of millions of women.

REFERENCES

1.   Bergström S, Diczfalusy E, Borell U, Karim S, Samuelsson B. Uvnas B. Wiqvist N. Bygdeman M. Prostaglandins in Fertility Control. *Science* 1972;175:1280-7

2.   WHO. In: Khanna J. Van Look PFA. Griffin PD. *Reproductive health a key to a brighter future*. Geneva. 1992.

3.   Milgrom E, Atger M, Baulieu EE. Progesterone in uterus and plasma. IV - Progesterone receptor(s) in guinea pig uterus cytosol. *Steroids* 1970;16:741-54.

4.   Baulieu EE. Antiprogesterone effect and midcycle (perioovulatory) contraception. *Eur J Obstet Gynecol Reprod. Biol.* 1975;4:161-6.

5.   Hospital M, Busetta B, Bucourt R, et al. X-ray crystallography of estrogens and their binding to receptor sites. *Mol Pharmacol* 1972;8:438-45.

6.   Sutherland RL, Mester J, Baulieu EE. Tamoxifen is a potent « pure » ant-oestrogen in chick oviduct. *Nature* 1977;267:434-5.

7.   Baulieu EE. 1993: RU486 - A decade on today and tomorrow. In: Donaldson MS. Dorflinger L, Brown SS, Benet LZ. *Clinical Applications of Mifepristone RU486 and Other Antiprogestins*. Washington: National Academy Press; 1993:71-119.

8.   Evans RM. The steroid and thyroid hormone receptor superfamily. *Science* 1988;240:889-95.

9.   Borgna JL, Rochefort H. High-affinity binding to the estrogen receptor of ^{3}H-4-hydroxytamoxifen, an active antiestrogen metabolite. *Mol Cell Endocrinol* 1980;20:71-85.

---

[*] For example basic studies on the physico-chemistry of receptors and receptor ligands.
[**] For example, studies on prostaglandin metabolism, which suggested synthesis of derivatives with decreased inactivation.

10. Binart N, Catelli MG, Geynet C, et al. Monohydroxytamoxifen: an antioestrogen with high affinity for the chick oviduct oestrogen receptor. *Biochem Biophys Res Commun* 1978;91:812-8.

11. Teutsch G. Analogues of RU486 for the mapping of the progestin receptor: synthetic and structural aspects. In: Baulieu EE, Segal SJ. *The Antiprogestin Steroid RU486 and Human Fertility Control.* New York: Plenum Press; 1985: 27-47.

12. Philibert D, Moguilewsky M, Mary I, et al. Pharmacological profile of RU486 in animals. In: Baulieu EE, Segal SJ. *The Antiprogestin Steroid RU486 and Human Fertility Control.* New York: Plenum Press; 1985: 49-68.

13. Herrmann W, Wyss R, Riondel A, et al. Effet d'un stéroïde anti-progestérone chez la femme : interruption du cycle menstruel et de la grossesse au début. *C.R. Acad Sci Paris* 1982;294:933-8.

14. Herrmann W, Schindler AM, Wyss R. Effects of the antiprogesterone RU486 in early pregnancy and during the menstrual cycle. *The Antiprogestin Steroid RU486 and Human Fertility Control.* New York: Plenum Press; 1985: 179-98.

15. Secchi J, Lecaque D, Tournemine C, Philibert D. Histopharmacology of RU486. *The Antiprogestin Steroid RU486 and Human Fertility Control.* New York: Plenum Press; 1985: 79-86.

16. Baulieu EE. Contragestion and other clinical applications of RU486, an antiprogesterone at the receptor. *Science* 1989;245:1351-7.

17. Cheng L, Kelly RW, Thong KJ, et al. The effects of mifepristone (RU486) on prostaglandin dehydrogenase in decidual and chorionic tissue in early pregnancy. *Human Reprod.* 1993;8:705-9.

18. Norman JE, Wu WX, Kelly RW, et al. Effects of mifepristone in vivo on decidual prostaglandin synthesis and metabolism. *Contraception* 1991;44:89-98.

19. Lobaccaro-Henri C, Saintot M, Laffargue F, et al. Effect of the progesterone antagonist-RU486 on human myometrial spontaneous contractility and PGI2 release. *Prostaglandins* 1992;44:443-55.

20. Brooks J, Holland P, Kelly R. Comparison of antiprogestin stimulation of uterine prostaglandin synthesis in vitro. *Prostaglandins, Leukotrienes and Essential Fatty Acids* 1990;40:191-7.

21. Bygdeman M, Swahn ML. Progesterone receptor blockade: effect on uterine contractility and early pregnancy. *Contraception* 1985;32:45-51.

22. Radestad A, Bygdeman M, Green K. Induce cervical ripening with mifepristone (RU486) and bioconversion of arachidonic acid in human pregnant uterine cervix in the first trimester. A double-blind, randomized biomechanical and biochemical study. *Contraception* 1990;41:283-92.

23. Csapo AI, Pulkkinen MO. Control of human parturition. In: Kaminetzky HA. Iffy L. Progress in Perinatology. Philadelphia:Stickley, 1977.

24. Ulmann A, Silvestre L, Chemama L, et al. Medical termination of early pregnancy with mifepristone (RU486) followed by a prostaglandin analogue: study in 16,369 women. *Acta Obstet Gynecol Scand* 1992;71:278-83.

25. Peyron R, Aubény E, Targosz V, et al. Early termination of pregnancy with mifepristone (RU486) and the orally active prostaglandin misoprostol. *New Engl J Med* 1993;328:1509-13.

26. Aubény E, Baulieu EE. Activité contragestive de l'association au RU486 d'une prostaglandine active par voie orale. *C.R. Acad. Sci. Paris* 1991;312:539-45.

27. Bygdeman M, Swahn ML. Antiprogestin drugs: research and clinical use in Sweden. *Law, Medicine and Health Care* 1992;20:157-60.

28. Swahn ML, Ugocsai G, Bygdeman M, Kovacs L, Belsey EM, Van Look PFA. Effect of oral prostaglandin E_2 on uterine contractility and outcome of treatment in women receiving RU486 (mifepristone) for termination of early pregnancy. *Hum Reprod* 1989;4:21-8.

29.   Norman JE, Thong KJ Baird DT. Uterine contractility and induction of abortion in early pregnancy by misoprostol and mifepristone. *Lancet* 1991;338:1233-6.

30.   Schönhöfer PS. Brazil: misuse of misoprostol as an abortifacient may induce malformations. *Lancet* 1991;337:1534-5.

31.   Coelho HLL, Misago C, da Fonseca WVC, Sousa DSC de Araujo JML. Selling abortifacients over the counter in pharmacies in Fortaleza, Brazil. *Lancet* 1991;338:247.

32.   Fonseca W, Alencar AJC, Mota FSB, Coelho HLL. Misoprostol and congenital malformations. *Lancet* 1991;338:56.

33.   Urquhart DR, Templeton AA. Mifepristone (RU486) for cervical priming prior to surgically induced abortion in the late first trimester. *Contraception* 1990;42:191-9.

34.   Rodger MW, Baird DT. Pretreatment with mifepristone (RU486) reduces interval between prostaglandin administration and expulsion in second trimester abortion. *Br J Obstet Gynecol* 1990;97:41-5.

35.   Haluska GJ, Stanczyk FZ, Cook MJ, et al. Temporal changes in uterine activity and prostaglandin response to RU486 in rhesus macaques in late gestation. *Am J Obstet Gynecol* 1987;157:1487-95.

36.   Haluska GJ, West N, Novy MJ, et al. Uterine estrogen receptors are increased by RU486 in late pregnant rhesus macaques but not after spontaneous labor. *J Clin Endocrinol Metab* 1990;70:181-6.

37.   Arkaravichien W, Kendle KE. Uterine contractile activity in rats induced by mifepristone (RU486) in relation to changes in concentrations of prostaglandins E-2 and F-2α. *J Reprod Fertil* 1992;94:115-20.

38.   Wolf JP Sinosich M, Anderson TL, et al. Progesterone antagonist (RU486) for cervical dilatation, labor induction, and delivery in monkeys: effectiveness in combination with oxytocin. *Am J Obstet Gynecol* 1989;160:45-7.

39.   Frydman R, Lelaidier C, Baton-Saint-Mleux C, et al. Labor induction in women at term with mifepristone (RU486): a double-blind, randomized, placebo-controlled study. *Obstet Gynecol* 1992;80:972-5.

40.   Dubois C, Ulmann A, Baulieu EE. Contragestion with late luteal administration of RU486 (mifepristone). *Fertil Steril* 1988;50:593-6.

41.   Lähteenmäki P, Rapeli T, Kääriäinen M, et al. Late postcoital treatment against pregnancy with antiprogesterone RU486. *Fertil Steril* 1988;50:36-8.

42.   Van Santen MR, Haspels AA. Failure of mifepristone (RU486) as a monthly contragestive, « Lunarette ». *Contraception* 1987;35:433-8

Advances in Prostaglandin, Thromboxane, and Leukotriene Research, Vol. 23,
edited by B. Samuelsson et al.
Raven Press, Ltd., New York © 1995

Prostaglandins as Ocular Hypotensive Agents; Development of an Analogue for Glaucoma Treatment

Johan Stjernschantz

Glaucoma Research Laboratories, Pharmacia Ophthalmics, S-751 82, Uppsala, Sweden

In experimental ophthalmology it has been known for a long time that cannulation of the anterior chamber of the rabbit eye frequently leads to acute inflammation. This acute ocular inflammation typically occurs after injury to the iris. In an attempt to identify the mediator of this acute inflammatory response Ambache (1957) prepared extracts from the rabbit iris containing the active substance(s), named irin (1). Injected into the cat eye irin caused pupillary constriction. Ambache was not able to identify the active principle of irin but suggested its structure to be an unsaturated hydroxy acid (2). In 1964 Änggård and Samuelsson demonstrated that extracts from sheep iris contained $PGF_{2\alpha}$ (3) and later several prostaglandins were identified in iris extracts (4,5).

When synthetic prostaglandins became available a large number of studies were performed in the 1960's and 1970's to investigate the ocular effects of prostaglandins. The results of these studies were difficult to interpret due to large doses used and to marked species differences. Prostaglandins administered to the eye caused increased intraocular pressure (IOP), breakdown of the blood-aqueous barrier and other signs of acute inflammation (6). Since at the same time aspirin was shown to block prostaglandin synthesis (7) and aspirin pretreatment of rabbits attenuated the inflammatory response to paracentesis of the anterior chamber and to argon laser treatment of the iris (8) it became generally accepted that prostaglandins were mediators of inflammation in the eye. However, a change was brought about by the discovery of the leukotrienes and other oxygenated metabolites of arachidonic acid, and of the neuropeptides which were shown to play a role in neurogenic inflammation of the eye (6).

A turning point was the study by Camras and Bito (1981) demonstrating that topically applied $PGF_{2\alpha}$ reduces IOP in monkeys with no or minimal intraocular side-effects (9). Since $PGF_{2\alpha}$, could reduce IOP without inflammation in primates it was proposed that prostaglandins potentially could be utilized as IOP reducing agents in glaucoma treatment (9). In 1983 a project was started by Pharmacia to determine whether prostaglandins could be developed into clinically useful drugs for glaucoma treatment.

ESTERS OF PGF$_{2\alpha}$ AS OCULAR HYPOTENSIVES

The first approach to develop prostaglandins into drugs for glaucoma treatment was based on esterification of the carboxylic acid moiety. The rationale for this was firstly, to reduce the superficial side-effects on the eye, secondly to reduce the amount of drug necessary to produce an effect, and thirdly to stabilize the prostaglandin molecule chemically. From animal experiments it was apparent that although the prostaglandins did not induce intraocular inflammation they nevertheless produced conjunctival hyperaemia and irritation. Since the cornea is rich in esterases, prodrugs containing ester bonds can be utilized. A large number of carboxylic acid esters, diesters and even tetraesters and lactones were prepared. Although some of the esters did improve the therapeutic index of PGF$_{2\alpha}$ in the eye, these compounds still caused too many side-effects. However, PGF$_{2\alpha}$-isopropyl ester (PGF$_{2\alpha}$-IE) was found to exhibit a side-effect profile acceptable for short term clinical trials and thus PGF$_{2\alpha}$-IE could be used for studying the mechanism of action of prostaglandins to reduce IOP and for the first clinical trials.

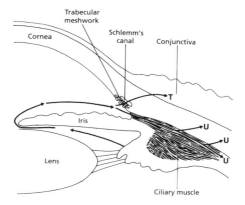

FIG. 1. Schematic picture of the uveoscleral outflow pathway (U). Trabecular outflow is denoted T.

Mechanism of Action

Surprisingly PGF$_{2\alpha}$ and PGF$_{2\alpha}$-IE were found to reduce IOP by increasing the uveoscleral outflow of aqueous humour and not by increasing the outflow through the trabecular meshwork or by reducing the production of aqueous humour (10-12). The uveoscleral outflow pathway was originally described by Bill (1966) but the physiological significance of this outflow pathway in man remained obscure (13). In experiments on human eyes to be enucleated it was estimated that the uveoscleral drainage accounts for 4-27% of the total outflow of aqueous humour (14). In the uveoscleral outflow pathway aqueous humour percolates through the ciliary muscle into the supraciliary and suprachoroidal spaces and leaves the eye through the sclera. Thus, the trabecular meshwork which is blocked in glaucoma is by-passed. The mechanism of the increased drainage of aqueous humour through the ciliary muscle is not known but it is possible that PGF$_{2\alpha}$ alters the extracellular matrix between the muscle bundles which reduces the resistance (15).

Clinical Studies with $PGF_{2\alpha}$-isopropyl ester

In the first study $PGF_{2\alpha}$-IE was used in topical doses of 0.1, 0.5, 2.5 and 10 µg in healthy volunteers (16). A good dose response in IOP was obtained but doses exceeding 0.5 µg caused too many side effects to be clinically acceptable. These comprised conjunctival hyperaemia, local irritation, foreign body sensation, photophobia and headache. However, signs of intraocular inflammation were not observed (16, 17). In subsequent studies in which a dose of 0.5 µg was used it was shown that $PGF_{2\alpha}$-IE reduced IOP in glaucoma patients (18,19). However, the therapeutic index of $PGF_{2\alpha}$-IE in the eye was not adequate, despite the fact that a dose at the lower end of the dose response curve was used.Thus, this prostaglandin ester could not be developed into a drug for glaucoma treatment.

PHENYL-SUBSTITUTED PROSTAGLANDIN ANALOGUES

A structure-activity program of different prostaglandin analogues was initiated by Pharmacia to investigate whether the therapeutic index of prostaglandins in the eye could be improved. Several stereoisomers and epimers of different prostaglandins, and other analogues including metabolites were synthesized and tested but without success. However, a group of omega chain phenyl-substituted analogues were unexpectedly shown to exhibit unique properties in that the IOP reducing property was retained or even improved while the irritating and hyperemic effects were largely reduced or eliminated (20,21). In particular substitution of carbons 18,19,20 with a phenyl ring proved advantageous. The compound 17-phenyl-18,19,20-trinor-$PGF_{2\alpha}$-isopropyl ester (PhDH100A) exhibited good IOP reducing effect in monkeys and little or no irritating effect as evaluated in the cat eye. This compound also caused less conjunctival hyperaemia in rabbits than $PGF_{2\alpha}$-IE (21).

The position of the terminal ring on the omega chain proved to be crucial. Attaching the terminal ring to C-16 of $PGF_{2\alpha}$ resulted in a compound which caused some irritation, and attaching the terminal ring to C-18 or higher resulted in decreased biologic activity (19). Thus, attaching the terminal ring to C-17 was optimal since most of the side effects were eliminated without compromising the IOP reducing effect (Fig.2). Various other ring structures such as cyclohexyl, thiophen, biphenyl, and furanyl were tested, and substitutions on the terminal ring structure, e.g. with methyl, methoxy, trifluormethyl, and fluoride were also tested but in general clear-cut improvements over the original compound (PhDH100A) could not be achieved (20).

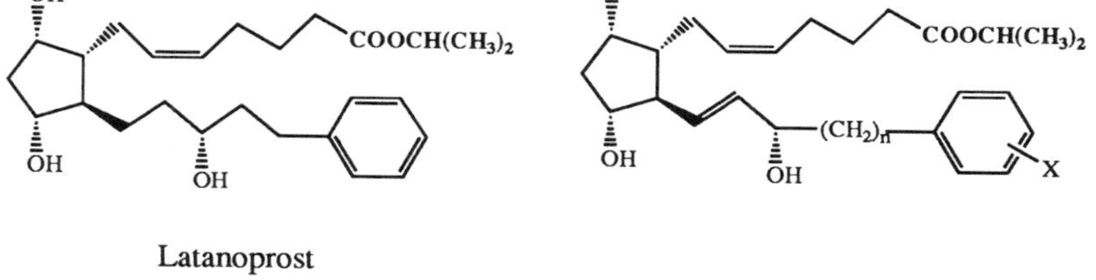

Latanoprost

FIG. 2. Latanoprost and different phenyl-substituted $PGF_{2\alpha}$ analogues tested in the eye (n=0-9; X=CH_3, OCH_3, F, CF_3 in different positions of the benzene ring when n=2).

Latanoprost

Saturation of the double bond between C-13-14 yielded a somewhat less potent compound but with a better therapeutic index in the eye than that of PhDH100A. The compound, 13,14-dihydro-17-phenyl-18,19,20-trinor-PGF$_{2\alpha}$-isopropyl ester (PhXA41; latanoprost) is the most promising of the phenyl-substituted PGF$_{2\alpha}$ analogues for a new glaucoma drug (Fig. 2). The receptor profile of latanoprost based on EC$_{50}$ values in different prostanoid receptor assay systems (21) is presented in Table I. Latanoprost is a relatively selective FP receptor agonist.

Table I.   Receptor profile of latanoprost based on EC$_{50}$ values in molar concentration.

FP	EP$_1$	EP$_2$	EP$_3$	DP/IP	TP
3.6×10^{-9}	6.9×10^{-6}	3.6×10^{-4}	1.7×10^{-5}	$>1.0 \times 10^{-2}$	1.1×10^{-4}

Kd values obtained in ligand binding experiments with latanoprost using cloned rat FP receptors expressed in CHO cells, and using bovine corpus luteum cells were 1.9×10^{-8} and 2.8×10^{-9} M, respectively. In experiments performed in monkeys latanoprost has been shown to reduce IOP mainly by increasing the uveoscleral outflow analogous to PGF$_{2\alpha}$ (23).

Several clinical dose-finding trials have been performed with latanoprost. Good IOP reduction is achieved with a dose of 1.5-2 µg applied once daily on the eye (24, 25). IOP reductions of 20-35% have been achieved depending on the starting pressure. Latanoprost has not been found to exert any effect on the blood-aqueous barrier or production of aqueous humour but was found to increase slightly outflow facility (26). However, most of the IOP reduction in man has also been found to be based on increased uveoscleral outflow (27). In the first phase III clinical trial, administration of 0.005% latanoprost once daily in the evening resulted in significantly better IOP reduction than administration of 0.5% timolol twice daily during a 6-month treatment period (28). The main side effect of latanoprost has been slight conjunctival hyperaemia and increased pigmentation of the iris, which seems to be a class effect of prostaglandins.

Our studies thus indicate that prostaglandins can be modified to become sufficiently selective for clinical use in the medical treatment of glaucoma.

ACKNOWLEDGEMENTS

I would like to thank Ms Iréne Aspman for help with preparation of the manuscript.

REFERENCES

1. Ambache N. Properties of irin, a physiological constituent of the rabbit iris. *J Physiol* 1957; 135: 114-32.

2. Ambache N. Further studies on the preparation, purification and nature of irin. *J Physiol* 1959; 146: 255-94.

3. Ånggård E and Samuelsson B. Smooth muscle stimulating lipids in sheep iris. The identification of prostaglandin $F_{2\alpha}$. Prostaglandins and related factors 21. *Biochem Pharmacol* 1964; 13: 281-3.

4. Ambache N, Brummer HC, Rose JG and Whiting J. Thin-layer chromatography of spasmogenic unsaturated hydroxy-acids from various tissues. *J Physiol* 1966; 185: 77-8.

5. Waitzman MB, Bailey WR and Kirby CG. Chromatographic analysis of biologically active lipids from rabbit irides. *Exp Eye Res* 1967; 6: 130-7.

6. Stjernschantz J. Autacoids and neuropeptides. In:Sears ML. *Pharmacology of the eye*. Berlin Heidelberg New York Tokyo: Springer Verlag; 1984: 311-65.

7. Vane JR. Inhibition of prostaglandin synthesis as mechanism of action for aspirin-like drugs. *Nature (New Biol)* 1971; 231: 232-5.

8. Neufeld AH, Jampol LM and Sears ML. Aspirin prevents the disruption of the blood-aqueous barrier in the rabbit eye. *Nature* 1972; 238: 158-9.

9. Camras CB and Bito LZ. Reduction of intraocular pressure in normal and glaucomatous primate (Aotus trivirgatus) eyes by topically applied prostaglandin $F_{2\alpha}$. *Curr Eye Res* 1981; 1: 205-9.

10. Crawford K and Kaufman PL. Pilocarpine antagonizes $PGF_{2\alpha}$-induced ocular hypotension: Evidence for enhancement of uveoscleral outflow by $PGF_{2\alpha}$. *Arch Ophthalmol* 1987; 105: 1112-6.

11. Nilsson SFE, Samuelsson M, Bill A and Stjernschantz J. Increased uveoscleral outflow as a possible mechanism of ocular hypotension caused by prostaglandin $F_{2\alpha}$-1-isopropyl ester in the cynomolgus monkey. *Exp Eye Res* 1989; 48; 707-716.

12. True Gabelt B'A and Kaufman PL. Prostaglandin $F_{2\alpha}$ increases uveoscleral outflow in the cynomolgus monkey. *Exp Eye Res* 1989; 49: 389-402.

13. Bill A. Conventional and uveoscleral drainage of aqueous humour in the cynomolgus monkeys (Macaca irus) at normal and high intraocular pressures. *Exp Eye Res* 1966; 5: 45-54.

14. Bill A and Phillips CI. Uveoscleral drainage of aqueous humour in human eyes. *Exp Eye Res* 1971; 12: 275-81.

15. Lindsey JD, Hoang, DT and Weinreb RN. Induction of c-Fos by prostaglandin $F_{2\alpha}$ in human ciliary smooth muscle cells. *Invest Ophthalmol Vis Sci* 1994, 35: 242-250.

16. Villumsen J and Alm A. Prostaglandin $F_{2\alpha}$-isopropyl ester eye drops: Effects in normal human eyes. *Br J Ophthalmol* 1989; 73: 419-26.

17. Kerstetter JR, Brubaker RF, Wilson SE and Kullerstrand LJ. Prostaglandin $F_{2\alpha}$-1-isopropyl ester lowers intraocular pressure without decreasing aqueous humor flow. *Am J Ophthalmol* 1988; 105: 30-4.

18. Villumsen J, Alm A and Söderström J. Prostaglandin $F_{2\alpha}$-isopropyl ester eye drops: effect on intraocular pressure in open angle glaucoma. *Br J Ophthalmol* 1989; 73: 975-79.

19. Camras CB, Siebold EC, Lustgarten JS, Serle JB, Frisch SF, Podos SM et al. Maintained reduction of intraocular pressure by prostaglandin $F_{2\alpha}$-1-isopropyl ester applied in multiple doses in ocular hypertensive and glaucoma

patients. *Ophthalmology* 1989; 96: 1329-36.

20. Stjernschantz J and Resul B. Phenyl-substituted prostaglandin analogs for glaucoma treatment. *Drugs of the Future* 1992; 17: 691-704.

21. Resul B, Stjernschantz J, No K, Liljebris C, Selén G, Astin M et al. Phenyl-substituted prostaglandins: Potent and selective antiglaucoma agents. *J Med Chem* 1993; 36: 243-8.

22. Coleman RA, Kennedy I, Humphrey PPA, Bunce K and Lumley P. Prostanoids and their receptors. In: Hansch C, Sammes PG and Taylor JB. *Comprehensive Medicinal Chemistry*. Oxford/New York; Pergamon Press: 1989; 3: 643-714.

23. Stjernschantz J, Selén G, Sjöquist B and Resul B. Preclinical pharmacology of latanoprost, a phenyl-substituted $PGF_{2\alpha}$ analogue. *This volume.*

24. Nagasubramanian S, Sheth GP, Hitchings RA and Stjernschantz J. Intraocular pressure-reducing effect of PhXA41 in ocular hypertension. *Ophthalmology* 1993; 100: 1305-11.

25. Rácz P, Ruzsonyi MR, Nagy ZT and Bito LZ. Maintained intraocular pressure reduction with once-a-day application of a new prostaglandin $F_{2\alpha}$ analogue (PhXA41). *Arch Ophthalmol* 1993; 111:657-661.

26. Ziai N, Dolan JW, Kacere RD and Brubaker RF. The effects on aqueous dynamics of PhXA41, a new prostaglandin $F_{2\alpha}$ analogue, after topical application in normal and ocular hypertensive human eyes. *Arch Ophthalmol* 1993; 111: 1351-8.

27. Toris CB, Camras CB and Yablonski ME. Effects of PhXA41, a new prostaglandin $F_{2\alpha}$ analog, on aqueous humor dynamics in human eyes. *Ophthalmology* 1993; 100: 1297-1304.

28. Alm A. Comparative phase III clinical trial of latanoprost and timolol in patients with elevated intraocular pressure. *This volume.*

Advances in Prostaglandin, Thromboxane,
and Leukotriene Research, Vol. 23,
edited by B. Samuelsson et al.
Raven Press, Ltd., New York © 1995

LEUKOTRIENE ANTAGONISTS AND INHIBITORS: CLINICAL APPLICATIONS

A.W. Ford-Hutchinson, Ph.D.

Merck Frosst Centre For Therapeutic Research
P.O. Box 1005, Pointe Claire (Dorval), Quebec H9R 4P8, Canada

Leukotrienes (LTs) are products of arachidonic metabolism derived through the action of the 5-lipoxygenase enzyme pathway. LTD_4 receptor activation is now thought to be an important event in the pathology of human bronchial asthma as well as possibly other related allergic diseases. The binding of LTB_4 with its receptor results in the activation of polymorphonuclear leucocytes and lymphocytes and has been postulated to be an important event in diseases in which neutrophil infiltration is a prominent pathological feature, such as inflammatory bowel disease and psoriasis. The present article summarize the current knowledge with regard to the therapeutic utilities of LT antagonists and inhibitors in the treatment of human bronchial asthma, inflammatory bowel disease, psoriasis and glumerulonephritis.

LEUKOTRIENE ANTAGONISTS AND INHIBITORS

Various therapeutic approaches have been used to block either the production or action of LTs. In an analogous fashion to the development of cyclooxygenase inhibitors, 5-lipoxygenase inhibitors have been developed which will inhibit the production of all products of the 5-lipoxygenase pathway. The most advanced of these compounds in clinical trials is zileuton which is being used in the treatment of bronchial asthma at a dose of 600mg q.i.d. In addition a class of compounds, termed LT biosynthesis inhibitors, have been discovered which also block the production of products of the 5-lipoxygenase pathway but have no effect on the 5-lipoxygenase enzyme. The first of these compounds to be studied mechanistically was MK-886 although subsequently other compounds with similar properties were discovered, including MK-0591 [2] and BAY X-1005. Through the use of MK-886-based photoaffinity probes and affinity columns, MK-886 [1] was shown to bind with high affinity to a novel 18kD protein localized in the nuclear envelope termed 5-lipoxygenase activating protein (FLAP)[3-5].

Although 5-lipoxygenase can function effectively as a purified enzyme in the test tube, FLAP has been shown to be essential for cellular LT biosynthesis. The current hypothesis for the mechanism of LT biosynthesis in cells is that 5-lipoxygenase, as well as possibly other components of the biosynthetic pathway, such as cytosolic phospholipase A_2, translocate from a site within the cell (the cytosol in the case of the polymorphonuclear leukocyte) to the nuclear envelope where FLAP is localized. The binding site for drugs such as MK-886 on FLAP is now thought to be an arachidonic acid binding site and FLAP is postulated to facilitate the transfer of arachidonic acid from phospholipases to 5-lipoxygenase, allowing 5-lipoxygenase to synthesize LTA_4 in an efficient fashion.

LTD_4 receptor antagonists have also been successfully used in the treatment of human bronchial asthma. Early antagonists were of limited potency and produced only small shifts in LTD_4 dose response curves in human subjects [6]. Such compounds also showed limited efficacy in the treatment of bronchial asthma. Subsequently compounds were developed which produced substantial shifts in LTD_4 dose response curves [6]. Many of the earlier studies pointing to an important role for LTD_4 receptor activation in asthma were carried out using MK-571 and one of its individual enantiomers, MK-679. Unfortunately, the development of MK-679 had to be discontinued, but more potent agents have since entered the clinical trials, including ICI 204219 (Acculast), which is an orally active agent in Phase III clinical trials. One of the most potent agents so far described is MK-0476, the structure of which is shown in Figure 1.

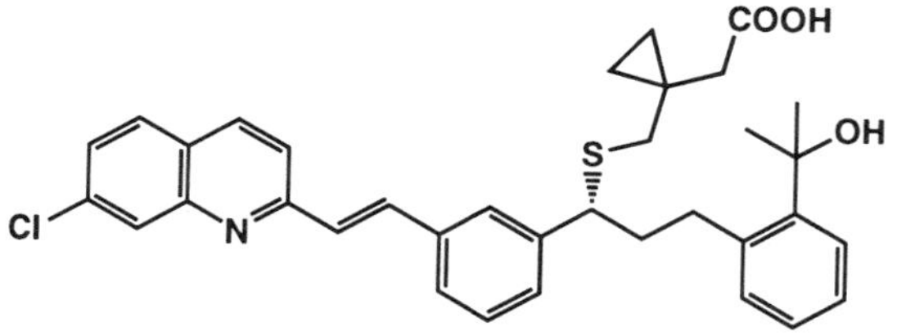

Biological Activity–Human Receptor (U–937 cell membranes)

IC_{50} vs. $[^3H]$–LTD_4	0.88 nM
IC_{50} vs. $[^3H]$–LTC_4	10 µM

Figure 1. Structure and Activity of MK-0476

MK-0476 is a potent and selective inhibitor of $[^3H]$-LTD_4 specific binding in guinea-pig lung, sheep lung and dimethylsulfoxide-differentiated U937 cell plasma membrane (human) preparations with respective Ki values 0.18 ± 0.03, 4 and $0.52 \pm 0.23nM^{[7]}$. The compound is also orally active to low doses (0.01-0.03mg/kg) in a variety of animal models including LTD_4-induced bronchoconstriction in conscious squirrel monkeys, antigen-induced bronchoconstriction in conscious sensitized rats and ascaris-induced early and late phase bronchoconstriction in conscious squirrel monkeys. In man, MK-0476 has been shown to cause prolonged, potent, LTD_4 receptor antagonism in the airways of asthmatics [8]. A dose of 200 mg administered orally 20h prior to LTD_4 challenge to the airways produced complete inhibition of the induced bronchoconstriction in 6 subjects. At a dose of 40 mg, only two of six patients demonstrated decreases in sGaw allowing PC_{50} values to be calculated. These results indicate that MK-0476 has all the characteristics of a once a day medication

LEUKOTRIENES IN BRONCHIAL ASTHMA

There area number of reasons why cysteinyl LTs might be important mediators of human bronchial asthma [6]. Firstly, LTs are produced both by constitutive cells (mast cells and alveolar macrophages) and induced infiltrating cells (eosinophils) within the lung. Consistent with this urinary levels of LTs are increased in asthmatics following provocation with either antigen or aspirin in appropriately sensitized individuals. In addition, LTs have been shown to be produced within the lung following antigen challenge of asthmatic subjects as assessed by bronchoalveolar lavage. Administration of LTD_4 to the lung induces a potent bronchoconstrictor response in both normal and asthmatic subjects. Cysteinyl LTs have also been shown to enhance airway hyperresponsiveness in asthmatic but not normal subjects. This enhanced responsiveness may be related to the ability of LTD_4 and LTE_4 to induce eosinophil recruitment into asthmatic airways *in vivo*. Finally LTD_4 may contribute to abnormal airway function in asthmatics by two other mechanisms, namely enhancement of vascular permeability in the lung and stimulation of mucus secretion resulting in mucus plug formation.

Clinical trials with LTD_4 receptor antagonists have supported the concept that cysteinyl LTs are important mediators of human bronchial asthma[6]. Many compounds have been tested against LTD_4-induced bronchoconstriction in either normal or asthmatic subjects and optimal responses has been obtained with compounds that produce greater than 20 fold shifts in the LTD_4 dose response curves. Such compounds inhibit both the early and late phase antigen-induced bronchoconstriction as well as the subsequent antigen-induced airway hyperresponsiveness in sensitive subjects. Such compounds have also been shown to substantially inhibit exercise-induced bronchoconstriction as well as bronchoconstriction induced by aspirin in patients sensitive to non-steroidal anti-inflammatory drugs. LTD_4 receptor antagonists will bronchodialate moderate to severe asthmatics, an effect additive with ß-agonists.   A number of chronic studies have also been carried with LTD_4 receptor antagonists. Improvements in objective parameters (FEV_1 and peak expiratory flow rates) as well as patient reported events (symptom scores, nocturnal asthma symptoms and usage of ß-agonists) have been observed with no evidence of mechanism-based side effects. Some studies have also been carried out with LT synthesis inhibitors but it is not clear whether such compounds have any advantages over LTD_4 antagonists suggesting that LTB_4 receptor activation has little or no role in the pathogenesis of bronchial asthma.

INFLAMMATORY BOWEL DISEASE

Inflammatory bowel disease is a disease characterized by extensive leukocyte infiltration and as such there has been some interest as to the nature of the major chemotactic factors in inflammatory bowel disease mucosa. It has been proposed that LTB_4 may be a major chemotactic factor in such patients and large amounts of LTs are found in the mucosa of patients with either ulcerative colitis or crohn's disease. There have also been suggestions that some of the drugs currently used in the treatment of inflammatory bowel disease (eg. 5-ASA derivatives) may be weak inhibitors of LTs synthesis and may exert their beneficial effects through this mechanism.

Some recent clinical trials have been reported with the 5-lipoxygenase inhibitor (zileuton). In one trial, zileuton (600mg q.i.d.) and zileuton (800mg b.i.d.) was compared with placebo[9]. The remission rate for zileuton (600mg q.i.d.) was 25%, 13% for zileuton (800mg b.i.d.) and 7% for placebo. A second study examined the effects of zileuton (600mg q.i.d.) compared with 5-ASA (400mg q.i.d.) and placebo on the maintenance of remission in patients with ulcerative colitis[10]. The relapse rates were 35% for the 5-ASA group, 42% for zileuton and 51% for placebo. These results suggests that zileuton has no significant advantage compared to current therapy. One possible explanation for these disappointing results was that zileuton was not fully effective at inhibiting LT synthesis within the ulcerative colitic mucosa. In this context administration of a single oral 250mg dose of MK-591 resulted in nearly complete blockade of rectal LTB_4 (>99%) and systemic LT (>95%) production in ulcerative colitis[11]. MK-591 will thus be of use to ascertain whether more complete inhibition of LT biosynthesis will produce superior efficacy to that seen with zileuton. However, the possibility that existing agents such as 5-ASA and its derivatives may be acting by mechanisms involving inhibition of LT biosynthesis may suggest that newer LT biosynthesis inhibitors approach will show no advantages over current therapy.

PSORIASIS

Psoriasis is another disease characterized by extensive leukocyte infiltration, albeit into the skin rather than the rectal mucosa. As with inflammatory bowel disease measurements have been made for the presence of various chemotactic agents in psoriatic lesions and the presence of LTB_4-like immunoreactive material has been described. There have also been suggestions that existing drugs may act by inhibiting the production of LTs. However, as recently reviewed[12], there is considerable circumstantial evidence to suggest that 5-lipoxygenase activation may not be a critical event in the pathology of psoriasis. The arguments presented to support this conclusion were as follows. 1) the LTB_4-like material found in psoriatic skin has never been shown to have the correct stereochemistry to indicate that it is derived through the 5-lipoxygenase enzyme pathway. 2) there is no convincing evidence presented to date to indicate that either 5-lipoxygenase or FLAP are present in human skin in cell types other than the polymorphonuclear leukocyte 3) drugs originally postulated to have some benefit in psoriasis through a 5-lipoxygenase inhibitory mechanism probably act through other mechanisms. 4) clinical trials have been carried out with both zileuton (topically and systematically) and MK-886. These agents were found not to decrease the amount of LTB_4-like material found in psoriatic skin lesions indicating that this material is not derived through the action of the 5-lipoxygenase pathway. In addition neither agent appear to have any therapeutic utility in the disease state.

GLOMERULONEPHRITIS

There have been suggestions that oxidative products of arachidonic acid metabolism, and in particular, LTs, may mediate the alterations in renal hemodynamics and glomerular filtration which occur in a variety of nephritides including nephrotoxic serum nephritis, murine lupus and passive Heymann nephritis. Studies in nephritic animals have demonstrated increase renal LTB_4 formation by isolated rat glomeruli and cortical hormogenates and a correlation between neutrophil infiltration and glomerular LTB_4 synthesis has been defined. Pharmacological blockade with either LT biosynthesis inhibitors or LTD_4 receptor antagonists has resulted in improvements in glomerular filtration rates and decreases in proteinuria supporting a causal role for cysteinyl LTs in the development of glomerulonephritis. Cysteinyl LTs may play a role in the pathogenesis and progression of glomerulonephritis not only through effects on renal blood flow and filtration but also through proliferative changes which are characteristic of this model. Thus proliferation of glomerular endothelial and mesangial cells has been shown *in vitro* in response to both LTC_4 and LTD_4 and *in vivo* inhibition of LT biosynthesis in nephritic rats with MK-886 was shown to prevent glomerular cell proliferation[13]. We have provided further support for a role for cysteinyl LTs in glomerulonephritis by demonstrating in a rat model of experimental glomeru-

-lonephritis enhanced urinary LTC_4 excretion into the urine, this enhancement of urinary LTC_4 excretion being paralleled by concomitant alterations in LTC_4 synthase activity in renal cortical microsomes[14]. These animal models suggest an early role for LTs in the development of subsequent functional changes and it will be of interest to see if similar results can be obtained in man.

CONCLUSIONS

Clinical data obtained to date support the conclusion that LTD_4 receptor activation is an important event in the pathology of human bronchial asthma and it seems likely that drugs such as LTD_4 receptor antagonists will have a useful role in the treatment of this disease. LTB_4 receptor activation has been postulated to play an important role in diseases where neutrophil infiltration is a predominant pathological feature such as psoriasis and inflammatory bowel disease. However, clinical data to support this concept has not been obtained. Another pathological state where LTD_4 receptor activation may be important is experimental glomerulonephritis in rats and it will be of interest to determine whether preclinical data obtained in rodent models will translate into therapeutic utility in man.

REFERENCES

1.   Gillard, J., Ford-Hutchinson, A.W., Chan, C., *et al.* Can. J. Physiol. Pharmacol. 1989; 67: 456-64.
2.   Brideau, C., Chan, C., Charleson, S., *et al.* Can.J.Physiol.Pharmacol. 1992; 70: 799-807.
3.   Miller, D.K., Gillard, J.W., Vickers, P.J., *et al.* Nature. 1990; 343: 278-81.
4.   Dixon, R.A.F., Diehl, R.E., Opas, E., *et al.* Nature. 1990; 343: 282-84.
5.   Woods, J.W., Evans, J.F., Ethier, D., *et al.* J. Exp. Med. 1993; 178: 1935-46.
6.   Ford-Hutchinson, A.W., (MacDonald, S.H., Ed.) Springer Series in Immunopathology, Springer-Verlag, Berlin. 1993; 15: 37-50.
7.   Jones, T.R., Champion, E., Charette, L., *et al.* Am. J. Resp. Crit. Care Med. 1994; 149: A463
8.   Botto, A., DeLepeleire, I., Rochette, F., *et al.* Am. J. Resp. Crit. Med. 1994; 149: A465
9.   Peppercorn, M., Das, K., Elson, K., *et al.* Gastroenterology 1994; 106: A751
10.   Hawkey, C., Gassull, M., Lauritsen, K., *et al.* Gastroenterology 1994; 106: A697
11.   Hillingsø , J., Kjeldsen, J., Laursen, L.S., *et al.* Gastroenterology 1994; 106: A698
12.   Ford-Hutchinson, A.W., Skin Pharmacol. 1993; 6: 292-97.
13.   Wu, S.H., Lianos, E.A., J. Lab Clin Med. 1993; 122: 703-10.

Advances in Prostaglandin, Thromboxane,
and Leukotriene Research, Vol. 23,
edited by B. Samuelsson et al.
Raven Press, Ltd., New York © 1995

Multiple Forms of Phospholipase A_2 in Macrophages Capable of Arachidonic Acid Release for Eicosanoid Biosynthesis

Edward A. Dennis, Elizabeth J. Ackermann, Raymond A. Deems, and Laure J. Reynolds

Department of Chemistry and Biochemistry, 0601
Revelle College and School of Medicine
University of California at San Diego
La Jolla, CA 92093-0601

Phospholipase A_2 (PLA$_2$) constitutes a very diverse family of enzymes with regard to sequence, structure, regulation, localization and Ca^{2+} role. Our current knowledge about the structure, function, and regulation of the most well-characterized PLA$_2$s has recently been summarized [Review: (1)]. Several forms of PLA$_2$ occur in individual cell types and tissues including the macrophage-like cell line P388D$_1$ (2). These include a Group II secretary or extracellular sPLA$_2$, a cytosolic high molecular-weight Group IV cPLA$_2$, and a Ca^{2+}-independent iPLA$_2$ (3). PLA$_2$ has been implicated as the control point in the generation of free arachidonic acid for eicosanoid biosynthesis [Review: (4)]. Each of the different PLA$_2$s in P388D$_1$ cells is potentially capable of releasing free arachidonic acid. We will first summarize the classification of PLA$_2$s, then discuss the newly purified and characterized Ca^{2+}-independent PLA$_2$ from macrophages (5) and finally summarize the recent findings on PAF receptor activation of PLA$_2$ (6) in LPS primed P388D$_1$ cells [Review: (7)] and our initial efforts utilizing antisense RNA technology to determine which of the PLA$_2$s is actually involved (3).

PHOSPHOLIPASE A₂ CLASSIFICATION

The best characterized PLA_2s are the secreted pancreatic and venom enzymes [Review: (8)]. These are soluble extracellular enzymes that have high disulfide bond content, low molecular mass (~14 kDa), and require mM levels of Ca^{2+} for catalysis. Traditionally these enzymes have been divided into three groups based on sequence homology and disulfide bond formation (9). The Group I enzymes are obtained from the venom of Elapidae snakes and various mammalian pancreases, the Group II enzymes from Viperidae snakes and the Group III from bee venom. Several human counterparts to these enzymes have now been identified. The best characterized is the Group II PLA_2 originally isolated from human synovial fluid. Group II enzymes are produced by many different cell types and are found in rat liver mitochondria [Review: (10)].

Recently, several other PLA_2s have been discovered that have quite different characteristics and clearly do not fit into these categories. One of the first enzymes found that did not fit into one of the three groups was the "cytosolic" PLA_2 [Review: (1)]. This enzyme has been identified in a variety of cells; it has a molecular mass of 85 kDa, an apparent preference for arachidonate containing phospholipids, and translocates from the cytosol to membranes in the presence of submicromolar levels of Ca^{2+}. Gross and coworkers (11) have purified another, apparently different, PLA_2 from canine myocardium. It is an intracellular, cytosolic PLA_2 that does not require Ca^{2+}, but does prefer arachidonyl-containing phospholipids. Its amino acid sequence has not been reported but it is a 40 kDa enzyme. This enzyme appears to be activated by ATP and associates with a large oligomeric protein thought to be phosphofructokinase.

We have discovered a similar enzyme in $P388D_1$ cells (5). While the $P388D_1$ enzyme does not require Ca^{2+} and is activated by ATP, it does differ from the myocardial enzyme in significant ways. Both enzymes, though, do not fit into the four groups mentioned above and, depending on their sequence, may define yet more groups.

There are numerous other Ca^{2+}-dependent and Ca^{2+}-independent intracellular PLA_2 activities described in the literature [Review: (10)]. These include: a phosphatidylserine specific Ca^{2+}-dependent PLA_2 and a 30 kDa dimeric PLA_2 purified from sheep platelets. Other Ca^{2+}-independent PLA_2 activities have also been reported such as a 97,000 kDa ectoenzyme found in guinea pig intestinal brush-border membranes. These enzymes have not been characterized sufficiently to allow their assignment to a particular group. PLA_2 may indeed be a much more diverse group of enzymes than had been previously believed.

As the list of PLA_2s increases, so too does the diversity in their characteristics. These enzymes, however, do share one important characteristic; they all must interact with large aggregated lipid structures. The nature of this interaction has been defined, in large part, by the studies carried out on the Group I and II PLA_2s. In this sense, the venom and pancreatic PLA_2s have stood as paradigms of enzymes acting on lipids. These enzymes continue to play an important role in understanding how soluble enzymes interact with phospholipid interfaces and in defining the parameters of this interaction. This knowledge is crucial if we are to understand how the new, more diverse PLA$_2$s are functioning (1).

Ca^{2+}-INDEPENDENT MACROPHAGE PHOSPHOLIPASE A$_2$

We reported the presence of a calcium-independent PLA$_2$ activity in P388D$_1$ cells in 1985 (2). This activity had a pH optimum of pH 7.5 and was shown to be cytosolic by sucrose density centrifugation. We (5) have subsequently purified this novel enzyme to apparent homogeneity and have identified several unique properties including its oligomerization. Its sensitivity to Triton X-100 and activation by ATP after purification on an ATP-agarose column is shown in Figure 1.

The purification procedure utilized an ammonium sulfate precipitation of P388D$_1$ whole cell homogenate, followed by sequential column chromatography on Octyl-Sepharose, ATP-Agarose, Mono-Q FPLC and Hydroxyapatite FPLC. Early in our studies, we found that the presence of Triton X-100 both stabilized the enzyme during the purification and increased the observed PLA$_2$ activity in a concentration dependent manner when included in the assay. Optimal activity was found at a Triton X-100/phospholipid molar ratio of 4:1. Under these assay conditions there is no apparent specificity for *sn-2* arachidonic acid nor for *sn-1* alkyl-ether containing phospholipids. Both crude and purified mixtures of the enzyme were also activated at least 2-6 fold by ATP and other di and triphosphate nucleotides. No activation was seen in the presence of AMP. Gel filtration chromatography carried out with the purified enzyme yielded a molecular weight estimate of roughly 400,000, even though SDS-PAGE yielded a single major band at a molecular weight of about 80,000. To clarify whether this oligomeric behavior was functionally significant, radiation inactivation experiments were carried out on the cell homogenate. These experiments yielded a target size of 337 ± 25 kDa suggesting that the active enzyme exists as a tetramer of 80 kDa subunits.

PAF/LPS ACTIVATION OF GROUP II PHOSPHOLIPASE A$_2$

Studies on P388D$_1$ cells in our laboratory have shown that LPS priming followed by PAF activation leads to the release of free arachidonic acid and the production of PGE$_2$ and other prostaglandins (12-15). Recent studies have shown that PAF activates a pertussis-sensitive G-protein which activates phospholipase C leading to the production of inositol-[1,4,5]-triphosphate and the mobilization of intracellular Ca^{2+} (6). However, we have found that in addition to Ca^{2+} mobilization, PAF causes a second undefined signal (6). Intracellular Ca^{2+} mobilization is necessary but not sufficient for arachidonic acid release. Further studies on the signaling mechanisms are summarized elsewhere (7).

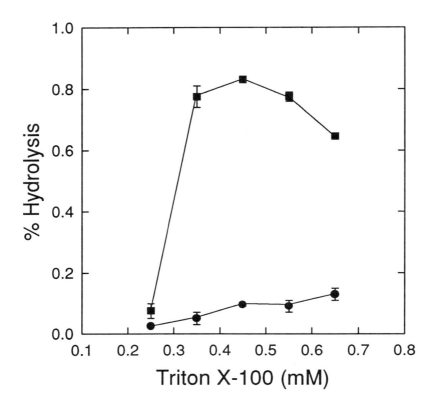

Fig. 1. Effects of Triton X-100 and ATP on Ca^{2+}-Independent PLA$_2$: Partially purified Ca^{2+}-independent PLA$_2$ (ATP agarose column fractions, purified ~26,000 fold (5)), were depleted of ATP and assayed with 100 µM dipalmitoyl-phosphorylcholine and increasing amounts of Triton X-100 (forming mixed micelles with molar ratios ranging from 2.5:1 - 6.5:1) in the presence (■) or absence (●) of 0.8 mM ATP.   Each point represents the average of duplicates.

In order to determine which PLA$_2$s in P388D$_1$ cells are responsible for arachidonic acid release, we (3) initiated the application of antisense RNA technology to block the production of specific PLA$_2$s. We initiated our studies by using antisense RNA technology to block the expression of sPLA$_2$ in P388D$_1$ cells using phosphorothioate oligonucleotides. In control cells, priming by LPS and activation by PAF leads to enhanced PGE$_2$ production. In antisense-treated cells, sPLA$_2$ expression as well as PGE$_2$ production and arachidonic acid release are dramatically reduced (3). These studies demonstrate a role for sPLA$_2$ in PGE$_2$ generation by these cells. Roles for the other PLA$_2$s (cPLA$_2$ and iPLA$_2$) present in these cells is now a subject of active investigation in our laboratory.

ACKNOWLEDGEMENTS

This work was supported by grants from the National Institutes of Health GM 20,501 and HD 26,171.

REFERENCES

1. Dennis, E. A. Diversity of Group Types, Regulation, and Function of Phospholipase A$_2$. *J. Biol. Chem.* 1994; 269: 13,057-13,060.
2. Ross, M. I., Deems, R. A., Jesaitis, A. J., Dennis, E. A., and Ulevitch, R. J. Phospholipase Activities of the P388D$_1$ Macrophage-Like Cell Line. *Arch. Biochem. Biophys.* 1985; 238: 247-258.
3. Barbour, S., and Dennis, E. A. Antisense Inhibition of Group II Phospholipase A$_2$ Expression Blocks the Production of Prostaglandin E$_2$ by P388D$_1$ Cells. *J. Biol. Chem.* 1993; 268: 21875-21882.
4. Dennis, E. A. The Regulation of Eicosanoid Production: Role of Phospholipases and Inhibitors, *Bio/Technology* 1987; 5: 1294-1300.
5. Ackermann, E. J., Kempner, E. S., and Dennis, E. A. Ca^{2+}-Independent Cytosolic Phospholipase A$_2$ from the Macrophage-Like P388D$_1$ Cells: Isolation and Characterization. *J. Biol. Chem.* 1994; 269: 9227-9233.
6. Asmis, R., Randrimampita, C., Tsien, R., and Dennis, E. A. Intracellular Ca^{2+}, Inositol-1,4,5-Trisphosphate and Additional Signaling in the PAF Stimulation of PGE$_2$ Formation in P388D$_1$ Macrophage-Like Cells. *Biochem. J.* 1994; 298: 543-551.
7. Asmis, R., and Dennis, E. A. Regulation of Prostaglandin E$_2$ Production in P388D$_1$ Macrophage-Like Cells. *Annals, New York Academy of Sciences* 1994; In press.
8. Dennis, E. A. Phospholipases. In: *The Enzymes, Third Edition, Vol. 16*, (Boyer, P., Edit.). New York: Academic Press; 1989: 307-353.

9. Davidson, F. F., and Dennis, E. A. Evolutionary Relationships and Implications for the Regulation of Phospholipase A_2: from Snake Venom to Human Secreted Forms. *J. Mol. Evol.* 1990; 31: 228-238.

10. Kudo, I., Murakami, M., Hara, S., and Inoue, K. Mammalian Non-pancreatic Phospholipases A_2. *Biochim. Biophys. Acta* 1993; 1170: 217-231.

11. Hazen, S. L., Stuppy, R. J., and Gross, R. W. Purification and Characterization of Canine Myocardial Cytosolic Phospholipase A_2- A Calcium-Independent Phospholipase with Absolute *sn*-2 Regiospecificity for Diradyl Glycerophospholipids. *J. Biol. Chem.* 1990; 265: 10622-10630.

12. Lister, M. D., Glaser, K. B., Ulevitch, R. J., and Dennis, E. A. Inhibition Studies on the Membrane-Associated Phospholipase A_2 *in vitro* and Prostaglandin E_2 Production *in vivo* of the Macrophage-Like $P388D_1$ Cells: Effects of Manoalide, 7,7-Dimethyl-5,8-eicosadienoic Acid, and *p*-Bromophenacyl Bromide. *J. Biol. Chem.* 1989; 264: 8520-8528.

13. Glaser, K. B., Asmis, R., and Dennis, E. A. Bacterial Lipopolysaccharide Priming of $P388D_1$ Macrophage-Like Cells for Enhanced Arachidonic Acid Metabolism, Platelet-Activating Factor Receptor Activation and Regulation of Phospholipase A_2. *J. Biol. Chem.* 1990; 265: 8658-8664.

14. Dennis, E. A. Modification of the Arachidonic Acid Cascade Through Phospholipase A_2 Dependent Mechanisms. *Adv. in Prostaglandin, Thromboxane and Leukotriene Res.* 1990; 20: 217-223.

15. Glaser, K. B., Asmis, R., and Dennis, E. A. PAF Receptor Mediated PGE_2 Production in LPS Primed $P388D_1$ Macrophage-Like Cells. *Adv. Prostaglandin, Thromboxane and Leukotriene Res.* 1991; 21: 249-255.

Advances in Prostaglandin, Thromboxane,
and Leukotriene Research, Vol. 23,
edited by B. Samuelsson et al.
Raven Press, Ltd., New York © 1995

AA-Release Is Under Control of PLA$_2$ and DAG Lipase in Rat Liver Macrophages

P. Ambs, E. Fitzke, and P. Dieter

Biochemisches Institut der Universität Freiburg c/o Klinik für
Tumorbiologie, Breisacherstr. 177, D-79106 Freiburg

The liberation of arachidonic acid (AA) from phospholipids by phospholipase (PL)A$_2$ and/or PLC + diacylglycerol (DAG) lipase is thought to be the rate-limiting step of eicosanoid synthesis.

RESULTS AND DISCUSSION

We could show that liver macrophages release AA upon treatment with PMA (phorbol ester), zymosan, A23187 (Ca^{2+}-ionophore), and fluoride (activator of G-proteins). We could furthermore demonstrate that PMA-induced liberation of AA is mediated by protein kinase (PK)C-ß, that PKC-δ is involved in the zymosan-induced formation of AA whereas A23187-elicited AA-release is not controlled by PKC isoenzymes [1,2].

DAG is formed upon addition of PMA, fluoride, and zymosan (Fig.1). The zymosan-induced formation of DAG is negatively controlled by PKC-δ while PKC-ß mediates the PMA-induced generation of DAG [1].

In order to investigate if DAG lipase is involved in AA-release we used the DAG lipase inhibitor RG 80267 (Rorer Central Research, Horsham, USA). RG 80267 inhibits almost totally the PMA- and fluoride-induced AA-release and by about 50% the zymosan-induced formation of AA but has almost no effect on the A23187-induced liberation of AA [2]. These data indicate that AA is released by the action of PLC/DAG lipase upon addition of zymosan, PMA, and fluoride but not with A23187.

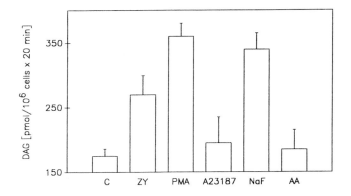

Fig.1: Formation of DAG mass in cells incubated for 30 min without (C) or with zymosan (ZY), PMA, A23187, fluoride (NaF) or AA [2].

Since it has been shown that release of AA has an absolute requirement for Ca^{2+} [1,2], the Ca^{2+}-dependence of PLA$_2$ and DAG lipase activity was measured. While DAG lipase activity shows no Ca^{2+}-dependence, PLA$_2$ activity is strictly dependent on the presence of Ca^{2+} (Fig.2). Furthermore, PLA$_2$ has been shown to translocate Ca^{2+}-dependently to membranes [4,6]. These data and the fact that only zymosan and A23187 induce an elevation of intracellular Ca^{2+}-concentration above 10^{-7} M [2] indicate that the PLA$_2$ pathway may be triggered by zymosan and A23187 but not by PMA or fluoride.

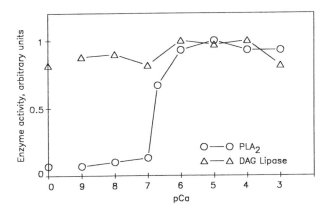

Fig.2: Ca^{2+}-dependence of PLA$_2$ (circles, [4]) and   DAG lipase activity (triangles, [3]). A value of 1 corresponds to a release of 180 (PLA$_2$) and 170 (DAG lipase) pmol AA/min x mg protein.

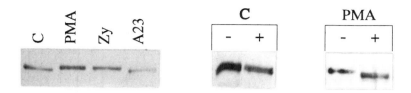

Fig.3: Western-blot analysis [1] of cPLA$_2$ from cells incubated for 10 min without (C) or with PMA (1µM), zymosan (Zy, 0,5 mg/ml) or A23187 (A23, 1µM). If indicated, homogenates were incubated without (-) or with potato acid phosphatase (+; 90 min, 6 units/ml). The antibodies against U937-cPLA$_2$ were a generous gift from Dr.J.D.Clark (Cambridge, USA).

It has been reported in other cell systems that upon stimulation cPLA$_2$ becomes phosphorylated which leads to increased enzymatic activity [5]. Treatment of liver macrophages with zymosan and PMA induces a phosphorylation of cPLA$_2$ reversable by treatment with potato acid phosphatase (Fig.3).

From these and previous results [1,2] we suggest the following hypothesis:
- Phorbol ester activates PKC-ß leading to activation of PLC and formation of DAG. Released AA arises predominantly from PLC/DAG lipase pathway.
- Zymosan activates via receptor(s) PIP$_2$-PLC which results in a formation of DAG and in an IP$_3$-mediated increase in intracellular free Ca^{2+}. PKC-δ exerts a negative control on the zymosan-induced PLC activation. Released AA arises from both, PLC/DAG lipase and PLA$_2$ pathway.

REFERENCES

1. Duyster J, Schwende H, Fitzke E, Hidaka H, Dieter P. Different roles of PKC-ß and PKC-δ in AA-cascade, superoxide formation and phosphoinositide hydrolysis. *Biochem J* 1993;292: 203-207.
2. Dieter P, Fitzke E. Formation of DAG, inositol phosphates, AA, and its metabolites in macrophages. *Eur J Biochem* 1993; 218: 753-758.
3. Xia T, Coleman RA. DAG metabolism in neonatal rat liver. *Biochim Biophys Acta* 1992; 1126: 327-336.
4. Krause H, Dieter P, Schulze-Specking A, Ballhorn A, Decker K. Ca^{2+}-induced reversible translocation of PLA$_2$ between the cytosol and the membrane fraction of rat liver macrophages. *Eur J Biochem* 1991; 199:355-359.
5. Lin LL, Wartmann M, Lin AY, Knopf JL, Seth A, Davis RJ. cPLA$_2$ is phosphorylated and activated by MAP-kinase. *Cell* 1993; 72: 269-278.
6. Ambs P, Fitzke E, Dieter P. Regulation of eicosanoid synthesis in macrophages. *Lipid mediators in health and disease*. Tel Aviv: Freund publishing house Ltd. 1994, in press.

Advances in Prostaglandin, Thromboxane, and Leukotriene Research, Vol. 23,
edited by B. Samuelsson et al.
Raven Press, Ltd., New York © 1995

Structural Characterization of Pancreatic Group I Phospholipase A₂ Receptor

Jun Ishizaki, Ken-ichi Higashino, Osamu Ohara, and Hitoshi Arita

Shionogi Research Laboratories, Shionogi and Co., Ltd., 5-12-4, Sagisu, Fukushima-ku, Osaka 553, Japan

Although mammalian pancreatic group I phospholipase A_2 (PLA$_2$-I) has been thought as a digestive enzyme, we have recently discovered the existence of a specific receptor for a mature form of PLA$_2$-I on a wide range of cell types (1) and identified various cellular responses, such as proliferation and prostaglandin E_2 synthesis, elicited by PLA$_2$-I in a receptor-mediated manner (2~4). For understanding molecular mechanisms leading to these cellular responses mediated by this PLA$_2$ receptor, we cloned cDNAs encoding bovine PLA$_2$ receptor on the basis of its partial amino acid sequences and characterized the structure of the receptor by using the recombinant DNA technology.

DOMAIN ORGANIZATION OF PLA₂ RECEPTOR

Interestingly, the deduced primary structure of the PLA$_2$ receptor (5) (1,463 amino acid residues) exhibits a close relatedness throughout the molecule to that of the macrophage mannose receptor, a unique member of Ca^{2+}-dependent (C-type) animal lectin family, in spite of their functional diversity. Based on this sequence similarity between these two receptors, the domain organization of the PLA$_2$ receptor could be assigned as shown in Fig. 1. The mature form of the receptor consists of ten extracellular domains (including eight tandemly repeated domains homologous to carbohydrate-recognition domains (CRDs) found in C-type animal lectins), a single transmembrane region, and a short cytoplasmic tail.

REGIONS RESPONSIBLE FOR THE LIGAND BINDING

In order to determine which domains are important for the PLA$_2$-I binding and internalization reactions, we synthesized several truncated forms of the receptor and analyzed their properties. The results indicated that the region responsible for

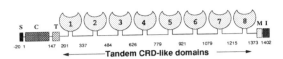

S: Signal sequence
C: Cys-rich region
T: Fibronectin type II repeat-like region
CRD: Carbohydrate-Recognition Domain
M: Membrane spanning region
I: Intracellular region

FIG. 1. Predicted overall domain structure of PLA$_2$ receptor. The numbers shown below the schematic drawing indicate the amino acid residue number located at the boundaries between domains (5).

the PLA$_2$-I binding is corresponding to CRD-like domains (CRD #1~8) and that the cytoplasmic tail is crucial for the internalization process (5). A further deletion analysis revealed that a mutant receptor carrying only three CRD-like domains (CRD #3~5) retained the PLA$_2$-binding capability (dissociation constant, 3.9 nM).

Amino acid sequence comparison of bovine PLA$_2$ receptor with rabbit (6) and mouse (7) counterparts showed that CRD #4 is the most highly conserved domain among CRD #1~8. Therefore, we next examined the importance of CRD #4 in the PLA$_2$ binding as follows. Each CRD-like domain in the PLA$_2$ receptor seems to have two disulfide bonds as in the case of CRD in animal lectins, since four cysteine residues involved in the disulfide bond formations are located in a highly conserved manner in all CRD-like domains in the PLA$_2$ receptor. A single amino acid substitution (Cys→Ser) introduced in one of those cysteine residues in CRD #4 resulted in the loss of the PLA$_2$-binding capability of the truncated mutant carrying CRD #3~5, indicating that CRD #4 plays a critical role in the PLA$_2$-I-recognition. In this respect, it is interesting to note that CRD #4 is experimentally shown to be a carbohydrate binding domain in the mannose receptor (8).

SEQUENCE HOMOLOGY WITH SNAKE PLA$_2$ INHIBITORS

Deletion mutant analyses showed that CRD-like domain(s) in the PLA$_2$ receptor is responsible for the PLA$_2$ binding. It is notable that the PLA$_2$ receptor is not the first example of PLA$_2$-binding protein belonging to the C-type lectin superfamily; Phospholipase A$_2$ inhibitors (PLIs), which are isolated from snake blood plasma and specifically bind and inhibit their own venom group II PLA$_2$, carry the CRD-like sequence motif (9, 10) (Fig. 2). Since overall three-dimensional structures of group I and II PLA$_2$s are almost superimposable (11), the PLA$_2$ recognition mechanisms of the PLA$_2$ receptor and PLIs might be similar. Actually, we recently observed that the PLA$_2$ receptor inhibited PLA$_2$-I catalytic activity (12).

Importantly, CRD-like domains in the PLA$_2$ receptor and PLI are structurally grouped into different C-type CRD subfamilies (13). Previous evolutional analyses concluded that these subfamilies were diverged early in evolution; genes encoding these proteins are thought to evolve individually from different ancestral genes arising from a common progenitor with a primordial CRD. Independent evolutional events appear to convert different ancestral CRD-carrying proteins into PLA$_2$ recognizing ones. This might be an indication of unknown, probably structural, relatedness between carbohydrates and PLA$_2$s as ligands.

A. *blomhoffii siniticus*	PLI	WAEGQPKKAD	GTCVKADTH	GLWHSTSCD DNLLVVCEF
T. *flavoviridis*	PLI-A	WAAGQPKEAD	GTCVKADTH	GSWHSASCD ENLLVVCEF
	PLI-B	WAAGQPKEAD	GTCVKADTH	GFWHSASCD EKLLVVCEF
PLA$_2$ Receptor	CRD-like 1	WKPEINFEPFVE	YHCGTFNAFMP	KAWKSRDCE STLPYVCKK
	CRD-like 2	WHTLEPHIFPNRS	QLCVSAEQSE	GHWKVKNCE ETLFYLCKK
	CRD-like 3	WNTRQPRYS	GGCVVMRGRSHP	GRWEVRDCRHFKAMSLCKQ
	CRD-like 4	YFGEDA	RNCAVYKAN	KTLLPSYCG SKREWICKI
	CRD-like 5	WDKGKERSMGLNES	QRCGFISSIT	GLWASEECS ISMPSICKR
	CRD-like 6	WSPFDTKNIPNHNTTEVQKRIPLCGLLSNNPNFHFTGKWYFEDCR EGYGFVCEK		
	CRD-like 7	WKDDESSFL	GDCVFADTS	GRWSSTACESYLQGAICQV
	CRD-like 8	WGIRKPEVYHFKP	HLCVALRIPE	GVWQLSSCQ DKKGFICKM
CRD	Invariant/Conserved	W ZPB	EOCØ Ω	G WND C Ω C

FIG. 2. Sequence alignment of carboxy-terminal regions of CRD-like domains in PLIs and bovine PLA$_2$ receptor. The conserved and invariant (bold) amino acid residues in C-type animal lectins (13) are given at the bottom line, and the residues directly involved in Ca^{2+}/carbohydrate interaction are underlined (14) (Z=E or Q; B=D or N; O=D, N, E or Q; Ø=aliphatic; Ω=aliphatic or aromatic). Most of the Ca^{2+}/carbohydrate-binding residues in animal lectins are substituted in PLIs and PLA$_2$ receptor, suggesting that these PLA$_2$-binding proteins do not have carbohydrate-binding activity.

REFERENCES

1. Arita H, Hanasaki K, Nakano T, Oka S, Teraoka H, Matsumoto K. Novel proliferative effect of phospholipase A$_2$ in Swiss 3T3 cells via specific binding site. *J Biol Chem* 1991;266:19139-41.
2. Hanasaki K, Arita H. Characterization of a high affinity binding site for pancreatic-type phospholipase A$_2$ in the rat. *J Biol Chem* 1992;267:6414-20.
3. Tohkin M, Kishino J, Ishizaki J, Arita H. Pancreatic-type phospholipase A$_2$ stimulates prostaglandin synthesis in mouse osteoblastic cells (MC3T3-E1) via a specific binding site. *J Biol Chem* 1993;268:2865-71.
4. Kishino J, Ohara O, Nomura K, Kramer RM, Arita H. Pancreatic-type phospholipase A$_2$ induces group II phospholipase A$_2$ expression and prostaglandin biosynthesis in rat mesangial cells. *J Biol Chem* 1994;269:5092-8.
5. Ishizaki J, Hanasaki K, Higashino K, *et al.* Molecular cloning of pancreatic group I phospholipase A$_2$ receptor. *J Biol Chem* 1994;269:5897-904.
6. Lambeau G, Ancian P, Barhanin J, Ladzunski M. Cloning and expression of a membrane receptor for secretory phospholipase A$_2$. *J Biol Chem* 1994;269:1575-8.
7. Higashino K, Ishizaki J, Kishino J, Ohara O, Arita H. Manuscript in preparation.
8. Taylor ME, Bezouska K, Drickamer K. Contribution to ligand binding by multiple carbohydrate-recognition domains in the macrophage mannose receptor. *J Biol Chem* 1992;267:1719-26.
9. Inoue S, Kogaki H, Ikeda K, Samejima Y, Omori-Satoh T. Amino acid sequence of the two subunits of a phospholipase A$_2$ inhibitor from the blood plasma of *Trimeresurus flavoviridis*. *J Biol Chem* 1991;266:1001-7.
10. Ohkura N, Inoue S, Ikeda K, Hayashi K. Isolation and amino acid sequence of a phospholipase A$_2$ inhibitor from the blood plasma of *Agkistrodon blomhoffii siniticus*. *J Biochem* 1993;113:413-9.
11. Wery J-P, Schevitz RW, Clawson DK, *et al.* Structure of recombinant human rheumatoid arthritic synovial fluid phospholipase A$_2$ at 2.2 Å resolution. *Nature* 1991;352:79-82.
12. Kishino J, Ishizaki J, Kawamoto K, Verheij HM, Ohara O, Arita H. Manuscript in preparation.
13. Drickamer K. Ca^{2+}-dependent carbohydrate-recognition domains in animal proteins. *Curr. Opin. Struct. Biol.* 1993;3:393-400.
14. Weiss WI, Drickamer K, Hendrickson WA. Structure of a C-type mannose-binding protein complexed with an oligosaccharides. *Nature* 1992;360:127-34.

Advances in Prostaglandin, Thromboxane,
and Leukotriene Research, Vol. 23,
edited by B. Samuelsson et al.
Raven Press, Ltd., New York © 1995

Inhibition Of CoA-Independent Transacylase Reduces Inflammatory Lipid Mediators

James D. Winkler, Alfred N. Fonteh *, Chiu-Mei Sung , Lisa Huang, Marie Chabot-Fletcher, Lisa A. Marshall and Floyd H. Chilton *

*Department of Pharmacology, SmithKline Beecham Pharmaceuticals, 709 Swedeland Rd., King of Prussia, PA, 19406, USA., * Department of Pulmonary and Critical Care Medicine, Bowman Gray School of Medicine, Medical Center Blvd., Winston-Salem, NC, 27157, USA.*

Evidence has accumulated that molecules of AA[1] move in an ordered path between different cellular phospholipids in inflammatory cells. This path involves a transfer of AA into the *sn*-2 position of PC and PE containing ether-linked fatty chains in the *sn*-1 position (1-3). This transfer reaction of AA into 1-ether-containing phospholipids has been hypothesized to be important for moving AA into specific phospholipid pools from which it can be released and to be mediated by the enzyme CoA-IT (3,4). To better understand the importantce of CoA-IT in AA transfer and lipid mediator generation, we developed an inhibitor of CoA-IT, SK&F 98625 (diethyl7-(3,4,5triphenyl-2oxo-2,3-dihydro-imidazol-1-yl)heptane-phosphonate), to block CoA-IT action in intact cells. Here we present evidence that CoA-IT is a key enzyme in AA movement between phospholipids as well as in the generation of lipid mediators of inflammation.

RESULTS AND DISCUSSION

In cell-free systems, SK&F 98625 inhibited CoA-IT activity (Fig 1) as well as 5-LO activity (IC_{50} 3 μM). SK&F 98625 failed to inhibit the activity of a variety of other enzymes which act at the *sn*-2 position of phospholipids, including pancreatic, synovial and cytosolic PLA_2 isozymes, cyclooxygenase and acetyltransferase.

[1] Abbreviations: arachidonic acid, AA; CoA-independent transacylase, CoA-IT; 5-LO, 5-lipoxygenase; phosphatidylcholine, PC; phosphatidylethanolamine, PE; phospholipase A_2; PLA_2; platelet-activating factor, PAF

Supported in part by National Institute of Health Grants AI24985 and AI26771.

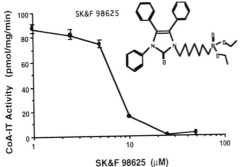

Fig 1 - Effect of SK&F 98625 on CoA-IT

The effects of SK&F 98625 on the transfer of AA into 1-ether phospholipids were measured. SK&F 98625 produced a concentration-dependent blockade of the movement of [^{3}H]AA into 1-ether-linked phospholipids in intact, unstimulated human neutrophils, at concentrations similar to that observed for inhibition of CoA-IT activity in microsomal preparations. It is important to note that SK&F 98625 could completely block AA movement, suggesting that not only can CoA-IT mediate this movement, but that no other enzyme is utilized within intact cells to compensate for the blockage of CoA-IT.

In inflammatory cells, transfer of AA into 1-ether phospholipids is markedly increased after stimulation and by cellular priming (5,6). We have postulated that this marked increase in phospholipid remodeling by CoA-IT is responsible for moving AA into the salient pools needed for release. Pretreatment of human neutrophils for 5 min with SK&F 98625 prior to challenge with A23187 produced a concentration-dependent and complete blockage of AA release (IC$_{50}$ 10 μM). This demonstrates the importance of CoA-IT action in maintaining AA levels in phospholipid pools during cell activation.

There has been increasing evidence over the last 3 years, in studies utilizing broken cell preparations, that CoA-IT, and not PLA$_2$, directly catalyzes the formation of lyso PAF and hence regulates PAF production (7-9). SK&F 98625 was therefore examined for its effects on the formation of PAF by activated neutrophils, which exibited a concentration-dependent inhibition of PAF production by SK&F 98625 (IC$_{50}$ 11 μM). As SK&F 98625 had no effect on acetyltransferase activity, this provides further support that CoA-IT activity plays a key role in PAF biosynthesis.

We compared the effects of zileuton, a compound that inhibits 5-LO activity (3 μM), but has no effects on CoA-IT activity (50 μM), with SK&F 98625. Zileuton increased the mass of free AA produced in stimulated neutrophils (10). In addition, it failed to completely block PAF production in neutrophils and had no effect on PAF production in mouse mast cells (10). This supports the claim that SK&F 98625 has an effect on AA release and PAF production by inhibition of CoA-IT activity.

The inhibition of AA release by SK&F 98625 could translate into decreases in eicosanoid production. To test this hypothesis, the effects of SK&F 98625 on prostaglandin and leukotriene production was examined in a number of settings (Table 1). SK&F 98625 was found to cause a concentration-dependent reduction in LT production, however, interpretation of these results is complicated by the observation that SK&F 98625 may have a direct effect on 5-LO activity. Importantly, SK&F 98625 fully inhibited prostaglandin and thromboxane production, while having no direct effect on cyclooxygenase activity.

Cell	Stimulus - Eicos.	SK&F 98625	Zileuton
Neutrophil	A23187 - LTB$_4$	1 µM	3 µM
Monocyte	Zymozan - LTC$_4$ - PGE$_2$	1 µM 3 µM	1 µM No effect 10 µM
Platelet	Thrombin - TxB$_2$	3 µM	
Mast cell	Antigen - PGD$_2$	3 µM	No effect 10 µM

Table 1 - Effects of SK&F 98625 and Zileuton on Eicosanoid Production. Inflammatory cells were treated with various concentrations of drugs, stimulated as shown and eicosanoids measured by EIA.

Using SK&F 98625 as a tool to explore the role of CoA-IT in inflammatory cells, we conclude that: 1) CoA-IT is responsible for the movement of AA into 1-ether phospholipids thereby making AA available for liberation; 2) CoA-IT is required for the production of lyso PAF thereby regulating PAF biosynthesis; and 3) inhibition of CoA-IT leads to blockade of inflammatory lipid mediator production. Taken together, these data reveal the importance of CoA-IT in inflammatory cell AA metabolism and demonstrate a novel therapeutic approach toward reducing lipid mediators of inflammation.

REFERENCES

1. Chilton, F.H. and R.C. Murphy. Remodeling of arachidonate-containing phosphoglycerides within the human neutrophil. *J. Biol. Chem.* 1986;261:7771-7777.
2. MacDonald, J.I.S. and H. Sprecher. Phospholipid fatty acid remodeling in mammalian cells. *Biochim. Biophys. Acta* 1991;1084:105-121.
3. Snyder, F., T.-C. Lee, and M.L. Blank. The role of transacylases in the metabolism of arachidonate and platelet-activating factor. *Prog. Lipid Res.* 1992;31:65-86.
4. Winkler, J.D. and F.H. Chilton. The role of CoA-independent transacylases in the production of platelet-activating factor and the metabolism of arachidonate. *Drug News Perspec.* 1993;6:133-138.
5. Fonteh, A.N. and F.H. Chilton. Rapid remodeling of arachidonate from phosphatidylcholine to phosphatidylethanolamine pools during mast cell activation. *J. Immunol.* 1992;148:1784-1791.
6. Winkler, J.D., C.-M. Sung, L. Huang, and F.H. Chilton. CoA-independent transacylase activity is increased in human neutrophils after treatment with tumor necrosis factor. *J. Immunol.* 1993;150:169A.
7. Venable, M.E., M.L. Nieto, J.D. Schmitt, and R.L. Wykle. Conversion of 1-*O*-[³H]alkyl-2-arachidonoyl-*sn*-glycero-3-phosphorylcholine to lyso platelet-activating factor by the CoA-independent transacylase in membrane fractions of human neutrophils. *J. Biol. Chem.* 1991;266:18691-18698.
8. Uemura, Y., T. Lee, and F. Snyder. A coenzyme A-independent transacylase is linked to the formation of platelet-activating factor (PAF) by generating the lyso-PAF intermediate in the remodeling pathway. *J. Biol. Chem.* 1991;266:8268-8272.
9. Winkler, J.D., C.-M. Sung, W.C. Hubbard, and F.H. Chilton. Evidence for different mechanisms involved in the formation of lyso platelet-activating factor and the calcium-dependent release of arachidonic acid from human neutrophils. *Biochem. Pharmacol.* 1992;44:2055-2066.
10. Winkler, J.D., C.-M. Sung, W.C. Hubbard, and F.H. Chilton. Influence of arachidonic acid on indices of phospholipase A$_2$ activity in the human neutrophil. *Biochem. J.* 1993;291:825-831.

*Advances in Prostaglandin, Thromboxane,
and Leukotriene Research, Vol. 23,*
edited by B. Samuelsson et al.
Raven Press, Ltd., New York © 1995

ON THE MECHANISM OF ACTIVATION OF PLA$_2$ AND PTDINS-PLC BY FLUORIDE IN MURINE MACROPHAGES

Rachel Goldman and Uriel Zor *

*Departments of Membrane Research & Biophysics and * Hormone Research
The Weizmann Institute of Science, Rehovot, Israel 76100*

Several second messengers regulate in concert the activity of cytosolic phospholipase A$_2$ (cPLA$_2$) and PtdIns-phospholipase C (PtdIns-PLC). We have previously shown that inactivation of protein tyrosine phosphatases (PTPs) by reactive oxygen species (ROS) (in combination with vanadate), is essential for the activation of cPLA$_2$ and PtdIns-PLC$_\gamma$ by TPA and zymosan (1,2). Here we probe the mechanism of activation phospholipases by fluoride (±aluminum). The activation of G-proteins by millimolar concentrations of fluoride was observed to depend on the addition of trace amounts of aluminum which presumably form multifluorinated complexes the major species being AlF$_4$- (3,4). AlF$_4$- is presumed to act as a phosphate analog that binds next to the GαGDP β phosphate and induces the switch to Gα(GDP AlFx)Mg which is analogous to Gα(GTP)Mg, and is the active form of the G-protein. AlF$_4$- was shown to activate and increase tyrosine phosphorylation of mitogen-activated protein kinase (MAPK) (5), to invoke protein kinase C (PKC) translocation (6) and to activate PLA$_2$ (6,7) and PtdIns-PLC (7,8) in intact cells.

PtdIns-PLC activity represents a family of subtypes of enzymes ($\alpha,\beta,\gamma,\delta$) differing in their structure as well as in their regulation. The β- subtype is activated via a GTP-binding protein (Gp), while the γ-subtypes are activated by tyrosine phosphorylation. Growth factors, hormones and antigen binding to the respective receptors induce protein tyrosine phosphorylation and activation of γ-type PtdIns-PLC. Platelet activating factor (PAF), vasopressin and AlF$_4$- activate the β- subtype of PtdIns-PLC (7,8,9).

cPLA$_2$ activation is regulated by free Ca^{2+}, GTP-binding proteins and phosphorylation by PKC and PTK culminating in the activation of the MAPK cascade and phosphorylation and activation of PLA$_2$ (1,7).

RESULTS AND DISCUSSION

NaF is a well known inhibitor of glycolysis (via inhibition of enolase), a major ATP providing route in phagocytes. In thioglycollate elicited mouse peritoneal macrophages (Tg-Mø; (1)) we found that NaF reduced cellular ATP in a time and dose dependent manner; 50% and 70 % reduction was observed after a 60 min incubation with 10 mM and 20 mM NaF, respectively. At 20 mM NaF, 50% reduction was achieved already at about 4 min. Tyrosine phosphorylation can be invoked in Tg-Mø by vanadate+zymosan, VOOH or vanadate+TPA (Fig. 1). Incubation of macrophages with NaF (or AlF$_4^-$) inhibits both in situ tyrosine phosphorylation (Fig. 1A&B) and the activation of PTK as assessed in cell lysates (Fig. 1C). NaF also inhibits up to 80 % of PTK activity when added to the assay system of PTK (which contains exogenous ATP) in cell lysates derived from Tg-Mø treated with the above stimuli. The phosphorylation of a partially purified insulin receptor was also shown to be inhibited by NaF and not to be due to the formation of complexes with aluminum (10). Thus *in situ* inhibition of tyrosine phosphorylation by NaF could stem from both reduction of cellular ATP and direct inhibition of PTK.

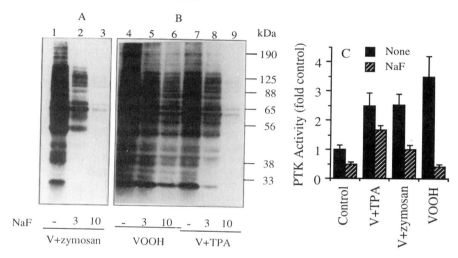

FIG. 1. Effect of NaF on *in situ* protein tyrosine phosphorylation (A & B) and PTK activation (C). (A)-Tg-Mø were incubated with or without 3 mM or 10 mM NaF as specified for 10 min. Vanadate (V, 0.25 mM), zymosan (500 µg/ml), VOOH (0.25 mM) or TPA (160 nM) were then added for additional 30 min of incubation as specified. The cells were lysed, SDS/PAGE (12 % gels) run, and the Western- blots analyzed as described (). Chemiluminescence from the blots treated sequentially with
rabbit anti-phosphotyrosine antibodies and protein A-horse radish peroxidase was recorded for 1 min (A) and 2 sec (B). (C)- Macrophages were treated as above (except for NaF, 20 mM, 30 min), cells were lysed and PTK activity assessed (1). Means of duplicate cultures±SD. None- incubation without NaF.

AlF$_4^-$ and/or NaF activate PtdIns-PLC in Tg-Mø in a dose (Fig. 2A) and time (not shown) dependent manner. Deferoxamine (DFO, a chelator of aluminum) partially inhibits (~ 30 %) the activation of PtdIns-PLC by either NaF or AlF$_4^-$. PKC has a negative regulatory role on PtdIns-PLC activity, since both an inhibitor of PKC (GF109203X) and PKC down regulation by an overnight incubation with TPA, enhance by 25% to 40% enzyme activity. The activation of

PtdIns-PLC is Ca^{2+} dependent; i.e. removal of exogenous Ca^{2+} by EGTA and chelation of internal Ca^{2+} by loading the cells with BAPTA/AM results in inhibition of *in situ* PtdIns-PLC activity (Fig. 2B).

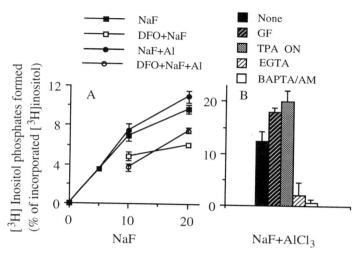

FIG. 2. *In situ* PtdIns-PLC activation by $NaF\pm AlCl_3$ and its sensitivity to deferoxamine (DFO) (A) and to modulation of PKC activity and $[Ca^{2+}]$ (B). (A)- Macrophages were incubated with or without 0.5 mM DFO for 30 min and then for additional 45 min with the specified concentrations of $NaF\pm 10$ μM $AlCl_3$. (B)- Macrophages were incubated with or without (None) the specified agents: GF109203X (GF, 10 μM); EGTA (3 mM) and BAPTA/AM (40 μM) for 30 min. TPA (160 nM, a 16 h treatment (ON)). AlF_4^- (20 mM NaF+10 μM $AlCl_3$) was then added for additional 45 min. The formed $[^3H]$inositol phosphates were assessed as described (2). Means of duplicate cultures±SD.

NaF activates MAPK and PLA₂ activities in Tg-Mø (Fig. 3 A&B). The activation of both enzymes was neither enhanced by addition of $AlCl_3$, nor was it prevented by the addition of DFO. A recent finding showed that NaF and AlF_4^- activate MAPK in BC_3H1 myocytes and in 3T3-L1 fibroblasts (5). It should be emphasized that MAPK is the final step in the cascade of protein kinases leading to activation of PLA_2.

NaF was shown to activate PtdIns-PLC, MAPK and PLA_2. Addition of 10 μM $AlCl_3$ did not lead to potentiation of the effectiveness of NaF. The lack of potentiation could stem in part from the fact that aluminum salts often contaminate solutions and tissue culture ware. To resolve this question we added DFO which indeed partially inhibited the activation of PtdIns-PLC, but did not prevent the activation of MAPK or PLA_2. This, could be interpreted as an indication that the activation of the latter enzymes stems from effects of NaF not related to G-protein activation, probably a result of its potent activity as a serine phosphatase inhibitor. Alternatively, it is possible that intracellular complex formation

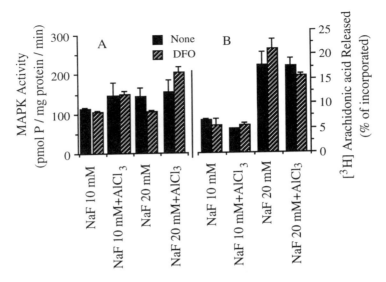

FIG. 3. Activation of MAPK and PLA$_2$ by NaF±AlCl$_3$ and its sensitivity to deferoxamine (DFO). Macrophages were incubated with 0.5 mM DFO or without (None) for 30 min and then for additional 30 min (A) or 60 min (B) with the specified concentrations of NaF ± 10 μM AlCl$_3$. Basal activity of MAPK was 33 pmol P/ mg protein / min. Basal activity of PLA$_2$ was 3.5 % and was subtracted from the results. Means of duplicate cultures±SD.

between fluoride and Mg^{2+} leads to activation of G-proteins in a manner analogous to that observed with Al^{3+} (11). This activation should not respond to DFO or added Al^{3+}. The apparent contradiction between reduction in cellular ATP and protein tyrosine phosphorylation and the activation of enzymes dependent on phosphorylation cascades, is of interest. Residual PTK activity and reduction in serine phosphatases may tilt the balance towards enzyme activation.

ACKNOWLEDGEMENTS

The study was partially supported by the German-Israel Foundation (GIF) for scientific research and development (Grant 1-156-040.0219)

REFERENCES

1. Zor U, Ferber E, Gergely P, Szücs K, Dombrádi V and Goldman R. Reactive oxygen species mediate phorbol ester-regulated tyrosine phosphorylation and phospholipase A$_2$ activation: potentiation by vanadate. *Biochem. J.* 1993; 295: 879-888.

2. Goldman R and Zor U. Activation of macrophage PtdIns-PLC by phorbol ester and vanadate: involvement of reactive oxygen species and tyrosine phosphorylation. *Biochem. Biophys. Res. Commun.* 1994; 199: 334-338.

3. Sternweis PC and Gilman AG. Aluminum: a requirement for activation of a regulatory component of adenylate cyclase by fluoride. *Proc. Natl. Acad. Sci. USA* 1982; 79: 4888-4891.

4. Chabre M. Aluminofluoride and beryllofluoride complexes: new phosphate analogs in enzymology. *TIBS*; 1990; 15: 6-10.

5. Anderson NG, Kilgour E and Sturgill TW. Activation of mitogen-activated protein kinase in BC$_3$H1 myocytes by fluoroaluminate. *J. Biol. Chem.* 1991; 266: 10131-10135.

6. Schulze-Specking A, Duyster J, Gebicke-Haerter PJ, Wurster S and Dieter P. Effect of fluoride, pertussis and cholera toxin on the release of arachidonic acid and the formation of prostaglandin E$_2$, D$_2$, superoxide and inositol phosphates in rat liver macrophages. *Cellular signalling* 1991; 3: 599-606.

7. Cockroft S. G-protein-regulated phospholipases C, D and A$_2$-mediated signalling in neutrophils. 1992; 1113: 135-160.

8. Fain JN. Regulation of phosphoinositide-specific phospholipase C. *Biochim. Biophys. Acta* 1990; 1053: 81-88

9. Cockroft S and Thomas GMH. Inositol-lipid-specific phospholipase C isoenzymes and their differential regulation by receptors. *Biochem. J.* 1992; 288: 1-14.

10. Viñals F, Testar X, Palacin M and Zorzano A. Inhibitory effect of fluoride on insulin receptor autophosphorylation and tyrosine kinase activity. *Biochem. J.* 1993;291: 615-622.

11. Antonny B, Sukumar M, Bigay J, Chabre M and Higashijima T. The mechanism of aluminum-independent G-protein activation by fluoride and magnesium. *J. Biol. Chem.* 1993; 268: 2393-2402.

Advances in Prostaglandin, Thromboxane,
and Leukotriene Research, Vol. 23,
edited by B. Samuelsson et al.
Raven Press, Ltd., New York © 1995

THE 3.1 Å X-RAY CRYSTAL STRUCTURE OF THE INTEGRAL MEMBRANE ENZYME PROSTAGLANDIN H₂ SYNTHASE-1

R. Michael Garavito, Daniel Picot, and Patrick J. Loll

Department of Biochemistry and Molecular Biology
The University of Chicago
920 E 58th Street
Chicago IL 60637 USA

The arachidonate cascade generates a number of important oxygenated derivatives of eicosanoids [1]. Major strides towards advancing our knowledge about the catalytic mechanisms involved in eicosanoid biosynthesis occurred with the recent X-ray crystal structure determinations of three major biosynthetic enzymes: soybean lipoxygenase [2], cyt-P450 BM [3] and prostaglandin H_2 synthase [4]. Prostaglandin H_2 synthase (PGHS; E.C. 1.14.99.1, MW 70 kDa/ subunit) is a membrane-bound enzyme that catalyzes the first step in the prostanoid pathway of the arachidonate cascade [5]. It is a bifunctional enzyme that converts arachidonic acid into prostaglandin G_2 (PGG_2) in the cyclooxygenase active site. The PGG_2 hydroperoxide product is then reduced in the second active site, the peroxidase, which yields the PGH_2.

In this preliminary report, we will focus on the cyclooxygenase (or COX) active site, the site of action of the nonsteroidal anti-inflammatory drugs (NSAIDs) [5]. The recent identification of a second inducible isoenzyme (PGHS-2) with slightly different properties regarding its inhibition [6,7] opens a new area in which drug-target interactions can be studied structurally. The spatial relationship of the COX active site with the enzyme's membrane-binding domain will also have mechanistic consequences for the binding of arachidonic acid.

STRUCTURE DETERMINATION

We have determined the crystal structure of the ovine isoform-1 enzyme co-crystallized with the NSAID flurbiprofen [4]. The phase determination was initially done at 3.5 Å resolution by multiple isomorphous replacement, using three heavy atom derivatives and the resulting atomic model was refined by simulating annealing [4]. The current stage of the resolution extension and structure refinement (simulated annealing implemented on the program XPLOR) is summarized in Table 1. The resolution has now been extended to 3.1 Å resolution and will be published elsewhere (D. Picot, P.J. Loll, and R. M. Garavito, manuscript in preparation).

Table 1: X-ray Refinement at 3.1 Å

Number of reflections	39540
Number of non-H atoms	2 x 4620 *
Free R factor	27.1 %
Rfactor	23.6
RMS distance	0.013 Å
RMS angle	1.74º

* Due to enforced strict non-crystallographic symmetry in the PGHS-1 dimer.

OVERALL FOLD

The asymmetric unit of the crystal contains a dimer, whose subunits are related by a non crystallographic twofold axis. The subunit structure is formed by three distinct folding units: an epidermal growth factor(EGF)-like module, a membrane-binding motif and an enzymatic domain (Figure 1).

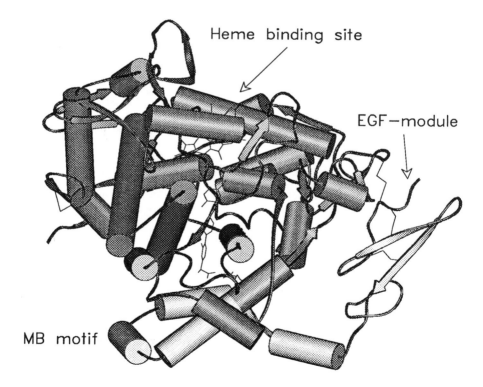

FIG. 1. A schematic of the PGHS-1 dimer showing the major features of the molecular including the membrane-binding (MB) motif.

EGF-like-module has a structure similar to the other known EGF hormones and EGF-like modules [8] and is localized in the dimer interface. Its C-terminus is directly connected with the membrane-binding motif, which it holds in place. It is further anchored to the catalytic domain by a disulfide bridge between Cys 37 and Cys 159.

The membrane-binding motif is formed by the amphiphilic α-helices A, B, C and the beginning of helix D. The helices A, B and C are roughly coplanar and form a unique monotopic membrane-binding motif (see below). In addition it forms also the entrance to the cyclooxygenase channel.

The catalytic domain contains the cyclooxygenase and the peroxidase activities as two spatially distinct active sites. The overall fold of the domain has a significant homology with myeloperoxidase, a mammalian peroxidase [4]. The core structure of PGHS-1 has also a similar topology to the other known structures of peroxidases, which suggests the existence of a super-family of peroxidases. The cyclooxygenase active site has therefore evolved within the existing fold of a peroxidase and not by the addition of an other domain.

THE COX CHANNEL

The cyclooxygenase active site is localized in a narrow channel that runs from the membrane-binding motif through an axis parallel to the molecular twofold. The helices from the membrane binding motif: B, C and D and to a lesser extend Helix A surround the lowest portion of the channel, and therefore offer a continuous path from the membrane to the active site. The channel is about 25 Å long, extending to the center of the enzyme, and is hydrophobic. The NSAID flurbiprofen binds in the upper portion of the channel next to Tyr 385 and Ser 530 (Figure 2).

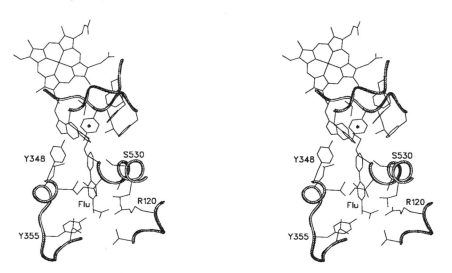

FIG. 2. A stereo view of the residues which form the cyclooxygenase active site and the hydrophobic channel. The putative radical acceptor Tyr 385 is denoted with an asterisk.

The upper portion of the cyclooxygenase channel is highlighted by residues that are in the vicinity (cutoff 4 Å) of Tyr 385, the residue which has been postulated to form a free radical during the catalytic mechanism [9,10]. Tyr 348 is the vicinity of Tyr 385 and the distance between the two hydroxyl oxygens is small (roughly 2.8 Å at the current stage of refinement), which raises the possibility of radical transfer and interaction between the two groups either as part of the catalytic mechanism or as part of the inactivation process. The other residues around Tyr 385 are Trp 387, Phe 205, Thr 206, Phe 209 and Phe 210. Ser 530 is near but at a larger distance (> 4 Å) from Tyr 385.

The middle portion of the cyclooxygenase channel is represented by the residues interacting with flurbiprofen (at a distance cutoff 4 Å). Arg 120 is in a good position to interact with the carboxylate group of flurbiprofen. Aspirin inhibits PGHS-1 by acetylation of Ser 530 by acetylation: Ser 530 is localized in a position compatible with the proposed mechanism of inhibition. All but one of the residues in this distance shell are conserved between PGHS-1 and PGHS-2. Ile 523, seen behind the flurbiprofen molecule in Figure 2, changes to Val. All the residues within a distance of 5 Å or less of Ser 530 are conserved between PGHS-1 and PGHS-2; this implies that the differences observed between these two isoenzymes either for the acetylated Ser 530 or for site-directed mutagenesis should have a quite subtle structural basis [11]. The following residues are seen on the middle portion of the COX channel surface: Val 349, Leu 352, Tyr 355, Leu 359, Met 522, Ile 523, Ala 527, Ser 530, Leu 531, Arg 120 and Val 116.

Reports have appeared [6,7] demonstrating that the PGHS isozymes can differ in their affinity towards NSAIDs, raising the possibility for designing ligands with high isozyme selectivity. From our current structure of the NSAID-inhibited holo-PGHS-1, we can not yet discern the structural basis for the observed differences in ligand binding between the isozymes. The sequence differences between ovine PGHS-1 and human PGHS-2 are minimal in the channel region. Thus, a crystal structure of PGHS-2 is necessary to understand better these phenomena.

THE INTERACTION WITH THE MEMBRANE

The x-ray crystal structure is incompatible with the enzyme models having a transmembrane domain, but rather strongly suggests that the protein is a monotopic and interacts with the membrane through the amphiphilic helices A, B, C and the amino terminal portion of helix D [12]. The three first helices are proposed to lie in a plane parallel to the plane of the membrane. The amino acid composition of the helices is in agreement with a face of the helices interacting directly with the hydrophobic core of the membrane. This is the first example of a monotopic membrane protein that is described structurally and demonstrates again that a membrane protein can interact in a far more complex way with a membrane than via a set of transmembrane helices. This implies that prediction of membrane-binding motif or transmembrane segment can be a quite daunting task [12]. The interaction with the membrane has two important consequences for the catalytic activity. First, the whole protein must be localized in the lumen and the potential physiological electron donors have to be found there. Second, the membrane-binding motif not only anchors the protein to the membrane but also offers a direct path from the membrane to the cyclooxygenase active site avoiding solvation and dessolvation of arachidonic acid. This should be taken into account in the kinetic analysis of the mechanism.

ACKNOWLEDGEMENTS

The work was supported by NIH Program Project grant HL30121. P. J. Loll was supported by a Damon Runyon-Walter Winchell Cancer Fund postdoctoral fellowship (DRG 1054). R. M. Garavito would like to acknowledge the support of the Martin D. and Virginia S. Kamen Sustaining Fund for Junior Faculty.

REFERENCES

1. Smith WL, Borgeat P, Fitzpatrick FA. The Eicosanoids: Cyclooxygenase, Lipoxygenase, and Epoxygenase Pathways. In:Vance DE, Vance J. *Biochemistry of Lipids, Lipoproteins and Membranes,*. Amsterdam: Elsevier; 1991:297-325.

2. Boyington JC, Gaffney BJ, Amzel LM. The Three-Dimensional Structure of an Arachidonic Acid 15-Lipoxygenase. *Science* 1993, **260**:1482-86.

3. Ravichandran KG, Boddupalli SS, Hasemann CA, Peterson JA, Deisenhofer J. Crystal Structure of Hemoprotein Domain of P450BM-3, a Prototype for Microsomal P450's. *Science* 1993, **261**: 731-36.

4. Picot D, Loll PJ, Garavito RM. The X-ray Crystal Structure of the Membrane Protein Prostaglandin H_2 Synthase-1. *Nature (London)* 1994, **367**:243-49.

5. Smith WL, Marnett LJ. Prostaglandin Endoperoxide Synthases. In:Sigal H, Sigel A. *Metal Ions in Biological Systems*. New York:Marcel Dekker, Inc.; 1994:163-99.

6. Meade EA, Smith WL, DeWitt DL. Differential Inhibition of Prostaglandin Endoperoxide Synthase (Cyclooxygenase) Isozymes by Aspirin and Other Non-steroidal Anti-inflammatory Drugs. *J Biol Chem* 1993, **268**:6610-14.

7. Mitchell JA, Akarasereenont P, Thiemermann C, Flower RJ, Vane JR. Selectivity of Nonsteroidal Antiinflammatory Drugs as Inhibitors of Constitutive and Inducible Cyclooxygenase. *Proc Natl Acad Sci USA* 1993, **90**:11693-97.

8. Campbell ID, Bork P. Epidermal Growth Factor-like Modules. *Curr Opin Struct Biol* 1993, **3**:385-92.

9. Karthein R, Dietz R, Nastainczyk W, Ruf HH. Higher Oxidation States of Prostaglandin H Synthase. An EPR Study of a Transient Tyrosyl Radical in the Enzyme During the Peroxidase Reaction. *Eur J Biochem* 1988, **171**:313-20.

10. Ruf HH, Raab-Brill U, Blau C. A Model for the Catalytic Mechanism of Prostaglandin Endoperoxide Synthase. *Biochem Soc Trans* 1993, **21**:739-44.

11. Lecomte M, Laneuville O, Ji C, DeWitt DL, Smith WL. *J Biol Chem* 1994, **269**:13207-15.

12. Picot D, Garavito RM. Prostaglandin H Synthase: Implications for Membrane Structure. *FEBS Lett* 1994, in press.

Advances in Prostaglandin, Thromboxane,
and Leukotriene Research, Vol. 23,
edited by B. Samuelsson et al.
Raven Press, Ltd., New York © 1995

Characterization of Human Prostaglandin H Synthase Genes

X-M Xu, A. Hajibeige, R. Tazawa,
D. Loose-Mitchell, L-H Wang and K.K. Wu.

Vascular Biology Research Center and Department of Medicine,
University of Texas Medical School, Houston, Texas 77030

Prostaglandin H synthase (PGHS) is a bifunctional enzyme which catalyzes the conversion of arachidonic acid (AA) to PGG_2 and PGG_2 to PGH_2. Two isoforms of PGHS have been identified. PGHS-1 is constitutively expressed in most mammalian tissues whereas PGHS-2 has a restricted tissue distribution and is expressed at a very low basal level but is highly inducible (1-5). Comparison of the sequence of these two isozymes reveals a high degree of homology and the conservation of heme ligand and catalytic active site (1). Despite the similarities in protein structure, the transcriptional regulation of these two isozymes is vastly different. Experimental data from murine, rat, rabbit and human cells provide strong evidence that PGHS-2 is highly inducible by mitogenic factors and cytokines (1-5). Inducibility of PGHS-1 is less clear and somewhat controversial. Our work with cultured endothelial cells indicate that PGHS-1 is stimulated by phorbol ester but the maximal stimulation is only 2-fold over the basal level. To understand the mechanism by which these two genes are differentially regulated, we have recently obtained human PGHS-1 and PGHS-2 genomic clones, determined the structure of these genes and characterized the 5'-flanking promoter structure and function.

Human PGHS-1 genomic DNA was cloned as described previously (6). This human genomic clone was 22 kb in length with a similar exon-intron structure as that reported previously (7). By primary extension and S1 nuclease mapping, multiple transcription start sites (TSS) were identified (6). Human PGHS-2 genomic clone was obtained by screening a bacteriophage P1 library using a 197-bp PCR fragment corresponding to the last exon of murine PGHS-2 genomic DNA (8). The structure of human PGHS-2 gene is similar to that of murine PGHS-2 gene. It is ~8 kb long with similar exon-intron

Promoters of PGHS genes

structure as that of mouse. A single TSS was identified. Analysis of the nucleotide sequence of the 2.4 kb 5'-flanking region shows several features: (1) no canonical TATA-box, (2) G & C rich and, (3) there are a number of regulatory elements, notably shear stress response element (SSRE). Comparison of the 5'-flanking sequence between human and murine PGHS-1 shows a high degree of sequencing identify in the 230-bp 5'-flanking region (6). By contrast, human PGHS-2 5'-flanking region contains a canonical TATA box and a cluster of regulatory elements including PEA3, C/EBP, GRE, MYB, MYC and ETS-1. Comparison of the 5'-flanking region among human, rat, chicken and murine PGHS-2 gene shows a high degree of homology. Hence, PGHS-2 5'-flanking region exhibits features of a primary response gene whereas PGHS-1 5'-flanking region exhibits features of a housekeeping gene.

To elucidate the mechanisms underlying the basal expression and the restrained stimulation of PGHS-1 gene, we prepared several restriction fragments from the 2.4-kb 5'-flanking region, linked them to luciferase reporter (luc) gene and expressed the chimeric plasmids in passage-2 HUVEC and NS-20 cells. We have also prepared a series of 5'-deletion and 3'-deletion mutants and expressed them in these cells. The AA metabolic pathway was similar between these two cells and expression patterns of these chimeric constructs were also similar except that the luciferase activity expressed in NS-20 cells was generally 7-10 fold higher than that expressed in HUVEC. As the NS20 cells can be more readily grown in sufficient numbers for transduction experiments, a majority of our transduction work was done in this cell. By restriction digestion and 5'-deletion, we identified the basal promoter to be located within the 113-bp of the transcription start site. We have also identified a distal promoter activity located between -593 and -428. This distal promoter is silenced by an adjacent repressor (-437, -106) and by the proximal promoter. In the absence of the proximal promoter, the activity from the distal promoter was about equivalent to that from the proximal promoter, indicating that the distal promoter may carry on basal expression when proximal promoter becomes defective. When p(MscI-PvuII)-Luc transfected NS-20 cells are treated with 50 nM of PMA for 16 h, the promoter activity was increased by 2-fold over the basal promoter activity. As (MscI-PvuII) construct extends beyond the major transcription start site and contains both promoter sites and the repressor, expression by this construct is considered to represent the overall 5'-promoter activity. Promoter stimulation by PMA, hence, matches the increase in PGHS-1 mRNA and protein levels stimulated by PMA. When the effects of PMA on several representative constructs were tested, the PMA stimulatory activity can be ascribed to its partial elimination of the repressor. These findings indicate that PGHS-1 expression is tightly controlled. Dual repression of the distal promoter ensures the restrained stimulation while providing a safeguard for constitutive expression of this housekeeping gene.

We have begun to evaluate the promoter activity of the 5'-flanking region of PGHS-2 gene. We obtained a 5'-flanking fragment, nucleotide -892 to +7, linked to the luc reporter gene and expressed in HUVEC by lipofection. The basal luciferase activity was very low but, upon stimulation with 50 nM of

Promoters of PGHS genes

PMA, the luciferase activity was increased by 5-fold.

These findings give some molecular clues to the differential promoter regulation of PGHS-1 and PGHS-2 genes. Further studies should provide important information regarding how these genes may be regulated by different transcription factors.

ACKNOWLEDGMENTS

The authors thank Teri Trevino for assistance in preparing the manuscript. This work is supported by grants from the National Institutes of Health P50 NS-23327, R01 HL-35387, HL-50675.

REFERENCES

1. Hla T, Neilson K. Human cyclooxygenase-2 cDNA. Proc Natl Acad Sci USA 1992;89:7384-88.
2. Jones DA, Carton DP, McIntyre TM, Zimmerman GA, Prescott SM. Molecular cloning of human prostaglandin endoperoxide synthase II and demonstration of expression in response to cytokines. J Biol Chem 1993;268:9049-54.
3. O'Sullivan MG, Chilton FH, Huggins EM, McCall CE. Lipopolysaccharide priming of alveolar macrophages for enhanced synthesis of prostanoids involves induction of a novel prostaglandin H synthase. J Biol Chem 1992;267:14547-50.
4. DeWitt DL, Meade EA. Serum and glucocortoid regulation of gene transcription and expression of prostaglandin H synthase-1 and -2 isozymes. Arch Biochem Biophys 1993;306:94-102.
5. O'Banion MK, Sadowski HB, Winn V, Young DA. A serum and glucocorticoid-regulated 4-kilobase mRNA encodes a cyclooxygenase related protein. J Biol Chem 1991;266:23261-7.
6. Wang L-H, Hajibeige A, Xu X-M, Loose-Mitchell D, Wu KK. Characterization of the promoter of human prostaglandin H synthase-1 gene. Biochem Biophys Res Comm 1993;406-11.
7. Yokoyama C, Tanabe T. Cloning of human gene encoding prostaglandin endoperoxide synthase and primary structure of the enzyme. Biochem Biophys Res Comm 1989;888-94.
8. Fletcher BS, Kujubu DA, Perrin DM, Herschman HR. Structure of the mitogen inducible TIS 10 gene and demonstration that the TIS 10-encoded protein is a functional prostaglandin G/H synthase. J Biol Chem 1992;267:4338-44.

Advances in Prostaglandin, Thromboxane,
and Leukotriene Research, Vol. 23,
edited by B. Samuelsson et al.
Raven Press, Ltd., New York © 1995

Structure and Expression of the Human Prostaglandin Endoperoxide Synthase 2 Gene

Hiroyasu Inoue, Tetsuya Kosaka, Atsuro Miyata, Shuntaro Hara, Chieko Yokoyama, Toyomichi Nanayama and Tadashi Tanabe

Department of Pharmacology, National Cardiovascular Center Research Institute, Suita, Osaka 565 Japan

Prostaglandin-endoperoxide synthase (PES) catalyzes the first committed step of the biosynthesis of prostaglandins and thromboxane as potent biological mediators. It is now evident that there exist two distinct isozymes for PES: a well-characterized and constitutive isozyme, designated PES-1 or cyclooxygenase-1; and a newly discovered and inducible isozyme, PES-2 or cyclooxygenase-2. Interestingly, the rapid induction of PES-2 mRNA was reported with inflammatory stimulants such as interleukin 1 and lipopolysaccharide. To investigate the contribution of PES-2 in inflammation it is important to elucidate the regulatory mechanism of PES-2 gene expression. As the initial step we have cloned and characterized the human PES-2 gene.[1, 2]

STRUCTURE OF HUMAN PES-2 GENE

The human PES-2 gene was isolated using a PCR generated cDNA fragment probe for human PES-2. Nucleotide sequence analysis of the entire human PES-2 gene demonstrated that it spans more than 8.3 kb and consists of 10 exons; this gene is very similar to the murine[3] and chicken[4] PES-2 genes. Human PES-1 gene has been isolated, characterized and shown to be approximately 22 kb in size and consist of 11 exons.[5] The structures of exons in the human PES-2 gene were also similar to those of the human PES-1 gene except the first and last exons. However, the sizes of introns in the human PES-2 gene were generally smaller than those of the human PES-1 gene. The human PES-2 gene possessed an AT-rich long 3'-flanking region containing 17 copies of the Shaw-Kamen's sequence (ATTTA) which are found in many proto-oncogenes and cytokines genes and have been shown to confer enhanced mRNA degradation.[6] Primer extension analysis with the RNA from differentiated U937 cells indicated the transcriptional start site is 134 bases

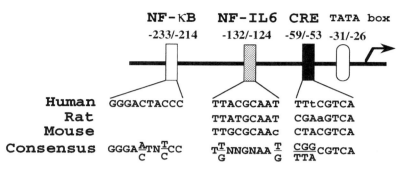

FIG. 1. Comparison of the proximal upstream regions of PES-2 genes. Lower case letters indicate different nucleotides from consensus sequences.

upstream of the translational initiation site. The nucleotide sequence of the 5'-flanking region of the human PES-2 gene contained a canonical TATA box and various transcriptional regulatory elements and showed no significant similarity to that of human PES-1 gene with no TATA box.[5] The nucleotide sequences of the human[1], mouse[3] and rat [7] PES-2 genes in their 5'-flanking regions share 60-63% similarities among the 275-bp nucleotide residues upstream of the transcriptional start site. As shown in Fig. 1, the sequences homologous to consensus NF-IL6 site and cyclic AMP response element (CRE) are conserved among them whereas the consensus sequence for NF-κB is found only in the human PES-2 gene. On the other hand, the upstream region of the chicken PES-2 gene[4] showed no significant similarity to that of the human PES-2 gene but contained both NF-κB site and CRE.

CRE AS A CIS-ACTING FACTOR IN HUMAN PES-2 GENE

The human monoblastoid U937 cells are differentiated into macrophage-like cells by incubation with TPA for 48 h. TPA-induced differentiation results in cessation of proliferation of cells and alterations in morphology from non-adherent cells to adherent cells. RNA blot analysis showed that human PES-2 mRNA was detected in differentiated U937 cells but not in undifferentiated U937 cells. To determine if the 5'-flanking region of the human PES-2 gene contains functional domains for its promoter, transient DNA transfection experiments using luciferase as a reporter in differentiated U937 cells were performed using deletion and site-specific mutants of the human PES-2 promoter (Fig. 2). The deletion or destruction of the CRE markedly reduced the promoter activity of this gene as shown with the expression vectors (-52/+59) and (CRM: -327/+59). These results suggested that the CRE (-59/-53) of the human PES-2 gene is essential for efficient transcription in differentiated U937 cells. To analyze trans-acting factors for CRE induced during monocytic differentiation of U937 cells, electrophoretic mobility shift assays were performed using the oligonucleotide coding for the CRE of the human PES-2 gene. These assays showed a nuclear binding protein(s) specific for CRE was induced during monocytic differentiation of U937 cells. These results suggested

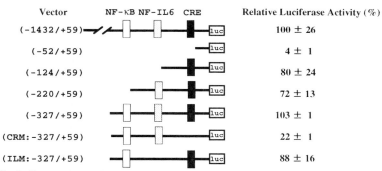

FIG. 2. Promoter activity of human PES-2 gene in TPA-differentiated U937 cells. Each construct was transfected by electroporation, together with pCMV-βgal used as the internal control of transfections. The relative luciferase activities of the constructs are expressed as percentages (means ± SD) of that of the reporter vector containing the DNA fragment -1432/+59.

that the CRE (-59/-53) plays an essential role in expression of the human PES-2 gene during differentiation of U937 cells.

REFERENCES

1. Kosaka T, Miyata A, Ihara H et al. Characterization of the human gene (PTGS2) encoding prostaglandin-endoperoxide synthase 2. *Eur J Biochem* 1994; in press.
2. Inoue H, Nanayama T, Hara S, Yokoyama C, Tanabe T. Cyclic AMP response element plays an essential role in expression of the human prostaglandin-endoperoxide synthase 2 gene in monocytic differentiated U937 cells. FEBS Lett 1994; in press.
3. Fletcher BS, Kujubu DA, Barnum BC, Lim RW, Herschman HR. Structure of the mitogen-inducible TIS10 gene and demonstration that the TIS-10 encoding protein is a functional prostaglandin G/H synthase. *J Biol Chem* 1992; 267:4338-44.
4. Xie W, Merrill JR, Bradshaw S, Simmons DL. Structural determination and promoter analysis of the chicken mitogen-inducible prostaglandin G/H synthase gene and genetic mapping of the murine homolog. *Arch Biochem Biophys* 1993;300:247-52.
5. Yokoyama C, Tanabe T. Cloning of human gene encoding prostaglandin endoperoxide synthase and primary structure of the enzyme. *Biochem Biophys Res Commun* 1989;165:888-94.
6. Sachs AB. Messenger RNA degradation in eukaryotes. *Cell* 1993;74:413-21.
7. Sirois J, Levy L, Simmons DL, Richards JS. Characterization and hormonal regulation of the promoter of the rat prostaglandin endoperoxide synthase 2 gene in granulosa cells. *J Biol Chem* 1993;268:12199-206.

Advances in Prostaglandin, Thromboxane, and Leukotriene Research, Vol. 23,
edited by B. Samuelsson et al.
Raven Press, Ltd., New York © 1995

EVALUATION OF PROSTAGLANDIN H SYNTHASE-1 MEMBRANE TOPOLOGY AND ENDOPLASMIC RETICULUM RETENTION SIGNALS

Y. Ren, K.-H. Ruan, C. Walker, and R.J. Kulmacz

Department of Internal Medicine, University of Texas Health Science Center at Houston, Houston, TX 77030 U.S.A.

Prostanoid synthesis involves the sequential actions of several enzymes, many of them membrane associated, on lipid substrates of varying polarity. The subcellular localization and orientation of these enzymes presumably influences their access to substrate, activators, and inhibitors. The enzyme catalyzing the first committed step in prostanoid synthesis, prostaglandin H synthase-1 (PGHS-1) has been localized to the endoplasmic reticulum (ER) membrane (1), and several models have been proposed for the arrangement of the PGHS-1 polypeptide in the ER membrane. The C-terminus of human PGHS-1 ends in the tetrapeptide -STEL, which is similar to the consensus sequence for the KDEL class of ER retention signals (2). We have examined the topology of PGHS-1 in the ER and the role of the C-terminus in targeting of the enzyme to the ER.

The topology of the PGHS-1 polypeptide with respect to the ER membrane was characterized by immunofluorescence microscopy using antibodies raised against several PGHS-1 peptide segments (see Table 1) or against the C3

TABLE 1: Peptide antigens used for preparation of site-specific antibodies.

Peptide	Residues
#1	25-35
#2	587-600
#3	377-390
#4	271-284
#5	483-496
#6	51-66
#7	156-170

poliovirus reporter epitope (3) inserted at the C-terminus of PGHS-1. Each peptide antigen produced antibodies which specifically recognized PGHS-1 on immunoblots of ovine seminal vesicle microsome proteins, except peptide #1, which appeared to be poorly immunogenic.

COS-1 cells expressing recombinant PGHS-1 or PGHS-1 with the C3 epitope inserted at the C-terminus were treated with streptolysin-O (SLO) to selectively permeabilize the plasma membrane (4) or with saponin for general permeabilization, before immunostaining with the antipeptide antibodies. Antibodies against peptides #2, #3, #4, #6, and #7 stained 9.4-11.4% of saponin-treated cells, reflecting consistent transfection efficiency and epitope availability. Antibodies against peptide #5 produced little staining even in saponin-treated cells, suggesting that this epitope becomes accessible only after PGHS-1 is extracted from the membrane. The two antibodies directed at the C-terminus (#2 and the C3 reporter epitope) stained 2.7 and 3.2%, and that targeted at the protease-sensitive R277 region (#4) stained 1.3% of the SLO-treated cells; antibodies for the #3, #6, and #7 peptides stained only 0.2-0.4% of these cells. Antibodies against protein disulfide isomerase (a marker for the ER lumen) stained only 0.3%, and FITC-labelled phalloidin (which binds cytosolic actin) stained 96.5% of the SLO-treated cells, confirming the selectivity of plasma membrane permeabilization by SLO.

The results indicate that the C-terminus and the R277 regions of PGHS-1 are accessible on the cytoplasmic side of the ER membrane in a significant fraction of cells expressing the recombinant enzyme. In all transfected cells the other peptides, which flank glycosylation sites and parts of the cyclooxygenase active site, are exposed to the ER lumen. One interpretation is that the recombinant PGHS-1 polypeptide adopts two arrangements in the ER: one with three transmembrane segments, and one with the entire polypeptide on the lumenal side of the ER membrane.

To evaluate C-terminus ER retention signals, cDNAs coding for PGHS-1 mutants with alterations designed to disrupt potential retention signals were used to transfect COS-1 cells. The mutations included: L600V to disrupt a KDEL-type signal; R595Q to disrupt signals based on positive charge; and deletion of the last six residues (Δ594). All three of the mutations resulted in expression of full-length recombinant protein as judged by immunoblotting, but only the R595Q mutant retained normal cyclooxygenase and peroxidase activities.

Double-label immunostaining with antibodies against PGHS-1 and protein disulfide isomerase produced essentially superimposable staining patterns for the two proteins in saponin-treated cells expressing wild type PGHS-1 and each of the C-terminal mutants. Thus, none of the C-terminal mutations tested altered the ER localization of PGHS-1. The results indicate that the C-terminus is important for functional integrity of PGHS-1, but it is not an essential part of its subcellular targeting mechanism.

ACKNOWLEDGMENTS

This work was supported in part by United States Public Health Service Grant GM 30509.

REFERENCES

1. Smith, W.L., DeWitt, D.L., and Allen, M.L. Bimodal distribution of the prostaglandin I_2 synthase antigen in smooth muscle cells. *J Biol Chem* 1983; 258:5922-5926.
2. Pelham, H.R.B. Control of protein exit from the endoplasmic reticulum. *Annu Rev Cell Biol* 1989; 5:1-24.
3. van der Werf, S., Charbit, A., Leclerc, C., et al. Critical role of neighbouring sequences on the immunogenicity of the C3 poliovirus neutralization epitope expressed at the surface of recombinant bacteria. *Vaccine* 1990; 8:269-277.
4. Bahkdi, S, and Tranum-Jensen. Damage to mammalian cells by proteins that form transmembrane pores. *Rev Physiol Pharmacol* 1987; 107:147-223.

Advances in Prostaglandin, Thromboxane,
and Leukotriene Research, Vol. 23,
edited by B. Samuelsson et al.
Raven Press, Ltd., New York © 1995

ENDOTHELIN REGULATES PGE$_2$ FORMATION IN RAT MESANGIAL CELLS THROUGH INDUCTION OF PROSTAGLANDIN ENDOPEROXIDE SYNTHASE-2

Emmanouel Coroneos, Mark Kester, Patrick Thomas and Michael J. Dunn
Departments of Medicine and Physiology/Biophysics
Case Western Reserve University, School of Medicine, Cleveland, Ohio 44106

Abstract   Endothelin-1 stimulates vascular smooth muscle and mesangial cells to release prostaglandin E$_2$ which attenuates the vasoconstrictor and mitogenic effects of endothelin. The role of endothelin-1 to regulate prostaglandin endoperoxide synthase (PGHS)-1 and -2 gene expression and protein synthesis was evaluated in cultured mesangial cells. Endothelin induced mRNA and protein expression for PGHS-2 but not for PGHS-1. A direct correlation was observed between the mass of immunoprecipitated PGHS protein and PGE$_2$ synthetic enzymatic activity.

Introduction   Endothelins (ET) are vasoactive and proliferative peptides that have well characterized actions upon glomerular mesangial cells (MC) (1). One of the important signaling cascades induced by ET-receptor activation in MC results in the formation of PGE$_2$, an autocoid linked to the attenuation of ET-stimulated contractility and mitogenesis. PGE$_2$ formation is the result of three sequential enzymatic activities; phospholipase A$_2$ (PLA$_2$), prostaglandin endoperoxide synthase (PGHS) and PGE$_2$ synthase (2). Recent studies have characterized and cloned two discrete PGHS gene products (2-4). PGHS-1 is constitutively expressed in most cell types in contrast to PGHS-2 which only expressed after stimulation by various growth factors and cytokines (5,6). We have previously reported that MC constitutively express PGHS-1 which can be regulated by serum through a protein kinase C (PKC)-dependent mechanism (7). In the present study, we investigate the mechanisms by which ET differentially regulates transcription and translation of PGHS-1 and PGHS-2 in MC.

Materials and Methods   ET-1 was purchased from Peptide Institude (Tokyo, Japan). Plasmids containing full length 2.8-kb and 4.2-kb of PGHS-1 and PGHS-2 cDNA inserts were kindly provided by Dr. Harvey Hershman (Los Angeles, CA). Purified bioactive preparations of PGHS-1 and PGHS-2 were purchased from Cayman Chemicals (Oxford, MI). Rabbit polyclonal anti-PGHS-1 and anti-PGHS-2 antisera were a generous gift from Dr. Jacques Maclouf (Paris). For the present experiments, cultured mesangial cells at 80% confluence were rendered quiescent (G$_0$) by holding them for 2 days in supplemented serum-free RPMI.

Analysis of PGHS mRNA and protein   Total cellular RNA was isolated and assessed by Northern blot analysis. PGHS-1 and PGHS-2 nick-translated hybridization signals were quantified by scanning densintometry . Western immunoblotting, using polyclonal antibodies to PGHS-1 and PGHS-2, was performed according to the methods of Habib et al. (8). Immunoprecipitation was done by using anti-PGHS-1 and anti-PGHS-2 antibodies bound to protein-A sepharose beads.

Assessment of PGHS Enzyme Activity   Immunoprecipitated PGHS-1 and PGHS-2 were asssyed for cyclooxygenase activity by measuring conversion of exogenous arachidonic acid to PGE$_2$ (8). RIA was used to quantify production of PGE$_2$ in the incubation mixture.

RESULTS   We have characterized and correlated the role of ET-1 to regulate PGHS-1 and PGHS-2 mRNA expression, protein formation and bioactivity in MC. MC were stimulated with 0.1 mM ET-1 for various times and PGHS-1 and PGHS-2 mRNA expression and protein formation were analyzed (Fig. 1). PGHS-2 mRNA expression, which was undetectable under basal conditions, was increased after 1 h, peaked at the second hour and returned to basal levels at the fourth hour. No further PGHS-2 induction was detected for up to 24 h of stimulation. In contrast, PGHS-1 mRNA was constitutively expressed in quiescent MC and was not augmented

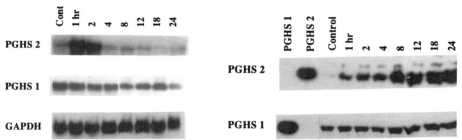

Fig. 1   *The effects of ET-1 , 0.1 uM,, upon PGHS-1 and PGHS-2 mRNA expression and protein formation : A) Northern blot analysis of 1 of 3 rexperiments B) Western blot analysis of 1 of 3 rexperiments using polyclonal anti-PGHS-1 and anti-PGHS-2 antibodies. On lane 1, PGHS-1 purified from sheep seminal vesicles and on lane 2, PGHS-2 isolated from sheep placenta were run as controls.*

with 0.1 mM ET-1 stimulation at any time point. We next correlated ET-1 stimulated protein expression and mRNA induction for PGHS-2. We observed that ET-1 induced PGHS-2 protein synthesis by the first hour of stimulation and this elevation was evident for up to 24 h compared to quiescent cells. PGHS-2 protein was still elevated at time points where PGHS-2 mRNA expression had returned to the basal levels. In contrast, ET-1 did not induce PGHS-1 protein synthesis above control levels at time points before 18 h. We also evaluated if the immunoprecipitated PGHS-1 and PGHS-2 proteins had enzymatic activity in vitro. We immunoprecipitated PGHS-1 and PGHS-2 and then exposed the immunoprecipitates to 50 mM AA and assessed PGE2 formation by RIA. Any increase in measured PGE_2 during the ET treatment was assumed to originate from increased formation of PGHS-1 or PGHS-2 protein followed by non-enzymatic conversion of resulting PGH_2 to PGE_2. Enzymatic activity of the immunoprecipitated PGHS-1 and PGHS-2 exhibited a time course parallel to the formation of PGHS-1 and PGHS-2 proteins as revealed by Western analysis (Fig. 2). In data not shown, actinomycin suppressed ET stimulated PGHS-2 but not PGHS-1 mRNA expression and protein

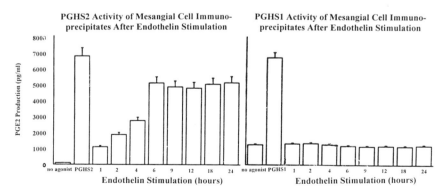

Fig. 2   *Correlation of the effects of ET-1 upon immunoprecipitated PGHS-1 and PGHS-2 protein formation and bioactivity. A time course of PGHS-1 and PGHS-2 enzymatic activity immunoprecipitated from ET-1 stimulated MC lysates is presented. PGHS-1 and PGHS-2 were immunoprecipitated from cell lysates (100 mg of protein) with specific polyclonal anti-PGHS-1 and anti-PGHS-2 antibodies and subsequently the enzymatic activity was assessed .*

synthesis. Cycloheximide prevented ET stimulated PGHS-2 protein synthesis but augmented both basal and ET stimulated PGHS-2 mRNA expression. Also, both dexamethasone and heparin suppressed ET induced PGHS-2 mRNA expression and protein formation.

Discussion   We have made parallel evaluations of PGHS-1 and PGHS-2 mRNA expression, protein formation and bioactivity in MC. ET-induced PGHS-2 mRNA expression but did not regulate PGHS-1 mRNA expression in MC. These results add GTP-binding protein-coupled receptors to the growing list of cytokine- (5,9), growth factor-(3,10) and gonadotropin-activated receptors (11) that upregulate PGHS-2 expression. ET-induced mRNA expression for PGHS-2 resembles the time course for an early-response gene. ET-induced PGHS-2 protein formation was still elevated at time points after which mRNA expression had returned to basal levels. PGHS-2 protein formation as assessed by Western analyses corresponded to bioactivity of the immunoprecipitated protein. These results suggest that newly synthesized MC PGHS-2 is biologically active and relatively stable. Moreover, we suggest that ET-induced release of PGE$_2$ from MC is predominantly a result of PGHS-2 and not PGHS-1 expression. These studies support earlier findings (1) that describe a role for released PGE$_2$ to serve as an autocrine negative regulator for inflammatory and mitogenic stimuli. ET may regulate PGHS-2 through both transcriptional and translational controls as actinomycin-D and cycloheximide reduced ET-stimulated mRNA expression and protein formation, respectively. Moreover, cycloheximide treatment reduced ET-stimulated PGHS-2 protein expression while potentiating mRNA levels, suggesting superinducibility of message, an observation previously reported in serum-treated fibroblasts (12). The apparent stability of the ET-induced PGHS-2 protein may reflect novel post-translational mechanisms. Also,we have confirmed studies that demonstrate that dexamethasone inhibits transcription and/or translation of IL-1, LPS or serum-stimulated PGHS-2 (12,13).   In addition to dexamethasone, we have demonstrated that heparin also reduces ET-stimulated PGHS-2 but not PGHS-1 mRNA expression and protein formation. It is reasonable to speculate that the anti-inflammatory and salutary effects of heparin in diverse models of inflammation including renal immunological injury (14) may be related to the capacity of heparin to transcriptionally regulate agonist-inducible PGHS-2, reducing the concentration of inflammatory and mitogenic eicosanoids.

References
1.   Simonson M. S. and Dunn M. J. (1993) Annu. Rev. Physiol. 55:249-265.
2.   Smith W. L. (1992) Am. J. Physiol. 263: F 181-F191.
3.   Kujubu, D. A. et al. (1991) J. Biol. Chem. 266:12866-12872.
4.   Xie W., Chipman J. G., Robertson D. L., Erikson R. L. and Simmons D. L. (1991) Proc. Natl. Acad. Sci. USA. 88:2692-2696.
5.   Baird N. R. and Morrison A. R. (1993) Am J. Kidney Dis. 21:557-564.
6.   Fletcher B. S., Kujubu D. A., Perrin D. M. and Herschman H. R. (1992) J. Biol. Chem. 267:4338-4344.
7.   Simonson M. S., Wolfe J. A., Konieczkowski M., Sedor J. R. and Dunn M. J. (1991) Molec. Endocrin. 5:441-451.
8.   Habib A., Creminon C., Frobert Y., Grassi J., Pradelles P. and Maclouf J. (1993) J. Biol. Chem. 268:23448-23454.
9.   Martin M. et al. (1994) Kid. Int. 45:150-158.
10.   Lin A. H., Bienkowski M. J. and Gorman R. R. (1989) J. Biol. Chem. 264:17379-17383.
11:   Sirois J., Levy L. O., Simmons D. L. and Richards J. S. (1993) J. Biol. Chem. 268:12199-12206.
12.   O'Banion M. K., Sadowski H. B., Winn V. and Young D. A. (1991) J. Biol. Chem. 266:23261-23267.
13.   O'Sullivan M. G., Huggins, Jr. E. M. and McCall C. E. (1993) Biochem. Biophys. Res. Commun. 191:1294-1300.
14.   Striker L. J., Peten E. P., Elliot S. J., Dol T. and Striker G. E. (1991) Lab. Invest. 64:446-456.

Advances in Prostaglandin, Thromboxane,
and Leukotriene Research, Vol. 23,
edited by B. Samuelsson et al.
Raven Press, Ltd., New York © 1995

Molecular Cloning and Expression of Prostacyclin Synthase from Endothelial Cells

Shuntaro Hara [a], Atsuro Miyata [a], Chieko Yokoyama [a],
Roland Brugger [b], Friedrich Lottspeich [c],
Volker Ullrich [b] and Tadashi Tanabe [a]

[a]*Department of Pharmacology, National Cardiovascular Center Research Institute,*
Suita, Osaka 565, Japan,
[b]*Department of Biology, University of Konstanz, Konstanz, Germany, and*
[c]*Max-Planck-Institute for Biochemistry, Genzentrum, Martinsried, Germany*

Prostacyclin synthase (PGIS) catalyzes the conversion of prostaglandin H_2 to prostacyclin, which is a powerful vasodilator and the most potent natural occurring inhibitor of platelet aggregation and counteracts the effects of platelet-derived thromboxane A_2. It has been postulated that an imbalance of prostacyclin and thromboxane A_2 causes several diseases such as myocardial infarction, stroke and atherosclerosis.[1] PGIS has been purified from porcine [2] and bovine aorta,[3] and it was reported that the molecular weight of the purified enzyme is 52 kDa, and that its spectral characteristics suggested that the enzyme is a hemoprotein of cytochrome P450 type. To better understand the primary structure and regulatory mechanism of the enzyme, we cloned the cDNA for the enzyme and deduced its primary structure.[4,5] Furthermore, it was found that several cytokines appears to regulate the gene expression of PGIS.

MOLECULAR CLONING AND EXPRESSION OF cDNA FOR BOVINE ENDOTHELIAL PROSTACYCLIN SYNTHASE

PGIS was purified and characterized from bovine aorta microsomes and the partial amino acid sequences were determined with the native enzyme and Lys-C-cleaved peptides. Using primers synthesized according to the amino acid sequences, cDNA coding for PGIS was amplified by polymerase chain reaction (PCR) with bovine aortic endothelial cell (BAEC) poly(A)+ RNA and cloned into

	-7	-3	0	+3	+6	+9	+13
bovine PGIS	WGA GHN QCL GKG YAVNS I KQF					
human PGIS	WGA GHN HCL GRS YAVNS I KQF					
human TXS	F GAGPR SCL GVRLGL LEVK LT					
human CYP1A1	F GMGKR KC I GET I ARWE VF LF					
human CYP2E1	F ST GKR VCAGEGL ARMEL FLL					
rabbit CYP4A4	F SGGARNC I GKQF AMREL KVA					
human CYP4F3	F SAGPRNC I GQA F AM AEMKVV					
human CYP7A	F GSGAT I CPGRL FA I HE I KQF					
human CYP19A1	F GF GPRGCAGKY I AM VMMK A I					

FIG. 1. Comparison of possible heme-binding peptide sequences around the active site cysteine in PGIS and several cytochrome P-450s.[9] Residues identical with those of bovine and human PGIS are indicated with shaded letters.

pBluescript.[4] The cloned cDNA inserts covered a 2206 bp sequence, which included a 1500-bp open reading frame coding for a 500-amino acid polypeptide with a molecular weight of 56,628.

The incubation of prostaglandin H_2 with microsomes prepared from the COS-7 cells transfected an expression plasmid harboring the PGIS cDNA clone formed 6-keto-prostaglandin $F_{1\alpha}$.[4] This result clearly demonstrated that our isolated cDNA encodes a functional PGIS.

PRIMARY STRUCTURES OF PROSTACYCLIN SYNTHASE

The deduced amino acid sequence of PGIS showed structural characteristics of cytochrome P450 superfamily. The highly conserved cysteine-containing sequence involved in the heme-binding site of P450[6] was found near the carboxy terminus of the enzyme (Fig. 1).[4] It is noteworthy that phenylalanine (7 amino acids amino terminus-side from the cysteine), which is conserved among all the sequenced mammalian P450s, is replaced by tryptophan (amino acid residue 434). Very recently, we have succeeded in cDNA cloning of human endothelial PGIS.[5] The tryptophan residue was conserved in the human enzyme, although the identity of the amino acid sequences between human and bovine enzyme was 88% over the entire region. The results of the homology search demonstrated that human cholesterol 7α-hydroxylase (CYP7A)[7] showed the highest identity with human and bovine PGIS (34 and 31%, respectively). However, the identity between the amino acid sequences of PGIS and thromboxane synthase (TXS)[8] was only 15-16%, and no P450 showed an identity higher than 40%, suggesting that PGIS represents a new family in the P450 superfamily.

INDUCTION OF PROSTACYCLIN SYNTHASE mRNA IN ENDOTHELIAL CELLS BY SEVERAL CYTOKINES

RNA blot analysis indicated that the mRNA for PGIS from BAEC showed a size of approximately 2.7 kb.[4] We further examined the effects of several cytokines (interleukin (IL)-1α, IL-1β, IL-6, tumour necrosis factor (TNF)-α and

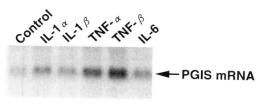

← PGIS mRNA

FIG. 2. Induction of PGIS mRNAs in endothelial cells by several cytokines. Total RNAs (20 μg) from BAEC treated with several cytokines for 24 h were analyzed.

TNF-β) on the induction of PGIS mRNA in BAEC, as the previous studies reported that several cytokines increased the production of prostacyclin.[10] All of these cytokines increased PGIS mRNA in BAEC (Fig. 2). TNF-α and TNF-β were the most potent cytokines to enhance the gene expression of PGIS, and the mRNA level increased about 3 fold and reached a plateau for about 4 h after the treatment of TNF-α.

REFERENCES

1. Moncada S, Vane JR. Arachidonic acid metabolites and the interactions between platelets and blood-vessel walls. *N Engl J Med* 1979;300:1142-7.
2. Graf H, Ullrich V. Prostacyclin synthase as a cytochrome P450 enzyme. In:Hietanen E, Laitinen M, Hänninen O. *Developmental Biochemistry, Vol. 23, Cytochrome P-450. Biochemistry, Biophysics and Environmental Implications.* Amsterdam: Elsevier Biomedical Press; 1982:103-6.
3. DeWitt DL, Smith WL. Purification of prostacyclin synthase from bovine aorta by immunoaffinity chromatography. Evidence that the enzyme is a hemoprotein. *J Biol Chem* 1983;258:3285-93.
4. Hara S, Miyata A, Yokoyama C et al. Isolation and molecular cloning of prostacyclin synthase from bovine endothelial cells. *J Biol Chem* 1994;in press.
5. Miyata A, Hara S, Yokoyama C, Inoue H, Ullrich V, Tanabe T. Molecular cloning and expression of human prostacyclin synthase. *Biochem Biophys Res Commun* 1994;in press
6. Nebert DW, Gonzalez FJ. P450 genes: structure, evolution, and regulation. *Ann Rev Biochem* 1987;56:945-93.
7. Noshiro M, Okuda, K. Molecular cloning and sequence analysis of cDNA encoding human cholesterol 7α-hydroxylase. *FEBS Lett* 1990;268:137-40
8. Yokoyama C, Miyata A, Ihara H, Ullrich V, Tanabe T. Molecular cloning of human platelet thromboxane A synthase. *Biochem Biophys Res Commun* 1991;178:1479-84.
9. Nelson DR, Kamataki T, Waxman DJ et al. The P450 superfamily: update on new sequences, gene mapping, accession numbers, early trivial names of enzymes, and nomenclature. *DNA Cell Biol* 1993;12:1-51.
10. Ristimäki A, Viinikka L. Modulation of prostacyclin production by cytokines in vascular endothelial cells. *Prostaglandins Leukot Essent Fatty Acids* 1992;47:93-9.

Advances in Prostaglandin, Thromboxane,
and Leukotriene Research, Vol. 23,
edited by B. Samuelsson et al.
Raven Press, Ltd., New York © 1995

Expression and Selective Inhibition of Constitutive and Inducible Forms of Cyclooxygenase

Karen Seibert, Jaime Masferrer, Yan Zhang, Kathleen Leahy,
Scott Hauser, James Gierse, Carol Koboldt, Gary Anderson,
Margaret Bremer, Susan Gregory, and Peter Isakson.
G.D. Searle, Monsanto Company, 800 N. Lindbergh,
St. Louis, Missouri 63167, U.S.A.

Non-steroidal anti-inflammatory drugs (NSAIDs) are widely used in the treatment of a number of inflammatory diseases and are believed to act via inhibition of the enzyme cyclooxygenase (COX). Commercially available NSAIDs are efficacious anti-inflammatory agents, but significant incidence of gastric side effects limit their use. The recent identification of two forms of COX - a constitutively expressed COX-1 and a cytokine-inducible COX-2 has led to the hypothesis that the gastric toxicities associated with NSAID therapy are due to inhibition of the non-regulated or constitutive form of COX (COX-1), whereas therapeutic benefit derives from inhibition of the inducible enzyme, COX-2. We have examined the relative distribution of COX-1 and COX-2 in both normal and inflamed tissues and report that COX-1 expression dominates normal tissues while COX-2 mRNA is induced at the inflammatory site. Furthermore, compounds that selectively inhibit COX-2 are anti-inflammatory without gastric toxicity.

Distribution of COX-1 and COX-2 in Normal and Inflamed Tissue

Prostaglandins are formed via the activity of the prostaglandin synthase or "cyclooxygenase" (COX) - present constitutively in most cells (for review see ref. 1). We have reported in a number of cell types and tissues, both *in vitro* and *in vivo*, that COX is induced following incubation with cytokines, growth factors, or endotoxin, a process that required new protein synthesis (2,3). The induction of *de novo* COX is inhibited by anti-inflammatory glucocorticoids, such as dexamethasone, (4-6). We hypothesized that there is an inducible form of the COX enzyme that differs from the constitutive enzyme originally cloned from sheep seminal vesicle (7-9); this "inducible" enzyme is selectively induced by cytokines and inhibited by antiinflammatory glucocorticoids. The hypothesis of a second cyclooxygenase gene was supported by the isolation of a second COX gene whose expression can induced by a number of inflammatory cytokines and whose mRNA expression is selectively blocked by dexamethasone (10-17).

We examined the distribution of COX-1 and COX-2 in normal rodent tissues by quantitative analysis of mRNA. In all tissues examined there was detectable mRNA for COX-1 including brain, liver, lung, spleen, kidney, stomach, and other tissues of the gastrointestinal tract. In particular we detected a significant amount of constitutive COX-1 mRNA in the renal medulla, consistent with the known abundant production of PGE2 in that tissue.   Virtually no mRNA encoding COX-2 was detectable, with the exception of normal rat brain, where a significant amount of mRNA was observed.

Non-steroidal anti-inflammatory drugs (NSAIDs) are antiinflammatory in a number of animal models. We evaluated the role of COX-2 expression in a rodent model of edema induced by injection of carrageenan into the footpad of the mouse. Following the administration of carrageenan to the footpad, there is a significant induction of edema over time that corresponds to the production of pro-inflammatory thromboxane (TxB2) extractable from the paw tissue, with TxB2 production and swelling both maximal at three hours. Quantitative analysis of mRNA by RNase protection from these paws showed that maximal induction of COX-2 mRNA was at three hours, coinciding with the maximal effect on edema and thromboxane production.

Pharmacology of a selective COX-2 inhibitor

The abundance of COX-2 at the inflammatory site provides impetus to generate selective non-steroidal anti-inflammatory drugs (NSAIDs) which could potentially provide useful improvement therapeutically in the treatment of chronic inflammatory disease via reduced mechanism-based side effects. Constitutive and inducible forms of human cyclooxygenase (hCOX-1 and hCOX-2) were cloned and expressed in insect cells utilizing a baculovirus expression system. COX-1 had a specific activity of 18.8 μmoles O_2/mg with a Km of 13.8 uM for arachidonate and Vmax of 1,500 nmoles O_2/nmole enzyme, while COX-2 had a specific activity of 12.2 μmoles O_2/mg with a Km of 8.7 μM for arachidonate and a Vmax of 1,090 nmoles O_2/ nmole enzyme.   Indomethacin and other commercially available NSAIDs inhibited both COX-1 and COX-2 while a Searle compound, SC-58125, potently and selectively inhibited the COX-2 enzyme (Table 1).

Table 1: Selective Pharmacology of NSAIDs *in vitro*

IC50 (uM)	H-COX1	H-COX2
Indomethacin	0.1	0.9
Flurbiprofen	0.1	0.4
Naproxen	1.1	36.
Diclofenac	.04	0.1
SC-58125	>100	.05

NSAIDs (.001-100uM) were preincubated with membranes containing COX-1 or COX-2   prior to the addition of arachidonic acid (10uM) for 10 min. COX activity was measured as PGE2 formed/min/mg protein.

The *in vivo* anti-inflammatory and analgesic properties of a non-selective NSAID, indomethacin, was evaluated against the COX-2 selective agent, SC-58125 (Table 2). Both indomethacin and SC-58125 were anti-inflammatory and analgesic in an acute model of inflammation (carrageenan-induced paw edema). Likewise, in a chronic model of adjuvant -induced arthritis, both indomethacin and SC-58125 potently inhibited swelling in a dose-dependent manner. The difference between the compounds rested in their relative GI toxicity where indomethacin caused gastric lesions in half the animals tested at 8mg/kg, while there was no demonstrable GI toxicity in animals treated with SC-58125 at doses up to 600 mg/kg.

Table 2: *In vivo* Pharmacology of COX Inhibitors

	ED50 (mg/kg, p.o.)		
	Analgesia	Arthritis	GI Toxicity
Indomethacin	2.0	0.1	8.0
SC-58125	10.	0.4	>600

In conclusion, normal tissue is dominated by expression of constitutive COX-1 while COX-2 is abundant at the site of inflammation. A selective inhibitor of COX-2 *in vitro* is anti-inflammatory *in vivo* without causing gastric lesions while non-selective commercial NSAIDs like indomethacin are both potent anti-inflammatory agents and ulcerogenic. Development of selective inhibitors of COX-2 that spare gastric PG production may represent a significant advance for the treatment of acute and chronic inflammatory disorders.

References

1. DeWitt, D. (1991) Biochim. Biophys. Acta. 1083: 121-134.
2. Raz, A., Wyche, A., Siegel, N., and Needleman, P. (1988). J. Biol. Chem.   263: 3022-3028.
3. Fu, J., Masferrer, J.L., Seibert, K., Raz, A., and Needleman, P. (1990) J. Biol. Chem., 265: 16737-16740.
4. Raz, A., Wyche, A., and Needleman, P. (1989) Proc. Natl. Acad. Sci., USA. 86: 1657-1661.
5. Masferrer, J.L., Seibert, K., Zweifel, B.S., and Needleman, P. (1992) Proc. Natl. Acad. Sci., USA 89: 3917-3921.
6. Masferrer, J.L., Zweifel, B.S., Seibert, K., and Needleman, P. (1990) J. Clin. Invest. 86: 1375-1379.
7. Merlie, J.P., Fagan, D., Mudd, J. and Needleman, P. (1988) J. Biol. Chem. 263, 3550-3553.
8. DeWitt, D.L. and Smith, W.L. (1988) Proc. Natl. Acad. Sci. USA 85, 1412-1416.
9. Yokoyama, C., Takai, T. and Tanabe, T. (1988) FEBS Lett/ 231. 347-351.
10. Xie, W., Chipman, J.G., Robertson, D.L., Erikson, R.L., and Simmons, D.L. (1991) Proc. Natl. Acad. Sci. USA 88: 2692-2696.
11. Kujubu, D.A., Fletcher, B.S., Varnum, B.C., Lim, R.W., and Herschman, H.R. (1991) J. Biol. Chem. 266: 12866-12872.
12. O'Banion, M.K., Sadowski, H.B., Winn, V., and Young, D.A. (1991) J. Biol. Chem. 266: 23261-23267.
13. Fletcher, B.S., Kujubu, D.A., Perrin, D.M., and Herschman, H.R. (1992) J. Biol. Chem. 267: 4338:4344.
14. Sirois, J., and Richards, J.S. (1992) J. Biol. Chem. 267: 6382-6388.
15. Kujubu, D.A., and Herschman, H.R. (1992) J. Biol. Chem. 267, 7991-7994.
16. O'Banion, M.K., Winn, V., and Young, D.A. (1992) Proc. Natl. Acad. Scit. USA 89: 4888-4892.
17. Kujubu, D.A., Reddy, S.T., Fletcher, B.S., and Herschman, H. (1993) J. Biol. Chem. 268: 5425-5430.

Advances in Prostaglandin, Thromboxane, and Leukotriene Research, Vol. 23,
edited by B. Samuelsson et al.
Raven Press, Ltd., New York © 1995

Characterization of the cyclooxygenase activity of human blood prostaglandin endoperoxide synthases

P. Patrignani, M.R. Panara, A. Greco, O. Fusco*, C. Natoli*, S. Iacobelli*, F. Cipollone, A. Ganci, C. Créminon#, J. Maclouf+, and C. Patrono

*Division of Clinical Pharmacology and *Oncology, University of Chieti "G. D'Annunzio" School of Medicine, 66013 Chieti, Italy, #Service de Pharmacologie et d'Immunologie, CE Saclay, 91191 Gif-sur-Yvette Cedex and +I.F.R. Biologie de la Circulation-Lariboisière, Institut National de la Santé et de la Recherche Médicale, Unité 348, Hopital Lariboisière, 75475 Paris, France*

Mammalian cells contain two related, but unique, isoforms of prostaglandin(PG) H synthase referred to as PGHS-1 and PGHS-2 (1). PGHS-1, constitutively expressed in most tissues and in blood monocytes and platelets, is likely involved in "housekeeping" prostanoid biosynthesis (1).

PGHS-2 expression is induced by serum, growth factors, phorbol esters and cytokines in fibroblasts and vascular smooth muscle and endothelial cells and by lipopolysaccharide (LPS) in monocytes/macrophages (2). Thus, prostanoid biosynthesis by the activity of PGHS-2 can mediate inflammation and mitogenesis.

Meade *et al.*(3), have recently demonstrated that murine PGHS-1 and PGHS-2 expressed in cos-1 cells are differentially sensitive to inhibition by common nonsteroidal anti-inflammatory drugs (NSAID)s.

Thus, the aim of our study was to characterize a model of human PGHS-2 expression allowing the assessment of pharmacological inhibition both *in vitro* and *ex vivo*.

METHODS

Peripheral venous blood samples were drawn from eight healthy volunteers (4F, 4M; aged 20-49 yr) before and 48 hours after the oral administration of aspirin 300 mg. One of these subjects was studied before, and after 7 days of oral dosing with nabumetone 500 and 1,000 mg/day. The induction of PGHS-2 was obtained by incubating one-ml aliquots of heparinized whole blood samples with LPS (0.1-50 µg/ml) for 0 to 24 hr at 37°C. The contribution of platelet PGHS-1 to eicosanoid production was suppressed by either pretreating the subjects with aspirin or adding aspirin (10 µg/ml) *in vitro* at time 0. Plasma was separated by centrifugation and assayed for PGE_2 by a previously described and validated radioimmunoassay (RIA) (4). The activity of platelet PGHS-1 was studied by allowing one-ml whole blood samples, drawn from non-aspirin-taking donors, to clot for 1 hour at 37°C. Serum was separated by centrifugation and assayed for TXB_2 by a previously described and validated RIA (4). Isolated monocytes, lymphocytes and neutrophils were lysed and 20 µg of proteins were analyzed by sodium dodecyl sulfate-polyacrylamide gel electrophoresis and immunoblotting techniques using rabbit polyclonal antibodies directed against PGHS-1 or against the 19-aminoacid peptide derived from a unique region of PGHS-2 protein near the carboxyl-terminal (5). Immunocomplexes were visualized by biotin conjugated anti-rabbit IgG and streptavidin-peroxidase.

RESULTS AND DISCUSSION

Incubation of heparinized whole blood with LPS resulted in a time- and concentration-dependent enhancement of PGE_2 production. LPS (10 µg/ml) did not significantly affect eicosanoid production at 1 hr while causing a 10-fold increase in PGE_2 production *vs* saline control at 24 hr. The contribution of platelet PGHS-1 activity to whole blood prostanoid production in response to LPS was largely suppressed by pretreating the subjects with 300 mg aspirin 2 days before sampling. After 24 hr at 10 µg/ml LPS, PGE_2 production averaged 12.1 ± 6.2 ng/ml (Mean$\pm$SD, n=7). Dexamethasone (2 µM) inhibited by $96 \pm 4\%$ LPS-induced PGE_2 production.

We studied prostanoid production and PGHS-2 biosynthesis by isolated human monocytes, lymphocytes and neutrophils incubated for 0-24 hours with LPS (10 µg/ml). Only monocytes responded to LPS by releasing large amounts of PGE_2 in a time-dependent fashion that correlated with the accumulation of a protein doublet of approximately 72 kDa analyzed by Western blot using antibodies specific for PGHS-2. Differently, the use of specific anti-PGHS-1 antibodies showed that monocytes not exposed to LPS contained PGHS-1 that was not increased at 24 hr. Altogether, these results suggest that enhanced cyclooxygenase activity in LPS-stimulated human whole blood was caused by the time-dependent selective expression of PGHS-2 in monocytes.

Four different cyclooxygenase inhibitors were tested *in vitro* on the cyclooxygenase activity of LPS-induced monocyte PGHS-2 and thrombin-stimulated platelet PGHS-1. IC_{50} values (μM) for inhibition of PGHS-1 and PGHS-2 were: indomethacin 0.70 ± 0.20 (Mean$\pm$SD) *vs* 0.36 ± 0.10 ($P<0.05$), S-indobufen 0.64 ± 0.22 *vs* 14.9 ± 8 ($P<0.05$), R-indobufen 38 ± 18 *vs* 230 ± 68 ($P<0.01$), 6-methoxy-2-naphthyl acetic acid (6-MNA, the active metabolite of the anti-inflammatory drug nabumetone) 278 ± 96 *vs* 187 ± 96.

We evaluated the effects of oral dosing with nabumetone on the cyclooxygenase activity of platelet PGHS-1 and LPS-induced monocyte PGHS-2. One healthy volunteer was treated with nabumetone 500 and 1,000 mg daily, each given for 7 days on two consecutive weeks. Platelet TXB_2 production was reduced by 63 and 72% after 500 and 1,000 mg, respectively. Similarly, LPS-induced PGE_2 production was inhibited by 55 and 78%, respectively.

We conclude that: 1) LPS-induced biosynthesis of PGHS-2 in human circulating monocytes accounts for the time-dependent expression of low-dose aspirin-insensitive cyclooxygenase activity in whole blood; 2) we have developed a relatively simple model of human PGHS-2 expression in LPS-stimulated whole blood allowing the assessment of pharmacological inhibition both *in vitro* and *ex vivo*.

REFERENCES

1. Smith WL. Prostanoid biosynthesis and mechanisms of action. *Am J Physiol*, 1992; 263: F181-91.
2. Hempel SL, Monick MM and Hunninghake GW. Lipopolysaccharide induces prostaglandin H synthase-2 protein and mRNA in human alveolar macrophages and blood monocytes. *J Clin Invest*, 1994; 93: 391-6.
3. Meade EA, Smith WL and DeWitt DL. Differential inhibition of prostaglandin endoperoxide synthase (cyclooxygenase) isozymes by aspirin and other non-steroidal anti-inflammatory drugs. *J Biol Chem*, 1993; 268: 6610-14.
4. Patrignani P, Filabozzi P and Patrono C. Selective cumulative inhibition of platelet thromboxane production by low-dose aspirin in healthy subjects. *J Clin Invest*, 1982; 69: 1366-72.
5. Habib A, Creminon C, Frobert Y, Grassi J, Pradelles P and Maclouf J. Demonstration of an inducible cyclooxygenase in human endothelial cells using antibodies raised against the carboxyl-terminal region of the cyclooxygenase-2. *J Biol Chem*, 1993; 268: 23448-54.

Advances in Prostaglandin, Thromboxane,
and Leukotriene Research, Vol. 23,
edited by B. Samuelsson et al.
Raven Press, Ltd., New York © 1995

HUMAN GENES FOR PROSTAGLANDIN ENDOPEROXIDE SYNTHASE-2, THROMBOXANE SYNTHASE AND PROSTACYCLIN SYNTHASE

Tadashi Tanabe,[a] Atsuro Miyata,[a] Toyomichi Nanayama,[a]
Yoshinori Tone,[a] Hayato Ihara,[a] Hiroyuki Toh,[b]
Ei-ichi Takahashi[c] and Volker Ullrich[d]

[a]Department of Pharmacology, National Cardiovascular Center Research Institute,
Suita, Osaka 565, [b]Department of Biochemical Engineering and Science,
Kyushu Institute of Technology, Iizuka, Fukuoka 820, [c]Division of Genetics,
National Institute of Radiological Sciences, Inage-ku, Chiba 263, Japan, and
[d]Department of Biology, Konstanz University, Konstanz M661·D-78434, Germany

The balance between the production of thromboxane (TX) A_2 and prostacyclin is important in the maintenance of vascular integrity.[1] TXA_2 has potent proaggregatory effects on platelets and strong vasocontricting properties and is synthesized from arachidonate by prostaglandin endoperoxide synthase (PES) and thromboxane synthase (TXS). The first step of the synthesis is catalyzed by two isozymes of PES, the constitutive (PES-1) and inducible forms (PES-2) of the enzyme. The following reaction is catalyzed by TXS showing a structural similarity to a cytochrome P450, CYP3A. To better understand the regulatory mechanism of TX synthesis, we isolated and characterized the genes for human PES-1[2] and -2,[3] and TXS[4] (PTGS1, PTGS2 and TBXAS1, respectively). The chromosomal localization of these three genes were determined by fluorescence *in situ* hybridization. Expression of these genes were studied with human monoblast U937 and erythroleukemia (HEL) cells. On the other hand, prostacyclin is the potent physiological antagonist of TXA_2 and is synthesized by prostacyclin synthase (PGIS). To isolate the human gene for PGIS, the cDNA encoding the human enzyme was cloned from cultured human aorta endothelial cells. Furthermore, the distribution of PGIS mRNA was determined using the cloned cDNA as a probe.

PROSTAGLANDIN ENDOPEROXIDE SYNTHASE-2

The human gene (PTGS2) encoding an inducible isozyme of PES (PES-2) was isolated using a cDNA fragment for human PES-2 generated by PCR as a probe.[3] The determined nucleotide sequence of the entire human PES-2 gene indicated that it spans more than 8.3 kb and consists of 10 exons, which is very similar to the murine and chicken PES-2 genes. The characterization of the human PES-2 gene is described by Inoue et al. (see this volume). The sequence of 1.69 kb nucleotides preceding the transcriptional start site and the 1st intron spanning 0.8 kb contained a canonical TATA box and various transcriptional regulatory elements such as NF-IL6, GATA-1, xenobiotic response element, cAMP response element (CRE), NF-κB, Sp-1 and AP-1. Fluorescence *in situ* hybridization study showed that the human genes coding for PES-1 (PTGS1) and -2 (PTGS2) were mapped to distinct chromosomes 9q32-q33.3 and 1q25.2-q25.3, respectively. The phylogenetic analysis of PES with available amino acid sequence data suggested that PES is a distantly related family of a peroxidase family and the evolution rate of PES-2 has increased after the divergence of PES-1 and -2.

THROMBOXANE SYNTHASE

The gene encoding human TXS (TBXAS1) was isolated using human platelet TXS cDNA as a probe.[4] The human TXS gene spans over 75 kb, and consists of 13 exons. The exon-intron boundaries of thromboxane synthase gene were quite similar to those of the human cytochrome P450 nifedipine oxidase gene (CYP3A4) except for introns 9 and 10, though the primary structures of these enzymes exhibited a 35.8% identity each other. The 1.2-kb of the 5'-flanking region sequence contained potential binding sites for several transcription factors (AP-1, AP-2, GATA-1, CCAAT box, xenobiotic-response element, PEA-3, LF-A1, myb, basic transcription element and cAMP-response element). Primer extension analysis indicated the multiple transcriptional start sites, and the major one was located 142 bases upstream of the translational-initiation site. However, neither typical TATA box nor CAAT box was found within 100 bases upstream of it. Furthermore, fluorescence *in situ* hybridization study revealed that the human gene for TXS (TBXAS1) was mapped to chromosome 7q33-q34. The TXS mRNA was widely expressed in human tissues and was particularly abundant in peripheral blood leukocyte, spleen, lung, and liver. Low levels of the mRNA were observed in kidney, placenta and thymus. Similar results were obtained with rat tissues.[5] On the other hand, we previously found that TXS mRNA in human erythroleukemia (HEL) cells induced by phorbol ester (TPA).[6] The results of the inhibition experiments with cycloheximide and actinomycin D, and run-off transcription assays showed that the induction of TXS mRNA by TPA in HEL cells is achieved by the stabilization of the mRNA depending on a newly-synthesized protein(s) (Ihara H et al., manuscript in preparation).

PROSTACYCLIN SYNTHASE

Recently, we cloned the cDNA coding for PGIS from bovine endothelial cells (Hara S et al., see this volume). On the basis of the nucleotide sequence of bovine PGIS cDNA, the cDNA for the human enzyme was cloned by PCR from cultured human aortic endothelial cells.[7] The cloned cDNA with a size of 1977 bp contained a 1500-bp open reading frame which encoded a 500-amino acid protein sharing an 88 % identity with bovine PGIS. RNA blot analysis with human aortic endothelial cells indicated a major PGIS mRNA with a size of approximately 6 kb and minor mRNAs with the sizes of 3.2, 2.5 and 1.7 kb differently from the bovine mRNA. Further, the mRNA level was increased by interleukin (IL)-1 or IL-6 treatment. Interestingly, PGIS mRNA is widely expressed in human tissues and is particularly abundant in ovary, heart, skeletal muscle, lung, and prostate.

GENE EXPRESSION OF PROSTAGLANDIN ENDOPEROXIDE SYNTHASE-1 AND -2, AND THROMBOXANE SYNTHASE

Human monoblastoid cell line U937 cells differentiated with 12-*O*-tetradecanoyl-phorbol-13-acetate (TPA) rapidly increased the activity of TXA$_2$ synthesis in response to the stimulation with lipopolysaccharide (LPS). RNA and immuno blot analyses showed that LPS increased both levels of PES-1 and -2 in a time-dependent manner without influencing the level of TXS; the mode of the induction was different between the two isozymes (Nanayama T et al., manuscript in preparation). The PES-1 and -2 mRNAs were maximally induced at 36 h of the stimulation (1.6 folds) and at 12 h (about 20 folds), respectively. The results indicate that TXA$_2$ synthesis induced by LPS in the differentiated cells is regulated at the levels of two PES isozymes, dominantly at the level of PES-2. By the stimulation of the cells with LPS for 48 h, unlike the differentiated U937 cells, the undifferentiated U937 cells did not express a detectable amount of PES-2 mRNA and hardly synthesized TXA$_2$. Notably, in the presence of both TPA and LPS the expression of PES-2 mRNA in the undifferentiated cells occurred after a longtime stimulation of about 8 h. These results suggested that the TPA-induced abilities of U937 cells to express the PES-2 enzyme and to synthesize TXA$_2$ in response to LPS were achieved probably by differentiation of the cells .

REFERENCES

1.   Moncada S, Vane JR. Arachidonic acid metabolites and the interactions between platelets and blood-vessel walls. *N Engl Med* 1979;300:1142-7.
2.   Yokoyama C, Tanabe T. Cloning of human gene encoding prostaglandin endoperoxide synthase and primary structure of the enzyme. *Biochem Biophys Res Commun* 1989;165:888-94.
3.   Kosaka T, Miyata A, Ihara H et al. Characterization of the human gene (PTGS2) encoding prostaglandin-endoperoxide synthase 2. *Eur J Biochem* 1994; in press.
4.   Miyata A, Ihara H, Bandoh S, Takeda O, Takahashi E, Tanabe T. Characterization of the human gene (TBXAS1) encoding thromboxane synthase. *Eur J Biochem* 1994; in press.
5.   Tone Y, Miyata A, Hara S, Yukawa S, Tanabe T. Abundant expression of thromboxane synthase in rat macrophages. *FEBS Lett* 1994;340:241-4.
6.   Ihara H, Yokoyama C, Miyata A et al. Induction of thromboxane synthase and prostaglandin endoperoxide synthase mRNAs in human erythroleukemia cells by phorbol ester. *FEBS Lett* 1992;306:161-4.
7.   Miyata A, Hara S, Yokoyama C, Inoue H, Ullrich V, Tanabe, T. Molecular cloning and expression of human prostacyclin synthase. *Biochem Biophys Res Commun* 1994; in press.

Advances in Prostaglandin, Thromboxane, and Leukotriene Research, Vol. 23,
edited by B. Samuelsson et al.
Raven Press, Ltd., New York © 1995

Genomic Organization and Regulation of The Human Thromboxane Synthase Gene

Rong-Fong Shen[1,2], Seung Joon Baek[1], Kuan-Der Lee[1], Liqun Zhang[1], and Tracey Fleischer[1]

[1]*Division of Human Genetics, Department of Obstetrics and Gynecology, Univ. of Maryland School of Medicine and* [2]*Medical Biotechnology Center, Univ. of Maryland Biotechnology Institute, Baltimore, MD 21201*

Thromboxane synthase (TS) is a membrane-bound, microsomal enzyme which catalyzes the formation of thromboxane A_2 (TxA_2). TxA_2 exerts its biological activity via the TxA_2 receptors and has been postulated to be involved in the etiologies of bleeding disorders (1,2) and other cardiovascular diseases (3,4). The enzyme exhibits interesting features in that it catalyzes the formation of both TxA_2 and HHT and undergoes self-inactivation during catalysis (5,6). The "suicide inactivation" results from a covalent modification of the enzyme by its substrate PGH_2 (7), which could be protected against by competitive inhibitors (4,7). TS cDNA has recently been cloned from three mammalian species (8-12). We demonstrated that TS protein sequences, as deduced from human, porcine and murine TS cDNAs, shared greater than 75% identity and that the TS gene was expressed primarily in the lung of all three species (12). A Cys^{480} residue in the consensus heme-binding domain of the human enzyme is essential for enzymatic activity, while *N*-glycosylation does not seem to be necessary for catalysis (10). To facilitate understanding of the genetic underpinning of TS in diseases and the regulation of its gene expression, we cloned the human TS gene and its flanking sequences.

MOLECULAR CLONING OF THE HUMAN TS GENE

Thirteen phage clones hybridized to a full-length human TS cDNA were isolated from a human genomic library constructed in a lambda vector. Restriction mapping and sequence analysis indicated that five of these clones contained exons encoding about two-third of the sequence of human TS cDNA. However, nucleotides 90-333 (exons II-IV) and 1135-1226 (exon XI) of the cDNA were not encoded by any of these phage clones. Since human TS gene has been mapped to chromosome 7q34-35 (13), a human chromosome 7-specific genomic library was screened. Four non-overlapping clones were isolated and found to contain the sequences not encoded by the phage clones. To establish the gene structure, sequence information of these exon-encoding clones was used to synthesize oligonucleotide primers for screening a P1 genomic library. Two over-lapping clones, 85 and 78 kb, respectively, were isolated, which contained the first through the fourth exons of the TS gene. Together, these genomic clones constitute the entire human TS gene, except for portions of introns 9 and 10. A schematic presentation of the human TS gene is shown in Fig. 1. The gene contains 13 exons and spans more than 130 kb. The first five exons are separated by large introns ($\geq$ 15 kb) and spread over 100 kb.

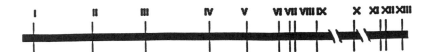

FIG. 1. *Genomic Organization of the Human TS Gene.*

REGULATION OF TS GENE EXPRESSION

We isolated a genomic phage clone hybridized to the 5' end of human TS cDNA. Sequencing analysis of a 1.7 kb subfragment revealed that it contained the entire 5' untranslated region and 46 bp of the coding sequence of TS cDNA, an upstream canonical TATA box (TATAAA), and several binding sites for transcription factors (AP1, PEA-3, PU.1, and GR), indicative of a promoter/first exon region of the TS gene. The transcription initiation site(s) were later determined by RNase protection and the RACE assays (14). To investigate the regulation of TS gene expression, constructs containing various lengths of human TS promoter cloned 5' to the luciferase (luc) reporter gene were used to transfect HL-60 cells. As shown in Table I, longer TS promoter significantly repressed luc gene expression, suggesting that a repression-derepression mechanism may be at work *in vivo* to regulate TS gene expression.

TABLE I. EXPRESSION OF LUCIFERASE ACTIVITY IN HL-60 CELLS CONTROLLED BY HUMAN TS PROMOTER

TS Promoter (kb)	5.3	3.8	1.1	0.3
Relative lucifer-ase activity (%)	15	17	65	100

ACKNOWLEDGMENTS

This work was supported by a Grant-in-Aid (to RFS) from the American Heart Association.

REFERENCES

1. Mestel F, Oetliker O, Bech E, Felix R, Imbach P, and Wafner H-P. *Lancet* 1980; i, 157.
2. Weiss HJ and Lages BA. *Lancet* 1977 ii, 760-761.
3. Moncada S and Vane JR. *Pharmacol Rev* 1982; 30:293-331.
4. Ogletree ML. *Fed Proc* 1987; 46:133-138.
5. Haurand M and Ullrich V. *J Biol Chem* 1985; 260:15059-15067.
6. Shen R-F and Tai HH. *J Biol Chem* 1986; 261:11592-11599.
7. Jones DA and Fitzpatrick FA. *J Biol Chem* 1991; 34:23510-23514.
8. Yokoyama C, Miyata A, Ihara H, Ullrich V, and Tanabe T. *Biochem Biophys Res Commun* 1991; 178:1479-1484.
9. Ohashi K, Ruan K-H, Kulmacz RJ, Wu KK, and Wang L-H. *J Biol Chem* 1992; 267:789-793.
10. Xia Z, Shen R-F, Baek SJ and Tai HH. *Biochem J* 1993; 295:457-461.
11. Zhang L, Chase M, and Shen R-F. *Biochem Biophys Res Commun* 1993; 194:741-748.
12. Shen R-F, Zhang L, Baek SJ, Tai HH, and Lee KD. *Gene* 1994; 140:261-265.
13. Chase MB, Baek SJ, Purtell D, Schwartz S, and Shen R-F. *Genomics* 1993; 16:771-773.
14. Lee K-D, Baek SJ, and Shen R-F. *Biochem Biophys Res Commun* 1994; 201:379-387.

Advances in Prostaglandin, Thromboxane, and Leukotriene Research, Vol. 23,
edited by B. Samuelsson et al.
Raven Press, Ltd., New York © 1995

11-Hydroxythromboxane B₂ Dehydrogenase from Porcine Kidney is Identical to Cytosolic Aldehyde Dehydrogenase

Pär Westlund[a], Ann Catrin Fylling[a], Anders Helander[b], Ella
Cederlund[c] and Hans Jörnvall[c]

a) Department of Woman and Child Health, Karolinska Hospital, L5, S-171 76 Stockholm,
Sweden, b) Department of Clinical Neuroscience, St. Göran's Hospital, Box 12500, S-112 81
Stockholm, Sweden, c) Department of Medical Biochemistry and Biophysics, Karolinska
Institute, S-171 77 Stockholm, Sweden

Urinary thromboxane B_2 metabolites are used as an index of thromboxane A_2 production in vivo. These metabolites are formed via two major metabolic pathways, β-oxidation and dehydrogenation at carbon atom eleven [1]. The metabolites are formed through one of the pathways or as combined products, and the metabolite used for quantitation is dependent on the studied species. In human and rabbit, where the blood and urinary profiles of the metabolites have been compared with each other [2, 3], 11-dehydrothromboxane B_2 seems to be the metabolite of choice if a metabolite is needed to cover measurements of thromboxane production in vivo in both species, in urine as well as in blood.

We have recently purified the 11-hydroxythromboxane B_2 dehydrogenase from porcine kidney to apparent homogeneity [4]. In the present paper we have characterized the enzyme further by amino acid sequence analysis and enzymatic studies. These studies clearly show that 11-hydroxythromboxane B_2 dehydrogenase from porcine kidney is identical to cytosolic aldehyde dehydrogenase (ALDH) (EC 1.2.1.3).

METHODS

The enzyme was purified by anion exchange chromatography, affinity chromatography on 5'-AMP Sepharose and gel permeation chromatography [4]. The purity and molecular mass of the enzyme was tested by SDS/PAGE, native PAGE and gel permeation chromatography.

The purified enzyme was carboxymethylated with ¹⁴C-iodoacetate and digested with a Lys-specific protease (Achromobactor) [5]. The total amino acid composition of the enzyme was analysed by acid hydrolysis [5].

The catalytic characterization of the enzyme was done using [1-^{14}C]TXB$_2$, 3,4-dihydroxyphenylacetaldehyde (DOPAL) [6], actealdehyde, propanal and p-nitrophenylacetate (substrate for esterase activity) as substrates, NAD as cofactor, and disulfiram, a well known inhibitor of cytosolic aldehyde dehydrogenase.

RESULTS

Attempts at direct sequence analysis did not produce any results, showing that the N-terminus is blocked like that of cytosolic aldehyde dehydrogenase. Cleavage with a Lys-specific protease of the ^{14}C-carboxymethylated protein and subsequent separations by HPLC, produced peptides suitable for analysis. 35 peptide sequences were determined, accounting for a total of 388 amino acid residues corresponding to 78% of the enzyme. Sequence comparison with known structures identify 11-hydroxy-thromboxane B$_2$ dehydrogenase as identical to cytosolic aldehyde dehydrogenase [5, 7]. The species' variability versus the corresponding human and horse enzyme was 7.5% and 9% respectively [7, 8], which is comparable to the horse/human variability of 9% [8]. Subunit molecular masses are identical, around 55 kDa by SDS/polyacrylamide gel electrophoresis.

The enzyme showed catalytic activity with all the tested aldehydes and with the esterase substrate p-nitrophenylacetate. DOPAL was used for further catalytic studies, recording the formed product 3,4-dihydroxphenylacetic acid (DOPAC) by HPLC and electrochemical detection, since the formation of NADH could not be used as an index of ALDH activity in this case. The formation of DOPAC was inhibited by TXB$_2$, see figure.

The inhibition was competitive, indicating that DOPAC and TXB$_2$ share the same active site. Using 10 μM DOPAL as substrate, 50% inhibition was obtained with 1 mM TXB$_2$ and 10 nM disulfiram. Furthermore 50% inhibition of the formation of 11-dehydro-TXB$_2$ from TXB$_2$ (final conc 500 μM) could be obtained by disulfiram (7μM) and propanal (700 μM). The catalytic data support that 11-hydroxythromboxane B$_2$ dehydrogenase is identical to ALDH. The data also indicate that TXB$_2$ binds to the same active site as the aldehydes.

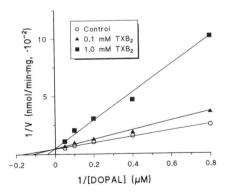

Inhibition of ALDH by thromboxane B$_2$ (TXB$_2$)

DISCUSSION

This study identifies the 11-hydroxy-thromboxane B$_2$ dehydrogenase as identical to cytosolic aldehyde dehydrogenase, proving additional important functions for the aldehyde dehydrogenase and supporting a possible catalytic mechanism of the 11-hydroxy-thromboxane B_2 dehydrogenase.

The catalytic mechanism of the conversion of TXB_2 to 11-dehydro-TXB_2 might be explained by the hemiacetal structure in the ring of TXB_2. TXB_2 can exist in three forms, two anomers with the 11-hydroxyl group in α or β-position, and the aldo form with an open ring structure. The conformation of TXB_2 is dependent on the nature of the solvent. Kotovych and Aarts [9] reported 76% 11α-OH TXB_2 and 24% 11β-OH TXB_2 in $CDCl_3$. However, in CD_3OD the predominant anomer is 11β-OH (80%). The same authors did not report any aldehyde form of the molecule. However, there is a continuous equilibrium between the two forms. If the aldo form of TXB_2 is the substrate, only minute amounts of the accurate substrate is expected to be present in solution as indicated by the relatively high K_m and low V_{max} values for TXB_2 [4].

The identification of 11-hydroxythromboxane B_2 dehydrogenase as cytosolic aldehyde dehydrogenase, highlights the possibility that several compounds might interfere with thromboxane metabolism and thus falsify recorded levels of thromboxane metabolites.

ACKNOWLEDGMENTS

This study was supported by grants from the Swedish Medical Research Council (Projects 10642, 9910 and 3532), the Swedish Tobacco Group and the Swedish Alcohol Research Found (Project 88/12:6 and 93/29).

REFERENCES

1. Jackson Roberts II L, Sweetman BJ and Oates JA. Metabolism of thromboxane B_2 in man. J Biol Chem 1981;256:8384-8393.
2. Westlund P, Granström E, Kumlin M and Nordenström A. Identification of 11-dehydro-TXB_2 as a suitable parameter for monitoring thromboxane production in the human. Prostaglandins 1986;31:929-960.
3. Westlund P, Kumlin M, Nordenström A, and Granström E. Circulating and urinary thromboxane B_2 metabolites in the rabbit: 11-dehydro-thromboxane B_2 as parameter of thromboxane production. Prostaglandins 1986;31:413-443.
4. Westlund P. Purification and some properties of 11-hydroxythromboxane B_2 dehydrogenase from porcine kidney. Eur J Biochem 1993;212:403-409.
5. Westlund P, Fylling AC, Cederlund E and Jörnvall H. 11-hydroxythromboxane B_2 dehydrogenase is identical to cytosolic aldehyde dehydrogenase. FEBS Lett 1994; in press.
6. Pettersson H. and Tottmar O. Aldehyde dehydrogenase in rat brain. Subcellular distribution and properties. J Neurochem 1982;38:477-487.
7. Hempel J, von Bahr-Lindström H and Jörnvall H. Aldehyde dehydrogenase from human liver. Eur J Biochem 1985;141:21-35.
8. von Bahr-Lindström H, Hempel J and Jörnvall H. The cytoplasmic isoenzyme of horse liver aldehyde dehydrogenase. Eur J Biochem 1984;141:37-42.
9. Kotovych G. and Aarts GHM. A high field proton magnetic resonance study of the solution conformation of thromboxane B_2. Can J Chem 1980;58:1111-1117

Advances in Prostaglandin, Thromboxane,
and Leukotriene Research, Vol. 23,
edited by B. Samuelsson et al.
Raven Press, Ltd., New York © 1995

Leukotriene-Deficient Mice Generated By Targeted Disruption Of The 5-Lipoxygenase Gene

Colin D. Funk, Xin-Sheng Chen, Usha Kurre, and Ginger Griffis

Department of Pharmacology, Vanderbilt University,
Nashville, TN 37232

5-lipoxygenase (arachidonate:oxygen 5-oxidoreductase, EC1.13.11.34) catalyzes the oxygenation of arachidonic acid to 5(S)-hydroperoxy-6,8,11,14-eicosatetraenoic acid and its subsequent rearrangement to the unstable allylic epoxide leukotriene A_4. This compound is then hydrolyzed to form leukotriene B_4 or conjugated with reduced glutathione to form the peptidyl leukotrienes by additional enzymes (leukotriene A_4 hydrolase and leukotriene C_4 synthase, respectively). The spectrum of biological effects elicited by the leukotrienes has led to the conclusions that these compounds are mediators of inflammation and allergic diseases (1). Although insights into the pathophysiologic consequences of leukotriene formation have been gleaned over the past decade there is no consensus on the physiologic importance of 5-lipoxygenase or the precise contribution of leukotrienes to various disease models. In the present study we disrupted the 5-lipoxygenase gene in mouse embryonic stem (ES) cells by homologous recombination to create leukotriene-deficient mice ($5LX^{-/-}$) and examined their phenotype.

METHODS

Construction of the targeting vector and isolation of targeted ES cell lines has been described (2). 5-Lipoxygenase gene-disrupted mice were generated by standard procedures (3). Experiments were performed on 6-9 week-old mice. All mice are C57BL/6J x 129 mixed genetic background.

Bone marrow-derived mast cells (BMMC) were isolated from the femurs and tibiae of mice and were cultured for 3 weeks. Purity was about 97 %. Resident macrophages were obtained by lavage of the peritoneal cavity with Dulbecco's modified Eagle medium containing 10 % serum and 5 U/ml heparin. Macrophages were allowed to adhere for 1-2 h at 37 °C in culture dishes, washed free of any contaminating cells and incubated either immediately with unopsonized zymosan (200 μg/ml) or opsonized Texas Red-conjugated yeast

BioParticles (Molecular Probes; 25:1 particles/cell). Macrophage purity was >
95 %.

To assess ear inflammation arachidonic acid (2 mg/ear) or phorbol myristate
acetate (2 μg/ear) in 20 μl acetone was topically applied to the inside surface of
the external ear of male or female age/sex matched mice. Vehicle was applied
to the contralateral ear. Edema was assessed by ear punch biopsy (6 mm
diameter) wet weight.

For shock experiments, platelet activating factor (1-O-alkyl-2-acetyl-sn-
glycero-3-phosphocholine; Sigma cat. #P-9525) in chloroform was dried down
under argon, resuspended in pyrogen-free normal saline containing 0.25 %
bovine serum albumin, and injected into the tail vein of conscious male and
female mice.

Male mice were pretreated with 5 mg iota carrageenan (Sigma; cat. #C-4014)
in 0.5 ml saline i.p. 24 h prior to injection (i.v.) of different doses of *E. coli
J5* lipopolysaccharide (mutant of *E.coli:0111:B4*; Calbiochem) and were
monitored over the course of 3 days.

For peritoneal cell influx studies, mice were injected intraperitoneally with
either: (i) 1 % sterile glycogen (2 ml); (ii) zymosan (2 mg in 0.5 ml saline); or
(iii) rat anti-ovalbumin IgG (800 μg diluted in normal saline; Cappel Research
Products) after prior i.v. injection of ovalbumin (20 mg/kg). At different time
points, the peritoneal cavity was lavaged and cells were counted
(hemocytometer) and prepared for differential analysis. Plasma protein leakage
was measured as described (4).

RESULTS AND DISCUSSION

Leukotriene-deficient mice were generated by targeted disruption of the 5-
lipoxygenase gene. Homozygous mice developed normally and showed no
observable abnormalities. They are fertile with a mean litter size of 7.3 ± 0.3
(n=66) compared to 6.6 ± 0.4 (n=44) for 5LX$^{+/+}$ mice. They are somewhat
more prodigious than wild-type mice (34 litters/250 pups vs. 22 litters/146 pups
recorded over the same period with equally matched mating pairs) with 5LX$^{-/-}$
mating pairs having 8-9 litters during their reproductive lifespan compared to
5-6 litters for wild-type mice.

BMMC from wild-type mice synthesize LTB$_4$, LTC$_4$, and 5-HETE when
stimulated with the calcium ionophore A23187. These products are absent in
5LX$^{-/-}$ mice. Prostaglandin D$_2$ synthesis is largely unaffected, however, and
there is no difference in the ability of these cells to release the granule
component, ß-hexosaminidase (Table 1). LTC$_4$ synthesis was absent in 5LX$^{-/-}$
macrophages but PGE$_2$ synthesis and functional capacity to phagocytose was not
substantially altered (Table 1).

Comparison of 5LX$^{+/+}$ and 5LX$^{-/-}$ mice

	5LX$^{+/+}$	5LX$^{-/-}$
macrophage		
LTC$_4$ (ng/10^6 cells)	22, 32	---, ---
PGE$_2$ (ng/10^6 cells)	54, 100	89, 110
phagocytosis (relative fluorescence units)	5.1$\pm$0.8 (n=9)	3.7$\pm$0.6 (n=8)
BMMC		
LTC$_4$ (ng/10^6 cells)	22, 25	---, ---
PGD$_2$ (ng/10^6 cells)	35, 27	32, 75
ß-hexosaminidase release (% of total)	47, 30	41, 33
spleen (mg)	79.1$\pm$6.2 (54.4-115.1)	*63.1$\pm$3.2 (46-75.3)

Table 1 Resident peritoneal macrophages were stimulated with zymosan and BMMC with 0.5 μM calcium ionophore A23187. Values obtained from two separate mice in each group are shown. ---, not detected. Phagocytosis assay was carried out as described[5]. Unstimulated BMMC release 9-11 % of ß-hexosaminidase, while failing to generate detectable leukotrienes. Spleens were from 8 week old male mice and are expressed as mean$\pm$SEM (range); n=11; *p<0.05, Student's t-test.

Blood analysis of 5LX$^{-/-}$ mice revealed no evidence of altered cell numbers or abnormal precursor cells of any lineage. 5-Lipoxygenase products, therefore, are not necessary for normal development nor do they appear to play strikingly significant biological actions in mice under usual physiological conditions. The 5LX$^{-/-}$ mice have shown no overt abnormalities up to ten months of age.

Two models of acute inflammation were examined for the involvement of 5-lipoxygenase products. 5LX$^{-/-}$ mice were found to exhibit a marked diminution of ear edema induced by topical application of arachidonic acid. However, these mice showed no difference from control mice in the phorbol ester-induced model of inflammation (Fig. 1). Histological analysis demonstrated evidence of edema, extensive disruption of the connective tissue layers of the dermis and dilated, congested vessels in sections from normal mice. The arachidonic acid-treated ear sections from 5LX$^{-/-}$ mice resembled more closely the vehicle-treated samples (data not shown). 5LX$^{-/-}$ mice can be used to selectively discriminate the role of leukotrienes in acute inflammatory models.

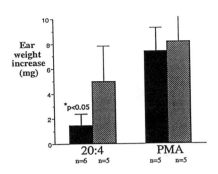

Figure 1   Ear inflammation induced by arachidonic acid or PMA.
Solid bars, 5LX$^{-/-}$; cross-hatched bars, 5LX$^{+/+}$.

Platelet activating factor is an important endogenous mediator of
inflammatory, systemic anaphylactic and shock states (6). Intravenous injection
of two different doses of PAF (140 and 175 μg kg^{-1}; Fig.2 left panel) causes
death in most conscious, unanesthetized 5LX$^{+/+}$ mice. The animals become
listless and usually die within 15-25 min. On the other hand, conscious 5LX$^{-/-}$
mice do not succumb to the lethal effects of PAF, even at doses up to 200 μg
kg^{-1} (Fig. 2). Although they exhibit the same behavior for the first 15 minutes,
these mice seem to recover quickly from the state of shock. By contrast, in a
septic shock model (7), leukotrienes do not appear to be involved in the
mortality caused by endotoxin (Fig.2 right panel).

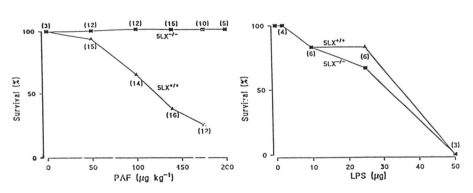

Figure 2   Survival curves after PAF or endotoxin injection. Numbers
of mice used for each point are shown in parentheses.

PAF is known to cause release of peptidyl leukotrienes from perfused rat lungs with subsequent pulmonary vasoconstriction and edema (8). It is known that the peptidyl leukotrienes are potent coronary vessel spasmogens released by PAF action in isolated perfused heart preparations (9,10). The interplay of complement activation (11), and the cytokine and leukotriene release caused by PAF may provoke enough tissue injury, vascular permeability changes and cardiac alterations to be lethal.

Leukotrienes are one of many compounds known to possess neutrophil chemotactic activity; others include interleukin-8, C5a, PAF, and f-Met-Leu-Phe. Three different challenges (glycogen, immune complex and zymosan) to induce an inflammatory chemotactic response in the peritoneal cavity were performed in order to assess the relative contribution of leukotrienes to this process. *In vivo* recruitment of leukocytes in 5LX$^{-/-}$ mice was dramatically diminished in an immune complex-induced peritonitis model (12) but not after a commonly used sterile challenge (glycogen) that is used to elicit recruitment into the peritoneal cavity (not shown). In a zymosan-induced peritonitis model significantly reduced plasma protein leakage into the peritoneal cavity was observed in the 5LX$^{-/-}$ mice 50 min after challenge (Fig.3).

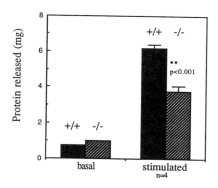

Figure 3   Plasma protein leakage in 5LX$^{+/+}$ and 5LX$^{-/-}$ mice induced by intraperitoneal zymosan challenge.

In conclusion, we have demonstrated that the phenotype of 5LX$^{-/-}$ mice can be markedly differentiated from 5LX$^{+/+}$ mice during certain defined challenged states. This first targeted disruption of a gene involved in the arachidonic acid cascade combined with future studies with cyclooxygenase-deficient mice will enable a thorough characterization of eicosanoid involvement in health and disease.

Acknowledgments

This work was supported by National Institutes of Health grant GM15431. C.D.F. is recipient of a Research Career Development Award HL02710.

References

1.   Samuelsson, B. Leukotrienes: mediators of immediate hypersensitivity reactions and inflammation. *Science* 1983;220:568-575.
2.   Chen, X-S, Sheller, J.R., Johnson, E.N., Nanney, L.B. and Funk, C.D. Role of leukotrienes as revealed by targeted disruption of the 5-lipoxygenase gene. (Manuscript submitted)
3.   Ramirez-Solis, R., Davis, A.C. and Bradley, A. Gene targeting in mouse embryonic stem cells. *Meth. Enzymol.* 1993;225:855-878.
4.   Doherty, N.S., Poubelle, P., Borgeat, P., Beaver, T.H., Westrich, G.L., and Schrader, N.L. Intraperitoneal injection of zymosan in mice induces pain, inflammation, and the synthesis of peptidoleukotrienes and prostaglandin E_2. *Prostaglandins* 1985;30:769-789.
5.   de Lanerolle, P., Gorgas, G., Li, Q., and Schluns, K. Myosin light chain phosphorylation does not increase during yeast phagocytosis by macrophages. *J. Biol. Chem.* 1993;268:16883-16886.
6.   Braquet, P., Touquit, L., Shen, T.Y., and Vargaftig, B.B. Perspectives in platelet activating factor research. *Pharmacol.* Rev. 1987;39:97-145.
7.   Ogata, M., Matsumoto, T., Kamochi, M., Yoshida, S.-I., Mizuguchi, Y., and Shigematsu, A. Protective effects of a leukotriene inhibitor and a leukotriene antagonist on endotoxin-induced mortality in carageenin-pretreated mice. *Inf. and Immunity*, 1992;60:2432-2437.
8.   Voelkel, N.F., Worthen, S., Reeves, J.T., Henson, P.M., and Murphy, R.C. Nonimmunological production of leukotrienes induced by platelet-activating factor. *Science* 1982;218:286-288.
9.   Piper, P.J., and Stewart, A.G. Coronary vasoconstriction in the rat isolated perfused heart induced by platelet-activating factor is mediated by leukotriene C_4. *Br. J. Pharmacol.* 1986;88:595-605.
10. Stahl, G.L., and Lefer, A.M. Mechanisms of platelet-activating factor-induced cardiac depression in the isolated perfused rat heart. *Circ. Shock* 1987;23;165-177.
11. Sun, X., and Hsueh, W. Platelet activating factor produces shock, in vivo complement activation, and tissue injury in mice. *J. Immunol.* 1991;147:509-514.
12. Zhang, Y., Ramos, B.F., and Jakschik, B.A. (1992) Neutrophil recruitment by tumor necrosis factor from mast cells in immune complex peritonitis. *Science* 1992;258:1957-1959.

Advances in Prostaglandin, Thromboxane,
and Leukotriene Research, Vol. 23,
edited by B. Samuelsson et al.
Raven Press, Ltd., New York © 1995

LOCALIZATION OF 5-LIPOXYGENASE TO THE NUCLEUS OF RESTING RAT BASOPHILIC LEUKEMIA CELLS

Thomas G. Brock and Marc Peters-Golden

Division of Pulmonary and Critical Care Medicine, Department of Internal
Medicine, University of Michigan, Ann Arbor, Michigan 48109 USA

Metabolism of free arachidonic acid to leukotrienes, initiated by 5-lipoxygenase (5-LO), is associated with translocation of 5-LO from a soluble to a particulate fraction, as determined in thoroughly disrupted granulocytic cells ((1, 2). The processing of arachidonate by 5-LO is facilitated by the 5-lipoxygenase activating protein (FLAP), which is always found in the particulate fraction (3).

Determining the intracellular locale of an enzyme is essential to understanding its full function. Recently, both 5-LO and FLAP were found in nuclear fractions in activated rat peritoneal macrophages (4). Similarly, both enzymes were localized at the nuclear membrane of activated peripheral blood leukocytes (PBL), by immunoelectron microscopy (5). However, 5-LO could not be detected in resting PBL by this technique, although the protein is abundant in PBL.

Based on these findings, it appears that 5-LO translocates to the nuclear membrane following stimulation of granulocytic cells. We asked whether the nucleus might also be the site for soluble 5-LO in unstimulated cells, and utilized rat basophilic leukemia (RBL) cells as model granulocytic cells to address this question. The 5-LO of RBL cells has been extensively studied in terms of its ability to metabolize arachidonate. The enzyme is found to be predominantly soluble in resting RBL cells and translocates to a pelletable fraction upon activation (2). However, its subcellular distribution has never been characterized.

MATERIALS AND METHODS

RBL-1 cells (ATCC(R) 1378-CRL) were seeded at 1×10^5 cells ml^{-1} in MEMα (with 10% fetal calf serum and penicillin/streptomycin), fed two days later and harvested the third day. PBS-washed-cells were resuspended in TKM buffer (50 mM Tris-HCl, pH 7.4, 25 mM KCl, 5 mM MgCl$_2$) with protease inhibitors at 10^7 cells ml^{-1} and broken by either detergent lysis (Triton-X 100, 0.1%) or Dounce homogenization. For both preparations, broken cells were then centrifuged at 1000 x g, 5 min. The low speed supernatant was ultracentrifuged to give cytosolic and non-nuclear membrane fractions. The low speed pellet was examined for total cell disruption by trypan blue exclusion, then overlayed on 2.3 M sucrose and ultracentrifuged to yield purified nuclei. Isolated nuclei were subsequently further separated into soluble and insoluble fractions by sonication followed by ultracentrifugation.

Samples of fractionated cells and nuclei were subjected to immunoblot analysis, loading identical protein amounts for all samples. Membranes were probed with antibodies to 5-LO (a rabbit polyclonal antibody raised against purified human leukocyte 5-LO (5), a generous gift from Dr. J. Evans, Merck Frosst Centre for Therapeutic Research, Pointe Claire-Dorval, Quebec, Canada) and FLAP (a rabbit polyclonal antibody against amino acid residues 41-52 of the human FLAP sequence (6), also a gift from Dr. J. Evans, Merck Frosst).

RESULTS AND DISCUSSION

In the present study, we used two techniques (detergent lysis and Dounce homogenization) to disrupt cells while sparing nuclei. Crude nuclei were subsequently centrifuged through high density sucrose to eliminate contaminants. Immunoblot analysis of the resulting purified nuclei from either technique indicated the presence of abundant antibody-detectable 5-LO (Fig. 1A). 5-LO was also detectable in both the cytosolic and membrane fractions. Slightly less 5-LO was found in membrane fractions derived from detergent lysis, presumably because detergent treatment released some membrane-associated 5-LO.

Within purified nuclei, 5-LO existed in both soluble and insoluble pools (Fig. 1B). Further analysis showed that some, but not all of the insoluble pool could be removed by high salt extraction (data not shown), indicating that some of the nuclear 5-LO was tightly bound. For comparison, FLAP was found exclusively in

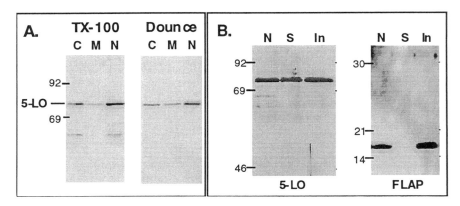

Figure 1. Evaluation of the subcellular distribution of 5-LO in unstimulated RBL cells by immunoblot analysis. **A.** 5-LO in cytosolic (C), membrane (M) or nuclear (N) fractions from cells disrupted by either detergent lysis (TX-100) or Dounce homogenization. **B.** 5-LO in soluble (S) or insoluble (In) fractions derived from purified nuclei (N). Comparable analysis of FLAP, a nuclear membrane-bound protein, is also presented.

the insoluble pool within the nucleus (Fig. 1B). Consistent with these findings, in studies using indirect immunofluorescent microscopy, abundant 5-LO was visualized within the nuclear compartment of resting RBL cells (7). The punctate pattern of fluorescence for 5-LO within the nucleus was very different from the pattern seen for FLAP, which was localized predominantly at the nuclear membrane.

Interestingly, 5-LO in dividing RBL cells was diffuse and cytosolic, with little 5-LO associated with the nuclear material. This suggested that some of the cytosolic 5-LO found by cell fractionation resulted from these dividing cells. When the contribution from dividing cells was minimized, either by overnight serum deprivation or by fractionating only cells susceptible to enucleation, 5-LO was prominent in the nuclear fraction but negligible in the cytosolic fraction (7).

These data provide the first evidence for the localization of 5-LO in resting granulocytic cells. The data support the idea that multiple pools of 5-LO exist in unstimulated RBL cells, and that these pools may be either soluble or bound. Which pools are directly involved in arachidonate metabolism upon cell activation, is unknown at present. It is possible that separate pools of 5-LO act on distinct pools of arachidonate. It is also likely that some pools are inactive with respect to arachidonate metabolism.

The surprising finding that a substantial proportion of enzyme is localized within the nucleus of resting RBL cells suggests potentially novel roles for 5-LO or its products within the nucleus. In particular, 5-LO protein or its enzymatic products may play direct roles in either gene regulation or intranuclear signaling.

REFERENCES

1. Rouzer CA, Kargman S: Translocation of 5-lipoxygenase to the membrane in human leukocytes challenged with ionophore A23187. *J Biol Chem* 1988; 263: 10980-8.
2. Wong A, Hwang SM, Cook MN, Hogaboom GK, Crooke ST: Interactions of 5-lipoxygenase with membranes: Studies on the association of soluble enzyme with membranes and alterations in enzyme activity. *Biochemistry* 1988; 27: 6763-9.
3. Reid GK, Kargman S, Vickers PJ et al.: Correlation between expression of 5-lipoxygenase-activating protein, 5-lipoxygenase, and cellular leukotriene synthesis. *J Biol Chem* 1990; 265: 19818-23.
4. Peters-Golden M, McNish R: Redistribution of 5-lipoxygenase and cytosolic phospholipase A_2 to the nuclear fraction upon macrophage activation. *Biochem Biophys Res Commun* 1993; 196: 147-53.
5. Woods J, Evans J, Ethier D et al.: 5-Lipoxygenase and 5-lipoxygenase activating protein are localized in the nuclear envelope of activated human leukocytes. *J Exp Med* 1993; 178: 1935-46.
6. Mancini J, Prasit P, Coppolino M et al.: 5-Lipoxygenase-activating protein is the target of a novel hybrid of two classes of leukotriene biosynthesis inhibitors. *Mol Pharmacol* 1992; 41: 267-72.
7. Brock TG, Paine R, Peters-Golden M: Localization of 5-lipoxygenase to the nucleus of unstimulated rat basophilic leukemia cells. *J Biol Chem* 1994; in press.

Advances in Prostaglandin, Thromboxane, and Leukotriene Research, Vol. 23,
edited by B. Samuelsson et al.
Raven Press, Ltd., New York © 1995

Properties of LTA$_4$ Synthase in Human Neutrophil Preparations

Elizabeth Hill, Denise MacMillan, Angelo Sala, Peter M. Henson, and Robert C. Murphy

National Jewish Center for Immunology and Respiratory Medicine
1400 Jackson Street
Denver, Colorado 80206

Following purification and cloning of mammalian 5-lipoxygenase (5-LO), biochemical studies revealed that this enzyme catalyzed the second step in the synthesis of leukotrienes which is the dehydration of 5(S)-HPETE into leukotriene A$_4$ (LTA$_4$) (1). Both enzymatic activities appear to have similar requirements for Ca^{2+} and ATP for maximal activity. While 5-LO is normally inactive as a cytosolic enzyme, elevation of intracellular calcium results in the translocation to a membrane compartment (2). The present investigations were undertaken to study LTA$_4$ synthase activity in terms of translocation and suicide inactivation.

METHODS

Granulocytes were prepared using plasma percoll gradients. Typical preparations yielded to polymorphonuclear leukocytes (95-97%) as well as the eosinophils (3-5%). Cell supernatants (cytosol) and membrane fractions were prepared as previously described (3). For some experiments cell suspensions were preincubated with 100 μM zileuton and 2 mM CaCl$_2$ and 1 μM A23187 for 30 min to stimulate 5-LO translocation. These cells were washed and then sonicated as described above.

The cytosol and membrane preparations were diluted 10-fold corresponding to an original concentration of 1 x 10^7 cells/mL. The standard assay for 5-LO contained 5 mL diluted cytosol to which was added ATP (2 mM) egg yolk glycerophosphocholine (100 μg/mL) and for certain experiments zileuton (100 μM). The mixture was prewarmed for 2 min following which time CaCl$_2$ (4 mM) and arachidonic acid (15 μM) was added. The LTA$_4$ synthase activity was employed in an identical assay mixture except that 5(S)-HPETE (15 μM) was added instead of arachidonic acid. The assay for 5-LO activity included

5(S)-HETE as well as all LTA_4 products (LTB_4, trans-LTB_4 isomers, and 5,6-diHETE).

RESULTS

Both enzymatic activities in the cytosol from the granulocyte preparation ceased after 10 min as can be seen in Figures 1A and 1B. Following this 10 min incubation, further products were not obtained when additional substrate was added. However, the addition of granulocyte cytosol to the incubations nearly doubled eicosanoid synthesis. The LTA_4 synthase activity was not observed following subsequent addition of 5(S)-HPETE (Figure 1B). Again, the addition of cytosol caused further LTA_4 biosynthesis.

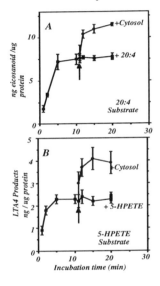

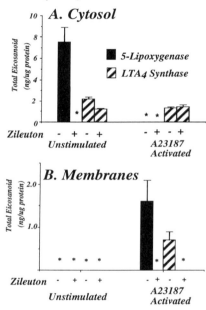

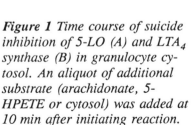

Figure 1 Time course of suicide inhibition of 5-LO (A) and LTA_4 synthase (B) in granulocyte cytosol. An aliquot of additional substrate (arachidonate, 5-HPETE or cytosol) was added at 10 min after initiating reaction.

Figure 2 5-LO and LTA_4 synthase activity in cytosol (A) and membrane (B) fractions from resting (unstimulated granulocytes) and cells treated with A23187 (stimulated). Zileuton was added to preparations prior to enzyme assay as indicated.

A dose dependent effect of zileuton, a reversible 5-LO inhibitor (4) on both enzymatic activities, 5-LO and LTA_4 synthase, confirmed a differential effect of this inhibitor on these two enzymatic activities. At 100 μM zileuton completely inhibited 5-LO activity, but only inhibited LTA_4 synthase activity by 47%. A similar difference in enzymatic activities was observed in response to incubation with fatty acid hydroperoxides which are known to inhibit lipoxygenases (5). When 1 μM of 13-HPODE, 12-HPETE, or 15-HPETE were incubated with granulocytes supernatants, 5-LO activity was completely inhibited, but LTA$_4$ synthase activity was reduced only by 55-64%. Hydrogen peroxide was a poor inhibitor of both activities.

Previous studies have shown that neutrophil 5-LO is a cytosolic enzyme that is rapidly translocated to membrane fraction during eicosanoid synthesis (2). In our studies, 100% of both 5-LO and LTA$_4$ synthase activities were present in the cytosol of resting cells and 100 μM zileuton completely inhibited cytosolic 5-LO activity while cytosolic LTA$_4$ synthase activity was reduced by 45% by zileuton (Figure 2A). When the cytosolic fraction from ionophore stimulated cells was assayed, all of the 5-LO activity had disappeared, but 59% of initial LTA$_4$ synthase activity (as measured by conversion of 5(S)-HPETE into LTA$_4$ products) remained. This LTA$_4$ synthase activity was not inhibited by 100 μM zileuton (Figure 2B). The small amount of membrane associated LTA$_4$ synthase and 5-LO activities present in the ionophore treated cells were completely inhibited by 100 μM zileuton.

DISCUSSION

This study shows that LTA$_4$ synthase activity present in the cytosol of human granulocyte preparations is not completely identical to 5-LO. 5-Lipoxygenase can be translocated to the membrane fraction of activated cells leaving significant LTA$_4$ synthase activity in the supernatant. Furthermore, this novel LTA$_4$ synthase activity is not inhibited by a known 5-LO inhibitor such as zileuton or MK886 (data not shown) or by fatty acid hydroperoxides. In many situations the production of 5-HETE is larger than the total production of LTA$_4$ products suggesting that some 5(S)-HPETE escapes conversion into LTA$_4$. This novel enzyme might assist in enhancing leukotriene biosynthesis within certain cells.

ACKNOWLEDGEMENT

This work was supported, in part, by a grant from the National Institutes of Health (HL34303).

REFERENCES

1. Shimizu T, Izumi T, Seyama Y, Tadokoro K, Radmark O, and Samuelsson B. *Proc Natl Acad Sci USA* 1986;83:4175-9.
2. Rouzer CA and Samuelsson B *Proc Natl Acad Sci USA* 1987;84:7393-7.
3. Hill E, Maclouf J, Murphy RC, and Henson PM *J Biol Chem* 1992;267: 22048-53.
4. Carter GW, Young PR, Albert DH, et al. *J Pharmacol Exp Ther* 1991;256:929-37.
5. Rapoport S, Hortel B, and Hansdorf G *Eur J Biochem* 1984;139:573.

Advances in Prostaglandin, Thromboxane,
and Leukotriene Research, Vol. 23,
edited by B. Samuelsson et al.
Raven Press, Ltd., New York © 1995

On the Interfacial Phenomena In Lipoxygenase Catalysis

Igor A. Butovich, Olga V. Kharchenko and Vitaliy M. Babenko

Laboratory for Chemical Enzymology, Institute of Bioorganic Chemistry, Ukrainian Academy of Sciences, 1 Murmanskaya Street, Kiev, 253660, UKRAINE (C.I.S)

Recently we have reported the preliminary results of our experiments aimed at investigation of the role of natural and synthetic amphiphiles in regulation of lipoxygenase (LO) activity [1-4]. Now we present the generalized scheme of lipoxygenation taking into account the physicochemical properties of polyunsaturated fatty acids (namely linoleic acid) and their derivatives.

The enzymatic activity of different lipoxygenases from plants (soybean LO-1 and LO-2, potato 5-LO, barley 5-LO) and porcine leukocyte 12-LO have been shown to be strongly dependent on the presence of a lipid phase regardless of its nature. Both natural and synthetic amphiphiles as phospholipids and detergents of varied nature influence the enzymatic activity. According to our results, we distinguished between two main classes of LOs, the first class prefers the water-soluble form of the substrate (ionized polyunsaturated fatty acid at concentration lower than it's CMC), and the second, oxidizes the aggregated form of the substrate (*e.g.*, membrane or micelle-bound ones).

The widely known representative of the first class of LOs is soybean LO-1, possessing the alkaline optimum of the enzymatic activity and oxidizing linoleate-ion in the form of a true molecular solution. The enzyme is inhibited by additions of any type of surface-active compounds (*e.g.*, Tween-20, Brij-35, Lubrol PX, Triton X-100, Aerosol OT, CTAB, *etc.*). This is mainly due to the effective absorption of the substrate from water phase into micellaric phase. The direct interaction of the enzyme with the detergents cannot be excluded as well.

The second proposed type of LOs prefers the aggregated form of the substrate. One of the best examples of this type of enzyme is potato 5-LO. The enzyme acts predominantly on the insoluble (aggregated or membrane-bound) form of the fatty acid and possesses maximal activity at pH 6.5. Potato 5-LO displays a sufficient activity even at pH 4.5 where the molar fraction of the water-soluble form of the substrate (linoleic acid, LA) is negligible. At the same time, the enzyme activity tends to zero with increases in pH. The kinetic properties of soybean LO-2 and barley 5-LO are very similar to those of potato 5-LO. Both enzymes can be activated by the addition of sufficient amounts of Lubrol PX forming the micellaric phase. Purified porcine leukocyte 12-LO is almost inactive in a system without the detergent at pH 7.5. The presence of 0.005-0.02% (w/v) of Lubrol PX or Brij-99 is crucial for the enzyme activity manifestation.

The following approach has been chosen to confirm the interfacial nature of lipoxygenase reaction. A solid-phase model of biological membrane based on nonporous silica modified with octadecyltrichlorosilane with phospholipid monolayer adsorbed on it has been synthesized. It has been determined that LA was almost completely bound with hydrophobic surface of the silica at pH<7 and significantly desorbed (up to 50%) at pH>10. The model composed of lecithin and LA in molar ratio 2:1 was much more stable. In this case the utmost desorption of LA (~8%) has been achieved at pH>10. At acidic and quasi-neutral pHs the partition coefficient of LA was higher than 10^5. The parameters of adsorption of potato 5-LO on the model biomembranes consisted of octadecyl-modified silica and individual phospholipid monolayer were virtually identical for lecithin- and phosphatidylinositol-containing particles. When a solution of LA was added to the adsorbed potato 5-LO, the reaction was also proceeding. This is evidence of the adsorption of the LO on the phospholipid surface in the native, catalytically active state. The most effective adsorption has been observed at pH 3–5 (pI of potato 5-LO is about 4.5). The increase in ionic strength up to 1M NaCl did not decrease the adsorption. These facts corroborate the significant role of hydrophobic interactions in the adsorption process.

Kinetics of the reaction have been investigated by using the Clark oxygen electrode. The biomembrane models consisted of phospholipids (lecithin or phosphatidylinositol) and LA in the molar ration 2:1 were used. The dependences of V_o (the reaction steady-state velocity) on pH for both phospholipids have had a specific plateau at pH 3.5–6.0, pH-optima at pH 6.5–7.0, and decreases at pH>8. Our investigations of the product partition showed that the major part of the reaction product (9-hydroperoxyoctadeca-10,12-dienoic acid) had also been localized in the membrane structure.

A mathematical model of the enzymatic oxidation of membrane-bound LA has been developed to separate and study individual steps of LO reaction. The following scheme:

$$ES_m \underset{S_m}{\overset{K_i}{\longleftrightarrow}} E \underset{S_{n-1}}{\overset{K_{ss}}{\longleftrightarrow}} ES_{n-1} \underset{S}{\overset{K_s}{\longleftrightarrow}} ESS_{n-1} \longrightarrow E + P$$

where E is free LO; S, S_{n-1}, and S_m are the substrate molecules in different aggregation states; ES_{n-1} is active adsorbed LO; ESS_{n-1} is adsorbed enzyme-substrate complex; ES_m is inactive adsorbed LO; and the corresponding kinetic equation:

$$V_o = V_m * S^n / (K_s * K_{ss} + K_s * K_{ss} * S^m / K_i + K_s * S^{n-1} + S^n)$$

have been proposed. The reaction scheme consists of the following steps: i) enzyme (E) adsorption at the surface of "supersubstrate"—aggregated fatty acid, phospholipid, or detergent (S_{n-1}); ii) substrate molecule (S) binding to the enzyme active center; iii) catalytical transformation of the substrate to product (P); iv) the substrate inhibition and/or activation of LO. Parameters K_s, K_{ss}, and K_i, represent the equilibrium constants of individual steps of the reaction; V_m is the reaction maximal velocity. The equation was successfully used to govern the substrate dependence of the enzymatic reaction.

Calcium ion has frequently been considered as a potent activator of LOs, but the reaction mechanism remained unknown. We have shown that Ca(II) can contribute to LO activation by reacting with the substrate (polyunsaturated *carboxylic* fatty acid, PUFA). Due to the formation of virtually insoluble salt—calcium carboxylate—the main part of the PUFA is removed from the solution and forms a separate phase that is crucial for the enzyme to be active. We have shown that neither plant lipoxygenases (potato 5-LO, soybean LO-1 and LO-2, barley LO), nor animal LO (porcine leukocyte 12-LO) do not require Ca(II) to be active in the reaction of PUFA oxidation if a sufficient amount of an appropriate surface-active compound (*e.g.*, non-ionic detergents Lubrol or Brij) has been added to the reaction mixture. In the presence of 0.02% Lubrol PX the addition of 0.1-2.0 mM $CaCl_2$ has not been capable of increasing the reaction steady-state velocity in the system at any pH (6–9) or LA concentration (25 to 100 µM). In the absence of Lubrol PX Ca(II) has slightly increased the reaction steady-state velocity. At the same time, the pronounced increase in optical density of the reaction solution without the detergent and the enzymes has been observed. Thus the resulting kinetic curves of the enzymatic reaction have been heavily distorted by high and variable turbidity. The latter is frequently misinterpreted as an increase of the enzyme activity while using the standard spectrophotometric assay.

In conclusion, we would like to state that data obtained in different experimental conditions by various research teams can be alternatively interpreted even with the same type of LO. The data clearly demonstrates the crucial role of the lipid phase in the lipoxygenase catalysis. Frequently interfacial phenomena are not taken into account while studying the enzymatic reaction *in vitro* and *in vivo* (*e.g.*, 5- and 12-LOs catalysis, translocation, or inhibition), that leads to the incorrect conclusions about the catalytic and regulatory properties of LOs. The latter can be—and must be—overcome by: i) choosing the correct experimental conditions; ii) taking into account physicochemical properties of all reaction components; and, iii) standardizing the enzyme assays.

REFERENCES

1. Butovich IA, Kukhar VP. Amphiphilic aliphatic acids as activators of 5-lipoxygenase. The adsorption-micellar regulatory mechanizm. Dokl Biochem. 1991: 316(1-6):33-37.
2. Butovich IA, Tsys' EV, Babenko VM, Kharchenko OV, Kukhar VP. In vitro activation of 5-LO caused by natural and synthetic amphiphiles. In:The 8th Int Conf Prostagland Rel Comp, Montreal, July 26-31, 1991:138.
3. Butovich IA, Tsys' EV, Mogilevich TV, Kukhar VP. The influence of physicochemical factors on linoleic acid oxidation by lipoxygenase. Bioorg. Khim 1991; 17(10):1273-1280.
4. Butovich IA, Parshikova TV, Babenko VM, Livarchuk LV, Kharchenko OV, Kukhar VP. Regulation of 5-lipoxygenase activity in the reaction of linoleic acid oxidation by phospholipids. Biol.Mem 1993, 6(6):791-800.

Advances in Prostaglandin, Thromboxane,
and Leukotriene Research, Vol. 23,
edited by B. Samuelsson et al.
Raven Press, Ltd., New York © 1995

OXYGENATION OF ARACHIDONYLETHANOLAMIDE (ANANDAMIDE) BY LIPOXYGENASES

N. Ueda, K. Yamamoto, Y. Kurahashi, S. Yamamoto, M. Ogawa*, N. Matsuki*, I. Kudo*, H. Shinkai[+], E. Shirakawa[+] and T. Tokunaga[+]

*Department of Biochemistry, Tokushima University, School of Medicine, Tokushima 770, *Faculty of Pharmaceutical Sciences, the University of Tokyo, Tokyo 113, and [+]Japan Tobacco Inc., Central Pharmaceutical Research Institute, Takatsuki, Osaka 569, Japan.*

Recently, an endogenous ligand for cannabinoid receptors was isolated from porcine brain by Devane and others (1). The compound was referred to as anandamide, and its chemical structure was determined as ethanolamide of arachidonic acid (Fig. 1). It is known that rabbit reticulocyte 15-lipoxygenase (2) and porcine leukocyte 12-lipoxygenase (3) are highly active not only with free arachidonic acid but also with unsaturated fatty acids of phospholipids and cholesterol ester. However, 12-lipoxygenase of human platelets is almost inactive (3). In view of these findings we were interested to examine whether the arachidonic moiety of anandamide could be oxygenated by various mammalian lipoxygenases.

We prepared ^{14}C-labeled anandamide, and incubated it with various lipoxygenases. The products were separated with thin-layer chromatography, and distribution of radioactivity was visualized by an imaging analyzer Fujix BAS 2000. Immunoaffinity-purified 5-lipoxygenase of porcine leukocytes was totally inactive with anandamide. In contrast, porcine leukocyte 12-lipoxygenase, which was also highly immunoaffinity-purified, produced a polar compound. Purified recombinant human platelet 12-lipoxygenase produced a faint, but significant band. Reticulocyte and soybean 15-lipoxygenases were highly active with anandamide. We should note that these bands were shifted slightly to more polar bands by sodium borohydride reduction, suggesting that the primary products were hydroperoxides. The reactivity with anandamide was also demonstrated by spectrophotometric assay. When absorption at 240 nm was monitored for a conjugated diene, the reaction of porcine leukocyte 12-lipoxygenase with anandamide proceeded as fast as arachidonic acid oxygenation. In contrast, the reaction of human platelet 12-lipoxygenase with anandamide was much slower.

We examined concentration-dependent lipoxygenase activities with free arachidonic acid and anandamide. For porcine leukocyte 12-lipoxygenase and rabbit reticulocyte and soybean 15-lipoxygenases, there were apparently no big differences in Km and Vmax between the two substrates. The reactivity of human platelet 12-lipoxygenase with anandamide was much lower than its arachidonic acid oxygenation. 5-Lipoxygenase was totally inactive with anandamide. These results indicated that lipoxygenases capable of oxygenating phospholipids could react actively with anandamide. These lipoxygenases had a wide substrate specificity in terms of carbon number of unsaturated fatty acids; namely, they react with C_{18} fatty acids such as linoleic acid as well as arachidonic acid (4).

For identification of the lipoxygenase products from anandamide, they were reduced with sodium borohydride, and analyzed by reverse-phase HPLC. As monitored at 235 nm, there was no significant peak with 5-lipoxygenase. Leukocyte and platelet 12-lipoxygenases produced a major peak which corresponded with synthetic 12-hydroxy derivative of anandamide (12-HAE). A minor peak corresponding to synthetic 15-hydroxy derivative (15-HAE) was also detected. On the other hand, by incubation with reticulocyte and soybean 15-lipoxygenases, a major peak cochromatographed with 15-HAE. The products were purified with reverse-phase HPLC and their ultraviolet spectra were recorded. Both the major products by leukocyte 12-lipoxygenase and soybean 15-lipoxygenase gave an absorption maximum around 235 nm, suggesting the presence of a *cis, trans*-conjugated diene. We also carried out electron ionization-mass spectrometry for the major product of leukocyte 12-

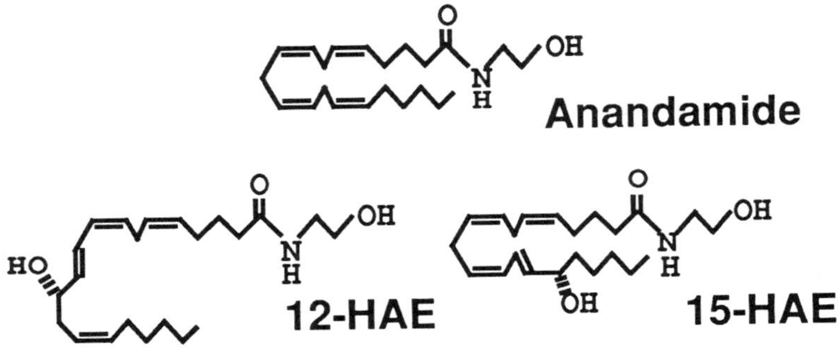

FIG.1. Structures of anandamide and its oxygenated derivatives.

lipoxygenase. Significant ion peaks included m/z 363 (M), 345 (dehydration peak of M), 252 (formed by cleavage between C_{12} and C_{13}), 234 (dehydration peak of 252, base peak) and 62 (protonated ethanolamine). Characteristic ions of the major product of soybean 15-lipoxygenase included m/z 363, 345, 292 (formed by cleavage between C_{15} and C_{16}), 274 (formed by dehydration of 292), 211 (produced by cleavage between C_{10} and C_{11}) and 62. Together with determination of molecular formulae by high-resolution FAB mass spectrometry and NMR spectra, these lipoxygenase products were identified as ethanolamides of 12- and 15-hydroxyeicosatetraenoic acids, respectively (Fig. 1). Thus, each lipoxygenase showed a regiospecificity of oxygenation with anandamide as substrate.

We were interested in pharmacological activities of these oxygenated derivatives of anandamide. Anandamide was reported to inhibit electrically-evoked contraction of vas deferens isolated from mice (1). We reproduced this inhibitory effect of anandamide with an IC_{50} value at 170 nM. 15-HAE also showed a significant activity, while 12-HAE was almost inactive. Thus, the biological activity of anandamide could be modulated by 12-lipoxygenase.

Previously, N-acylethanolamine phospholipids were found in the brain and infarcted myocardium, and a phospholipase D was shown to release N-acylethanolamine (5). Anandamide produced in this possible pathway may be hydrolyzed to free arachidonic acid and ethanolamine by a certain amidase. The lipoxygenase-catalyzed oxygenation of anandamide may lead to an alternative metabolic pathway to control the biological activity of this compound.

REFERENCES

1. Devane WA, Hanus L, Breuer A *et al.* Isolation and structure of a brain constituent that binds to the cannabinoid receptor. *Science* 1992; 258: 1946-49.
2. Murray JJ and Brash AR. Rabbit reticulocyte lipoxygenase catalyzes specific 12(S) and 15(S) oxygenation of arachidonoyl-phosphatidylcholine. *Arch. Biochem. Biophys.* 1988; 265, 514-23.
3. Takahashi Y, Glasgow WC, Suzuki H. *et al.* Investigation of the oxygenation of phospholipids by the porcine leukocyte and human platelet arachidonate 12-lipoxygenases. *Eur. J. Biochem.* 1993; 218, 165-71.
4. Yamamoto S. Mammalian lipoxygenases: molecular structures and functions. *Biochim. Biophys. Acta* 1992; 1128, 117-31.
5. Schmid PC, Reddy PV, Natarajan V, and Schmid HHO. Metabolism of N-acylethanolamine phospholipids by a mammalian phosphodiesterase of the phospholipase D type. *J. Biol. Chem.* 1983; 258, 9302-06.

Advances in Prostaglandin, Thromboxane,
and Leukotriene Research, Vol. 23,
edited by B. Samuelsson et al.
Raven Press, Ltd., New York © 1995

Molecular Cloning and Expression of Human Leukotriene C_4 Synthase

Dean J. Welsch, David P. Creely, Karl J. Mathis,
Scott D. Hauser, and Peter C. Isakson

Searle Research and Development, Monsanto Company,
700 Chesterfield Village Parkway, St. Louis, MO 63198

The peptidoleukotrienes (LTC_4, LTD_4, and LTE_4) are potent biological mediators derived from arachidonic acid in response to a variety of immunologic and inflammatory stimuli (1,2). They were first isolated and identified as the slow-reacting-substance of anaphylaxis (SRS-A) and are released from the lung tissue of asthmatics upon exposure to specific allergens (3). Additionally, exogenous application of these mediators results in many phenomena characteristic of asthma including pulmonary smooth muscle contraction, vasoconstriction, increased vascular permeability, increased mucus secretion, and eosinophil infiltration into airways (4-8). Furthermore, compounds that inhibit the production (5-lipoxygenase inhibitors and 5-lipoxygenase activating protein antagonists) or action (LTD_4 receptor antagonists) of the peptidoleukotrienes have been found to be efficacious in the treatment of asthma in clinical trials (3). Taken together, these data demonstrate that the peptidoleukotrienes play a prominent role in the pathogenesis of human bronchial asthma.

Leukotriene C_4 synthase (LTC_4S) is a unique membrane-bound enzyme that catalyzes the committed step in the biosynthesis of all of the peptidoleukotrienes. Specifically, LTC_4S conjugates reduced glutathione with the unstable epoxide LTA_4 to form LTC_4 and, as such, is a glutathione S-transferase activity. It has been reported that LTC_4S, like other known glutathione S-transferases, is enzymatically active as a multimer composed of low molecular mass subunits (9). However, unlike other members of the glutathione S-transferase multigene family, LTC_4S does not appear to be involved in cellular detoxification but rather appears to be exclusively committed to the biosynthesis of LTC_4 (10). Nicholson et al. reported the purification to homogeneity and amino-terminal sequence of human LTC_4S from THP-1 cells (9). They found LTC_4S to be a homodimer consisting of 18-kDa subunits.

To better understand the role that LTC_4S and it's products play in inflammation, an effort was initiated to clone and express the enzyme. We report here results from those efforts.

IMMUNOPRECIPITATION OF LTC₄S ACTIVITY

To immunologically characterize the association between LTC₄S biological activity and protein sequence, antisera was raised to a synthetic peptide of the partial sequence reported for LTC₄S. The antisera was used to immunoprecipitate LTC₄S activity from a crude detergent-solubilized preparation of LTC₄S enzyme prepared from THP-1 cells, a cell line that we and others have found to express high levels of LTC₄S biological activity. Following incubation of antisera (pre-immune sera control) with the crude enzyme preparation, the immune complexes generated were rendered insoluble by addition of excess protein A immobilized on agarose. Approximately 85% of the total LTC₄-biosynthetic activity was associated with the insoluble complex when peptide antisera was used. Contrastingly, roughly 95% of the activity remained in the soluble supernatant with control antisera. The results of this study provide independent immunological evidence that the reported sequence is associated with LTC₄S activity.

MOLECULAR CLONING AND PROPERTIES OF HUMAN LTC₄S

Oligonucleotides were designed based on the partial amino acid sequence of LTC₄S and a DNA fragment of the appropriate size was amplified from THP-1 poly A+ RNA using rt-PCR. The primer-independent DNA sequence that was amplified encoded amino acids identical to the published protein sequence. However, the amino acid at position 21, identified as glycine by protein sequencing, was found to be tyrosine based on the amplified DNA sequence. A 679 bp fragment of cDNA was obtained from a human THP-1 cDNA library using oligonucleotides based on the primer-independent rt-PCR amplified sequence. The nucleotide sequence contains an open reading frame that encodes a protein of 150 amino acids having an average molecular weight of 16,568 amu; this compares favorably with the molecular weight determined by SDS-PAGE for the purified protein (9). The deduced amino acid sequence contains 94 hydrophobic and 34 polar but uncharged amino acids. The calculated pI of 11.1 reflects the presence of 16 positively and 6 negatively charged residues in the protein. Analysis of the deduced sequence revealed two Ser-Ala-Arg consensus sequences for protein kinase C phosphorylation (11) at positions 28-30 and 111-113, suggesting that human LTC₄S may be a phosphoregulated enzyme. Additionally, the sequence contains a potential N-linked glycosylation site (Asn-Cys-Ser at positions 55-57). Finally, the sequence contains cysteine residues at positions 56 and 82; whether these residues are involved in forming enzymatically active LTC₄S homodimer has yet to be determined.

HOMOLOGY BETWEEN HUMAN LTC₄S AND 5-LIPOXYGENASE ACTIVATING PROTEIN (FLAP)

A search of the Swiss protein database (Version 28) using the Wisconsin Package indicated that the amino acid sequence for human LTC₄S was unique, and that it showed no homology to other glutathione S-transferases. Interestingly, LTC₄S is most similar to FLAP at the amino acid sequence level (32% identity, 53% similarity). Hydropathy analysis of LTC₄S identified three regions of 20-30 residues that are each predicted to form membrane-spanning domains (12). These membrane-spanning domains, as well as the two hydrophilic loops, can be closely aligned with those previously reported for FLAP (13).

EXPRESSION OF HUMAN LTC$_4$S

The cDNA encoding human LTC$_4$S was subcloned into appropriate vectors and subsequently expressed in bacterial, insect, and mammalian cell systems. The LTC$_4$S activity, relative to total cellular protein, was determined for mock- and cDNA-transfected cell lysates by quantitation of the LTC$_4$ produced in incubation mixtures containing LTA$_4$ and reduced glutathione (Table 1).

Table 1: Expression of Human LTC$_4$S

Expression system	LTC$_4$ Production (ng/µg total cell protein)	
	Mock transfected	cDNA transfected
Bacterial	≤ 0.002	1.5
Insect	≤ 0.5	275.4
Mammalian	≤ 0.05	21.7

In conclusion, we report the molecular cloning of LTC$_4$S from the human monocytic cell line THP-1 and expression of active enzyme in bacterial, insect, and mammalian cells. LTC$_4$S appears to be a unique glutathione S-transferase that is strikingly similar to FLAP, another protein involved in metabolism of arachidonic acid.

REFERENCES

1. Samuelsson B. *Science* 1983;220:568-75.
2. Ford-Hutchinson AW. *Crit Rev Immunol* 1990;10:1-12.
3. Margolskee DJ. *Ann NY Acad Sci* 1990;629:148-56.
4. Casale TB, Wood D, Richerson HB, Zehr B, Zabala DC, & Hunninghake GW. *J Clin Invest* 1987;80:1507-11.
5. Holroyde MC, Altounyan REC, Cole M, Dixon M, & Elliot EV. *Lancet* 1981;ii:17-8.
6. Griffin M, Weiss JW, Leitch AG, et al. *N Engl J Med* 1983;308:436-9.
7. Barnes NC, Piper PJ, & Costello JF. *Thorax* 1984;39:500-4.
8. Laitinen LA, Laitinen A, Haahtela T, Vilkka V, Spur BW, & Lee TH. *Lancet* 1993;341:989-90.
9. Nicholson DW, Ali A, Vaillancourt JP, et al. *Proc Natl Acad Sci USA* 1993;90:2015-9.
10. Nicholson DW, Ali A, Klemba MW, Munday NA, Zamboni RJ, & Ford-Hutchinson AW. *J Biol Chem* 1992;267:17849-57.
11. Woodget JR, Gould KL, & Hunter T. *Eur J Biochem* 1986;161:177-84.
12. Kyte J & Doolittle RF. *J Mol Biol* 1982;157:105-132.
13. Vickers PJ, Adam M, Charleson S, Coppolino MG, Evans JF, & Mancini JA. *Mol Pharmacol* 1992;42:94-102.

Advances in Prostaglandin, Thromboxane,
and Leukotriene Research, Vol. 23,
edited by B. Samuelsson et al.
Raven Press, Ltd., New York © 1995

CHARACTERIZATION OF HUMAN LTC$_4$ SYNTHASE

Ambereen Ali, Donald W. Nicholson and Anthony W. Ford-Hutchinson

Merck Frosst Centre for Therapeutic Research, Pointe Claire, Dorval, Quebec, Canada

LTC$_4$ synthase catalyzes the conjugation of LTA$_4$ with reduced glutathione, an enzymic activity now known to be distinct from other glutathione S-transferases (GSTs). Thus LTC$_4$ synthase is a microsomal enzyme separable from the soluble forms of GSTs (α, π, and μ) by differential centrifugation and chromatographic techniques (1). The enzyme was also separable from microsomal GST by differential detergent solubilization (1-4). LTC$_4$ synthase demonstrated high specific activity for the conjugation of glutathione to LTA$_4$ but not to any of the electrophilic GST substrates such as 1-chloro-2,4-dinitrobenzene, 4-nitrobenzyl chloride or 1,2-epoxy-3-(4-nitrophenoxy) propane (substrate for the θ class of GST). Microsomal GST activity was also activated by N-ethylmaleimide, whereas LTC$_4$ synthase activity was not (1,5). LTC$_4$ synthase and cytosolic GSTs also demonstrated large differences in sensitivity to inhibitors such as Rose Bengal (10-20-fold difference in IC$_{50}$ values). Diethylcarbamazine, a known SRS-A inhibitor, selectively inhibited LTC$_4$ synthase but not microsomal GST in RBL cells and Triton X-100 selectively solubilized and potentiated microsomal GST activity but inhibited LTC$_4$ synthase activity (5). Finally, the N-terminal sequence of LTC$_4$ synthase was not homologous to any sequence available in the databases including the GST sequences (3).

LTC$_4$ synthase may be subject to end-product inhibiton and thus a novel photoaffinity ligand was constructed based on LTC$_4$, to identify potential polypeptide candidates for LTC$_4$ synthase (1,4). The high affinity of the LTC$_4$-based photoaffinity ligand was then demonstrated by the ability of azido ^{127}I-LTC$_4$ to inhibit LTC$_4$ synthase activity (IC$_{50}$ value = 7.0 μM; (1)). The LTC$_4$-based photoaffinity ligand was used to probe U937, differentiated U937 (dU937) and THP-1 cell microsomal membranes. Two polypeptides (18 kDa and 27 kDa) were specifically labelled in dU937 microsomal membranes (1) and only one polypeptide (18 kDa) was specifically labelled in THP-1 cells (2). However, the possibility that this 18 kDa polypeptide was microsomal GST, an enzyme with a molecular mass of 17.2 kDa, had to be addressed. The 18 kDa polypeptide was determined to be the most probable candidate for being LTC$_4$ synthase or a subunit of this enzyme based on several observations. First, photolabelling of the 18 kDa polypeptide was specifically competed for by 100,000-fold lower concentrations of LTC$_4$ than reduced glutathione, whereas the opposite was observed for the specific labelling of the 27 kDa polypeptide. This 27 kDa polypeptide was most likely a contaminating cytosolic GST (1,2). Secondly, with the differentiation of U937 cells in the presence of Me$_2$SO there was a concomitant increase in the specific photolabelling of the 18 kDa polypeptide and LTC$_4$ synthase biosynthetic activity in the microsomal membranes of these cells (1). Thirdly, a comprehensive study of the specific photolabelling of this polypeptide in THP-1 cell microsomal membranes demonstrated that this polypeptide is unlikely to be microsomal GST (2). The specifically labelled 18 kDa polypeptide in THP-1 cell microsomal membranes was strongly competed for by LTC$_4$ but not at all by up to 1 mM GSH, indicating that this polypeptide had high affinity for the arachidonate backbone and not the glutathione moiety of LTC$_4$. Furthermore, the rank order of potencies of the structurally related leukotrienes and S-hexyl glutathione for competing for the specific labelling of the 18 kDa polypeptide corresponded exactly with their ability to attenuate LTC$_4$ synthase activity but not microsomal GST activity. Moreover, the specifically labelled 18 kDa polypeptide could be selectively solubilized by taurocholate consistent with the solubilization of LTC$_4$ synthase but not microsomal GST with this detergent. Fourthly, in a highly purified preparation of LTC$_4$ synthase (10,000-fold) from dU937 cells which contained three major polypeptide constituents with molecular masses of 18, 25 and 37 kDa, only the 18 kDa polypeptide was specifically photolabelled by azido ^{125}I-LTC$_4$ (4). These experimental approaches established that the photoaffinity ligand specifically labelled LTC$_4$ synthase and not microsomal GST.

Although several investigators have attempted to purify LTC$_4$ synthase from a variety of sources, the purification of this enzyme has been hampered by many factors. LTC$_4$ synthase is a hydrophobic, membrane-bound enzyme which loses activity when removed from its native membrane environment. LTC$_4$ synthase was also found to be very low in abundance in the human cells and leukemia cell lines tested. Furthermore, accurate measurement of LTC$_4$ synthase activity and storage of the enzyme required the presence of several cofactors including reduced glutathione, detergents, and lipids, particularly when the enzyme was in a highly purified state (4). A comprehensive analysis of LTC$_4$ synthase in U937 cells defined the several critical parameters that modulated the activity of the purified enzyme. LTC$_4$ synthase biosynthetic activity was stimulated by the presence of divalent cations, specifically, $Mg^{2+} > Ca^{2+}$ even in crude preparations (4). Once the enzyme was purified greater than 500-fold detection of its activity became dependent on both the presence of Mg^{2+} and phosphatidylcholine (4). The substrate, reduced glutathione (2-4 mM), stabilized LTC$_4$ synthase activity, particularly during storage, however, at concentrations greater than 5 mM, the presence of this substrate was toxic and irreversibly inactivated the enzyme (4).

Using the above information, LTC$_4$ synthase was purified to homogeneity from THP-1 cells in a 3-step procedure including anion-exchange, LTC$_2$ affinity and gel filtration chromatography (3). The latter step not only purified the enzyme to homogeneity but also determined a native molecular mass of approximately 39 kDa suggesting that LTC$_4$ synthase most likely functions as a homodimer (3). The 18 kDa polypeptide in inactive preparations of LTC$_4$ synthase eluted at a volume corresponding to 15-20 kDa indicating that the enzyme was only active in its dimeric form.

The N-terminal sequence of LTC$_4$ synthase had four notable features (3). First, LTC$_4$ synthase contains an N-terminal methionine residue indicating that the enzyme is most likely not proteolytically processed *in vivo*. Secondly, most of the 35 amino acids identified were hydrophobic, consistent with the membrane-bound localization of the enzyme. Thirdly, a consensus sequence for Protein Kinase C (PKC)-mediated phosphorylation was present in the N-terminal sequence (Ser-Ala-Arg) at position 28-30 suggesting that the activity of the enzyme may be phosphoregulated *in vivo*. Finally, the identified sequence was unique and not homologous to any known sequences contained in available databases.

The identification of a putative PKC consensus sequence in the N-terminal amino acid residues of LTC$_4$ synthase prompted a study which demonstrated that when neutrophilic or eosinophilic HL-60 cells were challenged with A23187 in the presence of PMA, the biosynthesis of LTC$_4$ and its metabolite LTD$_4$ were specifically attenuated whereas biosynthesis of the non-cysteinyl leukotrienes, LTA$_4$ and LTB$_4$, were unaffected (6,7). We investigated the involvement of other kinases in the regulation of LTC$_4$ biosynthesis with the use of selective inhibitors. The PMA-mediated inhibition of cysteinyl leukotriene biosynthesis was prevented only by PKC-specific inhibitors but not by any other kinase inhibitors (PKA, TK) excluding their involvement in this regulatory mechanism. Similar results were obtained when exogenous LTC$_4$ synthase substrates were added to the cells to measure the effect of PKC activation on LTC$_4$ synthase directly.These studies clearly demonstrated that the inhibitory effects of PKC activation were due to inhibition of the LTC$_4$ synthase enzyme itself and not upstream enzymes in the biosynthetic pathway (7). Kinetic analysis of LTC$_4$ synthase biosynthetic activity indicated that phosphorylation of LTC$_4$ synthase or a putative regulator of its activity causes a specific decrease in the V_{max} of the enzyme without any effect on the K_m, and thus demonstrates non-competitive inhibition which is typical for a phosphoregulatory mechanism (7).

Contrary to the effect on cysteinyl leukotriene biosynthesis, the formation of PGE$_2$ and TXB$_2$ was elevated 2 to 3-fold following PMA treatment and this too was prevented by staurosporine (7). Based on these studies, a model was proposed for the regulation of eicosanoid biosynthesis in eosinophils (7). First, activation of PKC can stimulate the release of arachidonic acid by stimulating cPLA$_2$ either directly or via MAP kinase (8). Secondly, PKC activation results in the induction of cyclooxygenase-2 (9). At the same time there is an attenuation of cysteinyl leukotriene biosynthesis (7), thus the net effect of PKC activation would be a shift in the profile of mediators synthesized by the eosinophil from leukotrienes to prostanoids.

References:

1. Nicholson DW, Ali A, Klemba MW, Munday NA, Zamboni RJ and Ford-Hutchinson AW. *J Biol Chem* 1992;267:17849-57.
2. Ali A, Zamboni RJ, Ford-Hutchinson AW and Nicholson DW. *FEBS Lett* 1993;317: 195-201.
3. Nicholson DW, Ali A, Vaillancourt JP, Calaycay J.R., Mumford RA, Zamboni RJ and Ford-Hutchinson AW. *Proc Natl Acad Sci USA* 1993;90: 2015-9.
4. Nicholson DW, Klemba MW, Rasper DM, Metters KM, Zamboni RJ and Ford-Hutchinson AW. *Eur J Biochem* 1992; 209: 725-734.
5. Bach MK, Brashler JR, Rebecca EP and Morton DR. *J Allergy Clin Immunol* 1984 ;74: 353-357.
6. Kargman S, Ali A, Vaillancourt JP, Evans JF and Nicholson DW. *Mol Pharmacol* 1994; In press.
7. Ali A, Ford-Hutchinson AW and Nicholson DW. *J Immunol* 1994; In press.
8. Lin L-L, Wartmann M, Lin AY, Knopf JL, Seth, A and Davis RJ. *Cell* 1993; 72: 269-278.
9. Kujubu DA, Fletcher BS, Varnum BC, Lim RW and Herschman HR. *J Biol Chem* 1991; 266:12866.

Advances in Prostaglandin, Thromboxane, and Leukotriene Research, Vol. 23,
edited by B. Samuelsson et al.
Raven Press, Ltd., New York © 1995

Human Umbilical Vein Endothelial Cells Contain Leukotriene A$_4$ Hydrolase Which Is Regulated by Phosphorylation

Irina V. Rybina, Willis Burton and Steven J. Feinmark

Department of Pharmacology, Columbia University, College of Physicians and Surgeons, New York, New York, USA 10032

Leukotriene (LT)A$_4$ hydrolase is a widely distributed enzyme which converts LTA$_4$ into LTB$_4$. This enzyme has recently been recognized as a member of the family of zinc metalloproteinases and, as such, possesses an aminopeptidase activity. Numerous studies have focussed on LT metabolism in endothelial cells (EC) since the LT have potent proinflammatory effects on the vasculature inducing leukocyte adhesion to EC, edema formation and vasoconstriction. Work from several labs including our own demonstrated that EC can take up LTA$_4$ from activated leukocytes and metabolize this lipid to LTC$_4$ but found no evidence that these same cells could convert LTA$_4$ to LTB$_4$ (1-3). In spite of these data, immunohistochemical analysis suggested that LTA$_4$ hydrolase was present in EC (4) and a subsequent biochemical report presented evidence that some human umbilical vein endothelial cell (HUVEC) cultures could convert LTA$_4$ to LTB$_4$ (5). Consequently, we decided to ask whether HUVEC contain LTA$_4$ hydrolase and if so, determine how the activity was regulated.

METHODS

Human umbilical vein endothelial cells were obtained and cultured using standard methods. Most experiments were carried out on cells after one passage. LTA$_4$ hydrolase activity in monolayer cultures was assessed by incubating the cells with LTA$_4$ (2-20 μM) in phosphate buffered saline with 0.5% human serum albumin (HSA) for 30 min. LT were analyzed by reverse phase HPLC after ethanol precipitation of the albumin (5).

Recombinant LTA$_4$ hydrolase was expressed in E. coli as described elsewhere
(6). HUVEC homogenates were prepared by sonication and in some cases
LTA$_4$ hydrolase was recovered from this preparation either by Mono-Q
chromatography or by immunoprecipitation. Activity of purified enzyme was
tested in 0.1 M Tris-HCl (pH 7.8) with HSA (0.2%). Aminopeptidase activity
was measured as reported by others (7).

Immunodetection of LTA$_4$ hydrolase in cell lysates was done with standard
methods of SDS-PAGE, electroblotting to nitrocellulose, incubation with anti-
LTA$_4$ hydrolase antibody and detection with a commercial alkaline phosphatase
detection kit (Amersham). In some experiments, the levels of LTA$_4$ hydrolase
were quantified by densitometery after immunoblotting. Levels of mRNA for
the LTA$_4$ hydrolase were measured by Northern blotting using standard
procedures.

RESULTS AND DISCUSSION

LTA$_4$ hydrolase was detected in EC lysates by both Northern and Western
blotting. In spite of these data, no LTA$_4$ hydrolase activity could be detected in
the crude cell lysate. LTA$_4$ hydrolase was purified by ion exchange
chromatography from EC lysates and detected by Western blot analysis of the
resulting fractions. The HUVEC enzyme was found to have similar
characteristics to the recombinant enzyme on Mono-Q and after SDS-PAGE
(Figure 1) but did not have detectable LTA$_4$ hydrolase activity. In contrast, the

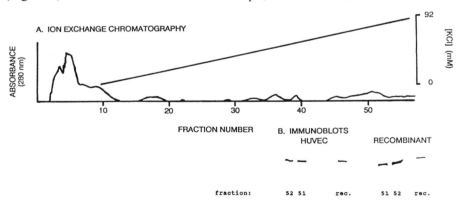

FIG. 1.   FPLC purification of HUVEC LTA$_4$ hydrolase.   HUVEC were
collected from monolayer cultures by scraping and centrifugation. A
homogenate was prepared and fractionated on a Mono-Q column eluted
at 2 ml/min, running 20 mM Tris on a linear gradient to 20 mM Tris,
0.15 M KCl over 75 min.   Protein was detected by UV absorbance
(panel A).   Recombinant LTA$_4$ hydrolase was purified in parallel and
fractions from each run were subjected to SDS-PAGE and
immunoblotting (panel B).

HUVEC enzyme was an active aminopeptidase with L-alanine-p-nitroanilide as substrate (specific activity, 2536 nmol/mg·min).

In order to determine whether HUVEC homogenates contained a factor which inhibited LTA$_4$ hydrolase activity, recombinant enzyme was incubated with LTA$_4$ in the presence or absence of cell homogenate and the production of LTB$_4$ was measured. In these studies, HUVEC homogenates significantly inhibited recombinant LTA$_4$ hydrolase ($24.8 \pm 2.4\%$, $p < 0.001$).

These data suggest that HUVEC contain LTA$_4$ hydrolase which under basal conditions functions solely as an aminopeptidase and cannot generate LTB$_4$. Regulation of this enzyme appears to be due to a post-translational modification rather than a soluble inhibitory factor since purification does not activate HUVEC LTA$_4$ hydrolase. We have also found that LTA$_4$ hydrolase is a substrate for PKC and propose that phosphorylation is responsible for the regulation of this enzyme.

ACKNOWLEDGMENTS

This work was supported by a grant from the NHLBI (HL-38312). Dr. Feinmark was a Boehringer-Ingelheim Established Investigator of the American Heart Association.

REFERENCES

1. Feinmark SJ, Cannon PJ. Endothelial cell leukotriene C$_4$ synthesis results from intercellular transfer of leukotriene A$_4$ synthesized by polymorphonuclear leukocytes. *J Biol Chem* 1986;261:16466-72.

2. Ibe BO, Campbell WB. Synthesis and metabolism of leukotrienes by human endothelial cells: Influence on prostacyclin release. *Biochim Biophys Acta* 1988;960:309-21.

3. Maclouf J, Murphy RC, Henson PM. Transcellular Sulfidopeptide Leukotriene Biosynthetic Capacity of Vascular Cells. *Blood* 1989;74:703-7.

4. Ohishi N, Minami M, Kobayashi J, et al. Immunological quantitation and immunohistochemical localization of leukotriene A$_4$ hydrolase in guinea pig tissues. *J Biol Chem* 1990;265:7520-5.

5. Claesson H-E, Haeggström J. Human endothelial cells stimulate leukotriene synthesis and convert granulocyte released leukotriene A$_4$ into leukotrienes B$_4$, C$_4$, D$_4$ and E$_4$. *Eur J Biochem* 1988;173:93-100.

6. Minami M, Minami Y, Emori Y, et al. Expression of human leukotriene A$_4$ hydrolase cDNA in Escherichia coli. *FEBS Lett* 1988;229:279-82.

7. Haeggström J, Wetterholm A, Vallee BL, Samuelsson, B. Leukotriene A$_4$ hydrolase: An epoxide hydrolase with peptidase activity. *Biochem Biophys Res Commun* 1990;173:431-7.

Advances in Prostaglandin, Thromboxane, and Leukotriene Research, Vol. 23,
edited by B. Samuelsson et al.
Raven Press, Ltd., New York © 1995

Metal Inhibition of LTA4 Hydrolase and Cellular 5-Lipoxygenase Activity

Anders Wetterholm, Luigi Macchia and Jesper Z. Haeggström

Department of Medical Biochemistry and Biophysics, Karolinska Institutet, S-171 77 Stockholm, Sweden.

Leukotriene (LT) A4 hydrolase is a zinc metalloenzyme which hydrolyzes LTA4 to LTB4. In addition to this epoxide hydrolase activity, the enzyme is also able to cleave peptide bonds (1). Treatment of the enzyme with the chelating agent 1,10-phenanthroline results in an apoenzyme which is devoid of zinc and exhibits significantly reduced catalytic activities (2, 3). It was possible to regain both activities by treating the apoenzyme with stoichiometric amounts of zinc, which demonstrated the catalytic role of the metal. Concentrations of zinc exceeding a 1:1 molar ratio (metal:enzyme) were inhibitory for the peptidase activity, a finding which prompted us to study the effects of metal ions on enzyme activities.

MATERIALS AND METHODS

A detailed description of materials and methods is reported in Ref. 4.

RESULTS AND DISCUSSION

Metal inhibition of purified LTA4 hydrolase

LTA4 hydrolase was inhibited by several divalent cations with different specificity and potency for the epoxide hydrolase and peptidase activities, respectively (Table 1). The epoxide hydrolase activity was inhibited by both zinc and cadmium with IC$_{50}$ of 10 µM, whereas the IC$_{50}$ value for nickel was 300 µM. Cobalt did not inhibit this enzyme activity at the highest concentration tested (1 mM). The peptidase activity was inhibited by all these cations with IC$_{50}$ ranging from 0.1 µM for zinc to 10 µM for cobalt. Thus, the peptidase activity was in general 100-fold more sensitive to inhibition by these metal salts. In contrast, copper was equally effective as an inhibitor of both catalytic activities with IC$_{50}$ of 2-3 µM.

Table 1. *Effects of metal ions on the catalytic activities of LTA$_4$ hydrolase.*

	Epoxide hydrolase activity (IC$_{50}$, µM)	Peptidase activity (IC$_{50}$, µM)
Zn	10	0.1
Cd	10	0.5
Ni	300	0.5
Co	>1000	10
Cu	3	2

A characteristic feature, which was only observed for copper, was that the peptidase substrate alanine-4-nitroanilide was able to prevent the inhibition by this metal salt suggesting that copper inhibition is an active site directed process.

The mechanism of zinc inhibition has been studied in some detail for certain other zinc hydrolases. For thermolysin, the inhibitory zinc ion presumably binds to His-231, a residue which is supposed to serve as a proton donor in the catalytic reaction (5). In the case of carboxypeptidase A, zinc inhibition is probably due to the formation of a zinc hydroxide bridge between Glu-270 and the catalytic zinc atom of the enzyme (6). Regarding LTA$_4$ hydrolase, we have no data to support either of the two mechanisms.

Effects of zinc on cellular leukotriene biosynthesis

Next we investigated if zinc could affect cellular leukotriene biosynthesis. Micromolar concentrations of zinc were found to inhibit LTB$_4$ formation in both intact human polymorphonuclear leukocytes stimulated by the calcium ionophore A23187 and homogenates of RBL-1 cells incubated with arachidonic acid.

Table 2. *Effects of zinc on enzymes involved in leukotriene biosynthesis.*

	IC$_{50}$ (µM)		
Celltype	5-LO	LTA$_4$ hydrolase	LTC$_4$ synthase
PMNL	2-3	>100	-
RBL-1	0.5-1.5	-	1000

5-Lipoxygenase activity in intact human polymorphonuclear leukocytes (PMNL) and homogenates of rat basophilic leukemia cells (RBL-1) was determined by incubating the respective preparation with the calcium ionophore A23187 (5 µM) and arachidonic acid (45 µM), respectively. LTA$_4$ hydrolase and LTC$_4$ synthase activities were analyzed from incubations with exogenous LTA$_4$ (6 µM). Product formation was analyzed by RP-HPLC.

However, in parallel to the inhibition of LTB$_4$ biosynthesis, both the formation of the nonenzymatic hydrolysis products of LTA$_4$ (Δ^6-*trans*-LTB$_4$ and 12-epi-Δ^6-*trans*-LTB$_4$) and 5-HETE were equally affected. In addition, when these preparations were incubated with exogenous LTA$_4$, formation of LTB$_4$ was not inhibited by zinc up to a concentration of 100 μM (Table 2). These findings suggested that the effect of zinc was not related to inhibition of LTA$_4$ hydrolase but rather to a direct or indirect inhibitory effect on the enzyme 5-lipoxygenase in isolated leukocytes or cell homogenates. This interpretation agrees well with a report in which purified recombinant 5-lipoxygenase was completely inhibited by 10 μM zinc (7).

The LTC$_4$ synthase activity in homogenates of RBL-1 cells was also analyzed in the presence of increasing amounts of zinc. In contrast to 5-lipoxygenase, this enzyme activity was found to be very resistant to zinc inhibition and IC$_{50}$ was in the range of 1 mM (Table 2).

Zinc has several anti-inflammatory activities both *in vitro* and *in vivo* (8-10) and it is possible that some of these effects are mediated through inhibition of leukotriene biosynthesis.

ACKNOWLEDGEMENTS

We thank Ms Eva Ohlson for excellent technical assistance. This project was financially supported by the Swedish Medical Research Council (O3X-217 and O3X-10350), Svenska Sällskapet för Medicinsk Forskning, Petrus & Augusta Hedlunds stiftelse, and Magnus Bergvalls stiftelse.

REFERENCES

1. Haeggström JZ, Wetterholm A, Medina JF, Samuelsson B. Leukotriene A$_4$ hydrolase: structural and functional properties of the active center. J. Lipid Mediators 1993;6:1-13.

2. Haeggström JZ, Wetterholm A, Shapiro R, Vallee BL, Samuelsson B. Leukotriene A$_4$ hydrolase: A zinc metalloenzyme. Biochem. Biophys. Res. Commun. 1990;172:965-970.

3. Haeggström JZ, Wetterholm A, Vallee BL, Samuelsson B. Leukotriene A$_4$ hydrolase: An epoxide hydrolase with peptidase activity. Biochem. Biophys. Res. Commun. 1990;173:431-437.

4. Wetterholm A, Macchia L, Haeggström JZ. Zinc and other divalent cations inhibit purified leukotriene A$_4$ hydrolase and leukotriene B$_4$ biosynthesis in human polymorphonuclear leukocytes. Arch. Biochem. Biophys. 1994;311:263-271.

5. Kester WR, Matthews BW. Crystallographic study of the binding of dipeptide inhibitors to thermolysin: Implications for the mechanism of catalysis. Biochemistry 1977;16:2506-2516.

6. Larsen KS, Auld DS. Carboxypeptidase A: Mechanism of zinc inhibition. Biochemistry 1989;28:9620-9625.

7. Percival MD, Denis D, Riendeau D, Gresser MJ. Investigation of the mechanism of non-turnover-dependent inactivation of purified human 5-lipoxygenase. Inactivation by H$_2$O$_2$ and inhibition by metal ions. Eur. J. Biochem. 1992;210:109-117.

8. Baginski B. Alterations of the oxidative metabolism and other microbicidal activities of human polymorphonuclear leukocytes by zinc. Free Rad. Res. Comms. 1990;10:227-235.

9. Cho CH, Dai S, Ogle CW. The effect of zinc on anaphylaxis *in vivo* in the guinea pig. Br. J. Pharmacol. 1977;60:607-608.

10. Chvapil M, Stankov L, Zukoski IV C, Zukoski I C. Inhibition of some functions of polymorphonuclear leukocytes by *in vitro* zinc. J. Lab. Clin. 1977;89:135-146.

Advances in Prostaglandin, Thromboxane,
and Leukotriene Research, Vol. 23,
edited by B. Samuelsson et al.
Raven Press, Ltd., New York © 1995

ENZYMATIC FORMATION OF HEPOXILIN A3

D. Reynaud, P.M. Demin and C.R. Pace-Asciak

Research Institute, Hospital for Sick Children, 555 University Avenue
Toronto, Ontario, CANADA M5G 1X8

We have previously shown that 12(S)-HPETE is converted into hepoxilins (Hx) A3 and B3 through a hemin-catalyzed intramolecular isomerization (2, 4) which was unaffected by heat treatment, hence suggesting a nonenzymatic route of formation. Preferential formation of HxB3 was observed. In the present study we demonstrate the conversion of both arachidonic acid and 12(S)-HPETE by intact pieces of pineal gland into mostly HxA3. HxA3 formation by the pineal was totally abolished from both substrates by boiling of the tissue, indicative of an enzymatic route. These findings lend support to a biological role of HxA3 in the pineal gland as a natural modulator of adenyl cyclase/melatonin formation in this tissue (5).

RESULTS and DISCUSSION

Pineal tissue was isolated as reported previously (5). 12(S/R)-HPETE was prepared through reaction of arachidonic acid with light catalyzed by methylene blue (1) and purified by straight phase HPLC. Incubations with arachidonic acid or 12(S/R)-HPETE were carried out with 1 pineal/tube for 60 min at 37°C. Samples were extractively esterified directly without acidification into the ADAM derivatives through a modification of the procedure of Yamaki and Oh-Ishi (6) and analyzed by HPLC with fluorescence detection. Typical straight phase chromatograms of an incubation of arachidonic acid (left panels) and 12(S/R)-HPETE (right panels) with pineal gland (middle panels) are shown in Figure 1. The corresponding chromatograms of samples derived from the incubation of arachidonic acid and 12(S/R)-HPETE with hemin are shown in the lower panels. The enzymatic process from both arachidonic acid and 12-HPETE greatly favoured HxA3 formation while HxB3 formation was favoured by the hemin-catalyzed pathway. Note that hemin does not catalyze the conversion of arachidonic acid.

Analysis of HxA3 formed from both the pineal experiments and those using hemin on straight phase HPLC revealed the presence of two enantiomers with 8(S) and 8(R)-hydroxyl groups (Figure 1). Figure 2 shows the effect of boiling of the pineal gland as well as hemin on the conversion of arachidonic acid and 12(S/R)-HPETE. It is clear from this data that boiling abolishes the conversion of both substrates *only* by pineal gland but not by hemin clearly demonstrating that pineal tissue contains a heat-sensitive pathway which is responsible for the formation of HxA3.

Further analysis on chiral phase HPLC of the HxA3 formed in these reactions revealed the presence of only *one* configuration of the 11,12-epoxide in the pineal

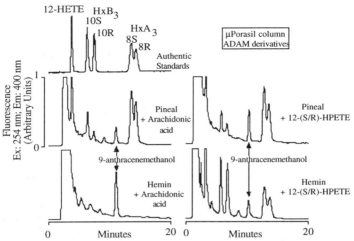

FIG. 1. Straight phase high performance liquid chromatograms of extracts of samples derived from the incubation of arachidonic acid (left panels) or 12(S/R)-HPETE (right panels) with intact pieces of pineal gland (middle panels) or hemin (lower panels). Retention times of authentic standards are shown in the top left panel. Peak labeled 9-anthracenemethanol is a product of the derivatization reagent. Note the different proportions of HxA3 and HxB3 by the pineal gland (which favours formation of the former) and by hemin (which favours formation of HxB3). Note that hemin does not convert arachidonic acid into hepoxilins (lower left panel).

experiments, i.e. 11(S), 12(S), indicating that a *trans* epoxide is formed from only 12(S)-HPETE (data not shown). In contrast, hemin catalyzes the conversion of both 12(S)- and 12(R)-HPETE into HxA3 having the 11,12-epoxide with both the S,S and R,R - *trans* configuration (data not shown). Further analysis by chiral phase also demonstrated the complete removal of 12(S)-HPETE in the pineal gland experiments (with the retention of 12(R)-HPETE) while both 12(S) and 12(R)-HPETE of the same ratio as in starting substrate were observed in the hemin experiments (data not shown).

In conclusion the following observations support an enzymatic process for the formation of HxA3 by the pineal gland: 1) pineal gland selectively utilizes 12(S)-HPETE for its conversion into primarily HxA3 having an 11S,12S-*trans*-configuration of the epoxide, while the nonenzymatic route with hemin catalysis forms mostly HxB3 with HxA3 having both the 11S,12S and 11R,12R-*trans*-epoxide configuration derived from both 12(S) and 12(R)-HPETE, 2) the hydroxyl group at C8 is racemic indicating its formation through a carbonium ion. Previous experiments with [18]oxygen gas have shown that this hydroxyl group originates from the hydroperoxy group of 12-HPETE (2, 4), 3) boiling of the pineal destroyed its ability to convert both arachidonic acid and 12-HPETE into the hepoxilins, and 4) HxA3 formation is favoured by the pineal. In fact our experiments suggest that HxA3 is an enzymatic product while HxB3 formation is probably nonenzymatic. Our present experiments lend support to a biological role for HxA3 in the pineal gland (5) and other tissues (3).

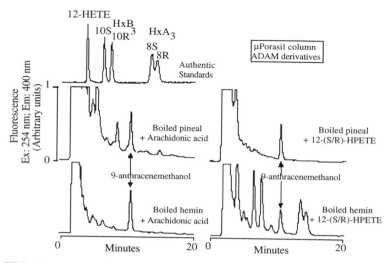

FIG. 2. Effect of boiling of pineal gland (middle panels) and hemin (lower panels) with arachidonic acid (left panels) and 12(S/R)-HPETE (right panels) on the formation of HxA₃ and HxB₃. Straight phase HPLCs are shown. Peak labeled 9-anthracenemethanol is a product of the derivatization reagent. Note that boiling of hemin retains its catalytic conversion of 12-HPETE into the hepoxilins while boiling of the pineal abolishes its 12-HPETE-converting ability indicative of an enzymatic process.

ACKNOWLEDGEMENTS

The financial support of the MRC and of ZymoGenetics is gratefuly acknowledged.

REFERENCES

1. Boeynaems JM, Oates JA, Hubbard WC. Preparation and characterization of hydroperoxy eicosatetraenoic acids. *Prostaglandins* 1980;19:87-98.
2. Pace-Asciak CR. Arachidonic acid epoxides. Demonstration through oxygen-18 labeled oxygen gas studies of an intramolecular transfer of the terminal hydroxyl group of 12S-hydroperoxy-eicosa-5,8,10,14-tetraenoic acid to form hydroxy epoxides. *J Biol Chem* 1984;259:8332-8337.
3. Pace-Asciak CR. Hepoxilins. *Gen Pharmacol* 1993;24:805-810.
4. Pace-Asciak CR, Granstrom E, Samuelsson B. Arachidonic acid epoxides: Isolation and structure of 2 hydroxy epoxide intermediates in the formation of 8,11,12-trihydroxy eicosatrienoic acid and 10,11,12-trihydroxy eicosatrienoic acid. *J Biol Chem* 1983;258:6835-6840.
5. Reynaud D, Delton I, Gharib A, Sarda N, Lagarde M, Pace-Asciak CR. Formation, metabolism, and action of hepoxilin A₃ in the rat pineal gland. *J Neurochem* 1994;62:126-133.
6. Yamaki K, Oh-Ishi S. 9-Anthryldiazomethane high-performance liquid chromatographic method for detection of prostaglandins and thromboxane. An application to the measurement of the products of stimulated rabbit platelets. *Chem Pharm Bull (Tokyo)* 1986;34:3526-3529.

Advances in Prostaglandin, Thromboxane,
and Leukotriene Research, Vol. 23,
edited by B. Samuelsson et al.
Raven Press, Ltd., New York © 1995

Pieces in the Puzzle:
Novel Arachidonate Metabolites

John C. McGiff, Mairead Carroll,
Bruno Escalante,* Nicholas R. Ferreri

*New York Medical College, Department of Pharmacology
Valhalla, New York 10595*
**Instituto Nacional de Cardiologia, Department Farmacologia
14080 Mexico D.F.*

Cytochrome P450 monooxygenases (P450) transform arachidonic acid (AA) to a wide range of products which are synthesized on demand and, in addition, can be released from storage in tissue phospholipids. These P450-AA metabolites possess diverse biological activities including inhibition of platelet and leukocyte activation/aggregation, stimulation of hormone production/release, and modulation of transport function and vasomotor tone (1). We will address the effects of P450-AA metabolites on a major component of the nephron, the cells of the thick ascending limb of Henle's loop.

Regulation of extracellular fluid volume and tonicity is dependent to a large extent on the reabsorptive function of the medullary segment of the thick ascending limb of the loop of Henle (mTALH). In cells isolated from the rabbit, AA is metabolized primarily by the cytochrome P450 monooxygenase pathway (2,3). Rabbit mTALH cells, when incubated with ^{14}C-AA for 30 min, form products that segregate into two peaks designated P_1 and P_2 based on their reverse phase HPLC retention times (Fig. 1), (4).

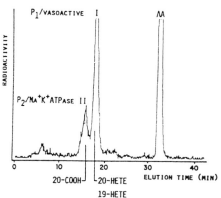

Fig. 1: Separation by reverse-phase HPLC of ^{14}C-labeled oxygenated metabolites of arachidonic acid (AA). Medullary thick ascending loop of Henle (mTALH) cells (3×10^6/ml) were incubated with ^{14}C-AA (0.4μCi) for 30 min.

187

Structural analysis by gas chromatography - mass spectrometry disclosed three AA products generated by the P450 pathway in the mTALH: 20-hydroxyeicosatetraenoic acid (20-HETE), 1,20-eicosatetraenedioic acid (20-COOH-AA), and 19-HETE (4). P_2, the more polar peak, was comprised of 20-COOH-AA, an inhibitor of Na^+-K^+-ATPase, that was devoid of vasoactivity. P_1 contained vasoactive material that was also capable of affecting Na^+-K^+-ATPase and yielded two products, 20-COOH-AA and 19-HETE. The final and crucial step in identifying novel AA metabolites was to compare the natural products of P_1 and P_2 with authentic standards (provided by J.R. Falck) in terms of their biological activity. Both P_2 and the standard, 20-COOH-AA, were potent inhibitors of Na^+-K^+-ATPase and neither exhibited vasoactivity. The lesser Na^+-K^+-ATPase inhibitory activity of P_1, presumably, reflects the presence of similar amounts of 19-HETE, the least active metabolite, and 20-HETE, which resembles 20-COOH-AA in its capacity to inhibit Na^+-K^+-ATPase. Thus, the biological activity of P_1 can be accounted for by 19- and 20-HETEs, and that of P_2, by 20-COOH-AA.

We next addressed the question as to whether these P450-AA metabolites affected ion transport in intact mTALH cells by testing their effects on ^{86}Rb uptake (5). As ^{86}Rb movement reflects that of K^+, ^{86}Rb uptake is a reliable index of changes in ion transport by the mTALH. Addition of 1 μM AA decreased the rate of ^{86}Rb uptake by ca 50%. This effect of AA was concentration-dependent, having a threshold of 10 nM AA, was unaffected by indomethacin but was prevented by either inhibition of P450-dependent AA metabolism or treatment of rabbits with $CoCl_2$ which induces the activity of heme oxygenase (6). Induction of this enzyme activity results in enhanced catabolism of cytochrome P450 and other heme-containing enzymes, thereby inhibiting cytochrome P450-dependent metabolism of AA (7). However, it was possible to bypass the blockade of P450-AA metabolism produced by $CoCl_2$ by substituting the relevant arachidonate metabolites (5,6). Either 20-HETE or 20-COOH-AA were able to inhibit ^{86}Rb uptake by mTALH cells despite $CoCl_2$ treatment (Fig. 2).

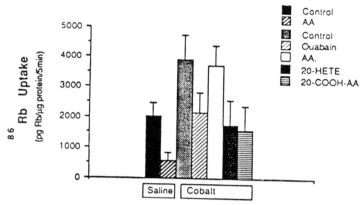

Fig. 2: Effects of 20-HETE and 20-COOH-AA on ^{86}Rb uptake in mTALH cells from CoCl$_2$-treated rabbits.   Cells from saline-treated rabbits and CoCl$_2$-treated rabbits were incubated with AA (1 μM).   Ouabain (1 mM), 20-HETE (1 μM), or 20-COOH-AA (1 μM) were added 5 min before addition of ^{86}Rb. Each bar represents the mean ± SE of three experiments.

At least three kinds of pathways for K$^+$ movement have been identified in the mTALH cells: Na$^+$-K$^+$-ATPase (Na$^+$ pump), the Na$^+$-K$^+$-2Cl$^-$ cotransporter and at least one variety of Ba^{2+}-sensitive K$^+$ channel (8).   The nature of the transport mechanism inhibited by P450-AA metabolites cannot be answered by studying their effects on K$^+$ movement, using ^{86}Rb uptake as an index of the latter.   Changes in ^{86}Rb movement produced by an agent will not discriminate between primary effects of a P450-AA metabolite on the cotransporter vs. the Na$^+$ pump as both furosemide (cotransporter inhibitor) and ouabain (Na$^+$ pump inhibitor) inhibit ^{86}Rb uptake (5).   It had been suggested that P450-AA metabolites blocked ^{86}Rb uptake by inhibiting Na$^+$-K$^+$-ATPase, based on ex vivo evidence that 20-HETE and 20-COOH-AA inhibited the activity of purified Na$^+$-K$^+$-ATPase obtained from the renal outer medulla. Because furosemide also reduced ^{86}Rb uptake in mTALH cells, inhibition of the Na$^+$-K$^+$-2Cl$^-$ cotransporter could also account for reduction of ^{86}Rb uptake.   An additional consideration is a possible direct effect of AA on K$^+$ channels, as AA as well as AA metabolites have been shown to block K$^+$ channels (9).

We addressed possible interactions involving P450-AA metabolites with the different pathways for K^+ movements in the mTALH by comparing the effects of AA and the principal P450-AA metabolites, 20-HETE and 20-COOH-AA, on ion content and ^{86}Rb uptake to those same effects produced by ouabain and furosemide (8). Ouabain increased Na^+ and decreased K^+ content in rabbit mTALH cells, whereas furosemide reduced both Na^+ and K^+ content. We found that 20-HETE and 20-COOH-AA resembled furosemide. Although the effects of AA and P450-AA metabolites on Na^+ and K^+ content of mTALH cells were furosemide-like and different from those of ouabain, we further tested the possibility of an additional effect of P450-AA metabolites on Na^+-K^+-ATPase in experiments carried out under conditions in which intracellular Na^+ concentration was not rate limiting for the Na^+ pump (8). Treatment of mTALH cells with monensin created these conditions, since incorporation of the ionophore into the mTALH cell membrane produced a parallel pathway for Na^+ entry. Under these conditions, furosemide, or a compound acting similarly to furosemide, would not affect ^{86}Rb uptake whereas ouabain would inhibit monensin-stimulated ^{86}Rb uptake. In contrast to ouabain, AA did not inhibit ^{86}Rb uptake in the presence of monensin, indicating that P450-derived AA metabolites do not modulate Na^+-K^+-ATPase of mTALH cells (7).

Finally, a third mechanism may also be involved in the inhibitory effect of P450-AA metabolites on transport in mTALH cells, one operating through K^+ channels. If this were the case, inhibition of K^+ efflux would have a secondary negative effect on the cotransporter. We explored this possibility by evaluating the effects of P450-AA metabolites on K^+ channels by measuring ^{86}Rb efflux from mTALH tubules loaded with ^{86}Rb (8). The addition of either AA or 20-COOH-AA to the mTALH incubate produced a transient increase in ^{86}Rb efflux which was prevented by blockade of K^+ channels with $BaCl_2$. These findings, then, did not support an inhibitory action of P450-AA products on the cotransporter, secondary to blockade of K^+ channels of the mTALH as AA and 20-COOH-AA increased K^+ efflux from mTALH cells (based on their effects on ^{86}Rb movement). The action of the P450-AA metabolites on regulation of Na^+ and K^+ movement in the mTALH segment, then, is similar to that of furosemide; viz, they affect the Na^+-K^+-$2Cl^-$ cotransporter.

Transcellular metabolism of P450-AA products is the basis for the hypothesis that cyclooxygenase has the capacity to metabolize certain P450-AA products, resulting in the acquisition of new properties (10). For example, either 20-HETE or 5,6-eicosatrienoic acid (EET), generated by segments of the nephron, affect transport function in the segment of origin. After their release into the extracellular space, they can be metabolized by mesenchymal or vascular cyclooxygenase which are contiguous to the nephron and are, thereby, converted into vasoactive agents. This metabolic sequence may serve a mechanism which couples changes in renal tubular function to changes in local blood flow. We have identified two components in the vasodilator action of 5,6-EET in the rabbit kidney (11). The first derives from the cyclooxygenase-dependent generation of vasodilator metabolites from 5,6-EET, chiefly 5,6-epoxy-PGE_1 and the second from the capacity of the epoxide to release the vasodilator prostaglandins, PGE_2 and PGI_2.

An immunomodulator function has also been ascribed to the TALH segment. Tamm-Horsfall (uromodulin) protein that coats the surface of mTALH cells binds interleukin-1 (IL-1) and tumor necrosis factor α (TNF) with high affinity (12). A relationship between cytokines and AA metabolism has been demonstrated and includes induction of cyclooxygenase expression and inhibition of cytochrome P450-related monooxygenases in response to cytokines (13,14). Synthesis of TNF by mTALH cells has been demonstrated to be low under basal conditions and subject to stimulation by lipopolysaccharide (LPS) (13,15). TNF, either endogenous (when stimulated by LPS) or exogenous, can affect transport function of mTALH cells, as evidenced by inhibition of ^{86}Rb uptake. This effect of TNF on ^{86}Rb uptake by mTALH cells required more than 4 h, presumably related to induction of cyclooxygenase synthesis as TNF mediated inhibition of ^{86}Rb uptake could be abolished by indomethacin. A reciprocal action of TNF on P450-monooxygenase activity in mTALH cells is under investigation. These findings support the following hypothesis: cytokines can promote cyclooxygenase-dependent AA metabolism increasing the formation of prostanoids that affect transport in the nephron segment of origin (autocrine function) and probably in other segments (paracrine function) as well.

ACKNOWLEDGMENTS

This work was made possible by National Institutes of Health Grant HL34300. We wish to thank Melody Steinberg for preparation of the manuscript and editorial assistance.

REFERENCES

1. Proctor KG, Capdevila JH, Falck JR, Fitzpatrick FA, Mullane KM, McGiff JC. In: *Blood Vessels* Bevan JA, Ed. Switzerland: S. Karger AG; 1989; 26:53-64.

2. Ferreri NR, Schwartzman M, Ibraham NG, Chander PN, McGiff JC. *J Pharmacol Exp Ther* 1984; 231:441-8.

3. Schwartzman M, Ferreri NR, Carroll MA, Songu-Mize E, McGiff JC. *Nature* 1985;314:620-2.

4. Carroll MA, Sala A, Dunn CE, McGiff JC, Murphy RC. *J Biol Chem* 1991; 266:12306-12.

5. Escalante B, Erlij D, Falck JR, McGiff JC. *Science* 1991; 251:799-802.

6. Escalante B, Erlij D, Falck JR, McGiff JC. *J Cardiovasc Pharmacol* 1993; 22:106-8.

7. Schwartzman ML, Abraham NG, Carroll MA, Levere RD, McGiff JC. *Biochem J* 1986; 238:283-90.

8. Escalante B, Erlij D, Falck JR, McGiff JC. *Am J Physiol* 1994; 266:C1775-82.

9. Clapham DE. *Biochem Pharmacol* 1990; 39:813-15.

10. McGiff JC. *Annu Rev Pharmacol Toxicol* 1991; 31:339-69.

11. Carroll MA, Balazy M, Margiotta P, Falck JR, McGiff JC. *J Biol Chem* 1993; 268:12260-6.

12. Hession C, Decker JM, Sherblom AP, et al. *Science* 1987; 237:1479-84.

13. Escalante BA, Ferreri NR, Dunn CE, McGiff JC. *Am J Physiol* 1994; 266:C1568-76.

14. Sujita K, Okuno F, Tanaka Y, et al. *Biochem Biophys Res Commun.* 1990; 168:1217-22.

15. Macica CM, Escalante BA, Conners MS, Ferreri NR. *Kidney International* 1994; 46:113-21.

Advances in Prostaglandin, Thromboxane, and Leukotriene Research, Vol. 23,
edited by B. Samuelsson et al.
Raven Press, Ltd., New York © 1995

Biosynthesis and Degradation of α-Paranaric Acid and Related Conjugated Tetraene Fatty Acids

Mats Hamberg

*Department of Medical Biochemistry and Biophysics,
Division of Physiological Chemistry II,
Karolinska Institutet, S-171 77 Stockholm, Sweden*

Seed oils from certain plants, *e.g. Parinarium laurinum* and *Impatiens balsamina*, contain large amounts of parinaric acid, a C_{18} fatty acid which is characterized by the presence of a conjugated tetraene structure located at $\Delta^{9,11,13,15}$ (1). Parinaric acid is used as a collective name for four geometrical isomers, *i.e.*, α-parinaric acid (9(Z),11(E),13(E),15(Z)-octadecatetraenoic acid), β-parinaric acid (9(E),11(E),13(E),15(E)-octadecatetraenoic acid), and two additional isomers recently characterized, 9(Z),11(E),13(E),15(E)-octadeca-tetraenoic acid and 9(E),11(E),13(E),15(Z)-octadecatetraenoic acid (2). Of these isomers, α-parinaric acid is the quantitatively predominant one is seed oils, and it is likely that the three other isomers are formed by chemical isomerization during storage and/or isolation. The conjugated *Z,E,E,Z* tetraene chromophore of α-parinaric acid gives rise to UV absorption with main bands at 291, 304, and 319 nm (2), and to strong fluorescence at 410-430 nm (3). Because of its fluorescence and its efficient incorporation into phospholipids of biological membranes, parinaric acid has found use as a fluorescent probe in membrane studies (3). Parinaric acid is easily peroxidized into non-fluorescent products and the decrease of parinaric acid fluorescence has been used as an index of lipid peroxidation in, *e.g.*, erythrocyte membranes and LDL particles (4). Low concentrations of parinaric acid suppress cell growth in culture (5). Interestingly, a number of malignant cell lines have been reported to be particularly sensitive in this respect (6). The mechanism of the growth inhibitory effect of parinaric acid has not yet been established, although a cytotoxic effect caused by oxidation products of parinaric acid seems likely (6).

Biosynthesis of α-parinaric acid from the corresponding non-conjugated trienoic acid, α-linolenic acid, has recently been realized using extracts of the red alga *Lithothamnion corallioides* (2). The present paper is a brief account of our biosynthetic studies of α-parinaric acid and related (7,8) conjugated tetraene fatty acids. In addition, recent data on the nonenzymatic oxygenation of parinaric acid, of relevance for the cytotoxic effect of the acid, will be described.

EXPERIMENTAL

α-Parinaric acid and its geometrical isomers were isolated from seed of *Impatiens balsamina* as described (2). [1-^{14}C]-γ-Linolenic acid and stereo-specifically deuteriated γ-linolenic acids were prepared by biological desaturation of the corresponding stearates (2,7).

Methyl 9(S),16(R)- and 9(S),16(S)-dihydroxy-10(E),12(E),14(E)-octadeca-trienoates were prepared by treatment of 9(S)-hydroperoxy-10(E),12(Z),15(Z)-octadecatrienoic acid (30 mg) with bovine hemoglobin (1 g) in 30 mL of 0.09 M potassium phosphate buffer pH 7.4 (9). Preparative straight-phase HPLC (solvent, ethanol-hexane (6:94 v/v); detection at 268 nm) of the esterified product afforded methyl 9(S),16(R)-dihydroxy-10(E),12(E),14(E)-octadecatrienoate (19.0-19.9 mL effluent) and methyl 9(S),16(S)-dihydroxy-10(E),12(E),14(E)-octadecatrienoate (20.7-21.7 mL); λ_{max} (CH$_3$OH/nm) 258, 268, 279; m/z (TMS ethers) 468 (1%, M$^+$), 453 (1, M$^+$ - CH$_3$), 439 (1, M$^+$ - C$_2$H$_5$), 437 (2, M$^+$ - OCH$_3$), 410 (2, M$^+$ - OHC-C$_2$H$_5$), 378 (42, M$^+$ - (CH$_3$)$_3$SiOH), 337 (7, M$^+$ - CH(OSi(CH$_3$)$_3$)-C$_2$H$_5$), 298 (7), 259 (10, (CH$_3$)$_3$SiO$^+$=CH-(CH$_2$)$_7$-COOCH$_3$), 221 (11, M$^+$ - (CH$_2$)$_7$-COOCH$_3$ - (CH$_3$)$_3$SiOH), 131 (31, (CH$_3$)$_3$SiO$^+$=CH-C$_2$H$_5$), 129 (35, (CH$_3$)$_3$SiO$^+$=CH-CH=CH$_2$), and 73 (100, (CH$_3$)$_3$Si$^+$). The absolute configurations of C-9 and C-16 of the two epimers were determined by oxidative ozonolysis of the di-propionyl derivatives followed by coupling of the resulting 2-propionoxy acids to the methyl ester of L-phenylalanine and steric analysis by GLC (Zhang, L.-Y., and Hamberg, M, to be published).

Procedures for incubation of polyunsaturated fatty acids with the red alga *Lithothamnion corallioides*, and techniques for isolation of oxidation products, were as described (2,7).

Hydrogen peroxide was determined by incubation of [1-^{14}C]oleic acid with a hydrogen peroxide-dependent peroxygenase from broad bean and determination of the percentage conversion into 9,10-epoxy-[1-^{14}C]stearic acid (7). Standard curves obtained by incubation of peroxygenase and [1-^{14}C]oleic acid showed a linear relationship using H$_2$O$_2$ concentrations up to 250 μM (Fig. 1A).

Non-enzymatic oxygenation of methyl parinarate (47 mg; a mixture of the methyl esters of α-parinaric acid (74%), Z,E,E,E- and E,E,E,Z-parinaric acids (22%), and β-parinaric acid)(4%)) were carried out at 37°C in 10 mL of either 1,2-dimethoxyethane-water (4:1 v/v) or methanol under an atmosphere of oxygen gas. The solutions contained 20 μg of the antioxidant 2,6-di-*tert*-butyl-4-methylphenol. Aliquots were removed at regular time intervals and analyzed by UV spectroscopy. The oxidation product (10-12 h) was subjected to SiO$_2$ chromatography followed by straight-phase HPLC (column, 250 x 4.6 mm of Nucleosil 50-5; eluted with ethanol-hexane (6:94 v/v) at 1.5 mL/min). Products isolate⸱ by HPLC were further characterized by physical and chemical methods.

RESULTS AND DISCUSSION

Incubation of α-linolenic acid.

Incubation of [1-^{14}C]α-linolenic acid with the enzyme preparation of *L. corallioides* yielded α-parinaric acid (13%), 11(S)-hydroxy-9(Z),12(Z),15(Z)-

octadecatrienoic acid (46%), and 14(R)-hydroxy-9(Z),12(Z),15(Z)-octadeca-trienoic acid (6%). The two bis-allylic hydroxy acids were dehydrated into parinaric acid isomers by acid in non-aqueous medium, however, no such conversion took place when labeled hydroxy acids were added to the enzyme preparation. Further evidence that α-parinaric acid was biosynthesized independently of the two hydroxy acids was provided by the finding that the conversion of α-linolenic acid into hydroxy acids was selectively blocked by 5 mM sodium azide. In the presence of azide, formation of α-parinaric acid increased slightly, presumably because of a shunting effect.

Incubation of γ-linolenic acid and arachidonic acid.

Enzymatic oxidation of γ-linolenic acid afforded a conjugated tetraene fatty acid, 6(Z),8(E),10(E),12(Z)-octadecatetraenoic acid (29%), and a bis-allylic hydroxy acid, 11(R)-hydroxy-6(Z),9(Z),12(Z)-octadecatrienoic acid (29%). Similarly, arachidonic acid was oxidized into a product that mainly consisted of 5,8,10,12,14-eicosapentaenoic acid and 13(R)-hydroxy-5,8,11,14-eicosatetra-enoic acid. As was observed in the α-linolenic acid incubations, 5 mM sodium azide selectively inhibited biosynthesis of the bis-allylic hydroxy acids from γ-linolenic acid and arachidonic acid.

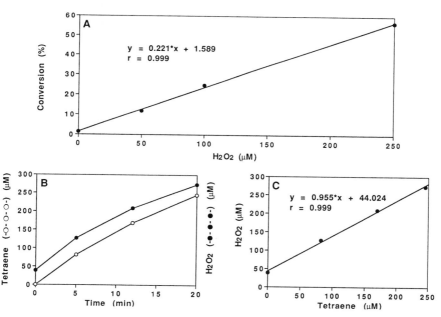

FIG. 1. Production of hydrogen peroxide. (A), standard curve; (B), time courses of formation of H_2O_2 and 6,8,10,12-octadecatetraenoic acid ("Tetraene") during incubation of γ-linolenic acid; (C), correlation between formations of H_2O_2 and 6,8,10,12-octadecatetraenoic acid during incubation of γ-linolenic acid.

Mechanism of formation of α-parinaric acid and other conjugated tetraene fatty acids.

Experiments where α-linolenic acid, γ-linolenic acid, and arachidonic acid were incubated with the enzyme preparation under anaerobic conditions revealed that conversion of the nonconjugated acids into the corresponding conjugated tetraenes was dioxygen-dependent. Interestingly, a number of artificial electron acceptors such as *p*-benzoquinone, phenazine methosulfate, and 2,6-dichlorophenol-indophenol were able to support biosynthesis of conjugated tetraenes under anaerobic conditions. *p*-Benzoquinone was most effective in this respect, and, when used in 2-5 mM concentration, was able to restore tetraene biosynthesis to the levels observed under aerobic conditions. It seemed possible that oxidation of the nonconjugated triene structure of the substrates into the conjugated tetraene of the products was coupled to reduction of O_2 to hydrogen peroxide. In order to test this hypothesis, varying concentrations of α- and γ-linolenic acids were incubated with the enzyme preparation, and hydrogen peroxide was determined by the enzymatic method described above. Sodium azide (5 mM) was included in these incubations in order to block hydroxy acid formation and to inhibit possible catalase activity. Oxidation of γ-linolenic acid occurred with a time- (Fig. 1B) and concentration-dependent formation of hydrogen peroxide. A plot of hydrogen peroxide formation *vs.* tetraene formation showed an essentially linear relationship (Fig. 1C). As shown by the slope of the line (k = 0.96), biosynthesis of tetraene was accompanied by a stoichiometrical production of hydrogen peroxide. Similar results were obtained with α-linolenic acid as the substrate. Lipoxygenase and cytochrome P-450 inhibitors did not block formation of conjugated tetraene fatty acids. This finding coupled with the facts that oxidation of triene to tetraene was supported by dioxygen and by artificial electron acceptors, and was accompanied by stoichiometric reduction of dioxygen to hydrogen peroxide, indicated that biosynthesis of conjugated tetraenes was catalyzed by a fatty acid oxidase (Fig. 2).

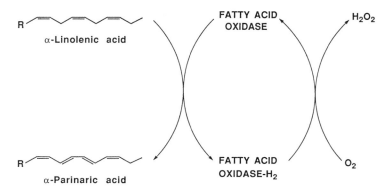

FIG. 2. Mechanism of formation of α-parinaric acid from α-linolenic acid. R = $(CH_2)_7$-COOH.

The steric course of the hydrogen removals was determined by incubation of γ-linolenic acid stereospecifically deuteriated in the 8(R)-, 8(S)-, 11(R)-, and 11(S)-positions. Mass-spectrometric analysis showed that 6,8,10,12-octadecatetraenoic acid lost the deuterium label when biosynthesized from the 8(S)- and 11(R)-deuterio acids and retained the label when formed from the 8(R)- and 11(S)-deuterio acids. Analysis of the isotopic contents of γ-linolenic acids recovered after incubation of 8(S)- and 11(R)-^{2}H-γ-linolenic acids in both cases showed isotope enrichments which increased at higher percentage conversions. The isotope enrichments observed with the 8(S)- and 11(R)-deuterio acids were of the same magnitude, and, accordingly, any conclusion as to which hydrogen was eliminated in the initial step could not be drawn.

Oxidation of parinaric acid.

UV spectroscopic analysis was used to monitor degradation of parinarate kept in aqueous 1,2-dimethoxyethane or methanol under oxygen gas. After a lag phase of ca. 6 h, presumably due to the presence of the antioxidant 2,6-di-*tert*-butyl-4-methylphenol, a rapid ($t_{1/2}$ = 2 h) degradation of parinarate took place as shown by the disappearance of the absorption bands at 291, 304, and 319 nm. Interestingly, oxidation was accompanied by the appearance of absorption bands at 260, 270, and 280 nm, suggesting the formation of compounds possessing a conjugated triene structure. The product obtained following oxidation of methyl parinarate for 10.5 h in aqueous 1,2-dimethoxyethane (>90% degradation of the methyl parinarate) was analyzed by straight-phase HPLC. Two major peaks of materials showing UV absorption bands typical for a conjugated triene, *i.e.*, Compounds A and B, appeared. Compound A was identified as an enantiomeric mixture of methyl 9(S),16(R)- and 9(R),16(S)-dihydroxy-10(E),12(E),14(E)-octadecatrienoates by chemical and physical methods using authentic methyl 9(S),16(R)-dihydroxy-10(E),12(E),14(E)-octadecatrienoate as reference. In the same way, Compound B was found to be due to the enantiomeric pair methyl 9(S),16(S)- and 9(R),16(R)-dihydroxy-10(E),12(E),14(E)-octadecatrienoates.

Experiments with $^{18}O_2$ and $H_2$$^{18}O$ showed that the oxygens of the two hydroxyl groups of 9,16-dihydroxyoctadecatrienoate had different origins, *i.e.*, one hydroxyl oxygen was derived from dioxygen and the other one from water. Oxidation of methyl parinarate in methanol afforded a mixture of 9-hydroxy-16-methoxy- and 9-methoxy-16-hydroxy-octadecatrienoates, thus supporting the notion that one of the oxygen functions was solvent-derived. On the basis of these data, it seemed likely that the initial event of one pathway of parinarate oxidation consisted of epoxidation of either of the terminal double bonds to produce a mixture of chemically unstable 9,10- and 15,16-epoxyoctadeca-trienoates. Opening of the epoxide function followed by double bond migrations and attack by water at C-16 and C-9, respectively, would result in the formation of 9,16-dihydroxyoctadecatrienoate (Fig. 3). Support for this pathway was provided by the isolation of small amounts of 9,10-dihydroxy-11,13,15- and 15,16-dihydroxy-9,11,13-octadecatrienoates, formed from the 9,10- and 15,16-epoxy-octadecatrienoates by solvent attack at C-10 and C-15, respectively.

9,16-Dihydroxyoctadecatrienoate, a relatively stable compound which is easily detected because of its strong absorption band at 268 nm, appears to be a suitable index of parinaric acid peroxidation in biological systems.

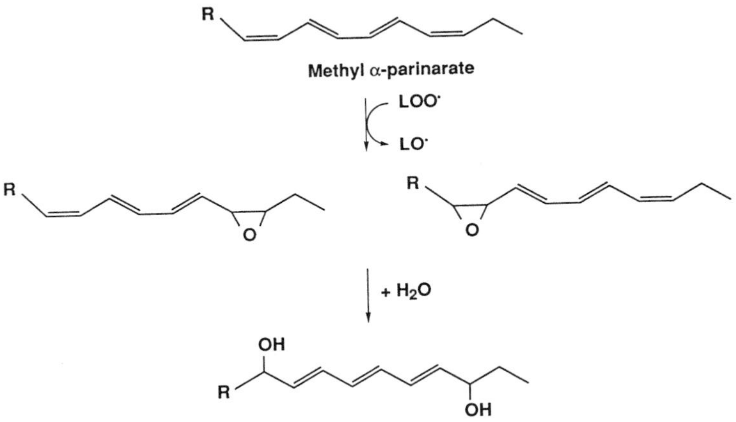

FIG. 3. Nonenzymatic oxygenation of methyl α-parinarate. The pathway involving epoxidation of either the Δ^9 or the Δ^{15} double bond into methyl 9,10- and 15,16-epoxyoctadecatrienoates followed by hydrolysis into methyl 9,16-dihydroxy-10,12,14-octadecatrienoate is shown. R = $(CH_2)_7$-$COOCH_3$.

REFERENCES

1. Farmer EH and Sunderland E. The highly unsaturated acid of the kernels of *Parinarium Laurinum. J Chem Soc* 1935;759-61.
2. Hamberg M. Oxidation of octadecatrienoic acids in the red alga *Lithothamnion corallioides. J Chem Soc, Perkin Trans 1*, 1993;3065-72.
3. Sklar LA, Hudson BS and Simoni RD. Conjugated polyene fatty acids as membrane probes. *Proc Natl Acad Sci USA* 1975;72:1649-53.
4. Kuypers FA, van den Berg JJM, Schalkwijk C, Roelofsen B and Op den Kamp JAF. Parinaric acid as a sensitive fluorescent probe for the determination of lipid peroxidation. *Biochim Biophys Acta* 1987;921:266-74.
5. Rintoul DA and Simoni RD. Incorporation of a naturally occurring fluorescent fatty acid into lipids of cultured mammalian cells. *J Biol Chem* 1977; 252:7916-18.
6. Cornelius AS, Yerram NR, Kratz DA and Spector AA. Cytotoxic effect of *cis*-parinaric acid in cultured malignant cells. *Cancer Res* 1991;51:6025-30.
7. Hamberg M. Metabolism of 6,9,12-octadecatrienoic acid in the red alga *Lithothamnion corallioides. Biochem Biophys Res Commun* 1992;188: 1220-27.
8. Gerwick WH, Åsen P and Hamberg M. Biosynthesis of 13R-hydroxy-arachidonic acid, an unusual oxylipin from the red alga *Lithothamnion corallioides. Phytochemistry* 1993;34:1029-1033.
9. Hamberg M. A novel transformation of 13-Ls-hydroperoxy-9,11-octadeca-dienoic acid. *Biochim Biophys Acta* 1983;752:191-197.

*Advances in Prostaglandin, Thromboxane,
and Leukotriene Research, Vol. 23,*
edited by B. Samuelsson et al.
Raven Press, Ltd., New York © 1995

IDENTIFICATION OF ARACHIDONATE EPOXIDES IN HUMAN PLATELETS

Michael Balazy, Elimor B. Schieber, John C. McGiff

*New York Medical College, Department of Pharmacology
Valhalla, New York 10595, USA*

Epoxides of arachidonic acid (EETs) are formed by cytochrome P450 epoxygenase and display a wide range of cardiovascular properties (1). In particular, these eicosanoids are blood platelet antagonists. Fitzpatrick et al. has shown that three epoxides (8,9-, 11,12-, and 14,15-EET) inhibit arachidonic acid (AA)-induced human platelet aggregation at concentrations from 1 to 10 μM with no evident stereospecificity and that platelet cyclooxygenase was inhibited by 14R,15S-EET and racemic 8,9-EET but not by the other EET isomers (2). Our research showed that 5,6-EET is a potent inhibitor of platelet cyclooxygenase (IC$_{50}$ 1.8 μM) and aggregation. However, the biosynthesis of EETs by platelets has not been demonstrated. We have been analyzing complex mixture of human platelet phospholipids using mass spectrometric techniques to address the hypothesis that platelets may contain EETs esterified within phospholipid stores.

MATERIALS AND METHODS

Human platelet phospholipids Human platelets were prepared as described (3). The pellet of cells was resuspended in phosphate buffered saline to the final concentration of 1×10^9 cells/ml and extracted by the method of Bligh and Dyer. Aliquots of this extract were hydrolyzed with phospholipase (PL)A$_2$ (*Naja mocambique*, Sigma). In control experiments the PLA$_2$ was omitted. The efficiency of extractions and PLA$_2$ hydrolysis was 40-50% as measured from recovery of AA from [^{3}H$_2$]AA-phosphatidylcholine added prior to extraction. 14,15-EET-d$_8$ (10 ng) was then added as internal standard and lipids were extracted twice with 1 ml of hexane. The extract was purified using reverse-phase HPLC column and a fraction containing EETs was collected and derivatized with pentafluorobenzyl (PFB) bromide (3) and finally analyzed by mass spectrometry. Separation of platelet phospholipids into major classes was accomplished using silica column (Spherisorb 3 μm, 150x4.6 mm) and eluted with hexane/isopropanol /ethanol/sodium acetate (400/200/100/30) at 1 ml/min.

Mass spectrometry GC/MS was performed on HP5989 instrument using methane electron capture ionization as described (3). The amount of the endogenous epoxides was determined from the standard curve obtained with 10 ng of 14,15-EET-d$_8$ (ion *m/z* 327) and various amounts of 14,15-EET (ion *m/z* 319).

PFB esters of endogenous platelet EETs were separated using silica column (Hypersil 200x4.6 mm) interfaced to the mass spectrometer via particle beam unit (PB-LC/MS) and eluted with 1% isopropanol in hexane at 1 ml/min (3).

RESULTS AND DISCUSSION

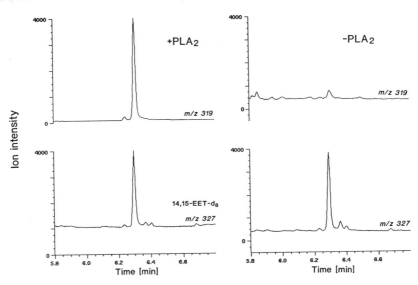

Figure 1. GC/MS analysis of human platelet phospholipid extract before (right) and after (left) hydrolysis with venom PLA$_2$. Ions m/z 319 and 327 correspond to endogenous EETs and internal standard (14,15-EET-d$_8$, 10 ng), respectively.

The hydrolysis of platelet phospholipid extract by PLA$_2$ followed by GC/MS analyses revealed the presence of endogenous EETs coeluting with the internal standard 14,15-EET-d$_8$ (Fig 1). The total amount of EETs released from human platelet phospholipids was 4.3±0.9 pmol/10^6 cells (n=4). The samples which were not treated with PLA$_2$ did not show measurable amounts of EETs. Separation of platelet EETs (as PFB esters) using a new method, PB-LC/MS, (Fig 2) revealed that all four EET regioisomers are represented in proportion (%) 37.1:30.8:25.3:6.8 (14,15-:11,12-:8,9-:5,6-EET). Fractionation of platelet phospholipid extract by normal-phase (NP)-HPLC (Fig 2) followed by PLA$_2$ hydrolysis and GC/MS analysis revealed that the EETs are esterified in phosphatidyl(P)-ethanolamine (PE), -choline (PC) and -inositol (PI) in proportion 31.1:39.6:9.8 (%). About half of the EETs associated with PC were in fractions containing 1-*O*-alkyl-PC.

We report a new finding that EETs are endogenous constituents of intact human platelet phospholipids. Data shown provide the link between the origin of platelet EETs (phospholipid stores) and their known biological activities in platelets (inhibition of cyclooxygenase, aggregation and Ca^{2+} influx).

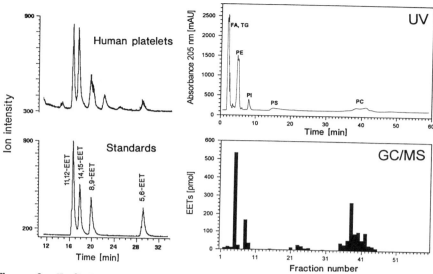

Figure 2. *(Left)* PB-LC/MS analysis of EETs (PFB esters) extracted from platelet phospholipids of four human donors *(top)* and separation of standard EETs *(bottom)* under the same conditions. Chromatograms represent selective monitoring of anion m/z 319. *(Right)* NP-HPLC of human platelet phospholipids (extracted from 5×10^8 cells) monitored by UV detector *(top)* and by GC/MS *(bottom)*, following hydrolysis by PLA_2.

These EETs may, therefore, play a role in modulating platelet responses when released intracellularly following activation of platelet PLA_2. The phospholipid-bound EETs may originate from processes other than platelet-mediated epoxidation of AA since it is uncertain whether EETs can be biosynthesized by platelets. We found that human platelets contain a pool of EETs esterified within phosphatidylinositols. During platelet activation, this pool may be available for hydrolysis by phospholipases C resulting in formation of diacylglycerols containing EETs. These epoxy-modified diacylglycerols may differ from 2-arachidonyl-diacylglycerols to alter activation of protein kinase C in platelets by transmembrane signals (4). We are currently investigating the implications of the above findings in relation to thromboxane A_2 formation and signal transduction in platelets. *This work was supported by the American Heart Association (Dallas, TX) 92013280 and by NIH HL34300.*

REFERENCES

1. McGiff JC (1991) *Annu. Rev. Pharmacol. Toxicol.* **31**, 339-369.
2. Fitzpatrick FA, Ennis MD, Baze ME, et al. (1986) *J. Biol. Chem.* **261**, 15334-15338.
3. Balazy M (1991) *J. Biol. Chem.* **266**, 23561-23567.
4. Kajikawa N, Kikkawa U, Nishizuka Y. (1989) *Methods Enzymol.* **169**, 430-442.

Advances in Prostaglandin, Thromboxane,
and Leukotriene Research, Vol. 23,
edited by B. Samuelsson et al.
Raven Press, Ltd., New York © 1995

Arachidonic Acid ω-hydroxylation and Cytochrome P450 4A Expression in the Rat Kidney

Fangming Lin*, Nader G. Abraham♦ and Michal Laniado Schwartzman*

*Department of Pharmacology, New York Medical College, Valhalla, NY, 10595
♦Department of Pharmacology, The Rockefeller University, New York, NY, 10021

Synthesis of 20-hydroxyeicosatetraenoic acid (20-HETE) from arachidonic acid (AA) is a reaction catalyzed by a cytochrome P450 4A (CYP4A). About 85% of 20-HETE synthesis along the nephron is localized to the proximal tubule. Biological activities of 20-HETE include regulation of renal vascular tone, modulation of tubular ion transport and stimulation of renal epithelial cell growth (1). In the rat kidney, CYP4A subfamily consists of three highly homologous isozymes, CYP4A1, CYP4A2 and CYP4A3, and all are believed to be capable of ω-hydroxylating AA (2). Both CYP4A1 and CYP4A3 are greatly induced by clofibrate whereas CYP4A2 is a constitutive enzyme in male and is undetectable in female. Sex-dependent expression and differential inducibility by chemicals suggest different sensitivity for the CYP4A isozymes to hormone/growth factor regulation and possibly different substrate specificity. We herein describe studies to examine the AA ω-hydroxylation and CYP4A expression in the kidney during the post-natal renal growth and functional maturation in Sprague Dawley rats.

METHODS

Renal cortical microsomes (RCM) were isolated from male Sprague Dawley rat kidneys (from 3 days before birth to 20-week-old). Clofibrate (10 mg/kg) or saline was given via i.p. injection for 3 days. RCM (0.3 mg) were incubated with ^{14}C-AA (0.4 μCi, 7 μM) in the presence or absence of NADPH generating system (0.4 mM glucose-6-phosphate, 1 U glucose-6-phosphate-dehydrogenase and 1 mM NADP) in a volume of 1 ml of 0.1 M potassium phosphate buffer for

30 min at 37°C. In some experiments, RCM were preincubated with 17-octadecynoic acid (17-ODYA, 3.6 μM) for 10 min prior to the addition of ^{14}C-AA. The reaction was terminated by acidification to pH 4.0 and metabolites extracted with ethyl acetate and separated by reverse phase HPLC. AA ω-hydroxylase activity was calculated based on the percent conversion of added ^{14}C-AA to 20-HETE and expressed as pmol/mg/min. For immunoblot analysis, 10 μg of RCM were reduced with 2-mercaptoethanol and separated on 8% SDS-PAGE at 20 mA for 20 hours. Di-(2-ethylhexyl)phthalate (DEHP)-treated rat liver microsomes (2.5 μg) were loaded on the same gel for identification of CYP4A1 (DEHP is an inducer of CYP4A1). Clofibrate-treated RCM were used to identify CYP4A1 and CYP4A3 and RCM of female rats were used to confirm the position of CYP4A2. After transfer, the nitrocellulose membrane was blocked in 10% milk/5% FCS for 2 hours and incubated with anti-rat liver CYP4A1 antibody (a generous gift from Dr. Okita, Washington State University) over night. The membrane was then incubated with alkaline phosphatase (AP)-conjugated secondary antibody and immunoreactive proteins were detected with AP color developing solution (Bio-Rad).

RESULTS

Incubation of RCM with ^{14}C-AA in the presence of NADPH resulted in the formation of 20-HETE as the major metabolite. No 20-HETE was formed in the incubation medium in the absence of NADPH. Preincubation of 17-ODYA caused 66±8.4% inhibition of 20-HETE synthesis. As seen in Figure 1, an age-dependent change of AA ω-hydroxylase activity was observed. 20-HETE synthesis displayed a striking increase from barely detectable levels in fetus to 159±3.2 pmol/mg/min in 5-week-old and reached a maximum of 165.2±6.1 pmol/mg/min in 7-week-old rats. AA ω-hydroxylase activity remained elevated through 13 weeks and decreased to about 50% of the maximal level at 20 weeks of age (74.8±4.5 pmol/mg/min).

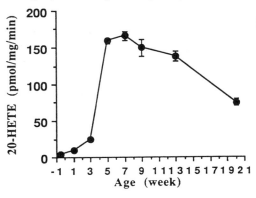

FIG. 1. Age-dependent 20-HETE synthesis in the rat kidney. RCM (0.3 mg) were incubated with ^{14}C-AA (7 μM) in the presence of NADPH generating system. Metabolites were separated by HPLC. 20-HETE was calculated from the percent conversion of ^{14}C-AA. Results are Mean±SE, n=4.

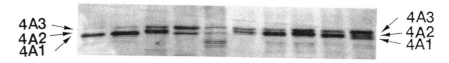

FIG. 2 Immunoblot of RCM with anti-rat liver CYP4A1 IgG.

Immunoblot analysis using anti-rat liver CYP4A1 antibody which cross reacts with CYP4A2 and CYP4A3 revealed the expression of all three isozymes in male Sprague Dawley rat kidney (Figure 2). The changes in protein levels corresponded to the changes in AA ω-hydroxylase activity. The most significant increase in CYP4A immunoreactive proteins was from 3-week-old to 7-week-old. CYP4A2 was not detected in 7-week-old female rat kidneys. Treatment with clofibrate caused an increase in CYP4A1 and CYP4A3 protein levels while treatment with DEHP induced mainly CYP4A1.

DISCUSSION

Synthesis of 20-HETE by RCM showed NADPH-dependency and was inhibited by 17-ODYA, suggesting a P450-mediated reaction. The greatest increase in AA ω-hydroxylase activity between 3 and 5 weeks of age correlated to post-natal kidney development and functional maturation of the nephron (3). A similar increase in CYP4A protein levels may be partially responsible for the enhanced formation of 20-HETE. Since 20-HETE stimulates proximal tubular cell growth in culture, we postulate that age-dependent changes of 20-HETE synthesis may play a role in renal epithelial cell growth during post-natal development and possibly in the recovery process following renal injury.

REFERENCES

1. Laniado-Schwartzman M., and Abraham NG. The renal cytochrome P-450 arachidonic acid system. *Pediatr. Nephrol.* 1992; 6:490-498.
2. Hardwick JP. CYP4A subfamily: Functional analysis by immunocytochemistry and *in situ* hybridization. *Meth. Enzymol.* 1991; 206:273-283.
3. Aperia A and Larsson L. Correlation between fluid reabsorption and proximal tubule ultrastructure during development of the rat kidney. *Acta. Physiol. Scand.* 1979; 105:11-22.

Advances in Prostaglandin, Thromboxane,
and Leukotriene Research, Vol. 23,
edited by B. Samuelsson et al.
Raven Press, Ltd., New York © 1995

Amiloride-Sensitive Ion Transport Inhibition by Epoxyeicosatrienoic Acids in Renal Epithelial Cells

Bruno A. Escalante,* Robert Staudinger, **
Michal Schwartzman,‡ and Nader Abraham**

Departments of Pharmacology of *Instituto Nacional Cardiologia,
Mexico DF14080, **The Rockefeller University, New York,
New York 10021, and ‡New York Medical College, New York 10595

Among the P450 Arachidonic Acid metabolites, the epoxyeicosatrienoic acids (EETs) have been extensively studied for their biological activities and their presence in tissues and biological fluids (1,2,). EETs inhibits Na and K transport, in isolated rabbit cortical collecting tubule (3), vasopressin-stimulated water reabsorption in the collecting duct (4) and renin release in cortical slices (5); and modulates angiotensin II-induced inhibition of Na transport in cultured proximal renal tubule cells (6). EETs have been reported to inhibit the activity of purified renal Na-K-ATPase (7), and to activate the Na/H exchanger of cultured mesangial cells (8).These studies were designed to further characterize the actions of EETs on ion transport in epithelial cells using LLC-PK1 cells.

METHODS

LLC-PK1cells ($10^5/100\mu l$) were incubated on ice for 20 min in K free Hank's balanced solution (HBS). 86Rb uptake was initiated by adding 86Rb ($1\mu Ci$) and K(5mM) and placing the cells in a shaking-water bath at 37C. Uptake was terminated by pipetting the cell suspension into a stop solution ($75\mu l$ HBS, $75\mu l$ silicone oil and $75\mu l$ dioctylphtalamate), and centrifugation at 13,000 g for 30 sec. The bottom of the tube containing the cell pellet was cut and radioactivity of the pellet was determined.

RESULTS

All four EETs significantly inhibited Rb uptake in a concentration-dependent manner. (figure 1).

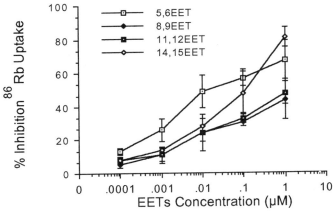

Figure 1.-Effect of Epoxyeicosatrienoic acids (EETs) on 86Rb uptake in LLC-PK1 cells, each curve represent the mean ± SE of 4 experiments

We compared the effects of ouabain and 14,15-EET on Rb uptake in LLC-PK1 cells treated with nystatin. Ouabain inhibited nystatin-stimulated Rb uptake, whereas 14,15EET did not affect Rb uptake (figure2). .

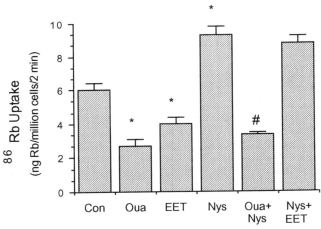

Figure 2.- Effects of 14,15EET on Nystatin-stimulated 86Rb uptake. Cells were incubated with vehicle (Con), Ouabain (Oua),14,15EET (EET), Nystatin (Nys), Ouabain + Nystatin (Oua+Nys) or Nystatin + 14,15EET (Nys+EET). Each bar represents the mean + SE of 6 experiments p<0.01 * vs control,# vs Nystatin

Amiloride (0.1mM) or ouabain (1mM) inhibited Rb uptake by 44±5 and 42±3%. Ouabain + amiloride inhibited Rb uptake by 58±3%. Whereas,14,15-EET (0.1μM) + amiloride produced 41±5% inhibition of Rb uptake.

DISCUSION

Rb uptake into LLC-PK1 can be regulated by the Na-K-ATPase directly, or indirectly by the Na/H exchanger and Na channels. First we determined wheter 14,15-EET act by inhibiting the Na-K-ATPase of the basolateral border, particularly, because it has been reported that EETs inhibited enzimatic activity of a purified preparation of the Na-K-ATPase (7). When Rb uptake was measured in cells that had been pretreated with nystatin to permeabilize them to Na, ouabain still inhibited Rb uptake and the effects of 14,15-EET were abolished, suggesting that the EETs act by limiting Na entry into the cells (9). If an important fraction of the Rb uptake is mediated by Na-K-ATPase, as suggested by the strong inhibitory effects of ouabain, reduced Na entry could markedly depress Rb uptake because Na-K-ATPase activity is driven by intracellular Na availability (10) Na channels and Na/H exchanger are important systems that allow Na entry into the cells. Indeed amiloride an inhibitor of these systems, markedly reduced Rb uptake. Moreover combination of amiloride and of 14,15-EET did not produce further inhibition of Rb uptake, suggesting that 14,15-EET and amiloride are affecting the same transport system in the cell membrane. Thus, EET inhibit ion transport via an amiloride-sensitive mechanism, suggesting a role of the EETs in the kidney function.

REFERENCES

1. McGiff JC. Cytochrome P450 metabolism of arachidonic acid. *Ann Rev Pharmacol Toxicol.* 1991;31:339-369.
2. Karara A. Dishman E. Glair I. Falck J. and Capdevila J. Endogenous epoxyeicosatrienoic acids. *J Biol Chem.* 1989;264:19822-19827.
3. Jacobson HR. Corona S. Capdevila J. et al. Effects of epoxyeicosatrienoic acids on ion transport in the rabbit collecting tubule. In:Braquet P. *Prostaglan and Membrane Ion Transport.* New York Raven Press; 1984:311-318.
4. Hirt DL. Capdevila J. Falck JR. Breyer MD. Jacobson HR. Cytochrome P450 metabolites of arachidonic acid are potent inhibitors of vasopressin action on rabbit cortical collecting duct. *J Clin Invest.* 1989;84:1805-1812.
5. Henrich WL. Falck JR. Campbell WB. Inhibition of renin release by 14,15-epoxyeicosatrienoic acid in renal slices. *Am J Physiol* 1990;258:E269-E274.
6. Romero MF. Madhun T. Hopfer V. Douglas JG. An epoxygenase metabolite of arachidonic acid 5,6epoxyeicosatrienoic acid mediates angiotensin-induced natriuresis in proximal tubular epithelium. *Adv Prostagl Thrombox Leuk Res.* 1990;31:205-208.
7. Schwartzman M. Ferreri NR. Carrol MA. Songe-Mize E. McGiff JC. Renal cytochrome P450 related arachidonate metabolites inhibit Na-K-ATPase. *Nature (London)* 1985;314:620-622
8. Harris RC. Homma T. Jacobson HR. Capdevila J. Epoxyeicosatrienoic acid activates Na+/H+ exchange and are mitogenic in cultured rat glomerular mesangial cells. *J Cell Physiol.* 1990;144:429-437.
9. Ribeiro CP. Mandel LJ. Parathyroid hormone inhibits proximal tubule Na+-K+-ATPase activity. *Am J Physiol.* 1992;262:F209-F216.
10. Grinstein S. Rothstein.A. Mechanisms of regulation of the Na/H exchanger *J Membr Biol.* 1986;90:1-12.

Advances in Prostaglandin, Thromboxane,
and Leukotriene Research, Vol. 23,
edited by B. Samuelsson et al.
Raven Press, Ltd., New York © 1995

Epoxyeicosatrienoic Acids Stimulate the Growth of Vascular Smooth Muscle Cells

H.L. Sheu, K. Omata, Y. Utsumi, E. Tsutsumi,
T. Sato, T. Shimizu, and K. Abe

*The 2nd Department of Internal Medicine,
Tohoku University School of Medicine, Sendai, Japan*

The proliferation of vascular smooth muscle cells (VSMC) play important pathophysiolgical roles in hypertension[1]. Recently, it is well focused on the non-cyclooxygenase arachidonic acid (AA) metabolites modulating the cell function involve proliferation of cell growth[2-4]. However, mechanisms responsible for stimulating the abnormal proliferation of VSMC are still precisely unknown.

We investigated the role of endogenous AA metabolites in the growth of VSMC cultured from spontaneously hypertensive rat(SHR) and Wistar-Kyoto rat(WKY).

Deisign and Methods:

Mesenteric VSMC were cultured from Sprague-Dawley rats (SD) , 4-wk-old SHR and WKY as previously described. Cells were grown in 0.1%, 10% FCS with or without cyclooxygenase inhibitor, indomethacin (10^{-5}M); epoxygenase inhibitor, ketoconazole (KETO) (10^{-5}M) or lipoxygenase inhibitor, baicalein (10^{-5}M) or PGI2 analoge, cicletanine (10^{-6}M). Cell numbers were counted on each subseqent day by coulter counter ZM model. After serum-depriving, cells were exposed to 10%FCS either in the presence or absence of inhibitors of AA metabolism. Then VSMC were homogenize and incubated with [^{14}C]AA (0.1μCi) and 40mM NADPH for 30 minites at 37℃. The reaction was terminated by acidification to pH 3.5 with 1M citric acid. AA metabolites were extracted with ethyl acetate and seperated by reverse-phase HPLC as previously described[3]. [^{3}H]-thymidine incorporation were measured after the stimulation of those agents.

Results and Discussion

VSMC of SD, SHR, WKY in synchronized quiescent stage and in asynchronous cycling stage represented arachidonate metabolites comigrated with epoxyeicosatrienoic acids (EETs) as non cyclooxygenase metabolites of AA. The production rate of EETs in quiescent stage of VSMC in SD was 3.58 pmol/mg protein and was increased lineally up to 455.17 pmol/mg protein after 8 hrs stimulation by serum. Similary we could detect EETs in human artherosclerotic vessels. Productions of prostaglandins and EETs in VSMC of SHR were higher than in that of WKY. [^{3}H]-Thymidine incorporation of VSMC in SHR were higher than in WKY, and only KETO inhibited the uptake of [^{3}H]-Thymidine dose dependently. Cell counts confirmed the above results, and only KETO inhibited the cell grouth both in SHR and WKY. Thus an enhanced proliferation of VSMC in SHR associate with the suprus production of EETs.

On the other hand cicletanine stimulated PGI$_2$ synthesis and inhibited the cell proliferation as well as [3H]-Thymidine incorporation in VSMC, suggesting that PGI$_2$ inhibited the cell growth. As like previous study[5], we firstly indicate that the P450 dependent epoxygenase is activated time-dependently in the quiescent cultured gflomerular mesangial cells by serum stimulation. Similarly the peak time of DNA synthesis is at about 24-36 h later than that of EETs synthesis in VSMC. Sellmayer et al[4] demonstrated that an endogenous cytochrome P450 or lipoxygenase product modulates c-fos and Egr-1 mRNA levels. However,the maximal induction of epoxygenase activity by serum appeared later than the maximum induction of c-fos (30 min) or c-myc (2 h) mRNA levels. These results elicit a possibility that EETs production may be related to the regulation of c-myc mRNA in DNA synthesis at a post-transcriptional step during the transition from the G$_0$ to G$_1$ stage.

The sesults of our investigation can be summarized as follows, (1) rat VSMC and human atherosclerotic vessels produced arachidonate metabolites comigrated with EETs as non cyclooxygenase metabolites, (2) productions of prostaglandins and EETs in VSMC of SHR were higher than in that of WKY, (3) only epoxygenase inhibitor, ketoconazole, inhibited the enhanced proliferation of hypertensive VSMC, (4) epoxygenase products of AA stimulated the growth of VSMC, (5) cicletanine stimulated PGI$_2$ synthesis, resulting the inhibition of the cell growth in VSMC.

When taken together PGI$_2$ antagonize to EETs in the the growth of the vascular smooth muscle cells (Fig.1). And inbalance between cyclooxygenase activity and epoxygenase activity of VSMC might cause vascular hypertrophy. Higher epoxy-

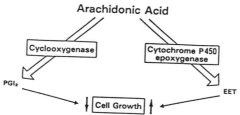

Fig.1. Modulation of the cell growth by AA metabolites.

-genase activity found in VSMC in SHR might associate the medial hypertrophy in resistence vessels.

Acknowledgments

This work was supported partly by a Grant-in-Aid for Scientific Reserch from the Ministry of Education, Science and Culture of Japan (03557031,03454246, 50194634), from Japan Reserch Foundation for Clinical Pharmacology, and from the Miyagi Prefecture Kidney Association.

References

1. Owens GK. and Reidy MA. Hyperplastic growth response of vascular smooth muscle cells following induction of acute hypertension in rats by aortic coarctation. *Circ Res* 1985;57:695-705.
2. Harris RC, Homma T, Jacobson HR, Capdevila J. Epoxyeicosatrienoic acids activate Na+/H+ exchange and are mitogenic in cultured rat glomerular mesangial cells. *J Cell Physiol* 1990;144(3):429-37.
3. Omata K, Abe K, Sheu HL, Yoshida K, Tsutsumi E, Yoshinaga K, Abraham NG, Schwartzman ML. Roles of renal cytochrome P450 dependent arachidonic acid metabolites in hypertension. *Tohoku J Exp Med.* 1992;166:93-106.
4. Alois S, Waltraud MU, Peter CW, Joseph VB. Endogenous non-cyclooxyge-nase metabolites of arachidonic acid modulate growth and mRNA level of immediated-early response genes in rat mesangial cells. *J Biol Chem* 1991; 266:3800-7.
5. Sato M, Abe K, Takeuchi K. Atrial natriuretic factor and cyclic guanosine 3', 5'-monophosphate in vascular smooth muscle. *Hypertension* 1986;8:762-71.
6. Sheu HL, Abe K, Omata K et al. Non-cyclooxygenase metabolites of arachi--donic acid modulate cell proliferation in rat mesangial cells. *Abstract* (The 8th international conference on prostaglandins and related compounds) 1992;pp51.

Advances in Prostaglandin, Thromboxane, and Leukotriene Research, Vol. 23,
edited by B. Samuelsson et al.
Raven Press, Ltd., New York © 1995

ACTIVATION OF XENOBIOTICS INTO FREE RADICALS BY PROSTAGLANDIN-H-SYNTHASE AND BY RAT LIVER MICROSOMES

P.F. Mannaioni, M.G. Di Bello, S. Raspanti, L. Mugnai,
V. Romano and E. Masini

*Department of Preclinical and Clinical Pharmacology, Florence University,
Viale G.B. Morgagni 65, 50134 Florence, Italy*

The generation of free radicals from xenobiotics or endogenous compounds is known to be mediated by the intervention of oxidative enzymes, in vivo (1). In vitro, oxidative enzymes have been used to detect the generation of free radicals by measuring the free radical-driven perturbation of cell membranes in target cells. We have recently proposed a free radical bioassay, in which the drug under study is incubated with isolated purified rat serosal mast cells, in the presence and in the absence of oxidative enzymes. The end point of the reaction is the free radical-driven release of histamine and of lactate dehydrogenase (LDH), the generation of markers of membrane lipoperoxidation, and the inhibition of these effects by free radical scavengers. Using this bioassay, we have recently shown that paracetamol, anthranilic antibiotics, arachidonic acid and linoleic acid evoke the release of mast cell histamine only in the presence of oxidative enzymes. The release of histamine was coupled with the generation of malonyldialdehyde (MDA), and abated by reduced glutathion and by a-tocopherol, thus fulfilling the criteria of a free radical-driven event (2, 3).

Here we report on the generation of free radicals from commonly abused drugs, using the same bioassay system.

MATERIALS AND METHODS

Mast cells of serosal phenotype were obtained by pleural and peritoneal lavage in Wistar rats, and purified by elutriation. Mast cells were incubated (Tyrode solution, pH 7.4, 37^0 C, gas phase, air) for 30 min. with a) cocaine, morphine or methadone, b) with oxidative enzymes, c) with cocaine, morphine, methadone in the presence of oxidative enzymes. The reaction was stopped by chilling the tubes. After centrifugation, histamine and LDH were analyzed in the supernatants and in the pellets (fluorimetric and spectrophotometric assays respectively) and expressed as percent of the total. MDA was measured by a colorimetric assay. Oxidative enzymes were prostaglandin-H-synthase (PHS) purified from ram seminal vesicles, and S10 Mix liver microsomes from phenobarbital or polychlorinated biphenyl treated rats.

RESULTS AND DISCUSSION

The results obtained are reported in Table I. Neither cocaine, morphine andmethadone, nor the oxidative enzymes, were capable of inducing any release of histamine in separate incubations. In the presence of the oxidizing systems, cocaine, morphine and methadone evoke the release of histamine as a function of both the concentrations of substrates and enzymes. The release of histamine by the activated xenobiotics is exocytotic in nature and triggered by the generation of free radicals, as shown by electronmicroscopic observation, LDH, MDA and diene determinations, and by the effect of free radical scavengers.

TABLE 1. Mast cell histamine release and MDA production by xenobiotics in the presence of oxidative enzymes: effect of free radical scavengers.

DRUGS		HISTAMINE RELEASE (%) BY DRUGS PLUS		MDA $nmol \cdot mg^{-1}$ protein (b)	INHIBITION OF HISTAMINE RELEASE (%) (b) BY	
		PHS (a)	S10 Mix (a)		GSH 10^{-4} M	α-TOCOPHEROL 10^{-4} M
Morphine	10^{-5} M	42.6	39.7	17.3	65.2	92.7
Cocaine	10^{-5} M	38.7	51.3	56.4	76.4	72.2
Methadone	10^{-5} M	22.2	34.2	21.9	69.8	90.9

a) PHS (25 mU) and s10 Mix (400 μl) did not produce any release of histamine when incubated alone.
b) The figures are from experiments carried out with mast cells incubated with drugs in the presence of PHS.

In mammals, including man, morphine and cocaine are detoxified by means of N-demethylation followed by conjugation with glicuronic acid (morphine) or by the intervention of ubiquitous esterases (cocaine). However, a small fraction of the metabolism of cocaine and morphine follows a toxifying pathway, leading to cocaine and morphine free radicals, after oxidation by P-from cocaine and morphine, lend further support to this hypothesis. Moreover, the PHS and S10 Mix activation of drugs of abuse into free radicals may explain organic injuries commonly observed among drug abusers.

REFERENCES

1. Mason RP, Chignell CR. Free radicals in pharmacology and toxicology. *Pharmacol. Rev.* 1982; 33:189-211.

2. Mannaioni PF, Masini E. The release of histamine by free radicals. *Free Rad. Biol. Med.* 1988; 5:177-197.

3. Masini E, Palmerani B, Gambassi F et al. Histamine release from rat mast cells induced by metabolic activation of polyunsaturated fatty acids into free radicals. *Biochem. Pharmacol.* 1989; 39: 879-889.

4. Evans MA. Microsomal activation of N-hydroxynorcocaine to a reactive nitoxide. *Toxicologist* 1981;1:1-6.

5. Misra AL, Vadlamani NL, Pontani RR et al. Evidence for a new metabolite of morphine-N-methyl-^{14}C in the rat. *Biochem. Pharmacol.* 1973; 22:2129-2139.

Advances in Prostaglandin, Thromboxane,
and Leukotriene Research, Vol. 23,
edited by B. Samuelsson et al.
Raven Press, Ltd., New York © 1995

THE ISOPROSTANES: NOVEL MARKERS OF LIPID PEROXIDATION AND POTENTIAL MEDIATORS OF OXIDANT INJURY

L. Jackson Roberts, II and Jason D. Morrow

Departments of Pharmacology and Medicine
Vanderbilt University School of Medicine
Nashville, TN 37232 U.S.A.

We reported in 1990 that there are a series of prostaglandin (PG)F_2-like compounds, termed F_2-isoprostanes, that are produced in vivo in humans by a non-cyclooxygenase mechanism involving the free radical catalyzed peroxidation of arachidonic acid.[1] This finding was novel in that it had previously been thought the cyclooxygenase was obligatory for the formation of prostaglandins in vivo. As shown in the figure below, the formation of these prostanoids proceeds through bicyclic endoperoxide intermediates that are reduced to F_2-isoprostanes. Four regioisomers of the F_2-isoprostanes are formed, each of which is comprised of 8 racemic diastereomers. Interestingly, in contrast to cyclooxygenase derived prostaglandins, F_2-isoprostanes are formed in situ esterified in phospholipids and are subsequently released preformed, presumably by phospholipases.[2]

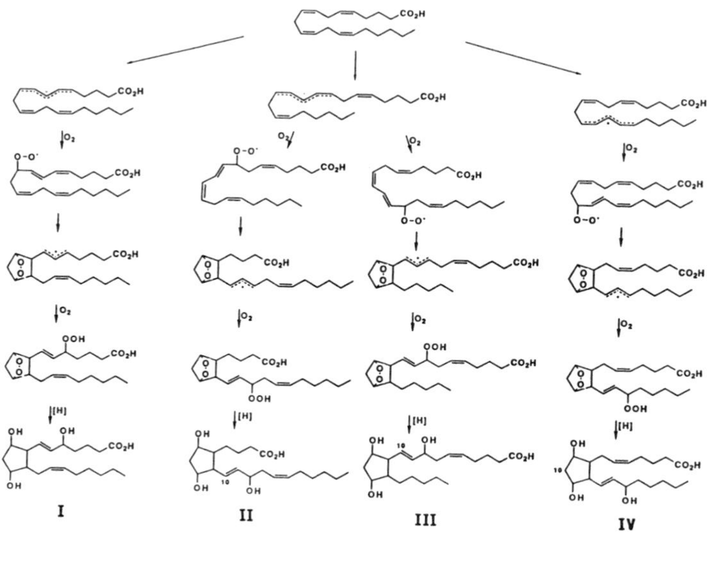

The fact that prostanoids can be produced in vivo independent of the cyclooxygenase is not only of considerable biochemical interest but may have important physiological ramifications because it has been shown that these compounds exert potent biological activity.[3,4] Interestingly, 8-iso-PGF$_{2\alpha}$, which was recently shown to be one of the more abundant F$_2$-isoprostanes produced in vivo, has been found to be an extremely potent renal vasoconstrictor with an EC$_{50}$ in the low nanomolar range.[1,3] Further, it is also a potent vasoconstrictor in the pulmonary vasculature.[4] These effects can be abrogated with SQ29548, a thromboxane receptor antagonist, suggesting that the isoprostanes may exert their effects by interaction with the thromboxane receptor. Surprisingly, however, 8-iso-PGF$_{2\alpha}$ is primarily an antagonist of the thromboxane receptor in the platelet.[5] Insight into this apparent paradox has been obtained from recent studies which suggest that 8-iso-PGF$_{2\alpha}$ interacts with a receptor in vascular smooth muscle which may be similar to, but distinct from, the thromboxane receptor.[6]

ISOPROSTANES ARE ACCURATE MARKERS OF ENDOGENOUS LIPID PEROXIDATION

Methods currently available to assess oxidant stress in vivo are generally unreliable. By contrast, we have obtained considerable evidence that measurement of isoprostanes represents an important advance in our ability to assess oxidant stress in vivo. Sufficient quantities of F$_2$-isoprostanes can be detected in human biological fluids from normal individuals, e.g. urine, plasma, etc., to define normal ranges.[1] Further, these compounds are very stable molecules. Nonetheless, precautions must be taken when analyzing F$_2$-isoprostanes in lipid containing biological samples since autoxidation ex vivo can lead to generation of these compounds.[7] Such precautions include either processing samples immediately after they are obtained or storing them at temperatures of -70°C or lower which appears to prevent autoxidation. It has been shown that in animal models of oxidant stress such as the administration of the herbicide diquat to selenium deficient rats or the administration of CCl$_4$ to normal rats, concentrations of free F$_2$-isoprostanes in the circulation increase up to 200-fold and levels of F$_2$-isoprostanes esterified in liver tissue increase up to 250-fold and correlate with the extent of tissue injury.[1,8] The fact that F$_2$-isoprostanes can be quantified in different organs provides a valuable method to localize endogenous lipid peroxidation to a particular site.

Quantification of F$_2$-isoprostanes also has proven to be a valuable tool to investigate the role of oxidant stress in human disease. Previously, we showed that circulating concentrations and urinary excretion of F$_2$-isoprostanes were markedly increased above normal in patients with the hepatorenal syndrome, implicating oxidant stress in the pathogenesis of this almost uniformly fatal disorder.[9] The syndrome is characterized by intense renal vasoconstriction in the setting of severe liver disease but the pathogenesis of the vasoconstriction that characterizes the disorder remains poorly understood.[10] It is of interest that the F_2-isoprostane, 8-iso-$PGF_{2\alpha}$, is a potent renal vasoconstrictor and thus isoprostanes may contribute, to some extent, to the renal vasoconstriction in this disorder.

More recently, we have examined the role of free radical generation and lipid peroxidation in association with heavy cigarette smoking. It has been postulated that the reason for the increased incidence of diseases such as atherosclerosis and lung cancer in smokers may be related to the large amounts of free radicals in cigarette smoke which could oxidize cellular biomolecules such as lipids and DNA.[11] Evidence that oxidative damage occurs in smokers, however, is poorly documented. For this study, we recruited 10 heavy smokers, (greater than 2 packs per day) and 10 age and sex match non-smokers and compared levels of free and esterified F_2-isoprostanes in the circulation. The majority of esterified F_2-isoprostanes in the circulation are likely carried in lipoproteins such as low density lipoprotein and oxidation of these protein lipid complexes has been implicated in the development of atheromatous plaques. Smokers, on average, had approximately a 200% increase in both free and esterified circulating F_2-isoprostane levels compared to non-smokers (p=0.03). In addition, after two weeks of smoking cessation, circulating levels of F_2-isoprostane levels in smokers fell a mean of 35% (p=0.03). These studies provide the first compelling evidence that smoking causes oxidative damage <u>in vivo</u>. These findings may explain the causative link between smoking and the enhanced risk of cancer and atherosclerotic cardiovascular disease.

DISCOVERY OF THE D_2/E_2-ISOPROSTANES

As mentioned, the formation of F_2-isoprostanes proceeds through the formation of bicyclic PGH_2-like endoperoxide intermediates that are reduced to form the F_2-isoprostanes. Factors involved in the reduction of the isoprostane endoperoxide intermediates <u>in vivo</u>, however, remain to be identified. Nonetheless, we hypothesized that the endoperoxide intermediates may, in part, escape reduction and rearrange to form PGE_2-like and PGD_2-like isoprostanes. Using a modified mass spectrometric assay for measurement of cyclooxygenase derived PGE_2, we initially found that D_2/E_2-isoprostanes were formed <u>in vitro</u> in plasma allowed to undergo autoxidation.[12] Abundant quantities of what appeared to be the same compounds could also be detected in the circulation and esterified to liver phospholipids following treatment of rats with CCl_4 to induce endogenous lipid peroxidation. Employing a variety of approaches including the use of deuteriated derivatives, catalytic hydrogenation, electron ionization mass spectrometry, and liquid secondary ion mass spectrometry, compelling evidence was obtained that these compounds are D-ring and E-ring isoprostanes. Levels of D_2/E_2-isoprostanes were found to increase dramatically in settings of oxidant stress. For example, in untreated rats, levels of D_2/E_2-isoprostanes present esterified to liver lipids were 0.90 ± 0.10 ng/g liver and increased to 85 ± 33 ng/g liver after administration of CCl_4 treated rats.[12]

We then examined the biological activity of the E-ring analogue of 8-iso-$PGF_{2\alpha}$, 8-iso-PGE_2. Interestingly, whereas cyclooxygenase derived PGE_2 is a vasodilator, 8-iso-PGE_2 was found to be a potent vasoconstrictor of the renal vasculature, with a potency very similar to 8-iso-$PGF_{2\alpha}$.[12] Like 8-iso-$PGF_{2\alpha}$, this effect can be blocked by the thromboxane receptor antagonist SQ29548. Interestingly, however, 8-iso-PGE_2 is an antagonist of the thromboxane receptor in platelets with a potency similar to 8-iso-$PGF_{2\alpha}$. Taken together, therefore, these findings suggest that 8-iso-PGE_2 may interact with the same "isoprostane" receptor as 8-iso-$PGF_{2\alpha}$.

More recently, we have begun to explore factors influencing the formation of D_2/E_2-isoprostanes relative to F_2-isoprostanes. Our interest in carrying out these studies was based on findings that relative levels of D_2/E_2-isoprostanes to F_2-isoprostanes esterified in lipids vary markedly in different tissues. For example, the ratio of esterified D_2/E_2-isoprostanes to F_2-isoprostanes in plasma lipids is significantly higher compared to the ratio in liver lipids. These data suggest that the efficiency of the reduction of isoprostane endoperoxides to F_2-isoprostanes varies in different tissues. Of note in this regard, we have found that the formation of D_2/E_2-isoprostanes to F-ring compounds can be enhanced in vivo in rats by depletion of endogenous glutathione. In addition, we have recently obtained evidence that the reduction of isoprostane endoperoxide intermediates is facilitated by a heat labile factor, presumably an enzyme, present in microsomes. Taken together, these studies suggest the formation of F_2-isoprostanes may modulated by glutathione and a reductive enzyme.

In spite of the fact that large quantities of D_2/E_2-isoprostanes can be detected esterified to tissue lipids which in some tissues exceeds levels of F_2-isoprostanes, D_2/E_2-isoprostanes cannot be detected freee in the circulation in the normal situation whereas levels of F_2-isoprostanes are easily measured (approximately 40 pg/ml). Thus, we questioned whether once released from tissue lipids, D_2/E_2-isoprostanes may be converted by cytosolic ketoreductases to F_2-isoprostanes. To examine this possibility, we incubated 8-iso-PGE_2 (100ng) with cytosol (2mg protein) from rat liver and kidney in the presence of NADH or NADPH (2mM). Products were analyzed and quantified by mass spectrometry. Interestingly, after a 1 hour incubation in the presence of NADPH, there was approximately an 80% conversion of 8-iso-PGE_2 to 8-iso $PGF_{2\alpha}$ in the presence of liver cytosol and a 24% conversion in kidney cytosol. Much less conversion occurred in the presence of NADH. These studies thus suggest that ketoreductases exist which can efficiently reduce E_2-isoprostanes to F-ring compounds. The extent to which this occurs in vivo, however, remains to be determined.

The discovery of D_2/E_2-isoprostanes extends our understanding of the biochemistry of the formation of isoprostanes in vivo. This discovery also indicates that the variety of novel prostanoids that can be produced by the non-enzymatic oxidation of arachidonic acid is greater than previously thought. Further the finding that D_2/E-isoprostanes, like F_2-isoprostanes, are capable of exerting biological activity also has important implications related to the possibility that isoprostanes may not only be accurate markers of oxidant injury but also mediators in the pathophysiology of oxidant injury.

ACKNOWLEDGEMENTS

Supported by NIH grants GM42056 and ES00267. J. Morrow is a Howard Hughes Medical Institute Physician Research Fellow and the recipient of a Career Development Award from the International Life Sciences Institute. The technical assistance of William Zackert, Gary Cunningham, Aping Wu and Vincent Daniel was apppreciated.

REFERENCES

1.   Morrow JD, Hill KE, Burk RE, Nammour TM, Badr KF, Roberts, LJ,II. A series of prostaglandin F_2-like compounds are produced in vivo in humans by a non-cyclooxygenase, free radical catalyzed mechanism. *Proc. Natl. Acad. Sci.* USA 1990;87:9383-9387.

2.   Morrow JD, Awad JA, Boss HJ, Blair IA, Roberts LJ,II. Noncyclooxygenase-derived prostanoids (F_2-isoprostanes) are formed in situ on phospholipids. *Proc. Natl. Acad. Sci.* USA 1990;89:10721-10725.

3.   Takahashi K, Nammour TM, Ebert J, Morrow JD, Roberts LJ,II, Badr KF. Glomerular actions of a free radical generated novel prostaglandin, 8-epi-prostaglandin $F_{2\alpha}$, in the rat: Evidence for interaction with thromboxane A_2 receptors. *J. Clin. Invest.* 1992;90:135-141.

4.   Banerjee M, Kang KH, Morrow JD, Roberts LJ,II, Newman JH. Effects of a novel non-cyclooxygenase derived prostaglandin, 8-epi-$PGF_{2\alpha}$, in rabbit lung in situ. *Am. J. Physiol.* 263(Heart Circ. Physiol. 32):H660-H663.

5.   Morrow JD, Minton TA, Roberts LJ,II. The F_2-isoprostane, 8-epi-prostaglandin $F_{2\alpha}$, a potent agonist of the vascular thromboxane/endoperoxide receptor, is a platelet thromboxane/endoperoxide receptor antagonist. *Prostaglandins* 1992;44:155-163.

6.   Fukunaga M, Makita N, Roberts, LJ, II, Morrow JD, Takahashi K, Badr KF. Evidence for the existence of F_2-isoprostane receptors on rat vascular smooth muscle cells. *Am. J. Physiol.* 263(Cell Physiol. 33):C1619-C1624.

7.   Morrow JD, Harris TM, Roberts LJ,II. Non-cyclooxygenase oxidative formation of a series of novel prostaglandins: Analytical ramifications for measurement of eicosanoids. *Anal. Biochem.* 1990;184:1-10.

8.   Morrow JD, Awad JA, Kato T, Takahashi K, Badr KF, Roberts LJ,II, Burk RF. Formation of novel non-cyclooxygenase derived prostanoids (F_2-isoprostanes) in carbon tetrachloride hepatotoxicity. An animal model of lipid peroxidation. *J. Clin. Invest.* 1992;90:2502-2507.

9.   Morrow JD, Moore KP, Awad JA, Ravenscraft MD, Marini G, Badr KF, Williams R, Roberts LJ. Marked overproduction of non-cyclooxygenase derived prostanoids (F_2-isoprostanes) in the hepatorenal syndrome. *J. Lipid Mediators* 1993;6:417-420.

10.   Schelling JR, and Linal SL. Hepatorenal syndrome. *Sem. Nephrol.* 1990;10:565-570.

11.   Chruch DF and Pryor WA. Free-radical chemistry of cigarette smoke and its toxicological implications. *Environ. Health Presp.* 1985;64:11-126.

12.   Morrow JD, Minton TA, Mukundan CR, Campbell MD, Zackert WE, Daniel VC, Badr KF, Blair IA and Roberts LJ,II. Free radical-induced generation of isoprostanes in vivo. Evidence for the formation of D-ring and E-ring isoprostanes in vivo. *J. Biol. Chem.* 1993; 269:4317-4326.

Advances in Prostaglandin, Thromboxane, and Leukotriene Research, Vol. 23,
edited by B. Samuelsson et al.
Raven Press, Ltd., New York © 1995

Formation of F₂-Isoprostanes during the oxidation of human low density lipoprotein by peroxynitrite

Kevin P Moore, Victor Darley-Usmar*,
Jason Morrow**, and LJ Roberts** II

*Department of Clinical Pharmacology,
Royal Postgraduate Medical School, London W12 0NN, UK*

**Biochemical Sciences, Wellcome Research Foundation,
Beckenham, Kent, UK*

***Department of Clinical Pharmacology,
Vanderbilt Medical Center, Nashville, Tennessee, USA*

Introduction

The oxidative modification of low density lipoprotein (LDL) is one of the key events in the pathogenesis of atherosclerosis. Oxidation of LDL is associated with the generation of a wide range of lipid derived oxidation products including hydroperoxides and aldehydes which ultimately converts the LDL particle to a form recognized by the macrophage scavenger receptor. It is well recognised that stereospecific oxidation of arachidonic acid by the lipoxygenase and cyclo-oxygenase enzymes, may contribute to the inflammatory component of atherosclerosis. Approximately 10% of the unsaturated fatty acid in LDL is arachidonic acid, which can form a multitude of oxidation products, the pharmacological properties of which are largely unknown. An important exception to this is the recently described F₂-isoprostanes, a family of compounds isomeric to PGF2α, formed by non-enzymic oxidation of arachidonyl-containing phospholipids (1,2). These are formed in animal models of oxidant stress, and during certain human pathological processes. More importantly, one of the F₂-isoprostanes, namely 8-epi-PGF2α is a potent renal, and pulmonary vasoconstrictor (3).

In the present study, we have investigated the hypothesis that oxidation of LDL is associated with the formation of F₂-isoprostanes, and may be initiated by the simultaneous production of the free radicals superoxide (O2-) and nitric oxide (NO).

225

Materials and Methods

Human LDL was isolated from plasma from individual donors by differential centrifugation. All oxidation experiments were carried out in duplicate at a final concentration of LDL of 200 μg/ml (total 50-100 μg LDL) in PBS. To initiate the oxidation reactions, peroxynitrite, or SIN-1 were added to the LDL, and incubated at 37°C for 24 hours. Esterified F_2-isoprostanes were quantitated following base hydrolysis as the free F_2-isoprostanes, after purification and derivitization, by selected ion monitoring gas chromatography negative ion chemical ionization/ mass spectrometry as previously described (1). Oxidation of LDL is associated with an increase in electrophoretic mobility, due to oxidation of the apoB. Electrophoretic mobility of LDL was determined using a Beckman system, and all results related to mobility of the control sample in each gel.

Results

Oxidation of LDL and formation of F₂-isoprostanes by peroxynitrite

Incubation of LDL with peroxynitrite overnight increased esterified F2-isoprostanes, and electrophoretic mobility in a concentration dependent manner, with a 2-13 fold increase of F_2-isoprostanes at 1.0 mM peroxynitrite (a typical LDL preparation is shown in the figure below). In contrast there was no increase in either the amount of F_2-isoprostanes formed or the electrophoretic mobility when LDL was incubated with peroxynitrite that had been allowed to decompose in PBS for 5 minutes.

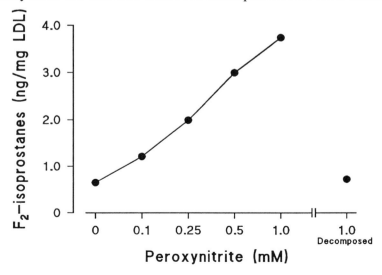

Oxidation of LDL and formation of F$_2$-isoprostanes by SIN-1

SIN-1 spontaneously decomposes to form both nitric oxide and superoxide anion in aqueous solution, and yields a continuous source of peroxynitrite over several hours. Incubation of LDL with SIN-1 (0.5mM-1mM) significantly increased formation of esterified F$_2$-isoprostanes by 8 to 31-fold and electrophoretic mobility by 1.8-fold. The formation of F2-isoprostanes was inhibited by coincubation with superoxide dismutase, consistent with the important role of superoxide in this oxidative process.

Discussion

The vascular endothelium produces significant concentrations of nitric oxide (NO), which causes vasorelaxation of smooth muscle, and concentrations of NO have been estimated to be of the order of up to 400nM. It now appears that superoxide attenuates the physiological action of NO, by enhancing its destruction, with the formation of peroxynitrite. The rate of reaction of NO with superoxide has been determined by flash photolysis to be 6.7×10^9 $M^{-1}S^{-1}$, which exceeds the rate of scavenging by superoxide dismutase (rate of reaction 2×10^9 $M^{-1}S^{-1}$), and recent evidence suggests that peroxynitrite dependent modification of proteins is a pathological feature of atherosclerotic plaques (4). This study demonstrates for the first time that peroxynitrite or the "peroxynitrite donor" SIN-1 oxidise human LDL with the formation of the F$_2$-isoprostanes. The continued production of NO and superoxide under physiological conditions may explain the normal, but significant, concentrations of F$_2$-isoprostanes observed in normal volunteers. Nitric oxide and superoxide production may be increased during pathophysiological processes such as sepsis, when there is induction of nitric oxide synthase. This may increase the formation of esterified, and presumably free F$_2$-isoprostanes. One of the F$_2$-isoprostanes, namely 8-epi-PGF$_{2\alpha}$ has potent biological actions. It is a potent renal and pulmonary vasoconstrictor. Both renal and pulmonary vascular resistance increase during sepsis, suggesting that increased formation of F$_2$-isoprostanes, perhaps by NO/superoxide dependent production of peroxynitrite, may occur *in vivo*.

1. Morrow, J.D., Hill, K.E., Burk, R.F., Nammour, T.M., Badr, K.F. & Roberts, L.J., II. *Proc. Natl. Acad. Sci. U.S.A.* 87, 9383-9387 (1990).
2. Morrow, J.D., Awad, J.A., Kato, T., Takahashi, K., Badr, K.F., Roberts, L.J., II, & Burk, R.F. *J. Clin. Invest.* 90, 2502-2507 (1992).
3. Takahashi, K., Nammour, T.M., Ebert, J., Morrow, J.D., Roberts, L.J., II & Badr, K.F. *J. Clin. Invest.* 90, 136-141 (1992).
4. Beckman, J.S., Zu Ye, Y., Anderson, G., Chen,J., Accavitti, M.A., Tarpey, M.M. and White, C.R. (1994) Biol. Chem. Hoppe Seyler. 375 81-88.

Advances in Prostaglandin, Thromboxane,
and Leukotriene Research, Vol. 23,
edited by B. Samuelsson et al.
Raven Press, Ltd., New York © 1995

Cyclooxygenase Dependent Formation of 8-ISO-Prostaglandin $F_{2\alpha}$ by Human Platelets

Domenico Pratico, John A. Lawson, and Garret A. FitzGerald

Centre for Cardiovascular Science,
Department of Medicine and Experimental Therapeutics
University College, Dublin 7.

F_2-isoprostanes are a family of prostaglandin F isomers formed in a free radical dependent manner from arachidonic acid. Using an assay to measure total F_2 isoprostanes, Morrow, Roberts and their colleagues have demonstrated exaggerated formation in plasma of animal models of free radical induced hepatic insult, such as diquat poisoning (1). This has led to the suggestion that measurement of F_2 isoprostanes might provide a quantitative index of free radical formation in vivo which would be useful in the assessment and targeting of putative antioxidant drugs.

Particular attention has focused upon one of the F_2-isoprostanes, 8-iso-PGF$_{2\alpha}$, as it has been shown to have biological activity as a vasoconstrictor and weak mitogen. These effects are blocked by thromboxane antagonists and it is being investigated whether the endogenous ligand might mediate such effects through the thromboxane receptor or a closely related receptor (2,3).

Given the particular interest in 8-iso-PGF$_{2\alpha}$ and its potential cardiovascular importance. We developed a method specifically to study its biosynthesis. We investigated its formation by human platelets, cells in which it induces shape change and a rise in intracellular calcium, but not aggregation (4,5).

RESULTS AND DISCUSSION

A quantitative assay for 8-iso was developed using an [$^{18}O_2$] -labelled internal standard and selected ion monitoring, using gas chromatography/mass spectrometry in the negative ion, chemical ionization mode. Chromatographic conditions were such that a peak corresponding to the retention time of the authentic standard was clearly separated from peaks corresponding to other F$_2$ isoprostanes and also from the peak corresponding to the authentic standard of PGF$_{2\alpha}$.

When platelets were activated with arachidonic acid, thrombin or collagen there was a time dependent increase in 8-iso, but not other F$_2$ isoprostanes. This was temporally related to the increase in the cyclooxygenase (COX) and lipoxygenase (LOX) products, TxB2 and 12-HETE. However, the quantity formed was considerably less than was the case for the other eicosanoids. Formation of 8-iso was completely blocked by aspirin and indomethacin and was independent of platelet aggregation per se.
The identity of the compound comigrating with the authentic 8-iso internal standard was further confirmed by an electron impact mass spectrum of d0 and d8 8-iso obtained after addition of d8 arachidonic acid to human platelets. This approach ruled out the presence of a heptadeuterated species, such as a PGD2 metabolite. Furthermore, the material cochromatographed with [^{3}H]-8-iso-PGF$_{2\alpha}$ over 4 HPLC columns after its formation by the purified COX.
Small amounts of 8-iso-PGF$_{2\alpha}$ are formed by human platelets in vitro and have now been shown to be formed ex vivo (6). The mechanism of formation remains to be defined precisely; however formation of 8-iso PGH2 by purified COX has been described (7). It is possible that COX dependent formation of this compound also occurs in other cells. Given the presence of platelet activation in many syndromes of human disease putatively associated with free radical generation, it would seem prudent to define the relative contribution of enzyme dependent and independent formation of 8-iso to levels measured in plasma, urine or other biological fluids.

ACKNOWLEDGEMENTS

Supported by grants from the Wellcome Trust, the European Union and a fellowship in Cardiovascular Disease from Bristol Myers Squibb to Dr. Pratico.

REFERENCES

1. Morrow JD, Hill KE, Burk RF, Nammour TM, Badr KF, Roberts LJ II. A series of prostaglandin F$_2$-like compounds are produced in vivo in humans by a non-cycooxygenase, free radical-catalysed mechanism. Proc Natl Acad Sci USA. 1990;87:9383-9387.

2. Fukunaga M, Makita N, Roberts LJ II, Morrow JD, Takahashi K, Badr KF. Evidence for the existence of F$_2$-isoprostane receptors on rat vascular smooth muscle cells. Am Phys Soc 1993;1619-1624.

3. Takahara K, Murray R, FitzGerald GA, Fitzgerald DJ. The response to thromboxane A$_2$ in human platelets: discrimination of two binding sites linked to distinct effector systems. J Biol Chem. 1990;265:6836-6844.

4. Morrow JD, Minton Ta, Roberts LJ II. The F$_2$-isoprostane, 8-epi-prostaglandin F$_{2\alpha}$, a potent agonist of the vascular thromboxane/endoperoxide receptor, is a platelet thromboxane/endoperoxide receptor antagonist. Prostaglandins. 1992, 44:155-163.

5. Lawson JA, Pratico D, FitzGerald GA. Cyclooxygenase dependent formation of 8-epi PGF$_{2\alpha}$ In: Cellular Generation, Transport and Effects of Eicosanoids (Goetzl E ed). Ann N.Y. Acad. Sci. (1994) in press.

6. Catella F, Reilly MP, Delanty N, et al. In vivo formation of 8-epi-PGF$_{2\alpha}$ physiological formation of 8-epi-PGF$_{2\alpha}$ in vivo is not affected by cyclooxygenase inhibition. Adv. Prostag. Thrombox Leuk Res, 1995 (in press).

7. Hecker M, Ullrich V, Fischer C, Meese C. Identification of novel arachidonic acid metabolites formed by prostaglandin H synthase. Eur J Biochem, 1987,169:113-123.

Advances in Prostaglandin, Thromboxane,
and Leukotriene Research, Vol. 23,
edited by B. Samuelsson et al.
Raven Press, Ltd., New York © 1995

Physiological Formation of 8-EPI-PGF$_{2\alpha}$ In Vivo is notAffected by Cyclooxygenase Inhibition

Francesca Catella, Muredach P. Reilly, Norman Delanty,
John A. Lawson, Niamh Moran, Emma Meagher, and Garret A. FitzGerald

*Centre for Cardiovascular Science, Department of Medicine and
Experimental Therapeutics, University College, Dublin,, Ireland*

Morrow et al. (1) have recently discovered a series of prostaglandin-like compounds that are produced by nonenzymatic free radical catalyzed peroxidation of arachidonic acid. These isoprostanes are formed in situ from arachidonic acid esterified to phospholipids and, once released in free form, are capable of biological activity. Potent renal vasoconstriction mediated through the TxA$_2$/PGH$_2$ receptor has been shown for 8-epi-prostaglandin (PG)F$_{2\alpha}$ (2) and also for 8-epi-PGE$_2$ (3).

The isoprostanes are potential markers of oxidant injury in vivo: they are chemically stable end-products of lipid peroxidation, their concentrations in biological fluids increase in animal models of free-radical induced injury (1) and they are formed in LDL exposed to oxidative stress in vitro (4).

We have developed a gas chromatography/negative ion chemical ionization-mass spectrometry (GC/NICI-MS) technique that enables us to quantitate in vivo formation of 8-epi-PGF$_{2\alpha}$.

We have recently shown that 8-epi-PGF$_{2\alpha}$, but not other F$_2$-isoprostanes, can be formed in a cyclooxygenase dependent manner by human platelets (5). The aim of the present study was to establish the relative contribution of enzymatic and non-enzymatic in vivo formation of 8-epi-PGF$_{2\alpha}$. To this end, we measured urinary excretion of 8-epi-PGF$_{2\alpha}$ in healthy volunteers, in patients with conditions putatively associated with free radical generation and after both acute and chronic inhibition of cyclooxygenase.

MATERIALS AND METHODS

In vivo formation of 8-epi-PGF$_{2\alpha}$ in humans. Urine for the measurement of 8-epi-PGF$_{2\alpha}$ was collected from apparently healthy smokers of > 15 cigarettes per day (n=12), from subjects with paracetamol overdose (n=8) and from patients with stable ischemic heart disease (n=9), from patients treated with lytic therapy for AMI (n=9) and from age-matched controls (n=21).

Effect of cyclooxygenase inhibition on endogenous production of 8-epi-PGF$_{2\alpha}$. Aspirin 325 mg, E5510 20 mg (a new reversible inhibitor of cyclooxygenase) and placebo were administered as single doses to 6 healthy volunteers in a cross-over, randomized, double-blind study. Four consecutive urine collections (-12-0 hours, 0-6 hours, 6-12 hours, 12-24 hours) were performed for the measurement of 8-epi-PGF$_{2\alpha}$ and 11-dehydro-thromboxane (Tx) B$_2$ before and after drug intake. Urinary excretion of 8-epi-PGF$_{2\alpha}$ was also measured in five apparently healthy smokers before and after the administration of aspirin 75 mg for ten days. Blood without anticoagulant was collected before and after aspirin administration for the measurement of TxB$_2$ and 8-epi-PGF$_{2\alpha}$ in serum.

Eicosanoid analysis. 8-epi-PGF$_{2\alpha}$ was measured by a stable isotope dilution/capillary gas chromatography/electron capture negative chemical mass spectrometry assay using an [^{18}O$_2$]-labelled internal standard developed in our laboratory. Samples were spiked with internal standard and glacial acetic acid, extracted on a solid phase extraction cartridge and then purified by silica gel thin layer chromatography (TLC). Following formation of the pentafluorobenzyl ester and further purification on TLC, derivatization of 8-epi-PGF$_{2\alpha}$ was completed by tertiary butyldimethylsilylation. Quantitative analysis was accomplished by GC/MS in NICI mode monitoring m/z 695 for the endogenous 8-epi and m/z 699 for the stable isotope labeled internal standard. 11-dehydro-TxB$_2$ and serum TxB$_2$ were also measured by GC/NICI-MS as previously described.

RESULTS AND DISCUSSION

Urinary 8-epi-PGF$_{2\alpha}$ was 159 ± 18 (mean ± SEM) pg/mg creatinine (creat) in healthy volunteers with no apparent diurnal variation. Excretion was increased in healthy smokers (336 ± 27 pg/mg creat; p < 0.0005) and in patients with paracetamol overdose (1,237 ± 407 pg/mg creat; p < 0.05). Urinary excretion of 8-epi-PGF$_{2\alpha}$ was also increased in patients treated with lytic therapy for acute myocardial infarction, as compared to patient with stable coronary artery disease and age matched controls.

Urinary excretion of 8-epi-PGF$_{2\alpha}$ was 162 ± 30 pg/mg creat at baseline and 186 ± 57, 173 ± 73 and 161 ± 29 pg/mg creat in the three urine collections performed after administration of a single doses of aspirin

325 mg. Similarly, E5510 had no effect on 8-epi-$PGF_{2\alpha}$ excretion in urine. Furthermore, aspirin 75 mg daily for ten days failed to suppress urinary 8-epi-$PGF_{2\alpha}$ (213 ± 57 and 250 ± 52 pg/mg creat before and after aspirin respectively). Urinary excretion of 11-dehydro TxB2 fell significantly after administration of both aspirin and E5510, as expected.

In contrast, the ex vivo formation of 8-epi-$PGF_{2\alpha}$ in serum was depressed in the volunteers given aspirin. While serum TxB2 was completely suppressed, 8-epi-$PGF_{2\alpha}$ fell by about 80%, suggesting a minor cyclooxygenase independent component to its formation, perhaps due to free radical generation, particularly by activated neutrophils.

These results indicate that 8-epi-$PGF_{2\alpha}$, in contrast to other F_2 isoprostanes, can be formed in a cyclooxygenase dependent manner by human platelets in vivo as well as in vitro. However, the contribution from this source to urinary 8-epi excretion in humans is trivial under physiological conditions. Nevertheless, circumstances in which we have demonstrated elevated 8-epi excretion, such as smoking, thrombolysis and reperfusion after bypass grafting, are all associated with platelet activation as well as putatively linked to free radical formation. The contribution of a cyclooxygenase dependent component to 8-epi excretion in urine in these circumstances remains to be established.

ACKNOWLEDGMENTS

Supported by grants from the Wellcome Trust, the Health Research Board, the Irish Heart Foundation and the European Union.

REFERENCES

1. Morrow JD, Hill KE, Burk RF, Nammour TM, Badr KF and Roberts LJ. A series of prostaglandin F_2-like compounds are produced in vivo in humans by a non-cyclooxygenase, free radical-catalyzed mechanism. *Proc. Natl. Acad. Sci.* USA 1990;87:9383-9387.
2. Takahashi K, Nammour TM, Fukunaga M et al. Glomerular actions of a free radical-generated novel prostaglandin, 8-epi-Prostaglandin $F_{2\alpha}$, in the rat. Evidence for interaction with Thromboxane A_2 Receptors. *J. Clin. Invest.* 1992;90:136-141
3. Morrow JD, Minton TA, Mukundan CR et al. Free radical-induced generation of isoprostanes in vivo. Evidence for the formation of D-ring and E-ring isoprostanes. *J. Biol. Chem.* 1994;269:4317-4326
4. Lynch SM, Morrow JD, Roberts LJ and Frei B. Formation of non-cyclooxygenase-derived prostanoids (F_2-isoprostanes) in plasma and low

density lipoprotein exposed to oxidative stress in vitro. *J. Clin. Invest.* 1994;93:998-1004

5. Praticó D, Lawson JA and FitzGerald GA. 8-epi-Prostaglandin F$_{2\alpha}$ but not other F-isoprostanes, is formed in a cyclooxygenase dependent manner by human platelets. *Adv. Prost. Thromb. Leuk. Res.* 1995 (in press)

Advances in Prostaglandin, Thromboxane,
and Leukotriene Research, Vol. 23,
edited by B. Samuelsson et al.
Raven Press, Ltd., New York © 1995

Molecular and Functional Evidence for the Distinct Nature of F2-Isoprostane Receptors from Those of Thromboxane A2.

Takafumi Yura, Megumu Fukunaga, Ryszard Grygorczyk*,
Naomasa Makita**, Kihito Takahashi[+], and Kamal F. Badr.

*Division of Nephrology, Department of Medicine, Emory University and
Veterans Administration Medical Center, Atlanta, Georgia 30033, USA,
*Department of Pharmacology, Merck Frosst Center for Therapeutic Research,
Pointe Claire-Dorval, Quebec H9R 4P8, Canada, **Division of Nephrology,
Vanderbilt University, Nashville, Tennessee 37232-2372, USA, and [+]Merck,
Sharp & Dohme Research Laboratories, Tokyo, 107, Japan*

8-epi-prostaglandin $F_{2\alpha}$ (8-epi-$PGF_{2\alpha}$) is an F_2-isoprostane produced in vivo by cyclooxygenase-independent, free-radial catalyzed lipid peroxidation mechanism. We have already reported that 8-epi-$PGF_{2\alpha}$ is a potent renal vasoconstrictor[1] and stimulates proliferation of cultured aortic smooth muscle cells (AoSMC) through enhancement of phosphoinositide turnover[2]. The vasoconstrictor effect of 8-epi-$PGF_{2\alpha}$ is abolished by thromboxane A_2 (TxA_2) antagonist[1] in spite of its very low binding capacity to TxA_2 binding sites[2]. This observation suggests the existence of specific isoprostane receptors, partially homologous to, but distinct from TxA_2 receptors. In this study, we demonstrate new evidence supporting our findings that the receptors of 8-epi-$PGF_{2\alpha}$ are distinct from those of TxA_2.

METHODS, RESULTS, AND DISCUSSION

Study of Glomerular Inulin Space

To examine the effect of 8-epi-$PGF_{2\alpha}$ on glomerular mesangial cells, we measured glomerular inulin space, as an index of intraglomerular capillary volume which decreases by mesangial contraction[3]. U46,619 (100nM) significantly decreased this index and this decrease was inhibited by coincubation with SQ29,548 (1μM), while 8-epi-PGF$_{2\alpha}$ (100nM) did not affect it, suggesting that 8-epi-PGF$_{2\alpha}$ receptor might be different from those of TxA$_2$ and that 8-epi-PGF$_{2\alpha}$ could not function through TxA$_2$ receptors at this concentration.

Study of Ins (1,4,5)P$_3$ Production by Rat Mesangial Cells

To confirm the hypothesis above, the effects of 8-epi-PGF$_{2\alpha}$ and U46,619 on the production of inositol 1,4,5-trisphosphate (Ins (1,4,5)P$_3$) were compared in cultured rat mesangial cells (MC). U46,619 (100nM) significantly increased Ins (1,4,5)P$_3$ production at 10 seconds, while 8-epi-PGF$_{2\alpha}$ was without effect. Since, in AoSMC, 8-epi-PGF$_{2\alpha}$ stimulated Ins (1,4,5)P$_3$ production with greater potency than that of TxA$_2$[2], these data provide further supportive evidence for the absence of functional 8-epi-PGF$_{2\alpha}$ receptors on MC.

Binding Studies of ^{3}H-8-epi-PGF$_{2\alpha}$ in Membrane Fractions of Mesangial cells and Aortic Smooth Muscle Cells

To identify 8-epi-PGF$_{2\alpha}$ receptor, competitive binding studies using 2.5nM ^{3}H-8-epi-PGF$_{2\alpha}$ as hot ligand was performed. In MC membrane fraction, cold 8-epi-PGF$_{2\alpha}$ displaced hot homoligand's binding in a pattern fitting the existence of a single class of binding sites but with much lesser binding potency than in the assay using ^{3}H-SQ29,548 (mean Kd=41.5nM); that is, mean Kd for 8-epi-PGF$_{2\alpha}$ was 0.47μM and mean Bmax was 18.0nmol/mg protein. These data strongly suggests that 8-epi-PGF$_{2\alpha}$ binds to TxA$_2$ receptors on MC and that MC have no specific isoprostane receptors. In AoSMC membrane, cold 8-epi-PGF$_{2\alpha}$ displaced ^{3}H-8-epi-PGF$_{2\alpha}$ binding in a pattern which suggested the existence of two component binding sites. Calculated mean Kd value for the putative low affinity binding site was 0.94μM, which was similar to the Ki value of 8-epi-PGF$_{2\alpha}$ in competing for ^{3}H-SQ29,548 binding in AoSMC[2], suggesting that this low affinity binding site may represent TxA$_2$ receptors. In contrast, the Kd value for the putative high affinity isoprostane binding sites (31.8nM) was about one thirtieth of that of the low affinity ones. These high affinity isoprostane binding sites were not found in MC. Since MC exhibit no functional responses to 8-epi-PGF$_{2\alpha}$, while, in AoSMC, both Ins (1,4,5)P$_3$ and DNA synthesis were increased by 8-epi-PGF$_{2\alpha}$ with a greater potency than TxA$_2$ agonists[2], we propose that the high affinity 8-epi-PGF$_{2\alpha}$ binding sites represent specific isoprostane receptors.

Luminometric Assay in Xenopus Oocytes Transfected with Human TxA$_2$ Receptor cDNA

In order to confirm the hypothesis that 8-epi-PGF$_{2\alpha}$ receptors are distinct from those of TxA$_2$, with functional experiments, we transfected human TxA$_2$ receptor cDNA cloned by Hirata et al. into Xenopus oocytes and compared the effects of U46,619 and 8-epi-PGF$_{2\alpha}$ by luminometric assay using Ca^{++}-sensitive photoprotein , aequorin[4]. Maximal responses were obtained with 1µM and 100nM U46,619 with a diminished response with 10nM of this agonist, while 8-epi-PGF$_{2\alpha}$ gave much weaker responses at 1µM and 100nM with no response at 10nM. These results suggest that 8-epi-PGF$_{2\alpha}$ did not act through TxA$_2$ receptor binding at physiologic concentrations, while at much higher concentrations, partial responses to 8-epi-PGF$_{2\alpha}$ are observed, likely through cross activation of TxA$_2$ receptors.

CONCLUSIONS

Taking all these results together with our previous finding that, in COS-7 cells transfected with human TxA$_2$ receptor cDNA, 8-epi-PGF$_{2\alpha}$ displaced ^{3}H-SQ29,548 binding with much lesser binding potency[2], we concluded the existence of a novel eicosanoid receptor subtype which specifically recognizes the F$_2$-isoprostanes and its heterologous localization. These findings provide further support for the potential pathophysiologic relevance of isoprostane in mediating vascular injury during oxidant stress .

ACKNOWLEDGMENTS

We thank Drs. Masakazu Hirata and Shuh Narumiya, Department of Pharmacology, Faculty of Medicine, Kyoto University, Kyoto, who kindly provided us with the cDNA for the TxA$_2$ receptor. This work was supported by National Institutes of Health Grants, 2P50 DK39261-06.

REFERENCES

1. Takahashi K, Nammour TM, Fukunaga M, et al. Glomerular actions of a free radical-generated novel prostaglandins, 8-epi-prostaglandin F$_{2\alpha}$, in the rat. Evidence for interaction with thromboxane A$_2$ receptors. *J Clin Invest* 1992;90:136-41.

2. Fukunaga M, Makita N, Roberts II LJ, Morrow JD, Takahashi K, Badr KF. Evidence for the existence of F2-isoprostane receptors on rat vascular smooth muscle cells. *Am J Physiol (Cell Physiol. 33)* 1993;264:C1619-24.

3. Fujiwara Y, Kitamura E, Ueda N, Fukunaga M, Orita Y, Kamada T. Mechanism of action of angiotensin II on isolated rat glomeruli. *Kidney Int* 1989;36:985-91.

4. Abramovitz M, Boie Y, Nguyen T, et al. Cloning and expression of a cDNA for the human prostanoid FP receptor. *J Biol Chem* 1994;269:1-5.

Advances in Prostaglandin, Thromboxane, and Leukotriene Research, Vol. 23, edited by B. Samuelsson et al. Raven Press, Ltd., New York © 1995

EP$_4$-Receptors and Cyclic AMP in Pig Venous Smooth Muscle: Evidence with Agonists and the EP$_4$-Antagonist, AH22921

Robert A.Coleman, Andrew Mallett and Robert L.G.Sheldrick.

Biology Division, Glaxo Research and Development Ltd, Ware, Herts, U.K.

It is has been known for some years that there are at least three subtypes of prostanoid EP-receptor, termed EP$_1$-EP$_3$(1). However, recently, a fourth subtype, termed EP$_4$, has been identified in the smooth muscle of piglet saphenous vein (PSV) (2), and there are now also reports of 'EP$_4$-like' receptors in hamster uterus, rabbit saphenous and jugular veins, rat trachea and rabbit ductus arteriosus (3-7). In the present study, we have gone on to investigate the presence of EP$_4$-receptors in another vascular preparation from the pig, the vena cava (PVC), as well as the role of cyclic AMP in EP$_4$-receptor mediated relaxations of PSV, and to discuss the implications of the findings.

METHODS

Ring preparations of piglet saphenous vein and vena cava were prepared and mounted for measurement of isometric tension measurement in organ baths containing oxygenated Krebs solution at 37°C, and containing indomethacin (2.8µM), as previously described (2). Preparations were contracted with histamine ($\simeq$EC$_{70}$,10µM), and cumulative relaxant concentration-effect curves to PGE$_2$ were repeated until constant, and then a further curve was constructed either to a test prostanoid, or to PGE$_2$ in the presence of antagonist (30 min equilibration). Agonist potency was expressed as EC$_{50}$, and antagonist potency as pA$_2$(8), as described previously (2).

For measurement of cAMP in PSV, vascular rings were placed in Krebs solution as above, containing IBMX (100µM). Preparations were then exposed to a range of different concentrations of the test prostanoids, and then cAMP levels determined. In each experiment, one ring served as an untreated control. After the incubation, preparations were frozen in liquid N_2, and then homogenised in 1ml of EtOH (0°C), centrifuged (1 min), the EtOH evaporated under N_2, and the sample resuspended in 100μl cAMP buffer, and 25μl taken for radioimmunoassay. The pellet was assayed for protein, and cAMP quantified as pmoles cAMP/mg protein. Measurements of cAMP were made using a cAMP assay kit (Amersham). EEC and CR values were determined at the EC_{100} (concentration to cause a doubling of cAMP).

RESULTS AND DISCUSSION

In preliminary experiments, in the absence of histamine, the TP-receptor agonist, U-46619 caused concentration-related contractions of both PVC and PSV ($EC_{50} \sim$ 5-10 nM). On PSV, these contractions were shown to be blocked by GR32191 (pA_2, 8.2-8.3; slope,0.91-0.98; n=2). All further studies were conducted in the presence of GR32191 (1μM).

PGE₂ caused concentration-related relaxation of both PVC (1.0-1,000nM, EC_{50}=40 nM) and PSV (0.1-10nM, EC_{50}=2.5 nM). In each case, PGD₂, PGI₂ and PGF₂α caused similar relaxant responses, but were at least 80-fold less potent than PGE₂. The TP-receptor agonist, U-46619, in concentrations up to 1μM, caused no relaxation of either preparation, and higher concentrations caused only further contractions. In contrast, the selective EP₃/EP₁-receptor agonist, sulprostone, and the selective EP₂-receptor agonist, AH13205, both caused concentration-related relaxation of PVC and PSV, but sulprostone was approximately 1,000-fold and more than 20,000-fold weaker than PGE₂, and AH13205 was 115 and 2,500-fold weaker than PGE₂ on PVC and PSV respectively. Mean concentration-effect curves are illustrated in Figure 1., and data are summarised in Table 1.

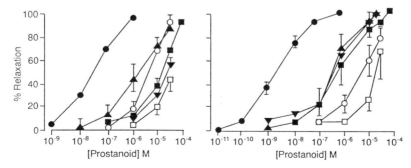

Figure 1.   Mean concentration-effect curves for relaxant responses to PGE₂ (●), PGI₂ (▲), PGF₂α (■), PGD₂ (▼), AH13205 (○) and sulprostone (□) on a. PVC and b. PSV.

Table 1.   Mean agonist potencies of prostanoids as relaxants of PVC and PSV

Agonist	PVC			PSV		
	EEC (PGE_2=1)	95% C.L.	n	EEC (PGE_2=1)	95% C.L.	n
PGE_2	1 (EC_{50}=40nM)		15	1 (EC_{50}=2.5nM)		25
PGI_2	82	77-171	4	174	95-320	6
PGD_2	475	102-2200	4	230	113-467	7
$PGF_2\alpha$	505	190-1670	5	376	198-713	7
U-46619	>3,000 (contraction only)		2	>20,000 (contraction only)		5
AH13205	115	77-171	6	2,500	1100-5600	6
Sulprostone	985	375-1700	3	>20,000	-	3

The EP_4-receptor blocking drug, AH22921 (3.0-30µM) (2) was tested for antagonist activity against relaxations of PVC and PSV to PGE_2. Although AH22921 antagonised responses to PGE_2 on both preparations with similar potency (pA_2 = 5.7), the slope of the Schild plot on PVC was shallow (0.35), whereas on PSV it was not significantly different from unity (0.89). Furthermore, when tested against relaxant responses of PVC to AH13205, AH22921 (30µM) was without effect. Data are summarised in Table 2.

Table 2.   Antagonist potency of AH22921 against prostanoid-induced relaxation of PVC and PSV

Agonist	PVC				PSV			
	pA_2	95% C.L.	Slope	n	pA_2	95% C.L.	Slope	n
PGE	5.74	5.21-6.14	0.35	4	5.74	5.22-6.26	0.89	3
AH13205	<4.5	-		5		Not tested		

Superficially therefore, PVC resembles PSV in its response to prostanoids, in that it contains both excitatory TP-receptors and inhibitory EP-receptors, but few if any inhibitory DP or IP-receptors. Furthermore, the inhibitory EP-receptors in PVC are similar to those in PSV in that the EP_1/EP_3-receptor agonist, sulprostone, is virtually inactive, and the EP_4-receptor blocking drug, AH22921, is ineffective against responses to PGE_2. However, it differs in two respects, firstly the relatively higher potency (~20-fold) of the EP_2-agonist, AH13205, and secondly, the shallow Schild plot for the interaction between AH22921 and PGE_2. The low slope of the Schild plot is consistent with a heterogeneous EP-receptor population, and the relatively high potency of AH13205 on PVC suggests that this preparation may contain not only EP_4-receptors, but also EP_2-receptors, both of which mediate smooth muscle relaxation. That the relatively high potency of AH13205 on PVC results from the additional presence of EP_2-

receptors is supported by its resistance to blockade by AH22921. The co-existence of these two EP-receptor subtypes in a single preparation is an important observation, as it rules out the possibility that the EP_4-receptor is simply the porcine variant of the EP_2-receptor.

The phosphodiesterase inhibitor, IBMX (0.1-1000µM, $EC_{50} \simeq 20µM$), the adenylate cyclase activator, forskolin (10-1000nM, $EC_{50} \simeq 200nM$) and dibutyryl cAMP (10-1000µM, $EC_{50} \simeq 120µM$) all caused concentration-related relaxation of PSV. When concentration-effect curves to PGE_2 were constructed on PSV in the presence of a concentration of IBMX (0.1µM) that caused little or no relaxation in its own right, they were displaced to the left in apparently parallel fashion by between 4 -18 fold (n = 3).

PGE_2 (0.01-10µM) caused concentration-related increases cAMP levels in PSV ($EC_{50} \simeq 40nM$), with a maximum of 4-5 fold over basal levels (~8-9 pmoles cAMP/mg protein). Of the other prostanoids, only PGI_2 and AH13205 appeared to elevate cAMP levels, but both were weaker than PGE_2 (EEC = 9- and 300-fold, respectively). PGD_2, $PGF_2\alpha$ and U-46619 (1-100µM, n=4) were without effect. Mean concentration-effect curves are illustrated in Figure 2.

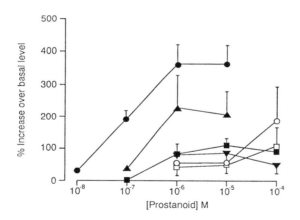

Figure 2. Prostanoid-induced increases in cAMP in DSV. a. Mean concentration-effect curves to PGE_2 (●), PGI_2 (▲), $PGF_2\alpha$ (■), PGD_2 (▼), AH13205 (○) and sulprostone (□).

AH22921 (3-30µM, n=7) was tested for antagonist activity against PGE_2-induced increases in cAMP. Although the results from these experiments were rather variable, AH22921 clearly inhibited PGE_2-induced increases in cAMP in a concentration-related fashion, and a pA_2 value of approximately 5.6 was calculated, with a Schild slope of approximately 1.3.

This study therefore provides several indications that an increase in adenylyl cyclase activity is the signal transduction system associated with EP_4-receptors in PSV. 1. The relaxant effects of dibutyryl cAMP, forskolin and IBMX, indicate a role for cAMP in relaxing the preparation. 2. The ability of a sub-threshold relaxant concentration of IBMX to cause an order of magnitude leftward shift of a concentration-effect curve to PGE_2 strongly supports a role for cAMP in EP_4-receptor mediated smooth muscle relaxation. 3. The demonstration that PGE_2 causes a concentration-related increase in cAMP that can be inhibited by AH22921 with a potency similar to that against PGE_2-induced smooth muscle relaxation further strengthens the association between PGE_2-induced relaxation of this preparation and increases in levels of cAMP.

Until recently, it was believed, on the basis of functional evidence, that were only three subtypes of EP-receptor. It has also been suggested that these three EP-receptor subtypes may be further characterised in terms of their cellular transduction mechanisms (9), with EP_1-receptors being associated with increases in phosphatidyl inositol (PI) turnover, EP_2-receptors with elevation of intracellular cAMP, and EP_3-receptors with both increases in PI turnover, and inhibition of intracellular cAMP. With the successful cloning of cDNAs for three separate EP-receptors (10-12), the functional system of subclassification of EP-receptors appeared to be justified, as convincing evidence has been presented for the identity of one of the recombinant receptors as EP_1, and another as EP_3. Indeed, the identification of isoforms of the recombinant EP_3-receptor (13) has provided an explanation for the observed heterogeneous G_q/G_i-protein coupling of this subtype of EP-receptor. However, the third recombinant EP-receptor, when transfected into COS cells was identified as EP_2 on the basis of the low affinities of various EP_1 and EP_3-receptor ligands, and its coupling to a G_s-protein, and hence to an elevation of intracellular cAMP. However, two factors cast some doubt on this interpretation, the rather high affinity of PGE_2 (PGE_2 has a rather low absolute potency on native EP_2-receptors), and the low affinities of two EP_2-receptor agonists, misoprostol, and more importantly, butaprost. Therefore, the more recent discovery of a fourth subtype of EP-receptor, EP_4, presents the possibility that the recombinant EP-receptor initially classified as EP_2, may in fact be EP_4. The present results provide some a degree of support for this suggestion, in that the EP_4-receptor in PSV, like the EP_2-receptor, appears to be positively linked to adenylyl cyclase. Also, unlike EP_2-receptors, EP_4-receptors have a consistently high sensitivity to PGE_2 (2-7), which is more consistent with the affinity recorded in the recombinant 'non-EP_1/EP_3'-receptor. However, in order to positively identify the recombinant receptor as either EP_2, EP_4 or perhaps some further EP-receptor subtype, it will be necessary to perform functional studies with a wider range of agonists and antagonists on native EP_2 and EP_4-receptors, and with the recombinant receptor.

REFERENCES

1. Coleman RA Kennedy I Humphrey PPA Bunce KT and Lumley P. Prostanoids and their receptors. In:Emmett JC. *Comrehensive Medicinal Chemistry, Vol. 3, Membranes and Receptors.* Oxford: Pergamon Press; 1990:643-714.

2. Coleman RA Grix SP Head SA Louttit JB Mallett A and Sheldrick RLG. A novel inhibitory prostanoid receptor in piglet saphenous vein. *Prostaglandins* 1994; 47: 151-68.

3. Yeardley H Coleman RA Marshall K and Senior J. The effects of PGE_2, sulprostone and AH13205 on hamster uterus *in vitro*. *Br J Pharmacol Proc Suppl1992;*105:241P.

4. Lawrence RA and Jones RL. Investigation of the prostaglandin E (EP-) receptor subtype mediating relaxation of rabbit jugular vein. *Br J Pharmacol 1992;* 105:817-24.

5. Lydford SJ and McKechnie K. Classification of the prostaglandin EP-receptor located on the rat isolated trachea. *Br J Pharmacol Proc Suppl* 1993;108: 72P.

6. Lydford SJ and McKechnie K. Characterisation of the prostanoid receptors located on the rabbit isolated saphenous vein. *Br J Pharmacol Proc Suppl* 1994; in press.

7. Smith GCS Coleman RA and McGrath JC. Characterisation of dilator prostanoid receptors in fetal rabbit ductus arteriosus. *J Pharmacol Exp Ther* 1994; in press.

8. Arunlakshana O and Schild HO. Some quantitative uses of drug antagonists. *Br J Pharmacol Chemother* 1959;14: 48-58.

9. Coleman RA and Humphrey PPA. Prostanoid receptors: their function and classification. In: Vane JR and O'Grady J. *Therapeutic Applications of Prostaglandins.* London: Edward Arnold; 1993:15-36.

10. Watabe A Sugimoto Y Honda A *et al.* Cloning and expression of cDNA for a mouse EP_1 subtype of prostaglandin E receptor. *J Biol Chem* 199;268: 20175-8.

11. Honda A Sugimoto Y Namba T *et al.* Cloning and expression of a cDNA for mouse prostaglandin E receptor EP_2 subtype. *J Biol Chem* 1993;268: 7759-62.

12. Sugimoto Y Namba T Honda A *et al.* Cloning and expression of a cDNA for mouse prostaglandin E receptor EP_3-subtype. *J Biol Chem* 1992;267: 6463-6.

13. Namba T Sugimoto Y Negishi M *et al.* Alternative splicing of C-terminal tail of prostaglandin E receptor subtype EP_3 determines G-protein specificity. *Nature* 1993;365: 166-70.

Advances in Prostaglandin, Thromboxane,
and Leukotriene Research, Vol. 23,
edited by B. Samuelsson et al.
Raven Press, Ltd., New York © 1995

Regulated Expression of the Gene Coding for the Human Thromboxane A$_2$ Receptor

B.T. Kinsella, D.J. O'Mahony, F. Griffin, and G.A. FitzGerald

Centre for Cardiovascular Science, Department of Medicine and Experimental Therapeutics, University College, Dublin, Ireland

The eicosanoid thromboxane A$_2$ (TxA$_2$) is a potent stimulator of vascular and bronchial smooth muscle contraction, platelet aggregation, and is crucial to hemostasis (1). In addition, TXA$_2$ amplifies the response to powerful platelet agonists, such as collagen and thrombin (1). The synthesis of TXA$_2$ is increased in a number of cardiovascular diseases, including myocardial infarction. TxA$_2$ binds to the TxA$_2$ receptor which is expressed on a number of cell types, including brain, thymus, vascular and bronchial smooth muscle cells and platelets (2). In platelets, receptor activation results in platelet shape change and aggregation (1). Both the cDNA and the gene coding for the human TxA$_2$ receptor have been cloned (3,4,5). The cDNA is deduced to code for a G protein-coupled, heptahelical receptor. Point mutations in the human TxA$_2$ receptor discriminate between agonist and antagonist binding sites in competition and saturation binding experiments (6). Both in vitro and in vivo studies have confirmed that the receptor is a phosphoprotein (7). The gene, which can be alternatively spliced (4,5) spans 15kb on chromosome 19p13.3 as determined by Fluorescence in situ hybridizations, and comprises of 2 promoters (P1 and P2), four exons and three introns.

The structural organization of the gene coding for the human TXA$_2$ receptor is shown in Figures 1, together with the deduced mRNA transcripts which differ in the 5' untranslated region, but which code for an identical TXA$_2$ receptor. Comparison of our restriction map of the human TXA$_2$ receptor gene with the published restriction map indicates variation, as indicated by the arrow symbol in Figure 1A. Sequence polymorphism in the gene sequence has also been found (5), including sequence variation in the proposed binding site for the myc transcription factor located in promoter 2 (5).

The promoter control elements found in promoters P1 and P2 (Figure 1B) may potentially regulate the expression of the TXA₂ receptor gene. These include a phorbol ester response element or TRE in promoter 1, and a glucocorticoid response element (GRE) and acute phase response elements (APRE) in promoter 2 (Figure 1B).

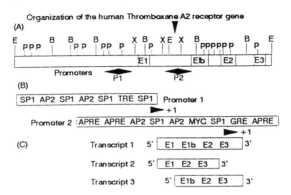

Figure 1. Structural organization of the TXA₂ receptor gene. [A] Restriction map and exon organization of the TXA₂ receptor gene, including the location of promoters 1 and 2. The arrow indicates difference with the published restriction map (4). B=BamH1, E=EcoR1, P=Pst1, X=Xho1. [B] The putative transcription factor binding sites and transcription initiation sites (+1) in promoters 1 and 2. [C] The 3 mRNA transcripts coded by the human TXA₂ receptor gene.

We are particularly interested in determining whether there is differential utilization of promoters 1 and 2, and whether there is coordinated regulated expression of the TXA₂ receptor gene with the genes coding for the enzymes involved in the biosynthesis of TXA₂ in vivo. The synthesis of TXA₂ is regulated by the enzyme TXA₂ synthase and it is reported that the expression of its mRNA is increased 4 fold in HL-60 cells in response to the phorbol ester TPA in vivo, suggesting that up-regulation of TXA₂ synthase is controlled at the transcription level.

We have analysed the synthesis of the mRNA coding for the TXA₂ receptor in control human erythroleukemia (HEL) cells, a tumor cell which expressed platelet markers, and in HEL cells treated with the phorbol ester PMA for 4 hours. This analysis was performed by Northern Blot studies, using a riboprobe complementary to the human TXA₂ receptor-encoding mRNA. In control HEL cells we observe a single transcript hybridizing to the probe (Figure 2). This band comigrates with 18S rRNA and also hybridizes to a radiolabelled oligo probe complementary to 18S rRNA. In contrast, in the HEL cells treated with 100nM PMA for 4 hours we detected the 18S rRNA comigrating band and an inducible transcript at 2.3kb (Figure 2). These results demonstrate that the expression of the mRNAs coding for both TXA$_2$ synthase and the TXA$_2$ receptor is regulated in response to phorbol esters. In the case of the HEL cells probed with the TXA$_2$ receptor riboprobe, it is formally possible that the band comigrating with 18S rRNA, is a constitutively expressed mRNA coding for the TXA$_2$ receptor, and that the larger transcript is an inducible form. Indeed, the TXA$_2$ receptor cDNA probe cross-hybridizes with 2 mRNA bands found in polyA$^+$ mRNA isolated from human placenta and megakaryocytes (3). We could not induce expression of the TXA$_2$ transcript from the control elements in promoter 2.

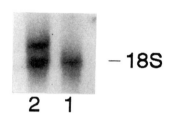

2   1

Figure 2. Northern blot analysis. Total RNA isolated from control HEL cells (lane 1) or HEL cells treated with 100nM PMA for 4 hours (lane 2) was fractionated by electrophoresis on 1.1% agarose/formaldehyde gels, blotted to nylon membrane and probed with a riboprobe complementary to the human TXA$_2$ receptor mRNA. The position of the RNA standards is not shown.

Acknowledgements. This research was funded by a programme grant from the Wellcome Trust (to GAF), by project grants from The Irish Heart Foundation (to BTK and D'OM) and a President's Research Award (to BTK).

References.
1. FitzGerald, G.A. (1991) Am J Cardiol. **68**, 11B-15B.
2. Borg, C., Lim, C.T., Yeomans, D.C., Dieter, J.P., Komiotis, D., Anderson, E.G. and Le Breton, G.C. (1994) J. Biol. Chem. **269**, 6109-6116.
3. Hirata, M., Hayashi, Y., Ushikubi, F., Yokota, Y., Kageyama, R., Nakanishi, S. and Narumiya, S. (1991) Nature **349**, 617-620.
4. Nusing, R.M., Hirata, M., Kakizuka, A., Eki, T., Ozawa, K. and Narumiya, S. (1993) J. Biol. Chem. **268**, 25253-25259.
5. Kinsella, B.T., O'Mahony, D.J., Lawson, J.A., Pratico, D. and FitzGerald, G.A. (1994) Annals. New York Acad. Sci. **714**, 270-279.
6. Funk, C.D., Furci, L., Moran, N., and FitzGerald, G.A. (1993) Mol. Pharm. **44**, 934-939.
7. Kinsella, B.T.; O'Mahony, D.J. and FitzGerald, G.A. (1993) Blood **82**, 610 (Abstract).

Advances in Prostaglandin, Thromboxane,
and Leukotriene Research, Vol. 23,
edited by B. Samuelsson et al.
Raven Press, Ltd., New York © 1995

ANDROGEN REGULATION OF THROMBOXANE A_2 RECEPTORS

A.A. Ajayi, K.Matsuda, K.Schrör, A.Masuda, R.Mathur* and P.V.Halushka.

*Departments of Pharmacology and Medicine, and * Obstetrics and Gynecology, Medical University of South Carolina, Charleston, SC.*

Thromboxane A_2 (TXA_2), a major arachidonic acid metabolite of platelets, produces platelet aggregation and vasoconstriction (1). Both the synthesis of TXA_2 and the density of its receptor, are increased in thrombotic cardiovascular disorders (2), and the inhibition of TXA_2 synthesis by aspirin therapy reduces mortality in ischemic heart disease(3). Thus, TXA_2 and its receptor may play a pathophysiological role in cardiovascular disease. The prevalence and mortality burden of ischemic heart disease is higher in men than in premenopausal women. This gender difference has been attributed both to a cardioprotective effect of estrogens in women, and/or thrombogenicity of androgens in men (4). Indeed, there are many reports of premature myocardial infarctions, strokes or pulmonary embolism in young male atheletes abusing anabolic steroids (5,6) and in non-atheletes administered androgens therapeutically (7). Collectively, these observations suggest that androgenic steroids may regulate platelet reactivity, a notion supported by experimental evidence in animals. It has been reported that rats pretreated with testosterone had higher mortality rates, and greater clot size than untreated controls (8). This is consistent with the observation that testosterone enhances platelet aggregation *in vitro* (9), and increases the mortality and aortic contractile response to intravenous arachidonic acid in mice (10). We have undertaken a series of investigations, using ^{125}I-BOP or U46619, TXA_2-mimetics, to test the hypothesis that androgenic steroids regulate vascular and platelet TXA_2 receptor expression.

VASCULAR THROMBOXANE A_2 RECEPTORS.

The effects of testosterone and 17β-estradiol treatment *in vitro* on TXA_2 receptors were studied in cultured rat aortic smooth muscle cells, RASMC (11). Incubation with testosterone for 24 or 48 hrs significantly increased TXA_2 receptor density

B_{max} without changing the affinity, K_d (11). By contrast, estradiol (100nM) affected neither the K_d nor the B_{max}. Concurrent incubation of testosterone with hydroxyflutamide (1μM), an androgen receptor antagonist, significantly inhibited the testosterone induced increase in B_{max}. The I-BOP induced increase in cytosolic free calcium was significantly greater in testosterone treated RASMC compared with the controls. Testosterone, but not estradiol, significantly increased the inositol triphosphate (IP$_3$) formation, compared to the control group. The EC$_{50}$ values for the I-BOP induced increases in cytosolic calcium or IP$_3$ were not affected by testosterone. The *in vivo* regulation of vascular TXA$_2$ receptors by testosterone was studied in male rats treated with testosterone cypionate for 2 weeks, in castrated or sham operated rats, and castrated rats treated with testosterone (12). Testosterone significantly increased the TXA$_2$ receptor density in rat aortic membranes, by 77%, while castration caused a significant reduction (-47%) in the receptor density, which was restored by testosterone replacement. The K_d values were unaffected. The testosterone induced increase in TXA$_2$ receptor density was associated with a significant increase in the maximum aortic contractile response to U46619. Castration reduced the maximum aortic contractile response, which was restored to control values by testosterone replacement.

The treatment of guinea pigs with testosterone for 2 weeks on coronary artery vascular reactivity to TXA$_2$ mimetics was examined in isolated, perfused guinea pig heart (Langendorff preparation) (13). Coronary perfusion pressure increased dose dependently with U46619. Testosterone significantly augmented the maximum vasoconstrictor response to U46619, by 300% in comparison to controls.

Human Erythroleukemia (HEL) cell and Platelet TXA$_2$ receptors.

Platelets are terminally differentiated fragments of megakaryocytes, lacking transcriptional and translational mechanisms. Owing to this limitation, platelet TXA$_2$ receptors have been studied *in vitro* using HEL cells as surrogates (14). HEL cells are a megakaryocyte- like tumor cell line, with platelet marker proteins. In HEL cells, testosterone(200nM), but not estradiol, significantly increased the TXA$_2$ receptor B_{max} without changing the K_d. The U46619 and I-BOP induced increases in cytosolic free calcium were significantly higher in testosterone treated cells compared to the controls. The testosterone enhancement of second messenger calcium fluxes were blocked by hydroxyflutamide(1μM). Actinomycin D (10ng/ml) or cycloheximide (0.1μg/ml) inhibitors of transcription and translation, respectively, inhibited the effects of testosterone to increase HEL cell TXA$_2$ receptor density. The K_d was unaltered. *In vivo,* testosterone treatment of rats significantly increased the platelet TXA$_2$ receptor density by 69% and significantly lowered the threshold for U46619 induced platelet aggregation(12).

Conclusion

Testosterone administration *in vitro, in vivo,* and recently in man (15) was associated consistently with increased TXA$_2$ receptor density, enhanced TXA$_2$-mimetic induced increases in second messengers, IP$_3$ and cytosolic calcium. These effects were blocked by a specific androgen receptor blocker, hydroxyflutamide. Functionally, there was an augmentation of TXA$_2$-mimetic induced aortic and coronary vasoconstriction and platelet aggregation. These results collectively indicate that androgenic steroids regulate the expression of TXA$_2$ receptors. This may provide a potential mechanism for anabolic steroid induced thrombotic events in man. Since the recently cloned, human TXA$_2$ receptor gene posseses a glucocorticoid responsive element, GRE (16), it is likely that the androgenic regulation of TXA$_2$ receptors is at the genomic level. It remains to be determined whether manipulation of endogenous androgens will influence TXA$_2$ receptors.

References

1. Halushka P.V., Mais D.E., Mayeux P.R., Morinelli T.A. Thromboxane, prostaglandin, and leukotriene receptors. *Annu. Rev. Pharmacol. Toxicol.* 1989, 29, 213-239.
2. Dorn G.W., Liel W., Trask J.L., Mais D.E., Assey M.E., Halushka P.V. Increased platelet TXA$_2$/PGH$_2$ receptors in patients with acute myocardial infarction. *Circulation.* 1990, 81, 212-228
3. Patrono C. Aspirin as an antiplatelet drug.*N. Engl. J. Med.* 1994,330, 1287-94.
4. Wingard. D.L. The sex differential in morbidity, mortality and life style. *Annu. Rev. Public. Health.* 1984, 5, 433-458.
5. Rockhold R.W. Cardiovascular toxicity of anabolic steroids. *Annu. Rev. Pharmacol. Toxicol.* 1993, 33, 497-520.
6. Ferenchick G.S. Androgen / anabolic steroids abuse and thrombosis. is there a connection ? *Medical hypothesis* 1991, 35, 27-31.
7. Nagelberg S.B.,Laue L., Loriaux D.L.,Liu L, Sherins R.J. Cerebrovascular accident associated with testosterone therapy in a 21 year old hypogonadal man.*N. Engl. J. Med.* 1986, 314, 649-50.
8. Uzunova A.D., Ramey E.R., Ramwell P.W. Gonadal hormones and pathogenesis of acute arterial thrombosis. *Am. J. Physiol.* 1978, 234, H 454-H459.
9. Johnson M., Ramey E., Ramwell P.W. Androgen mediated sensitivity in platelet aggregation. *Am. J. Physiol..* 1977, 232, H 381- H 385.
10. Myers A.J., Penhos E., Ramey E., Ramwell P. Thromboxane agonism and antagonism in a mouse sudden death model. *J. Pharmacol. Exp. Ther.* 1982, 224,369-72.
11. Masuda A., Mathur R., Halushka P.V. Testosterone increases Thromboxane A$_2$ receptors in cultured rat aortic smooth muscle cells. *Circ. res.* 1991, 69, 638-643.
12. Matsuda K., Ruff A., Morinelli T.A., Mathur R., Halushka P.V. Testosterone increases thromboxane A$_2$ receptor density in rat aortas and platelets. *Am. J. Physiol.* (in press).
13. Schrör K., Morinelli T.A., Masuda A., Matsuda K., Mathur R., Halushka P.V. Testosterone treatment enhances thromboxane A$_2$-mimetic induced coronary artery vasoconstriction in guinea pigs. *Eur. J. Clin. Invest.* 1994, 24, suppl 1, 50-52.
14. Matsuda K., Mathur R., Duzic E., Halushka P.V. Androgen regulation of Thromboxane A$_2$/Prostaglandin H$_2$ receptor expression in human erythroleukemia cells. *Am. J. Physiol.* 1993, 265, E928-E934.
15. Ajayi A.A., Mathur R., Halushka P.V. Testosterone increases human platelet thromboxane A$_2$ receptor density. *Clinical Research.* 1994, 42, 252A.
16. Nusing R.M., Masakazu H., Kakizuka A., Eki T., Ozawa K., Narumiya S. Characterization and chromosomal mapping of the human thromboxane A$_2$ receptor gene. *J. Biol. Chem.* 1993, 268, 25253-25259.

Advances in Prostaglandin, Thromboxane,
and Leukotriene Research, Vol. 23,
edited by B. Samuelsson et al.
Raven Press, Ltd., New York © 1995

Signal Transductions of Three Isoforms of Mouse Prostaglandin E Receptor EP3 Subtype

Manabu Negishi.[1], Yukihiko Sugimoto[1], Tsunehisa Namba[2], Atsushi Irie[1], Shuh Narumiya[2] and Atsushi Ichikawa[1]

[1]*Department of Physiological Chemistry, Faculty of Pharmaceutical Sciences;*
[2]*Department of Pharmacology, Faculty of Medicine, Kyoto University, Sakyo-ku, Kyoto 606, Japan*

Prostaglandin (PG) E_2 has a wide spectrum of physiological and pharmacological actions in diverse tissues through specific receptors on plasma membranes for maintenance of local homeostasis in the body (1). PGE receptors are pharmacologically divided into at least three subtypes, EP1, EP2 and EP3, on the basis of their responses to various agonists and antagonists (2). Among these subtypes, EP3 has been most well characterized and suggested to be involved in the diverse actions of PGE_2, such as contraction of the uterus, and inhibition of gastric acid secretion, neurotransmitter release, lipolysis in adipose tissue, sodium and water reabsorption in kidney tubules, and modulation of catecholamine release from adrenal chromaffin cells (3). These actions of PGE_2 through the EP3 have been thought to be mediated mainly by inhibition of adenylate cyclase, but the dose dependency varies with the tissues. Furthermore, some of the PGE_2 actions appears to be mediated by another second messenger pathway. These different properties of the EP3 imply heterogeneity of this type receptor. We report here identification of three isoforms of the mouse EP3 with different COOH-terminal tails produced by alternative splicing, which differ in G protein coupling.

RESULTS AND DISCUSSION

We found three isoforms of mouse EP3 (EP3α, β and γ), which are produced through alternative splicing and differ only in COOH-terminal tail (4, 5, 6). Fig. 1 schematically show the structures of these three isoforms. The EP3α and β cDNAs only differ in the deletion of a 89-bp sequence in the coding region of the COOH-terminal tail, resulting in the generation of two different COOH-terminal peptides. EP3γ cDNA has an identical sequence to those of EP3α and β

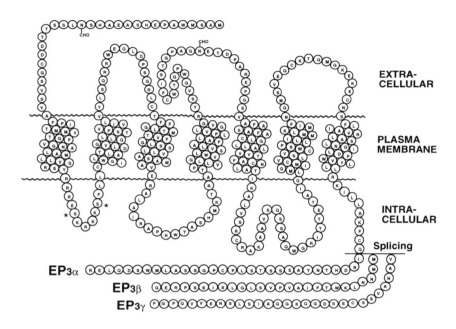

FIG. 1. Seven transmembrane-spanning model of the mouse EP3 isoforms. The transmembrane domains were defined by hydropathicity analysis. Potential sites of *N*-linked glycosylation are indicated by CHO. Stars indicate potential phosphorylation sites for cAMP-dependent protein kinase.

upstream of this junction, followed by a distinct nucleotide sequence, creating a new COOH-terminal peptide.

These isoforms display identical agonist binding properties, indicating that the COOH-terminal tail does not contribute to agonist binding. However, these isoforms are functionally different. EP3α and β were exclusively coupled to inhibition of adenylate cyclase via Gi, but EP3α caused adenylate cyclase inhibition more efficiently than EP3β, the IC50 of EP3α with the inhibition being three orders lower than that of EP3β. The difference in agonist potency of adenylate cyclase inhibition is due to the difference in agonist-induced G protein activation. On the other hand, EP3γ was coupled to both Gs and Gi, causing the inhibition of adenylate cyclase in a low concentration range of PGE₂ and stimulation in a high concentration range. Thus, in the EP3 the COOH-terminal tail plays an important role not only in the efficiency of G protein activation but also in the specificity of G protein coupling. The interaction of receptors with G proteins is modulated by guanine nucleotides, and they usually reduce agonist binding affinity, due to elevation of dissociation rate of agonist binding without a change of association rate. In the case of EP3 isoforms, guanine nucleotides increased the

PGE$_2$ binding affinity of both EP3α and γ, while they decreased that of EP3β. This unique guanine nucleotide-induced increase in the affinity of EP3α is due to elevation of association rate of PGE$_2$ binding without a change of dissociation rate of bound PGE$_2$ from the receptor.

To further assess the role of the COOH-terminal tail in G protein coupling, we truncated the COOH-terminal tail at the alternative splicing site. The truncated receptor failed not only to inhibit the forskolin-stimulated adenylate cyclase activity but also to stimulate the basal activity. Furthermore, the receptor could not stimulate the GTPase activity. In contrast, the truncated receptor retained the ability to physically associate with Gi, forming an agonist-receptor-Gi ternary complex, and to undergo the unique conversion of its agonist-binding affinity mediated by a guanine nucleotide from a low-affinity state to a high-affinity one. Therefore, EP3 forms the stable ternary complex with G protein in a region other than the COOH-terminal tail and then activates G protein with the COOH-terminal tail.

This study will be of help in understanding the diversity of cellular responses to PGE$_2$ and elucidating the molecular mechanism underlying interaction of receptors with G proteins and subsequent activation of G proteins.

REFERENCES

1. Samuelsson B, Goldyne M, Granström E, Hamberg M, Hammarström S and Malmsten C. Prostaglandins and thromboxanes. Ann Rev Biochem 1978; 47: 997-1029.
2. Coleman RA, Kennedy I, Humphrey PPA, Bunce K and Lumley P. Prostanoids and their receptors. In: Hansch C., Sammes PG, Taylor JB, Emmett JC. *Comprehensive Medicinal Chemistry, Vol. 3.* Oxford: Pergamon Press; 1989: 643-714.
3. Negishi M, Sugimoto Y and Ichikawa A. Prostanoid receptors and their biological actions. Prog Lipid Res 1993; 32: 417-434.
4. Sugimoto Y, Namba T, Honda A, Hayashi Y, Negishi M, Ichikawa A and Narumiya S. Cloning and expression of a cDNA for mouse prostaglandin E receptor EP$_3$ subtype. J Biol Chem 1992; 267: 6463-6466.
5. Sugimoto Y, Negishi M, Hayashi Y, Namba T, Honda A, Watabe A, Hirata M, Narumiya S and Ichikawa A. Two isoforms of the EP$_3$ receptor with different carboxyl-terminal domains. J Biol Chem 1993; 268: 2712-2718.
6. Irie A, Sugimoto Y, Namba T, Harazono A, Honda A, Watabe A, Negishi M, Narumiya S and Ichikawa A. Third isoform of the prostaglandin-E-receptor EP$_3$ subtype with different C-terminal tail coupling to both stimulation and inhibition of adenylate cyclase. Eur J Biochem 1993; 217: 313-318.

Advances in Prostaglandin, Thromboxane,
and Leukotriene Research, Vol. 23,
edited by B. Samuelsson et al.
Raven Press, Ltd., New York © 1995

Molecular Cloning and Expression of a cDNA of the Bovine Prostaglandin $F_{2\alpha}$ Receptor

Kazuichi Sakamoto[a], Toshihiko Ezashi[a], Keiko Miwa[a], Emiko Okuda-Ashitaka[a], Takeshi Houtani[b], Tetsuo Sugimoto[b], Seiji Ito[a,c] and Osamu Hayaishi[a]

[a]Department of Cell Biology, Osaka Bioscience Institute, Suita 565, Japan, and Departments of [b]Anatomy and [c]Medical Chemistry, Kansai Medical University, Moriguchi 570, Japan

It has been well recognized that prostaglandin (PG) $F_{2\alpha}$ is involved in the initiation of luteolysis of corpus luteum. It is also well accepted that $PGF_{2\alpha}$ conducts the signal transduction by increasing phosphoinositide metabolism and following elevation of intracellular Ca^{2+} concentration. For further understanding of molecular mechanism of $PGF_{2\alpha}$, we recently isolated the functional cDNA clone for bovine $PGF_{2\alpha}$ receptor(1).

RESULTS

Cloning and Characterization of $PGF_{2\alpha}$ Receptor cDNA

We have used a PCR approach to isolate a cDNA fragment encoding the $PGF_{2\alpha}$ receptor from a bovine corpus luteal cDNA library. PCR by using several pairs of degenerated primers created from common motif of transmembrane domains of known prostanoid receptors, gave a clone SN463 carrying the homologous sequence which covered transmembrane motif IV to VI of thromboxane (TX) A_2 receptor. This PCR

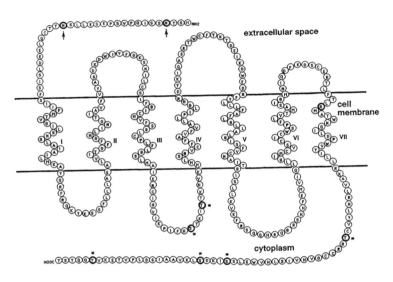

Fig.1. The deduced amino acid sequence for the bovine PGF$_{2\alpha}$ receptor. Positions of the seven putative transmembrane segments I-VII are tentatively assigned by hydropathy analysis. The *arrows* indicate potential *N*-glycosylation sites in the amino-terminal region; *, the potential phosphorylation sites by protein kinase C.

product was utilized as a probe DNA for following cross hybridization and a clone BC2211 carrying a 2.2-kbp insert DNA was isolated. As shown in Fig.1, this clone encodes a protein of 362 amino acid residues (Mr 40,983) with seven potential transmembrane domains and represented significant overall sequence homology to other prostanoid receptors including human TXA$_2$ receptor (34% in amino acid). The N-terminal region contains two potential N-glycosylation sites, and there are some serine or threonine residues which could be potentially subjected to phosphorylation by protein kinase C. The transmembrane segment VII contains Arg 291 at the fourth residue, as commonly conserved in the prostanoid receptor family.

Functional Assay of PGF$_{2\alpha}$ Receptor

Injection of the sense-mRNA synthesized *in vitro* from the cloned cDNA into a *Xenopus* oocyte elicited electro-physiological response to PGF$_{2\alpha}$, representing BC2211 encodes a functional full-length cDNA. Then the ligand-binding properties of the receptor were examined in COS-7 cells transfected with the cloned cDNA. The Scatchard plot analysis indicated the presence of a single binding site with a Kd value of 12.4 nM and the ligand-binding displacement experiment indicated the affinity of the receptor to PGs in the order of $PGF_{2\alpha} > PGD_2 > PGE_2 > STA_2$. We further examined that $PGF_{2\alpha}$ activated total InsP formation in COS-7 cells transfected with receptor cDNA.

Expression Assay of $PGF_{2\alpha}$ Receptor mRNA

Northern blot analysis demonstrated that 5-kb mRNA is abundantly expressed and accumulated in the corpus luteum, but not in the ovary devoid of corpus luteum and other organs examined. Next we analyzed bovine ovary tissue for $PGF_{2\alpha}$ receptor mRNA by *in situ* hybridization and the great majority of large luteal cells in the corpus luteum exhibited specific hybridization signals with the anti-sense riboprobe.

Identification of G-protein Coupled to $PGF_{2\alpha}$ Receptor

Then we examined intracellular signal transduction of $PGF_{2\alpha}$ receptor in CHO cells transfected by the cloned cDNA(2). In whole-cell clamp recordings, $PGF_{2\alpha}$ induced an outward current in the presence of external Ca^{2+}, but it induced a long-lasting inward Ca^{2+} current in a Na^+-free solution containing K^+ channel blockers. $Gq\alpha$ antibody applied intracellularly blocked both outward and inward currents induced by 1 μM $PGF_{2\alpha}$. These results demonstrate that the $PGF_{2\alpha}$ recepotr is coupled to phosphoinositide metabolism in CHO cells via Gq.

REFERENCES

1. Sakamoto, K., Ezashi, T., Miwa, K., Okuda-Ashitaka, E., Houtani, T., Sugimoto, T., Ito, S., and Hayaishi, O. (1994) *J. Biol. Chem.* **269**:3881-3886.
2. Ito, S., Sakamoto, K., Mochizuki-Oda, N., Ezashi, T., Miwa, K., Okuda-Ashitaka, E., Shevchenko, V. I., and Hayaishi, O. (1994) *Biochem. Biophys. Res. Comm.* 200, 756-762.

Advances in Prostaglandin, Thromboxane, and Leukotriene Research, Vol. 23,
edited by B. Samuelsson et al.
Raven Press, Ltd., New York © 1995

PROSTACYCLIN EFFECTS ON ADENYLATE CYCLASE IN PLATELETS AND VASCULAR SMOOTH MUSCLE: INTERACTION WITH AN INHIBITORY RECEPTOR OR PARTIAL AGONISM?

G. Enrico Rovati, Serenella Giovanazzi,
Anna Negretti and Simonetta Nicosia.

Laboratory of Molecular Pharmacology
Institute of Pharmacological Sciences, University of Milan
Via Balzaretti 9, 20133 Milan, Italy

We have shown that (5E) and (5Z)-carbacyclin, two PGI_2 analogs, displayed the same efficacy as PGE_1, and hence PGI_2, in stimulating adenylate cyclase activity in membranes from human platelets. On the contrary, (5Z)-carbacyclin failed to produce the same maximal degree of enzyme stimulation in cultured myocytes from rabbit mesenteric artery (1). It was, therefore, concluded that (5Z)-carbacyclin could discriminate between PGI_2 receptors in platelets and vascular smooth muscle cells and that, having a lower intrinsic activity (2-3), displayed a partial agonist properties (1). More recently it has been postulated that there are separate stimulatory and inhibitory prostaglandin receptors on platelet membranes (4). In fact, it is well known that some biological systems are regulated by stimulatory (R_s) and inhibitory (R_i) receptors, and this has been clearly demonstrated in the adenylate cyclase system (5).

METHODS

Adenylate cyclase assay, cell cutures and membrane preparation were performed as previously described (1).

Starting from the classical four parameter logistic equation (6) we developed the following model to describe the interaction of R_s and R_i (7):

$$Y = \left[\frac{a_1 - d}{1 + (X/c_1)^{b_1}} + d \right] - \left[d - \left(\frac{a_2 - d}{1 + (X/c_2)^{b_2}} + d \right) \right] \qquad \text{eq. 1}$$

where 'Y' is the response, 'X' the arithmetic dose, 'a_1' the response of R_s when 'X' = 0, 'a_2' is the response of R_i for an infinite dose, 'b_1' is the slope that determines the steepness of the ascending part of the bell, 'b_2' is the slope that determines the steepness of the descending part of the bell, 'c_1' is the EC_{50}, i. e. the dose resulting in half the maximal response, 'c_2' is the IC_{50}, i. e. the dose resulting in half the maximal inhibition and 'd' the response for an infinite dose of R_s.

RESULTS AND DISCUSSION

On the basis of the previous considerations, we have developed a mathematical model and a computer program to describe the interaction of a drug with two different receptors with opposite effects. We have demonstrated that this model can account for both the apparent reduction in efficacy of some members of a series of related compounds and the downward curvature of the upper plateau of some dose-response curves, as the ones obtained with the (5Z)-carbacyclin. Our model, therefore, can give both a biological and a mathematical explanation to the bell-shaped dose-response curves obtained with (5Z)-carbacyclin in myocytes and its apparent lower efficacy compared to PGE₁ (Tab. 1). Moreover, it can explain how an agonist interacting with stimulatory and inhibitory receptors can be mistaken for a partial agonist.

TABLE 1

	PGE$_1$	(5E)-Carbacyclin	(5Z)-Carbacyclin
R$_{min1}$	50	31	41
Slope$_s$	1.1	.64	1
EC$_{50}$	1.9×10^{-5}	7.9×10^{-6}	3.2×10^{-4}
R$_{max}$	194	230	217
Slope$_i$	--	--	-1.1
IC$_{50}$	—	--	1.4×10^{-3}
R$_{min2}$	—	--	40

REFERENCES

1. Corsini A, Folco GC, Fumagalli R, Nicosia S, Noè MA, Oliva D. (5Z)-Carbacyclin discriminates between prostacyclin-receptorscoupled to adenylate cyclase in vascular smooth muscle and platelets. *Br. J. Pharmacol.* 1987;90:255-261

2. Ariëns EJ. Affinity and intrinsic activity in the theory of competitive inhibition. Part 1. *Arch. Internat. Pharmacodyn. Therap.* 1954;99:32-49

3. Stephenson RP. A modification of receptor theory. *Br. J. Pharmacol.* 1956;11:379-393

4. Ashby B. Comparison of Iloprost, Cicaprost and Prostacyclin in effects on cyclic AMP metabolism in intact platelets. *Prostaglandins* 1992;43:255-261

5. Gilman AG. G-Proteins and dual control of Adenylate-Cyclase.*Cell* 1984;36: 577-579

6. De Lean A, Munson PJ, Rodbard D. Simultaneous analysis of families of sigmoidal curves: application to bioassay, radioligand assay, and physiological dose-response curves. *Am. J. Physiol.* 1978;235(2):E97-E102

7. Rovati GE and Nicosia S. Lower Efficacy: Interaction with an Inhibitory Receptor or Partial Agonism? *Trends Pharmacol. Sci.* 1994;15:140-151

Advances in Prostaglandin, Thromboxane,
and Leukotriene Research, Vol. 23,
edited by B. Samuelsson et al.
Raven Press, Ltd., New York © 1995

RECEPTORS FOR CYS-LEUKOTRIENES IN HUMAN LUNG PARENCHYMA: CHARACTERIZATION BY COMPUTER MODELLING AND PHOTOAFFINITY LABELLING OF BINDING SITES

S. Nicosia, V. Capra, D. Ragnini, S. Giovanazzi, M. Mezzetti*,
D. Keppler§, M.Müller§ and G. E. Rovati

*Institute of Pharmacological Sciences and *IV clinic of surgery, University of Milan, Milan, Italy; §Div. Tumor Biochemistry, DKFZ, Heidelberg, Germany*

The number and subtypes of receptors for cysteine-containing leukotrienes (cys-LTs) in the airways are still a matter of debate. The evidence available at present suggests that in guinea pig airways two different classes of receptors exist, one that recognizes LTD_4 and LTE_4, while the other one is specific for LTC_4. On the contrary, the LT receptors in human airways seem to be different from both those present in guinea pig airways, inasmuch as the classical LT antagonists, such as FPL 55712, ICI 198,615 and SKF 104353, are unable to discriminate between the contractile action of LTD_4 and of LTC_4.

Given the potential role of cys-LT receptor antagonists as novel anti-asthma drugs, it is important to understand in more detail the precise nature of such receptors in human airways, in order to design specific and selective antagonists. Aim of the present work was to clarify whether the three cys-LTs interact with a single homogeneous class of receptors or with heterogeneous subtypes in human airways.

We have addressed this problem by performing both classical binding studies and photoaffinity labelling with various LT agonists and antagonists in membranes from human lung parenchyma. Binding data have been interpreted by means of computer modelling with an objective mathematical approach, using the computer program LIGAND (1).

METHODS

Membranes from macroscopically normal specimens of human lung parenchyma were prepared as previously described (2) and incubated with either ^{3}H-LTC$_4$ or ^{3}H-LTD$_4$ for 30 min at 25°C, in the presence or absence of antagonists. For photoaffinity labelling, after incubation the samples were photolysed under UV light (300 nm) for 5 min and the distribution of radioactivity was investigated by SDS-polyacrylamide gel electrophoresis (3).

RESULTS AND DISCUSSION

Self- and cross-displacement curves were performed and analyzed with the computer program LIGAND, which revealed the presence of at least two classes of binding sites for both ligands. Binding parameters were: for LTD$_4$, $K_{d1} = 0.57$ nM, $K_{d2} = 7.2$ µM, $B_{max1} = 0.01$ and $B_{max2} = 20$ pmol/mg prot.; for LTC$_4$, $K_{d1} = 0.08$ nM, $K_{d2} = 440$ nM, and B_{max} values were very similar to those of LTD$_4$. Unlabelled LTC$_4$ inhibited ^{3}H-LTD$_4$ binding, suggesting that the two cys-LTs shared the same binding sites, but unexpectedly LTD$_4$ was unable to displace ^{3}H-LTC$_4$.

Photoaffinity labelling studies showed that ^{3}H-LTD$_4$ labelled two different peaks (molecular mass 55 and > 100 kDa), while ^{3}H-LTC$_4$ labelled two peaks with the same molecular mass as those of ^{3}H-LTD$_4$, plus an extra peak at 32 kDa. Labelling of the peak at 55 kDa could be inhibited by both unlabelled LTD$_4$ and LTC$_4$, and by the classical antagonists ICI 198,615 and SKF 104353, while labelling of the 32 and > 100 kDa peaks by ^{3}H-LTC$_4$ was inhibited only by LTC_4. While a more extensive study will be necessary in order to assign a function to these proteins labelled by ^3H-LTD_4 and ^3H-LTC_4, the results obtained suggest that the protein at 55 kDa is a good receptor candidate; we have not established whether the protein at 32 kDa might be a LTC_4 synthase not separated into subunits (4) and whether the one at > 100 kDa represents a biologically significant protein (an export carrier?).

These data can be reconciled by the hypothesis that at least two different sub-classes (or affinity states) of cys-LT receptors exist, both recognized by LTD_4; LTC_4 might bind to the same two classes labelled by LTD_4. To take into account the lack of displacement of ^3H-LTC_4 by LTD_4, we suggest that either the interaction with one of the sites is allosteric with respect to LTD_4, or binding to a receptor site is masked by the presence of other specific LTC_4 sites (carrier? enzyme?). The latter should display an affinity and density similar to the LTD_4 low affinity site, thus becoming indistinguishable from it simply by means of binding studies. Photoaffinity labelling studies seem to confirm the existence of these extra sites for LTC_4.

All the antagonists tested bind to a homogeneous class of sites, either to the higher- or to the lower-affinity one. Therefore, both sites or states might be important for the development of cys-LT antagonists.

REFERENCES

1. Munson PJ, Rodbard D. LIGAND: A versatile computerized approach for characterization of ligand binding systems. *Anal Biochem* 1980;107:220-239.
2. Rovati GE, Giovanazzi S, Mezzetti M, Nicosia S. Heterogeneity of binding sites for ^3H-ICI 198,615 in human lung parenchyma. *Biochem Pharmacol* 1992;44:1411-1415.
3. Falk E, Müller M, Huber M, Keppler D, Kurz G. Direct photoaffinity labeling of leukotriene binding sites. *Eur J Biochem* 1989;186:741-747.
4. Leier I, Jedlitschky G, Buchholz U, Keppler D. Characterization of the ATP-dependent leukotriene C_4 export carrier in mastocytoma cells. *Eur J Biochem* 1994;220:599-606

Advances in Prostaglandin, Thromboxane,
and Leukotriene Research, Vol. 23,
edited by B. Samuelsson et al.
Raven Press, Ltd., New York © 1995

SYNERGISM EXHIBITED BY LTD₄ AND PAF RECEPTOR ANTAGONISTS IN DECREASING ANTIGEN-INDUCED AIRWAY MICROVASCULAR LEAKAGE

Martin A. Wasserman, Ann F. Welton, and Louis M. Renzetti

Department of Bronchopulmonary Research, Hoffmann-La Roche, Inc.,
Nutley, New Jersey 07110

A variety of substances have been identified as potential mediators of the symptomatology and sequelae of complex inflammatory diseases. In particular, LTD₄ and PAF are involved in respiratory diseases with a large inflammatory component. In addition to bronchoconstriction, LTD₄ and PAF have also been shown to increase airway microvascular permeability. The purpose of the present investigation was to examine the effects of Ro 24-5913, (E)-4-[3-[2-(4-cyclobutyl-2-thiazolyl)ethenyl]phenyl-amino]-2,2-diethyl-4-oxobutanoic acid and Ro 24-4736, (5-{3-[4-(2-chloro-phenyl)-9-methyl-6H-thieno[3,2-f][1,2,4]triazolo[4,3-a][1,4]diazepin-2-yl]-2-propynyl}phenanthridin-6(5H)-one), selective LTD₄ and PAF receptor antagonists, respectively, alone and in combination in a guinea-pig model of antigen-induced airway microvascular leakage (1,2). It is possible that for optimal therapy, a combination of LTD₄ and PAF antagonists may be most useful.

METHODS

Male guinea pigs (200-300 g) of the Hartley strain were sensitized subcutaneously with ovalbumin (OA; 10 μg plus 1 mg Al(OH)₃ in 0.5 ml saline) on days 1 and 14 and used for study 21-35 days later. On the day of the experiment, the animals were anesthetized with urethane (2 g/kg, i.p.), the jugular vein was cannulated and the animals were allowed to stabilize for 15 min. Pyrilamine (2 mg/kg, i.v.) and indomethacin (10 mg/kg, i.v.) were then administered; 14 min later an Evans blue dye injection (30 mg/kg, i.v.) followed. Airway microvascular leakage was induced by a single injection of OA (1 mg/kg, i.v.) given 1 min after the dye. The airways were removed and divided into the trachea (T;distal 5 mm), main bronchi (MB) and the intrapulmonary airways (IA). All tissues were blotted between filter paper, then weighed. Dye was extracted in formamide (37°C, 24 hr) and quantified by absorbance at 620 nm with a spectrophotometer. Dye content was expressed in ng/mg of tissue wet weight. Guinea pigs were dosed orally with Ro 24-5913, Ro 24-4736, a combination of these antagonists or vehicle 1 hr prior to OA challenge. Baseline or background plasma leakage was measured in a group of sensitized animals that were given only i.v. saline.

RESULTS AND DISCUSSION

Ovalbumin challenge induced a substantial leakage of dye into the T, MB and IA (Fig. 1). Both Ro 24-5913 (0.1, 0.3, 1 mg/kg) and Ro 24-4736 (1 mg/kg) significantly blocked this effect (Fig. 1; Table 1), but it was not affected by pretreatment with 0.03 mg/kg Ro 24-5913 or 0.3 mg/kg Ro 24-4736. However, leakage in the T, MB and IA was significantly decreased by ~79, ~69 and ~60%, respectively, when these two doses of the antagonists were administered in combination (Fig. 1; Table 1).

These results suggest that both LTD_4 and PAF may contribute to OA-induced airway microvascular leakage. The ability of a combination of Ro 24-5913 and Ro 24-4736 to inhibit this response at doses that had no effect when used alone suggests that there may be synergy between LTD_4 and PAF antagonists. The use of both LTD_4 and PAF receptor antagonists may offer greater therapeutic potential for the treatment of airway diseases such as asthma.

REFERENCES

1. O'Donnell, M., Crowley, H.J., Yaremko, B., O'Neill, N. and Welton, A.F. Pharmacological actions of Ro 24-5913, a novel antagonist of leukotriene D_4. *J. Pharmacol. Exp. Ther.* 1991; 259: 751-8.

2. Crowley, H.J., Yaremko, B., Selig, W., Janero, D., Burghardt, C., Welton, A.F. and O'Donnell, M. Pharmacology of a potent platelet-activating factor antagonist: Ro 24-4736. *J. Pharmacol. Exp. Ther.* 1991; 259: 78-85.

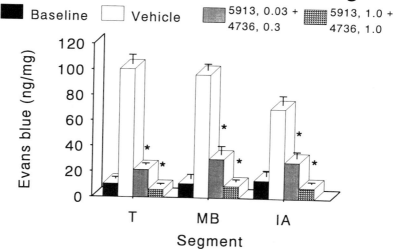

FIG. 1. Effect of Ro 24-5913 and Ro 24-4736 on OA-induced airway leakage in the guinea pig. Animals were dosed orally with vehicle or Ro 24-5913 + Ro 24-4736 1 hr prior to OA challenge. Each bar represents the mean ± SEM for determinations made on at least n=4 animals per group. *p < 0.05 vs. vehicle-treated group.

TABLE 1. Effects of Ro 24-5913 and Ro 24-4736 alone and in combination on OA-induced airway microvascular leakage in the guinea pig. *p < 0.05

Treatment (mg/kg)	Evans blue dye (ng/mg)		
	Trachea	Main Bronchus	Intrapulmonary Airway
Baseline	12 ± 2	12 ± 2	13 ± 3
Vehicle	99 ± 7	96 ± 4	71 ± 7
Ro 24-5913 (0.03)	72 ± 12	70 ± 19	55 ± 18
Ro 24-4736 (0.3)	81 ± 13	88 ± 9	85 ± 17
Combination	*21 ± 2**	*30 ± 7**	*28 ± 5*
Ro 24-5913 (1.0)	27 ± 7*	32 ± 6*	33 ± 8*
Ro 24-4736 (1.0)	53 ± 16*	58 ± 12*	39 ± 6*
Combination	*6 ± 1**	*9 ± 2**	*9 ± 1**

*Advances in Prostaglandin, Thromboxane,
and Leukotriene Research, Vol. 23,*
edited by B. Samuelsson et al.
Raven Press, Ltd., New York © 1995

SB 209247, A HIGH AFFINITY LTB4 RECEPTOR ANTAGONIST DEMONSTRATING POTENT ANTIINFLAMMATORY ACTIVITY

H.M. Sarau, J.J. Foley, D.B. Schmidt, M.N. Tzimas, L.D. Martin
R.A. Daines, P.A. Chambers, W.D. Kingsbury and D.E. Griswold

SmithKline Beecham Pharm., King of Prussia, PA, 19406

In hyperproliferative skin disorders, like psoriasis, there are several arachidonic acid (AA) proinflammatory metabolites present in abnormally high concentrations, including LTB4 and 12(R)-HETE (1). These eicosanoids have been postulated to contribute significantly to the pathophysiology of skin disorders. An antagonist that will block the activity of both mediators may be more useful for the treatment of skin disorders than an agent that selectively blocks only one of them. We have found that SB 209247, (E)-3-[6-[[2,6-dichlorophenyl]thio]methyl]-3-(2-phenylethoxy)-2-pyridinyl]-2-propenoic acid, is a high affinity LTB4 receptor antagonist which blocks the functional activity of both LTB4 and 12(R)-HETE and demonstrates potent antiinflammatory activity in animal models

IN VITRO PHARMACOLOGY

Methods used in this study were described previously, for binding and Ca^{2+} mobilization (2) and for the murine inflammation models (3,4).

SB 209247 is a high affinity competitive antagonist of [^{3}H] LTB4 binding to human PMNs with an apparent K_i of 0.88 ± 0.20 nM. It appears selective in that it competes with [^{3}H] fMLP and [^{3}H] LTD4 with IC50s of 3250 nM and 16,800 nM, respectively, and for another 14 ligands evaluated in binding assays the IC50 was >10,000 nM.

To evaluate the functional antagonist activity at the cellular level, agonist-induced Ca^{2+} fluxes in PMNs and human U 937 cells were blocked. SB 209247 is a potent competitive antagonist of LTB4-induced Ca^{2+} mobilization with an IC50 of 6.6 ± 1.5 nM (Fig. 1) and 4.3 ± 0.5 nM in U 937 cells. Additionally, it potently inhibited the 12(R)-HETE-induced Ca^{2+} mobilization in PMNs with an IC50 of 1.3 ± 0.3 nM and weakly antagonized the fMLP Ca^{2+} response with an IC50 of 623 nM (Fig. 1). In the Ca^{2+} functional assay, it demonstrated weaker activity for LTD4, PAF, C5a and IL-8 than for fMLP, for all agonists the IC50s were >10,000 nM.

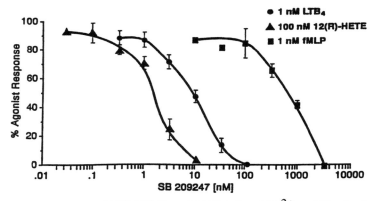

Fig. 1. *Inhibition of LTB4-, 12(R)-HETE- and fMLP-induced Ca²⁺ mobilization by SB 209247. Values are the mean ± SEM for at least 3 experiments.*

Some LTB4 functional responses require higher concentrations of agonist, e.g., PMN degranulation. SB 209247 blocked LTB4-induced degranulation with an IC_{50} of 117 ± 39 nM. The compound was selective for LTB4 since it required at least 25 fold higher concentrations to block the responses to fMLP, C5a and PAF.

IN VIVO PHARMACOLOGY

SB 209247 was evaluated for antiinflammatory activity in a number of murine dermal inflammation models. It blocked the topically applied LTB4-induced neutrophil influx by 74% at 250 μg/ear. The topical antiinflammatory activity of SB 209247 was examined using the AA-induced inflammation in mouse ear (3). In this assay, SB 209247 markedly inhibited the neutrophil infiltration induced by 1 mg of AA with an ED_{50} of 8 μg/ear and the edematous component of the response with an ED_{50} of 20 μg/ear. This is one of the most potent compounds ever tested in this assay system.

A more protracted and intense dermal inflammatory response is obtained with the topical application of phorbol ester (PMA, 4). In this murine model, topical application of SB 209247 dose dependently inhibited the neutrophil influx and the edematous responses with ED_{50}s of 114 μg/ear and 106 μg/ear, respectively. Additional studies were designed to examine the effect of SB 209247 on the long lasting PMA-induced response. At 300 μg/ear the inflammatory response was still inhibited by >50% at 24 hours.

Oral antiinflammatory activity of SB 209247 was also demonstrated in the murine AA ear model. The model involves the application of 1 mg AA to the skin of the mouse ear with the drug administered orally 30 min before the AA (3). In this model SB 209247 dose dependently inhibited AA-induced neutrophil influx and edema with ED_{50}s of 14.8 mg/kg and 18.7 mg/kg, respectively. The AA-induced inflammatory response was utilized to evaluate the oral duration of action. Oral administration of SB 209247 at 21 mg/kg for various pretreatment times showed >50% inhibition with up to 4 hours pretreatment (Fig. 2). These data indicate a substantial duration of activity after oral administration.

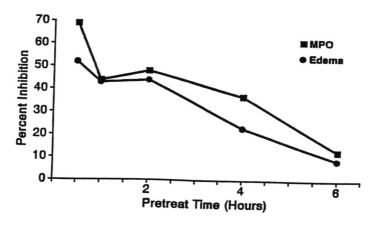

Fig. 2. *Duration of action of oral SB 209247 on AA-induced ear inflammation. All data points , except the 6 hr pretreat, were significat from control at a p<0.001.*

The data show that SB 209247 is a selective high affinity antagonist of LTB4 receptors. It selectively blocks the actions of LTB4 and 12(R)-HETE *in vitro* and *in vivo* it demonstrates potent and long lasting topical and oral antiinflammatory activity in murine dermal models of inflammation.

References

1. Duell EA, Ellis CN and Voorhees JJ. Determination of 5-, 12-, and 15-lipoxygenase products in keratomed biopsies of normal and psoriatic skin. J. Invest. Dermatol. 1988; 91: 446-450.

2. Daines RA, Chambers PA, Pendrak I "et.al.". Trisubstituted pyridine leukotriene B4 receptor antagonists: Synthesis and structure-activity relationships. J. Med. Chem. 1993;36: 3321-3332.

3. Griswold DE, Webb E, Schwartz L and Hanna N. Arachidonic Acid-Induced Inflammation: Inhibition by dual inhibitor of arachidonic acid metabolism, SK&F 86002. Inflammation 1987;11:189-199.

4. Carlson RP, O'Neill-Davis L, Chang J and Lewis AJ. Modulation of mouse ear edema by cyclooxygenase and lipoxygenase inhibitors and other pharmacological agents. Agents and Actions 1985;17:197-204.

*Advances in Prostaglandin, Thromboxane,
and Leukotriene Research, Vol. 23,*
edited by B. Samuelsson et al.
Raven Press, Ltd., New York © 1995

Estimation of Antagonistic Activity of ONO-4057 against Leukotriene B4 in Humans

Katsuya Kishikawa, Shintaro Nakao, Shigeru Matsumoto,
Kigen Kondo and Nobuyuki Hamanaka

*Bioscience Division of Discovery Research Laboratories , Minase Research Institute,
Ono Pharmaceutical Co., Ltd., Shimamoto, Mishima, Osaka 618, Japan.*

Leukotriene B4 (LTB4), a 5-lipoxygenase product of arachidonic acid, is considered to be one of the important inflammatory mediators. The regulation of the activity of LTB4 may provide a novel therapeutic approach for the treatment of inflammatory diseases such as ulcerative colitis, psoriasis and asthma (1). We have reported ONO-4057 is a selective, potent and orally active antagonist of LTB4 receptor in vitro and in vivo (2). The development of a sensitive ex vivo assay for LTB4 antagonistic activity will be useful in the clinical evaluation of ONO-4057. In the present study, we have developed a useful assay for the estimation of clinical efficacy of LTB4 antagonists by measuring LTB4-induced neutrophil [Ca^{2+}]i increase in plasma.

METHODS

LTB4-induced neutrophil [Ca^{2+}]i increase in tisolated plasma

The guinea pig plasma was prepared 5 min before and 60 min after oral administration of ONO-4057 (3-30 mg/kg)or vehicle. The human plasma was prepared before and 1,2,3,4 and 6 hrs after oral administration of ONO-4057 (300 mg/person) in Phase I study. Neutrophils were prepared from the venous blood of healthy volunteers or the peritoneal fluid of casein-treated guinea pigs. The neutrophils (2×10^7/ml) were incubated for 30 min at 37°C with 2 µM of flou-3 AM and washed with HBSS-0.5% BSA. Fluo-3 loaded neutrophils (5×10^7/ml) were resuspended in HBSS-0.5% BSA (3).

One hundred µl of the fluo-3 loaded neutrophil suspensions was added to 890 µl of each isolated plasma sample followed by the addition of 10 µl of LTB4. The fluorescence intensity was measured at 37°C at 505 nm excitation, 530 nm emission, and neutrophil $[Ca^{2+}]i$ increase was expressed as changes of fluorescence intensity.

LTB4-induced transient neutropenia in guinea pigs

ONO-4057 was administered orally 1 hour before the injection of LTB4 (300 ng/kg). The blood was collected 1 min before and 30 sec after the injection of LTB4 to count numbers of neutrophils using a multi-blood cell counter.

RESULTS AND DISCUSSION

LTB4 concentration-dependently increased $[Ca^{2+}]i$ of fluo-3-loaded neutrophils suspended in the guinea pig plasma The isolated plasma from guinea pigs treated with ONO-4057 (3-30 mg/kg, p.o.) inhibited LTB4 (30 nM)-induced neutrophil $[Ca^{2+}]i$ increase in a dose-dependent manner (FIG. 1-a). Intravenous injection of LTB4 caused a transient and profound neutropenia in guinea pigs. ONO-4057 (3-30 mg/kg, p.o.) also inhibited LTB4 (300 ng/kg, i.v.)-induced transient neutropenia in a dose-dependent manner (FIG. 1-b). The inhibitory effect of ONO-4057 on LTB4-induced neutrophil $[Ca^{2+}]i$ increase closely paralleled that seen in vivo LTB4-induced neutropenia . In addition, plotting these effects of ONO-4057 against plasma concentrations of ONO-4057 determined by the HPLC methods, there was a good correlation between ex vivo and in vivo assays (FIG. 2). Therefore, these results suggest that in vivo antagonistic activity of ONO-4057 against LTB4 can be estimated by the measurement of neutrophil $[Ca^{2+}]i$ increase in plasma.

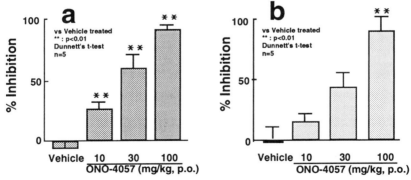

FIG. 1. a : Effect of the isolated plasma from guinea pigs treated with ONO-4057 on LTB4 (30 nM)-induced neutrophil $[Ca^{2+}]i$ increase. **b :** Effect of ONO-4057 on LTB4 (0.3 µg/kg, i.v.)-induced neutropenia in guinea pigs. Results were expressed as the mean values ± S.E.

LTB4 (1-100nM) concentration-dependently increased $[Ca^{2+}]i$ of fluo-3-loaded neutrophils suspended in human plasma. In Phase I study, the plasma from healthy volunteers orally administered with 300 mg/person of ONO-4057 inhibited LTB4 (3 nM)-induced neutrophil $[Ca^{2+}]i$ increase. As shown in FIG. 3,

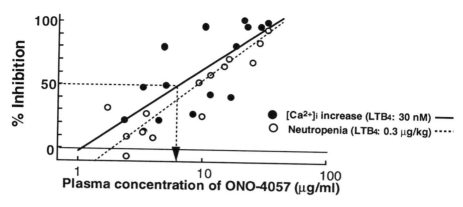

FIG. 2. Correlation of [Ca^{2+}]i increase with neutropenia in guinea pigs.

the plasma concentration of ONO-4057 to show 50% inhibition of this response was approximately 1 μg/ml. From this result, the plasma concentration of ONO-4057 to show <u>in vivo</u> antagonistic activity against LTB4 is estimated to be approximately more than 1μg/ml in humans.

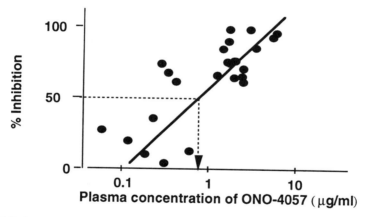

FIG. 3. Effect of the isolated plasma from volunteers treated with ONO-4057 on LTB4 (3 nM)-induced neutrophil [Ca^{2+}]i increase.

REFERENCES

1. Noal C. Recent progress in the development of leukotrieneB4 antagonists. Curr. Opin. Invest. Drug 1994;3:13-22.
2. Kishikawa K. ONO-4057, a novel, orally active leukotrieneB4 antagonist: Effects on LTB4-induced neutrophil functuions. Prostaglandins 1992;44:261-275.
3. Merritt JE. Use of fluo-3 to measure cytosolic Ca^{2+} in platelets and neutrophils. Biochem. J. 1990;269:513-519.

*Advances in Prostaglandin, Thromboxane,
and Leukotriene Research, Vol. 23,
edited by B. Samuelsson et al.
Raven Press, Ltd., New York © 1995*

Prostanoid and Leukotriene Receptors: A Progress Report from the IUPHAR Working Parties on Classification and Nomenclature

Robert A. Coleman[1], Richard M. Eglen[2], Robert L. Jones[3],
Shuh Narumiya[4], Takao Shimizu[5], William L. Smith[6],
Sven-Erik Dahlén[7], Jeffrey M. Drazen[8], Phillip J. Gardiner[9],
William T. Jackson[10], Thomas R. Jones[11], Robert D. Krell[12] and
Simonetta Nicosia[13].

[1]*Glaxo Research and Development, Ware, Hertfordshire, U.K.;* [2]*Syntex Research, Palo Alto, California, U.S.A.;* [3]*The Chinese University of Hong Kong, Shatin, Hong Kong;* [4]*Kyoto University, Kyoto, Japan;* [5]*University of Tokyo, Bunkyo-ku, Tokyo, Japan;* [6]*Michigan State University, East Lansing, U.S.A.;* [7]*Karolinska Institutet, Stockholm, Sweden;* [8]*Brigham and Woman's Hospital, Boston, U.S.A.;* [9]*Bayer plc, Slough, U.K.;* [10]*Eli Lilly & Co., Indianapolis, U.S.A.;* [11]*Merck Frosst, Pointe Claire Dorvall, Canada;* [12]*Pharmakon, Waverly, U.S.A.;* [13]*Institute of Pharmacological Science, Milan, Italy.*

Although prostanoids and leukotrienes are all products of arachidonic acid metabolism, their biological activities are distinct, and are produced through interaction with distinct families of receptor. It is of great importance to those working in the field that there are systems of classification and nomenclature for these receptors. Such systems should be rational, comprehensive and easy to use; and should be sufficiently flexible to allow for a degree of extension as more information becomes available. Finally, of course, they must be acceptable by all those who work in the area. For prostanoid receptors, a system was proposed by Kennedy *et al.* in 1982 (1), and this has now gained widespread acceptance, albeit in a somewhat extended form. For leukotrienes, however, no such generally accepted system of classification and nomenclature exists. Recently, the International Union of Pharmacologists (IUPHAR) set up working parties to identify and recommend systems of classification and nomenclature for hormone receptors. The present chapter, therefore, outlines proposed systems of classification and nomenclature for both classes of receptor, recommended to IUPHAR by these working parties.

PROSTANOID RECEPTORS

Prostanoid receptors are classified into five types on the basis of their sensitivity to the naturally-occurring prostanoids, prostaglandin (PG) D_2, PGE_2, $PGF_2\alpha$, PGI_2 and thromboxane (TX) A_2. These receptors are termed P-receptors, with a preceding letter indicating which of the naturally-occurring prostanoids is the most potent; thus they are DP, EP, FP, IP and TP respectively. However, within EP-receptors there is further subdivision, thus there are at least four subtypes of EP-receptor, termed arbitrarily, EP_1, EP_2, EP_3 and EP_4. There is at present, no conclusive evidence of such subdivision of any of the other four types of prostanoid receptor.

The original classification was based on functional data obtained with a range of agonists and some antagonists. There are examples of agents which exhibit some degree of selective agonist activity at each of the prostanoid receptors, except EP_4, for which no selective agonist has yet been identified. In contrast, while there are selective antagonists at DP, EP_1, EP_4 and TP-receptors, there are none for any of the other prostanoid receptor types.

Of the above receptor types, the DP, EP_1, EP_3, EP_4, FP, IP and TP-receptors have now been cloned, all are of the seven-transmembrane domain type, and there is a moderate degree of conservation across them. Cloning experiments have revealed that the EP_3-receptor may exist in a variety of different isoforms, resulting from alternative splicing at the C-terminus. These are tentitively termed EP_{3A}, EP_{3B}, EP_{3C} etc. However, as such splicing appears to be species specific, it is necessary to also quote the species when referring to such isoforms.

It appears that DP, EP_2, EP_4 and IP-receptors couple to adenylyl cyclase via a G_s-protein, and receptor activation results in increases in intracellular levels of cAMP. In contrast, EP_1, EP_3, FP and TP-receptors appear to couple to phospholipase C (PLC) via a G_q-protein, and receptor activation results in increases of both inositol trisphosphate production and intracellular levels of free Ca^{2+}. EP_3-receptors are also believed to couple to adenylyl cyclase via a G_i-protein. It is now known that the different isoforms of the EP_3-receptor differ in their G-protein coupling.

The functional characteristics, signal transduction and molecular biology of prostanoid receptors have recently been comprehensively reviewed (2).

LEUKOTRIENE RECEPTORS

Although there is no doubt that leukotrienes act through a range of distinct receptors, the classification and nomenclature of these receptors are not established. Leukotrienes (LTs) are of two types, the simple hydroxy-LTs, e.g. LTB_4, and the cysteine-containing LTs, e.g. LTC_4, LTD_4 and LTE_4, and there are distinct receptors for each of these types. There appears to be no ligand cross-reactivity between these receptors. While there is no evidence for subdivision of the receptors for the hydroxy-LTs, there appear to be at least two subtypes of the receptors for the cysteinyl-LTs. To date there is no accepted nomenclature for LT receptors, and they are commonly referred to in terms of the natural ligand, ie 'LTB-receptor', 'LTC-receptor' and 'LTD-receptor'. However, this is misleading, as: 1. it suggests three distinct classes of receptor, whereas in fact, there are two classes, one of which may be subdivided, 2. it suggests that there is a receptor at which LTC is more potent than LTD, and another at which LTD is more potent than LTC, which is incorrect, and 3. it does not allow for any further subdivision of receptors for the cysteinyl-LTs. We now propose a more rational, yet simple system of nomenclature within which, receptors for the hydroxy-LTs are termed BLT-receptors, and those for the cysteinyl leukotrienes are termed CysLT-receptors.

The classification of the LT-receptors is based on functional data, obtained mainly with antagonists; there being few agonists for either BLT- or CysLT-receptors. There are now many antagonists, both at BLT- and at CysLT-receptors, however, of this latter group, virtually all selectively block one subtype, termed arbitrarily, $CysLT_1$. At present it is assumed that all CysLT-receptors that are not of the $CysLT_1$ type form a homogeneous group, termed $CysLT_2$. However, it may subsequently prove necessary to further subdivide this group on the basis of new evidence.

As yet, there are no reports of successful cloning of either BLT- or CysLT-receptors, so there is no information as to the structural class to which they belong. However, BLT-receptors appear to be coupled via a G-protein to PLC, and CysLT-receptors probably via a G_q-protein to IP_3 turnover, and increases in levels of intracellular free Ca^{2+}.

ACKNOWLEDGEMENTS

We wish to acknowledge the valuable assistance of Professors PPA Humphrey, R Paoletti and PW Ramwell in the development of these systems of classification and nomenclature.

REFERENCES

Kennedy I, Coleman RA, Humphrey PPA *et al.* Studies on the characterisation of prostanoid receptors: a proposed classification. *Prostaglandins* 1982;24:667-89.

Coleman RA, Smith WL and Narumiya S. International Union of Pharmacology Classification of Prostanoid Receptors: Properties, distribution and structure of the receptors and their subtypes. *Pharmacol Rev* 1994;46:205-29.

Advances in Prostaglandin, Thromboxane,
and Leukotriene Research, Vol. 23,
edited by B. Samuelsson et al.
Raven Press, Ltd., New York © 1995

Cytokines and Eicosanoids Regulate PAF Receptor Gene Expression

Marek Rola-Pleszczynski, Maryse Thivierge,
Sylvie Ouellet, Pierre Dagenais, Jean-Luc Parent and Jana Stankova

*Immunology Division, Department of Pediatrics, Faculty of Medicine,
Université de Sherbrooke, Sherbrooke, QC Canada J1H 5N4*

Platelet-activating factor (PAF) is a potent phospholipid mediator of inflammation and immunoregulation (1). It is produced by many cell populations, including monocytes, macrophages, neutrophils, eosinophils, basophils, platelets and vascular endothelial cells in response to a variety of cell-specific stimuli. These same cell populations, as well as other cells such as B lymphocytes, NK cells and vascular smooth muscle cells, can become targets of PAF bioactivity. In recent years, we and others have shown PAF to modulate immune cell functions and, in particular, up-regulate their production of cytokines, such as interleukin (IL)-1, IL-6, IL-8 and tumor necrosis factor-alpha (TNFα) (2-8). Most if not all biological actions of PAF are thought to be mediated via specific receptors in the plasma membranes of responsive cells (9). A PAF receptor (PAFR) was first cloned from the guinea pig lung by Honda et al. (10), and this was followed by the cloning of a human (h)PAFR by the same group as well as several other groups soon afterwards (11-13).

Because of the potential for modulating cellular responses to PAF by modulating PAFR expression, we designed a series of experiments to address this topic. Most of these experiments were carried out on human monocytes, but they also involved other cell types, as indicated. They were greatly facilitated by the production of polyclonal antibody to the hPAFR which was used in flow cytometry studies (14). Moreover, in studies of transcriptional and post-transcriptional regulation of PAFR gene expression, a 0.7 kb cDNA fragment of the hPAFR was cloned and used as probe.

RESULTS AND DISCUSSION

Down-regulation of PAFR gene expression   by cAMP-augmenting agents.

In a first series of studies, we examined the effects of increasing intracellular cyclic AMP levels on the expression of hPAFR. Peripheral blood monocytes constitutively express hPAFR mRNA transcripts. Transiently elevated intracellular concentration of cyclic AMP induced either with prostaglandin E_2, cholera toxin or forskolin were a sufficient signal to inhibit PAFR expression. To determine the mechanisms of this inhibition, human monocytes were treated with dibutyryl cAMP, a cell-permeable cAMP analogue. cAMP reduced the expression of hPAFR in a concentration- and a time-dependent manner (15). The effect was seen as early as 1h and was essentially total by 4h. Stability of hPAFR mRNA was not markedly decreased by cAMP, as assessed by measuring half-life of the transcripts. Moreover, the nuclear transcription rate of the hPAFR gene was reduced as early as 30 min after stimulation with cAMP. The inhibition of hPAFR mRNA accumulation was associated with diminished responsiveness to PAF, as assayed by intracellular Ca^{2+} fluxes, decreased number of binding sites and decreased hPAFR protein expression on the cell surface, as assessed by flow cytometry using the polyclonal anti-hPAFR antibody (15).

Concentrations of 0.1 μM to 10 μM PGE_2 or the PGE_1 analog, misoprostol, induced concentration-dependent reductions in hPAFR mRNA expression of up to 75%. Moreover, the combination of pentoxifylline, a phosphodiesterase inhibitor, and the β-adrenergic agonist, salbutamol, similarly reduced hPAFR mRNA expression as early as 1h after treatment (16). These studies were the first demonstration that PAFR expression could be regulated at the transcriptional level by elevation of intracellular cAMP.

Upregulation of hPAFR gene expression by cytokines.

IFNγ has been demonstrated to synergistically enhance PAF-stimulated IL-1 production in human monocytes (17). Moreover, we had previously shown that priming with IFNγ was necessary to observe an enhancing effect of PAF on

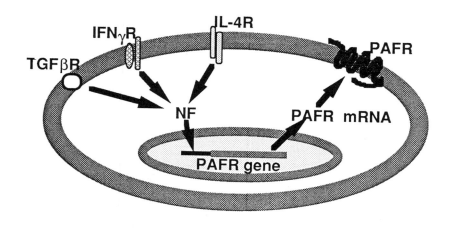

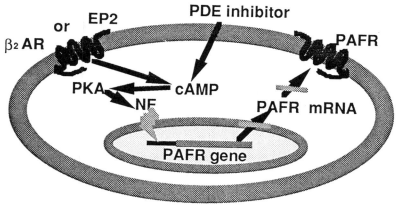

Fig. 1. Positive (upper) and negative (lower) modulation of hPAFR gene expression in monocytes by selected cytokines and cAMP-augmenting agents, respectively.

muramyl dipeptide (MDP)-driven TNF production in the human promyelocytic cell line HL-60 differentiated toward the monocyte lineage with vitamin D_3 (18). We had also observed that human monocytes pretreated with IFNγ and then stimulated with PAF produced more TNFα than non-treated cells (19). This led us to investigate the modulation of hPAFR gene expression by IFNγ. Treatment of monocytes with IFNγ caused a time- and concentration-dependent accumulation of hPAFR mRNA (20). In contrast, IFNα was inactive. The effect of IFNγ was rapid, being already evident after 1 h of stimulation and reaching a maximum after 2 h. The high level of hPAFR mRNA was maintained for at least 24 h. Flow cytometry analysis revealed that monocytes treated with IFNγ had a 2- to 6-fold increase in PAFR expression at the cell surface, when compared to untreated cells. The increase in hPAFR expression was associated with an augmented response of IFNγ-treated cells to PAF in terms of cytosolic calcium ($[Ca^{2+}]_i$) variations. Mechanisms of this up-regulation were investigated. The IFNγ-dependent accumulation of hPAFR mRNA was not due to the stabilization of hPAFR mRNA, as shown by assays done in the presence of the transcription inhibitor actinomycin D. Pretreatment of monocytes with actinomycin D, however, completely abrogated the effect of IFNγ, suggesting a transcriptional regulation. Moreover, the up-regulation of hPAFR mRNA by IFNγ was independent of *de novo* protein synthesis since cycloheximide, an inhibitor of protein synthesis, did not affect this up-regulation. These studies are the first report showing that IFNγ regulates hPAFR gene expression in human monocytes, by a mechanism suggesting transcriptional regulation. This may represent a prototypic example of regulation by lymphocyte-derived cytokines of lipid mediator receptors in myeloid cells, thus adding a novel element in the interrelationship between immune and inflammatory responses.

In this context, IL-4, a cytokine which is produced by a T helper cell subset (Th2) distinct from the one producing IFNγ (Th1), was also investigated. Somewhat to our surprise, IL-4 induced a similar, albeit smaller upregulation of hPAFR gene expression (21). IL-4 could not, however, modify the effect of IFNγ, suggesting common elements in the signal transduction pathways. In contrast, IL-10 was capable of blocking the up-regulation of hPAFR mRNA by IFNγ.

On the other hand, transforming growth factor (TGF)β, a pleiotropic cytokine with immunosuppressive properties, was found to markedly upregulate hPAFR mRNA expression in the myeloid leukemia cell line U937 as well as in the B cell lines Raji (EBV-positive) and Ramos (EBV-negative) (22).

ACKNOWLEDGMENTS

This work was supported in part by grants to M.R.-P. and a studentship to S.O. from the Medical Research Council of Canada. The authors wish to thank Suzanne Bédard, Denis Gingras, Marie-Josée Poirier and Sylvie Turcotte for excellent technical assistance.

REFERENCES

1. Braquet P and M Rola-Pleszczynski. Platelet-activating factor and cellular immune responses. *Immunol. Today* 1987; 8:345-352.

2. Dubois C, Bissonnette E and Rola-Pleszczynski M. Platelet-activating factor (PAF) stimulates tumor necrosis factor production by alveolar macrophages: prevention by PAF receptor antagonists and lipoxygenase inhibitors. *J Immunol* 1989; 143:964-971

3. Rola-Pleszczynski M. Priming of human monocytes with PAF augments their production of tumor necrosis factor. *J Lipid Mediators* 1990; 2:S77-S82

4. Pignol B, Hénane S, Sorlin B, Rola-Pleszczynski M, Mencia-Huerta J-M and Braquet P. Effect of long-term treatment with platelet-activating factor on IL 1 and IL 2 production by rat spleen cells. *J Immunol* 1990; 145:980-984

5. Poubelle P, Gingras D, Demers C, Dubois C, Harbour D and Rola-Pleszczynski M. Platelet activating factor (PAF-acether) enhances the concomitant production of tumor necrosis factor alpha and interleukin 1 by subsets of human monocytes. *Immunology,* 1991; 72:181-187

6. Thivierge M and Rola-Pleszczynski M. Platelet-activating factor (PAF) enhances interleukin-6 production by alveolar macrophages. *J Aller Clin Immunol* 1992; 90:796-802

7. Rola-Pleszczynski M and Stankova J. Differentiation-dependent modulation of TNF production by PAF in human HL-60 myeloid leukemia cells. *J Leuk Biol* 1992; 51:609-616

8. Denault S, M-J April, S Kocsis and J Stankova. Platelet-activating factor (PAF) up-regulates IL-8 gene expression in human monocytes: transcriptional and post-transcriptional mechanisms. *J Immunol* 1993;150 (II):125a. (Abstr.)

9. Hwang S-B. Specific receptors of platelet-activating factor, receptor heterogeneity, and signal transduction mechanisms. *J Lipid Mediators* 1990; 2:123.

10. Honda Z-I, M Nakamura, I Miki, M Minami, T Watanabe, Y Seyana, H Okado, H Toh, K Ito, T Miyamota and T Shimizu. Cloning by functional expression of platelet-activating factor receptor from guinea-pig lung. *Nature* 1991; 349:342.

11. Nakamura M, Z-I Honda, T Izumi, C Sakanaka, H Mutoh, M. Minami, H Bito, Y Seyama, T Matsumoto, M Noma and T Shimizu. Molecular cloning and expression of platelet-activating factor receptor from human leukocytes. *J Biol Chem* 1991; 266:20400.

12. Ye R, ER Prossnitz, A Zou and CG Cochrane. Characterization of a human cDNA that encodes a functional receptor for platelet-activating factor. *Biochem Biophys Res Commun* 1991; 180:105.

13. Kunz D, NP Gerard and C Gerard. The human leukocyte platelet-activating factor receptor. *J Biol Chem* 1992; 267:9101.

14. Müller E, P Dagenais, N Alami and M Rola-Pleszczynski. Identification and functional characterization of platelet-activating factor receptors in human leukocyte populations using polyclonal anti-peptide antibody. *Proc Natl Acad Sci USA* 1993; 90:5818-5822.

15. Thivierge M, N Alami, E Müller, AJ deBrum-Fernandes and M Rola-Pleszczynski. Transcriptional modulation of platelet-activating factor receptor gene expression by cyclic-AMP. *J Biol Chem* 1993; 268:17457-17462.

16. Thivierge M and M Rola-Pleszczynski. Regulation of platelet-activating factor receptor gene expression by β_2-adrenergic stimulation. *FASEB J* 1994; A220.

17. Barthelson R and F Valone. Interaction of platelet-activating factor with interferon-γ in the stimulation of interleukin-1 production by human monocytes. *J Allergy Clin Immunol* 1990; 86:193.

18. Rola-Pleszczynski M and J Stankova. Differentiation-dependent modulation of TNF production by PAF in human HL-60 myeloid leukemia cells. *J. Leukocyte Biol.* 1992; 51:609.

19. Ouellet S, D Gingras, S Turcotte and M Rola-Pleszczynski. Priming of monocytes with interferon-gamma is associated with upregulation of expression of the receptor for platelet-activating factor. In: Goetzl E, Lewis R, Rola-Pleszczynski M. *Cellular generation, transport and effects of eicosanoids: Biological roles and pharmacological intervention.* Ann NY Acad Sci. 1994; in press.

20. Ouellet S, E Müller and M Rola-Pleszczynski. Interferon-gamma upregulates platelet-activating factor receptor gene expression in human monocytes. *J Immunol* 1994; 152:5092-5099.

21. Ouellet S and M Rola-Pleszczynski. Interleukin-4 modulates the expression of platelet-activating factor (PAF) receptor gene in human monocytes.*FASEB J* 1994; A220.

22. Parent J-L and J Stankova. *Biochem Biophys Res Commun* 1993; 197:1443-1449.

Advances in Prostaglandin, Thromboxane, and Leukotriene Research, Vol. 23,
edited by B. Samuelsson et al.
Raven Press, Ltd., New York © 1995

The 5-lipoxygenase pathway in normal and malignant human B lymphocytes

P.-J. Jakobsson*, P. Larsson*, S. Feltenmark*, B. Odlander*,
G. Runarsson#, M. Björkholm# and H.-E. Claesson*

*Department of Medical Biochemistry and Biophysics, Karolinska Institutet, S-17177 Stockholm and
#Division of Medicine, Section of Hematology and Medical Immunology, Karolinska Hospital, S-17176
Stockholm, Sweden

The ability of human lymphocytes to synthesize 5-lipoxygenase products has been a matter of controversy. Earlier studies claimed that human T lymphocytes synthesized 5-HETE and LTB$_4$ (1-4). However, several groups could not repeat these initial findings (5-7). Later, one group actually retracted their original reports concerning LTB$_4$ synthesis in T cells, since they were unable to reproduce their own published results (8, 9). Recently, evidence was provided for 5-HETE production by certain B cell lines (10). However, no LTA$_4$ products were demonstrated. As a result of these reports, the consensus before our present investigation was that human lymphocytes were not able to synthesize leukotrienes from arachidonic acid.

LEUKOTRIENE BIOSYNTHESIS IN CELL HOMOGENATES

A modified homogenate assay was utilized in order to study leukotriene formation in sonicated cells. Applying this assay in studies on the regulation of 5-lipoxygenase activity in monocytes, it was shown that the activity found in sonicated cell preparations did not correspond well to the activity found in ionophore A23187 stimulated intact monocytes. These findings led to re-evaluation of the presence of 5-lipoxygenase activity in human lymphocytes and it was discovered that homogenates of several monoclonal B cell lines, as well as normal human B lymphocytes, converted arachidonic acid to LTB$_4$ (11). In contrast, no leukotriene formation was detected in peripheral blood T lymphocytes or monoclonal T cell lines.

The fact that no 5-HETE or LTB_4 were detected in intact B lymphocytes after stimulation with the calcium ionophore A23187, regardless of the presence or absence of exogenous arachidonic acid, strongly suggests a different regulation of cellular leukotriene formation in B lymphocytes as compared with myeloid cells.

STIMULATION OF INTACT B LYMPHOCYTES WITH THIOLREACTIVE AGENTS

It had previously been reported that the glutathione depleting agents, azodicarboxylic acid bis(dimethylamide) (diamide) and 1-chloro-2,4-dinitrobenzene (Dnp-Cl), stimulated the formation of 5-HETE and LTB_4 in neutrophils incubated with exogenous arachidonic acid (12, 13). The mechanism of action for Dnp-Cl was suggested to be mediated by decreased glutathione peroxidase activity due to the lack of reduced glutathione, resulting in higher intracellular levels of fatty acid hydroperoxides. These fatty acid hydroperoxides in turn could stimulate the 5-lipoxygenase. Treatment of intact B lymphocytes with these compounds, followed by stimulation with arachidonic acid and ionophore A23187, led to leukotriene formation (14, 28). Table 1 summarizes the relative importance of EDTA, Ca^{2+}, arachidonic acid, and calcium ionophore A23187 in sonicates versus intact cell assays. No LTC_4 formation was detected, even in the presence of 1 mM glutathione. However, a three-fold increase of 5-HETE formation was observed in intact cells after treatment with diamide in the presence of glutathione (1 mM).

Table 1. Relative effects of various compounds on leukotriene biosynthesis in B cells.

Assay	EDTA	ATP	Diamide	Ca^{2+}	AA	Ionophore A23187	GSH	LTB_4	5-HETE
								\(pmol / 10^6\) cells)	
Sonicated cells	+	+		+	+			16	218
	+	+		+	-			nd	nd
	+	+		-	+			< 1	4
	-	+		+	+			1.5	9
Intact cells			+	+	+	+		26	74
			-	+	+	+		< 1.5	10
	+		+	-	+	+		nd	3
	+		+	+	-	+		nd	nd
	+		+	+	+	-		< 2	6
	+		+	+	+	+	+	28	201

BL41-E95-A cells (10 x 10^6 cells / ml) were suspended in PBS without Ca^{2+} and Mg^{2+}. Under standard conditions the cells were sonicated for 3 x 5 s, in the presence of EDTA (1 mM). Subsequently, the cells were prewarmed to 37°C, followed by the addition of ATP (1 mM), Ca^{2+} (2 mM) and arachidonic acid (40 µM). Intact cells were stimulated with diamide (500 µM) for 10 min, followed by addition of Ca^{2+} (1 mM), arachidonic acid (AA, 40 µM), and ionophore A23187 (5 µM).
+ = added compounds; - = not added; blank = not considered; nd = not detectable.

Interestingly, diamide and two additional compounds, methyl methanethiosulfonate (MMTS) and *N*-ethylmaleimide, were found to instantaneously induce leukotriene formation by BL41-E95-A cells stimulated with the calcium ionophore

A23187 and arachidonic acid. In contrast, the stimulatory action of Dnp-Cl on leukotriene biosynthesis by B cells was dependent on a five minutes incubation period before the additions of arachidonic acid and ionophore A23187.

Dnp-Cl acts as a substrate for glutathione-*S*-transferase (15), but diamide oxidizes reduced glutathione to its disulfide form (GSSG) (16). *N*-etylmaleimide has also been reported to reduce the cellular contents of glutathione (17), with subsequent increase of LTB$_4$ formation in alveolar macrophages challenged with arachidonic acid. Methyl-methanethiosulfonate quantitatively delivers CH$_3$S-groups to cysteinyl sulfhydryl groups in both proteins and glutathione (18). In addition to these four compounds which all induce leukotriene biosynthesis by intact B lymphocytes, other "thiolreactive" compounds, including diethylmaleate, iodoacetate, iodoacetamide and monobromobimane, were tested and found not to stimulate cellular leukotriene biosynthesis. Diethylmaleate, like Dnp-Cl, is a substrate for glutathione transferease (19), but monobromobimane (20), iodoacetate and iodoacetamide all react with thiol groups exposed on either glutathione or proteins (18). This promotes the formation of thiol adducts, *i.e.*, a mechanism of action similar to that of N-etylmaleimide and MMTS. The reason for the different effects of these compounds on leukotriene biosynthesis is not known. One possible explanation may be different degrees of plasma membrane penetration. However, monobromobimane readily penetrates the cell membrane and reacts with all exposed thiols (20). Therefore, it is at present not clear why *N*-ethylmaleimide and MMTS activates the cells but not monobromobimane.

In order to investigate the role of glutathione in 5-lipoxygenase regulation, we cultivated B cells in the presence of buthioninesulfoximine (BSO), an inhibitor of γ-glutamylcysteine synthase (19). This treatment reduced the intracellular content of total glutathione from ~ 6 to 0.5 nmol glutathione / 10^6 cells. However, the glutathione depleted BL41-E95-A cells did not synthesize leukotrienes after stimulation with arachidonic acid and calcium ionophore (14). This finding argues against a primary glutathione inhibition of 5-lipoxygenase. Of importance, leukotriene formation in homogenates of glutathione-depleted cells was not affected by the BSO treatment, while the stimulatory effect of diamide on intact cells was abolished.

These results indicate that diamide mediates its effect through immediate modulation of glutathione levels, resulting in 5-lipoxygenase activation as a secondary event. Furthermore, all thiol-reactive compounds that stimulate 5-lipoxygenase activity in intact cells acted as inhibitors of 5-lipoxygenase in sonicates, which excluded the possibility of a direct stimulatory effect on 5-lipoxygenase.

HYDROGEN PEROXIDE AND 5-LIPOXYGENASE ACTIVITY

Treatment of granulocytes with the glutathione depleting agent Dnp-Cl for five minutes led to impaired ability to reduce lipid hydroperoxides (13). Also, in granulocyte homogenates, glutathione was found to inhibit leukotriene biosynthesis. Addition of glutathione peroxidase in the sonicate assay caused a rapid cessation of 5-lipoxygenase activity (13). These data suggested that hydroperoxides stimulated

5-lipoxygenase activity. This was supported by the observation that addition of different lipid hydroperoxides (10 μM) to intact cells, stimulated leukotriene synthesis in the presence of arachidonic acid (13). However, no effect with hydrogen peroxide (10 μM) was observed. Interestingly, granulocytes from selenium-deficient rats, with impaired GSH peroxidase activity, produced sevenfold more 5-lipoxygenase metabolites above control levels (21). These reports, and the stimulatory effect of the glutathione depleting agent, N-ethylmaleimide, on LTB_4 biosynthesis in alveolar macrophages, (17), supports the contention that depletion of glutathione increases the levels of hydroperoxides. However, the low efficiency by which diamide reduced the cellular glutathione content (12), as well as our own data with BSO treated cells (see above), does not entirely fit this model. Consequently, other mechanisms may still operate. Nevertheless, it is likely that Dnp-Cl and diamide and the other thiol-reactive agents may mediate their effects through increased hydro / hydrogen peroxide formation.

To test this assumption, B lymphocytes were incubated with different concentrations of hydrogen peroxide. It was demonstrated that hydrogen peroxide (1 - 5 μM) stimulated B lymphocytes to produce LTB_4 after stimulation with arachidonic acid and ionophore A23187. This positive effect of hydrogen peroxide agrees with studies on soybean lipoxygenase activity, demonstrating that subnanomolar concentrations of hydrogen peroxide activate this enzyme (22). At higher concentrations (>1 nM), no stimulatory effect was observed on soybean lipoxygenase (22).

EFFECT OF PROTEIN TYROSINE KINASE INHIBITORS ON LEUKOTRIENE BIOSYNTHESIS

Thiol-oxidizing agents like diamide as well as various alkylating agents have been shown to stimulate protein tyrosine kinase (PTK) activity in the B cell line, A20 (23). Several research groups, investigating the regulation of prostaglandin and leukotriene formation in different cells claim that PTK inhibitors block the formation of eicosanoids (24-26). We investigated the effects of several PTK inhibitors on 5-lipoxygenase activity, both in chronic lymphocytic leukemia of B cell type (B-CLL) cells and granulocytes (Table 2), in order to investigate if this was the mechanism of action by which diamide activated B lymphocytes.

Table 2 demonstrates the approximate IC_{50} values obtained for erbstatin A, tyrphostin 23, genistein and RG-13022 on leukotriene synthesis in granulocytes, B-CLL cells and recombinant 5-lipoxygenase. Tyrphostin (Tyr) 1 was included as a negative control. Erbastatin A and tyrphostin 23 inhibited leukotriene synthesis in intact B-CLL cells, stimulated with diamide, arachidonic acid and the ionophore A23187, in a dose-dependent fashion. Since B-CLL cells in contrast to granulocytes require exogenous archidonic acid to produce leukotrienes, the higher IC_{50} values obtained for genistein and RG-13022 might be due to the presence of exogenous arachidonic acid. Therefore, the effects of the PTK inhibitors was tested on granulocytes stimulated only with the calcium ionophore A23187. Under these conditions the IC_{50} of genistein and RG-13022 was

Table 2. Apparent IC_{50} of protein tyrosine kinase inhibitors on 5-lipoxygenase activity.

	Erb A	Tyr 23	Tyr 1	Genistein	RG-13022
Granulocytes	3*	10*	>100	30*	10*
B-CLL	20	10	>100	100	100
r 5-LO	3	3	>250	25	250

Granulocytes were incubated with 0.5 µM A23187. B-CLL cells were stimulated with diamide (500 µM), arachidonic acid (40 µM) and A23187 (2,5 µM). Recombinant 5-lipoxygenase (0.1 µg / 100 µl/ assay) was incubated with arachidonic acid (160 µM). The values depict the apparent IC_{50} (µM) from one representative experiment.
* Inhibition was competitive with arachidonic acid.

reduced. However, genistein as well as Erbstatin A and Tyrphostin 23 also blocked the activity of recombinant 5-lipoxygenase (table 2)

In conclusion, the involvement of PTK in the activation process of cellular leukotriene formation is difficult to evaluate, due to the non-specificity of the available PTK inhibitors. The data in the literature concerning the involvement of PTK activity in leukotriene formation, is therefore hard to interpret.

EXPRESSION OF ENZYMES INVOLVED IN EICOSANOID METABOLISM IN LEUKOCYTES

Table 3 summarizes the results obtained using reverse transcription (RT)-PCR analysis of the gene expression of various proteins involved in the metabolism of eicosanoids in different types of cells. Normal tonsillar B-lymphocytes, as well as B-CLL cells expressed enzymes obligatory for leukotriene synthesis. However, these cells did not express the cytosolic phospholipase A_2 (cPLA$_2$, 85 kDa) gene. Four of eight investigated acute pre B lymphocytic leukemia (pre-B-ALL) clones expressed cPLA$_2$ but not 5-lipoxygenase mRNA, while the other four clones expressed 5-lipoxygenase but not cPLA$_2$ (27). This inverse expression of cPLA$_2$ and 5-lipoxygenase mRNA suggest that the transcriptional regulation of these two genes are different and that their cellular functions are not linked to each other.

Table 3. RT-PCR analysis of the gene products coding for the enzymes involved in leukotriene and prostaglandin biosynthesis in different cell types.

Cells	cPLA$_2$	5-LO	FLAP	LTA$_4$ hydrolase	PGHS-1	PGHS-2
B lymphocytes (tonsils)	-	+	+	+	-	-
B-CLL	-	+	+	+	+	-
B-ALL group 1	+	-	+	+	+	+
B-ALL group 2	-	+	+	+	+	+[#]
PMNL	-	+	+	+	n.d.	n.d.
Monocytes	+	+	+	+	+	+
Peripheral T cells	-	-	+	+	+	+
HUVEC	-	-	-	+	+	-
platelets	-	-	-	-	+	-

n.d., not determined. [#](3 out of 4). HUVEC, human umbilical vein endothelial cells.

All pre B-ALL clones expressed genes coding for 5-lipoxygenase activating protein, leukotriene A_4 hydrolase and prostaglandin (PG)H synthase 1. Seven of the eight pre B-ALL clones expressed PGH synthase 2. Normal B cells isolated from tonsils did neither express PGH synthase 1 nor PGH synthase 2.

ACKNOWLEDGMENT

The authors are greatly indebted to Ms Hélène Ax:son-Johnson for excellent technical assistance and to Dr. Rådmark for recombinant 5-lipoxygenase. This work was supported by grants from King Gustaf V´s 80-year Fund, the Funds of Karolinska Institutet and Cancerfonden (3519).

REFERENCES

1. Parker, CW, Stenson, WF, Huber, MG, Kelly, JP. 1979. *J. Immunol.* 122: 1572-1577.
2. Goetzl, EJ. 1981. *Biochem. Biophys. Res. Commun.* 101: 344-350.
3. Atluru, D, Goodwin, JS. 1986. *Cell. Immunol.* 99: 444-452.
4. Goodwin, JS, Atluru, D, Sierakowski, S, Lianos, EA. 1986. *J. Clin. Invest.* 77: 1244-1250.
5. Goldyne, ME, Burrish, GF, Poubelle, P, Borgeat, P. 1984. *J. Biol. Chem.* 259: 8815-8819.
6. Goldyne, ME, Rea, L. 1987. *Prostaglandins.* 34: 783-795.
7. Poubelle, PE, Borgeat, P, Rola-Pleszczynski, M. 1987. *J. Immunol.* 139: 1273-1277.
8. Goodwin, JS, Behrens, T. 1988. *Ann. NY. Acad. Sci.* 524: 201-7.
9. Behrens, TW, Lum, LG, Lianos, EA, Goodwin, JS. 1989. *J. Immunol.* 143: 2285-2294.
10. Schulam, PG, Shearer, WT. 1990. *J. Immunol.* 144: 2696-2701.
11. Jakobsson, P-J, Odlander, B, Steinhilber, D, Rosén, A, Claesson, H-E. 1991. *Biochem. Biophys. Res. Commun.* 178: 302-308.
12. Hatzelmann, A, Ullrich, V. 1987. *Eur. J. Biochem.* 169: 175-184.
13. Hatzelmann, A, Schatz, M, Ullrich, V. 1989. *Eur. J. Biochem.* 180: 527-533
14. Jakobsson, P-J, Steinhilber, D, Odlander, B, Rådmark, O, Claesson, H-E, Samuelsson, B. 1992. *Proc. Natl. Acad. Sci. USA.* 89: 3521-3525.
15. Habig, WH, Pabst, MJ, Jakoby, WB. 1974. *J. Biol. Chem.* 249: 7130-7139.
16. Kosower, EM, Kosower, NS. 1969. *Nature.* 224: 117-120.
17. Peters-Golden, M, Shelly, C. 1987. *J. Biol. Chem.* 262: 10594-10600.
18. Kenyon, GL, Bruice, TW. 1976. *Methods Enzymol.* 47: 407-430.
19. Meister, A. 1985. *Methods. Enzymol.* 113: 571-585.
20. Cotgreave, IA, Moldéus, P. 1986. *J Biochem. Biophys. Methods.* 13: 231-249.
21. Weitzel, F, Wendel, A. 1993. *J. Biol. Chem.* 268: 6288-6292.
22. Kulkarni, AP, Mitra, A, Chaudhuri, J, Byczkowski, JZ, Richards, I. 1990. *Biochem. Biophys. Res. Commun.* 166: 417-423.
23. Bauskin, AR, Alkalay, I, Ben-Neriah, Y. 1991. *Cell.* 66: 685-696.
24. Glaser, KB, Sung, A, Bauer, J, Weichman, BM. 1993. *Biochem. Pharmacol.* 45: 711-721.
25. Atluru, D, Gudapaty, S. 1993. *Vet. Immunol. Immunopathol.* 38: 113-122.
26. Olsen, S, Atluru, D, Erickson, H, Ames, T. 1994. *Biochem. Arch.* 10: 11-16.
27. Feltenmark, S, Runarsson, G, Larsson, P, Jakobsson, P-J, Björkholm, M, Claesson, H-E, 1994. to be published.
28. Claesson, H-E, Jakobsson, P-J, Steinhilber, D, Odlander, B, Samuelsson, B. 1993. J. Lip. Med. 6: 15-22.

Advances in Prostaglandin, Thromboxane,
and Leukotriene Research, Vol. 23,
edited by B. Samuelsson et al.
Raven Press, Ltd., New York © 1995

Characterization of Prostaglandin E$_2$ Receptors on Normal and Malignant B Lymphocytes

Deborah M. Brown and Richard P. Phipps

University of Rochester Cancer Center, 601 Elmwood Ave., Rochester, New York 14642 USA

Prostaglandin E$_2$ (PGE$_2$) is a pleiotropic molecule synthesized by macrophages, fibroblasts and follicular dendritic cells in response to inflammatory stimuli including TNF-α, IL-1 and bacterial LPS. PGE$_2$ is a potent immunoregulatory molecule because of its effects on B and T lymphocyte functions such as antibody production and cytokine synthesis. The differential effects of PGE$_2$ on B lymphocytes include the down-regulation of IgM, production while enhancing immunoglobulin class switching. For example, PGE$_2$ can inhibit hapten-specific IgM responses, but can augment immunoglobulin class switching to IgE by B lymphocytes cultured with IL-4 and LPS. PGE$_2$ also differentially affects murine and human T helper lymphocyte cytokine production. In studies employing both human and murine T lymphocyte subsets, PGE$_2$ inhibited TH1 synthesis of IL-2 and IFN-γ, while enhancing TH2 synthesis of IL-5. TH2 synthesis of IL-4 was unaffected by treatment with PGE$_2$. These studies indicate that PGE$_2$ is not solely an immunosuppressive agent, but has potent regulatory effects on cells of the immune system (1).

To further characterize the dual modulatory role of PGE$_2$ in the immune system, it has become important to identify the putative PGE$_2$ receptor on cells of hematopoietic origin. Cell surface receptors for PGE$_2$ have been identified on many tissue preparations including kidney, intestine and liver. PGE$_2$ receptors have also been characterized on selected cell types such as macrophages and T lymphocytes. To date, the PGE$_2$ receptor has not been identified on cells of the B lineage.

Our laboratory has used B cell lymphomas as models for normal B cell function. These lymphomas can be separated into "immature" (CH31) and "mature" (CH12) phenotypes based on their response to treatment with anti-Ig reagents. CH31 mimics immature B lymphocytes in that it is growth inhibitable by treatment with anti-μ. CH12 is indicative of mature B lymphocytes since it is resistant to anti-μ-mediated growth inhibition. We have further characterized these lymphomas into PGE$_2$-sensitive (CH31) and PGE$_2$-resistant (CH12) subsets based on their ability to undergo apoptosis in response to μM concentrations of PGE$_2$ (1). The differential susceptibility of B cell lymphomas to treatment with PGE$_2$ is an attractive model system to study PGE$_2$ receptors since sensitivity to PGE$_2$ may be a consequence of distinct receptor profiles.

RESULTS

Normal and Malignant B Lymphocytes Display PGE2 Receptors

PGE2 is a small molecular weight, lipophilic molecule consisiting of a carbon backbone and alkyl side chains. Classic receptor-binding studies employ ^{125}I-lableled proteins because of their high specific activity, however, iodination of PGE2 is impractical since the native molecule contains no tyrosines. Therefore, a receptor binding assay utilizing ^{3}H-PGE2 was employed. Figure 1 demonstrates Scatchard analysis of ^{3}H-PGE2 binding to normal and malignant B lymphocytes. Figure 1 indicates that cells of the B lineage bind PGE2 in a single high affinity state with dissociation constants in the 0.5-0.8 nM range. The PGE2 resistant CH12 B cell lymphoma has more PGE2 receptors on its surface than the PGE2-sensitive CH31 lymphoma, with CH12 possessing 350 receptors/cell compared to 125 receptors/cell on CH31. Normal murine splenic B lymphocytes also display PGE2 receptors with a K_d of 0.8 nM and a B_{max} of 1.2 pM, or, 50 sites/cell.

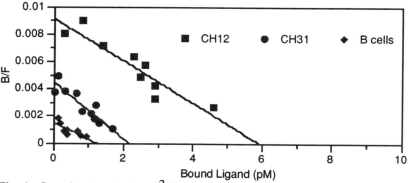

Fig. 1. Scatchard analysis of ^{3}H-PGE2 binding to normal and malignant B lymphocytes. PGE2 binding assays were performed by incubating 1 x 10^7 cells with varying concentrations of ^{3}H-PGE2. Nonspecific binding was determined by incubating duplicate wells with 1000-fold molar excess of cold PGE2.

LPS Upregulates PGE2 Receptor Numbers on CH12 and CH31 Cells

Bacterial LPS can upregulate activation antigens such as Class II MHC and the low affinity receptor for IgE (CD23) on normal B lymphocytes. LPS also has a regulatory effect on B cell lymphomas by abrogating anti-μ-mediated growth inhibition. We were interested in determining whether LPS could regulate PGE2 receptor numbers or affinity on B cell lymphomas. Figure 2 demonstrates that a 20 h treatment with 5 μg/ml LPS upregulates PGE2 receptor numbers on both CH12 and CH31 B cell lymphomas while having no effect on the affinity of the PGE2 receptor. Scatchard analysis demonstrates a 2.5-fold increase in PGE2 receptor numbers on CH12 from 5.9 pM or 350 sites/cell to 14.2 pM, or 850 sites/cell. Similarly, PGE2 receptor capacity increased on CH31 from 2.2 pM or 125 sites/cell to 4.7 pM or 280 sites/cell.

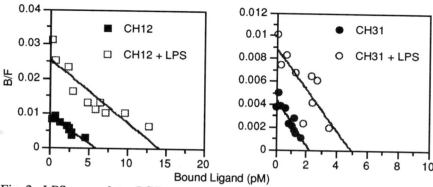

Fig. 2. LPS upregulates PGE2 receptor numbers on CH12 and CH31 B cell lymphomas. Scatchard analysis was performed as in legend to Fig. 1.

DISCUSSION

We have demonstrated that the PGE2 receptor exists in a single high affinity state on cells of the B lineage. Normal and malignant B lymphocytes can bind PGE2 with an affinity in the 0.5-0.8 nM range. This is in agreement with reported Kd's for the high affinity site on the macrophage-like cell line P388D1 (3 nM) as well as Kd's reported for a cloned murine T cell hybridoma (0.7 nM) and activated human T lymphocytes (0.5 nM). LPS, which upregulates activation antigens on murine B lymphocytes, can upregulate PGE2 receptors on B cell lymphomas. This suggests that activation of B lymphocytes with mitogens or cytokines may make them more susceptible to regulation by PGE2 by increasing cell surface receptors for PGE2. Studies are underway to address this hypothesis by assaying receptor levels on normal B lymphocytes after treatment with LPS or IL-4.

Normal and malignant B lymphocytes elevate intracellular cAMP in response to treatment with PGE2. Based on the classification scheme for the PGE2 receptor described by Coleman, these data suggest the presence of an EP2 receptor subtype on B lineage cells. Recent data has demonstrated that the EP3 subtype of the murine PGE2 receptor can exist in three different isoforms generated by alternative splicing mechanisms. Two of these isoforms, α and β, are linked to an inhibitory G-protein and can inhibit cAMP formation. The third isoform, γ, can be coupled to either a stimulatory or inhibitory G-protein, which can stimulate or inhibit formation of cAMP, respectively (2). By using subtype specific agonists, we will be able to determine which PGE2 receptor subtype is present on cells of the B lineage and which subtype is responsible for increases in cAMP.

REFERENCES

1. Borrello, M. A., Fedyk, E. R., Brown, D. M. and Phipps, R. P. Strategies for studying the regulation of B lymphocytes by PGE2. *Immunomethods*. 1993;2:261-72.
2. Irie, A., Y. Sugimoto, T. Namba, A. Harazono, A. Honda, A. Watabe, *et al.*. Third isoform of the prostaglandin-E-receptor EP3 subtype with different C-terminal tail coupling to both stimulation and inhibition of adenylate cyclase. *Eur. J. Biochem.* 1993;217:313-18.

Advances in Prostaglandin, Thromboxane, and Leukotriene Research, Vol. 23,
edited by B. Samuelsson et al.
Raven Press, Ltd., New York © 1995

Production of PGE$_2$ and 15-HETE by Fibrosarcoma Cells

Keyvan Mahboubi and Nicholas R. Ferreri

Department of Pharmacology, New York Medical College, Valhalla, New York 10595

Tumors metabolize arachidonic acid (AA), by either the lipoxygenase or cyclooxygenase pathways, to different eicosanoids. Prostaglandin E$_2$ (PGE$_2$) has been shown to play a role in the growth and metastasis of tumors (1). Further, PGE$_2$ and 15-hydroxyeicosatetraenoic acid (15-HETE), a lipoxygenase product, have multiple effects on immune cells such as T lymphocytes (2, 3). Since MCA-101 is a fibrosarcoma cell line which is not killed by CD8$^+$ cytotoxic T cells (4), we assessed the production of eicosanoids from these cells in response to cytokines. Both interleukin-1 (IL-1) and tumor necrosis factor-α (TNF-α) have been shown to increase PGE$_2$ release from normal fibroblasts (5, 6). Induction of the cyclooxygenase enzyme (COX-2) by IL-1 and TNF-α increased the conversion of AA to PGE$_2$. Also, cells transfected with the COX-2 gene converted AA to 15-HETE in the presence of aspirin, a COX inhibitor (7) . The purpose of our study was to examine the conversion of AA by MCA-101 cells in response to TNF-α and IL-1, in order to determine whether these tumor cells have characterstics of the COX-2 pathway similar to those previously reported for normal fibroblasts.

METHODS

MCA-101 cells were seeded in RPMI 1640 plus 10% FCS and incubated at 37°C and 5% CO$_2$. After 24 hr, media were removed and cells incubated in RPMI plus 0.1% BSA, in the presence or absence of appropriate cytokine treatment. After 24 hr, media were removed and cells incubated with ^{14}C-AA (2μM) for 90 min followed by addition of calcium ionophore (A23187, 5 μM) for 30 min. Products released into the media were acidified to pH 4.0 with formic acid, and the metabolites were extracted with ethyl acetate and separated by reverse phase HPLC (RP-HPLC). In order to measure 15-HETE production, cells were seeded in 6-well plates in RPMI plus 10% FCS. At confluency, cells were incubated with new media in the absence or presence of aspirin (100 μM) or indomethacin (10 μM) for

30 min. After incubation, cells were harvested and incubated with 1X PBS containing ^{14}C-AA (0.3 μCi, 21 μM) for 15 min at 37°C. The reaction was terminated and analyzed by RP-HPLC, as described above.[14]C-labeled 15-HETE was used as a standard. Specific activity was calculated based on the percent conversion of added ^{14}C-AA to 15-HETE and expressed as μg/hr/mg protein.

RESULTS

Unstimulated MCA-101 cells did not metabolize AA to any eicosanoid products that could be detected by HPLC (Fig 1a). Addition of AA followed by A23187 resulted in the release of a radioactive product from unstimulated cells (data not shown). Stimulation with IL-1 (10 [-9] M) plus TNF-α (10[-9] M) for 24 hr prior to the addition of AA and A23187 resulted in the release of a radioactive peak with a retention time (8-10 min) similar to that for PGE₂ (Fig 1b).

MCA-101 cells did not convert exogenous AA to 15-HETE, as there was no radioactive peak corresponding to 15-HETE on the HPLC chromatogram. Addition of aspirin, but not indomethacin, prior to AA, resulted in the release of a radioactive peak with the same retention time as authentic 15-HETE. The specific activity was determined to be 18.85±2.0 (μg/ hr/ mg) in the presence of aspirin (Table 1).

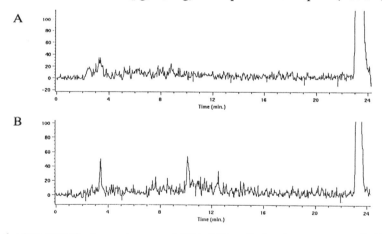

FIG.1.: RP-HPLC chromatogram. MCA-101 cells in the presence of: (A) 2 μM AA alone, or (B) 24 hr preincubation with IL-1 (10[-9] M) + TNF-α (10[-9]M).

Treatment	15-HETE (μg/hr/mg)
Control	0
Indomethacin	0
Aspirin	18.85±2.0

Table 1: 15-HETE production by MCA-101 cells. Cells were preincubated with indomethacin (10 μM) or aspirin (100 μM), prior to addition of AA (21 μM), (n=3).

DISCUSSION

We have found that PGE$_2$ is the major prostaglandin released from MCA-101 cells stimulated with IL-1 and TNF-α. IL-1 and TNF-α increased COX-2 mRNA and COX-2 protein in a time-dependent manner in MCA-101 cells (unpublished data). Thus, AA metabolism via COX-2 may be responsible, in part, for the increase in PGE$_2$ production by these cells. In human lung fibroblasts, IL-1 induces the accumulation of cPLA2 and PGE$_2$ without affecting the levels of cyclooxygenase (6), whereas in human dermal fibroblasts IL-1 has been shown to increase synthesis of cyclooxygenase (5). Further experiments will elucidate the mechanisms by which IL-1 and TNF-α stimulate PGE$_2$ synthesis in MCA-101 cells. Conversion of AA to 15-HETE by COX-2 in the presence of aspirin is one of the characteristics of COX-2. This effect has been shown to be specific for aspirin since other non-steriodal antiinflammatory drugs did not exhibit such an effect (7). For example, MCA-101 cells converted AA to 15-HETE only in the presence of aspirin, but not indomethacin. These data suggest that MCA-101 cells express COX-2. Production of 15-HETE was potentiated when cells were treated with IL-1 plus TNF-α prior to the addition of aspirin (unpublished data). Cytokine-mediated production of 15-HETE, in the presence of aspirin, may be due to induction of COX-2 protein by these cytokines. 15-HETE released from MCA-101 in response to aspirin and cytokines may modulate various *in vivo* effects of aspirin. Future studies will investigate the role of 15-HETE released from MCA-101 in response to cytokines and aspirin.

REFERENCES

1) Kenneth V. Honn, Richard S. Bockman and Lawrence J. Marnett. Prostaglandins and cancer: A review of tumor initiation through tumor metastasis. *Prostaglandins,* May 1981, vol 21, No 5, 833-864.

2) Nicholas R. Ferreri, Bardia Askari, Keyvan Mahboubi and Nancy H. Ruddle. Tumor necrosis factor-α and Lymphotoxin: Regulation by PGE$_2$ in T-cell subsets. *Immunomethods,* Vol 2, No3, 1993, 245-254.

3) Jack Y. Vanderhoek. Role of 15-lipoxygenase in the immune system. *Ann.NY Acad.Sci.,* 524, 1988, 240-251.

4) Nicholas P. Restifo, Paul J. Spiess, Stephen E. Karp, James J. Mule, and Steven A. Rosenberg. A nonimmunogenic sarcoma transfected with the cDNA for interferon γ elicits CD8$^+$ T cells against the wild type tumor: Correlation with antigen presentation capability. *The Journal of Experimental Medicine,* Vol. 175, June 1992, 1423-1431.

5) Amiram Raz, Angela Wyche, Ned Siegel, and Philip Needleman. Regulation of fibroblast cyclooxygenase synthesis by interleukin-1. *The Journal of Biological Chemistry,* 1988, Vol. 263, No. 6, 3022-3028.

6) Lin Lin-Ling, Alice Y. Lin, and David L. Dewittt. Interleukin-1α induces the accumulation of cytosolic phospholipases A$_2$ and the release of prostaglandin E$_2$ in human fibroblasts. *The Journal of Biological Chemistry,* 1992, Vol. 267, No. 33, 23451-23454.

7) Elizabeth A. Meade, William L. Smith, and David L. Dewitt. Differential inhibition of prostaglandin endoperoxide synthesis (cyclooxygenase) isozymes by aspirin and other non-steroidal anti-inflammatory drugs. *The Journal of Biological Chemistry,* 1993, Vol. 268, No. 9, 6610-6614.

Advances in Prostaglandin, Thromboxane,
and Leukotriene Research, Vol. 23,
edited by B. Samuelsson et al.
Raven Press, Ltd., New York © 1995

Evidence For Reciprocal Regulation Of Pro- And Anti-inflammatory Lymphokines In Rat Nephrotoxic Serum (NTS) Nephritis

Fadi G. Lakkis, Eddie N. Cruet, Megumu Fukunaga, and Karen A. Munger

Renal Division, Emory University School of Medicine & Veterans Administration Medical Center, Atlanta, Georgia, U.S.A.

Based on the pattern of lymphokine secretion, helper T lymphocytes (Th) are divided into at least two subsets: Th1 and Th2 (1). Interleukin 4 (IL-4), IL-10, and IL-13, produced by Th2 cells, suppress production of inflammatory mediators by macrophages whereas IFNγ, secreted by Th1 lymphocytes, promotes tissue inflammation (1). *In vitro* and *in vivo* cross-regulation between Th lymphocytes suggests that the outcome of an inflammatory response can be influenced by the net balance of Th1 and Th2 lymphokines (1).

Although T lymphocytes have been implicated in the pathogenesis of human and experimental glomerulonephritis (GN), their role is not clearly defined (2). In this report, we studied glomerular expression of Th1 and Th2 lymphokine genes during the first 48 hours of passive anti-glomerular basement membrane (anti-GBM) GN in the rat. The data demonstrate reciprocal expression of pro- and anti-inflammatory cytokine genes suggesting that Th lymphocyte subsets play a regulatory role in inflammatory renal disease.

METHODS

Male Sprague-Dawley rats (200-250 gms) (Charles River, MA) were injected intravenously with 150 μl of rabbit anti-rat GBM nephrotoxic serum (kind gift of George F. Schreiner, CV Therapeutics, Palo Alto, CA). Control animals were injected with an equal volume of normal rabbit serum (Sigma, St. Louis,

MO). Rats were sacrificed at 2, 16, 24 and 48 hours post-injection (n=4 per time point). Kidneys were excised and glomeruli were isolated by graded sieving.

Total cellular RNA was purified from isolated glomeruli by the Chomczynski method (3). Two μg of glomerular RNA was reverse transcribed (RT) and 40 cycles of PCR amplification were performed in a DNA Thermal Cycler 480 (Perkin-Elmer, CT) using oligonucleotide primers specific for rat cytokines. PCR parameters were optimized for each cytokine to achieve maximum specificity. Amplified products were electrophoresed on 2% agarose (American Bioanalytical, MA) and stained with ethidium bromide. DNA band corresponding to the target cytokine was identified by its predicted size.

Electrophoresed products of the IL-4 and IL-10 RT-PCR reactions were transferred to Hybond-N+ nylon membranes (Amersham, IL) by capillary Southern blotting, covalently linked by UV-irradiation, and probed with chemiluminescent (Amersham, U.S.A.) rat IL-4 and rat IL-10 cDNA probes, respectively.

RESULTS

Figure 1 summarizes the time course of glomerular Th1 and Th2 lymphokine mRNA detected by RT-PCR during the first 48 hours of passive anti-GBM GN. IL-4 mRNA increases at 2 hours following induction of disease, peaks at 16 hours and declines rapidly thereafter. IL-10 mRNA follows a similar temporal pattern except that increased levels persist at 24 and 48 hours. IL-2 and IFNγ mRNA levels also increase very early in the course of GN but are relatively suppressed at 16 hours. This time point corresponds to the period during which IL-4 and IL-10 gene expression is maximal. Production of lymphokine mRNA in glomeruli of control rats injected with normal rabbit serum is minimal and does not vary over time (figure not shown). Southern blot analysis confirmed the

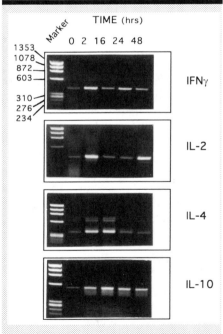

FIGURE 1: RT-PCR analysis of Th1 and Th2 lymphokine gene expression during the first 48 hours of GN.

identity of the IL-4 and IL-10 bands visualized by ethidium bromide staining (figure not shown).

Because IL-4 and IL-10 inhibit IL-1 and induce IL-1 receptor antagonist (IL-1RA) production by monocytes *in vitro* (4), we studied IL-1α and IL-1RA mRNA production during the first 48 hours of disease (figure not shown). The results demonstrate significant decline in IL-1α mRNA at the 16 and 24 hour time points after an initial increase at 2 hours. When compared to the time course of IL-4 mRNA (Figure 1), IL-1α mRNA is low during peak expression of IL-4 and increases again only after IL-4 mRNA level has declined. IL-1RA mRNA is also induced in the glomerulus 2 hours following injection of anti-GBM antibodies. IL-1RA mRNA level declines afterwards and is back to baseline by 48 hours. IL-1α and IL-1RA gene expression in glomeruli of control rats is minimal and remains constant over time (data not shown).

DISCUSSION AND CONCLUSION

In this report, we demonstrated for the first time that anti-inflammatory lymphokine, IL-4 and IL-10, mRNA is increased in glomeruli following induction of immune injury. We also provided evidence for reciprocal regulation of Th2 (IL-4 and IL-10) and Th1 (IFNγ and IL-2) lymphokines in antibody-induced GN. Moreover, gene expression of an inflammatory mediator, IL-1, was inversely related to that of IL-4. The data suggest that the role of T-lymphocytes in experimental GN is not limited to mediating tissue injury. Instead, we hypothesize that Th-lymphocyte subsets modulate glomerular inflammation by producing lymphokines with opposing actions. The net balance between pro-inflammatory (Th1) and anti-inflammatory (Th2) lymphokines could then determine the outcome of the inflammatory process.

REFERENCES

1. Powrie F, Coffman RL. Cytokine regulation of T cell function: Potential for therapeutic intervention. *Immunol Today* 1993; 14:270-4.
2. Main IW, Nikolic-Paterson DJ, Atkins RC. T cells and macrophages and their role in renal injury. *Seminars in Nephrology* 1992; 12:395-407.
3. Chomczynski P, Sacchi N. Single-step method of RNA isolation by acid guanidinium thiocyanate-phenol-chloroform extraction. *Anal Biochem* 1987; 162:156-9.
4. Wong HL, Costa GL, Lotze MT, Wahl SM. IL-4 differentially regulates monocyte IL-1 family gene expression and synthesis in vivo and in vitro. J Exp Med 1993; 177:775-81.

Advances in Prostaglandin, Thromboxane,
and Leukotriene Research, Vol. 23,
edited by B. Samuelsson et al.
Raven Press, Ltd., New York © 1995

Crosstalk in Signal Transduction via EP Receptors: Prostaglandin E$_1$ Inhibits Chemoattractant-induced Mitogen-activated Protein Kinase Activity in Human Neutrophils

Michael H. Pillinger, Mark R. Philips, Aleksander Feoktistov and
Gerald Weissmann

Department of Medicine, Division of Rheumatology
New York University Medical Center, New York, NY 10016

Whereas most prostaglandins have proinflammatory effects, several classes of prostaglandins have distinctly antiinflammatory effects. In particular, stable prostaglandins of the E series (PGEs) have been shown *in vivo* to suppress the development of adjuvant arthritis in rats (1), prevent the development of glomerulonephritis in NZB/NZW F$_1$ hybrid mice (2), and inhibit the reverse passive Arthus reaction in rats (3). These effects of PGEs may be due, at least in part, to the action of PGEs on neutrophils. Our laboratory has previously demonstrated that the PGE$_1$ analog misoprostol inhibits neutrophil superoxide anion generation in response to the chemoattractant formyl methionyl-leucyl-phenylalanine (FMLP) and enhances the inhibitory effect of non-steroidal antiinflammatory drugs on other neutrophil functions including degranulation, aggregation and global rises in cytosolic calcium (4). However, the intracellular mechanisms whereby PGEs exert their effects on neutrophils remain incompletely elucidated. We have demonstrated that PGEs stimulate increases in neutrophil intracellular cAMP levels, and that elevations in [cAMP]$_i$ inhibit neutrophil degranulation, suggesting that PGEs may act through their effect on cAMP (5). However, the mechanism by which cAMP exerts an almost global inhibitory effect on neutrophil function and release of inflammatory substances remains unexplained.

The mitogen-activated protein kinases (MAPKs) ERK1 and ERK2 mediate cellular responses to epidermal growth factor (EGF), nerve growth factor (NGF) and platelet-derived growth factor (PDGF) in cultured cells (FIG. 1). Autophosphorylation of a tyrosine-kinase receptor leads, through a series of steps, to the activation of the low molecular weight GTP-binding protein p21^{ras} via the promotion of GDP/GTP exchange. p21^{ras} in turn activates Raf-1 by interacting with its amino-terminal regulatory region, possibly in conjunction with an as-yet unidentified Raf-1-directed serine/threonine kinase (6,7). Raf-1 is itself a serine/threonine kinase which phosphorylates and activates MEK (Map or

Erk Kinase) (8-10). MEK, a dual specificity tyrosine/threonine kinase, phosphorylates and thereby activates MAPK (11,12).

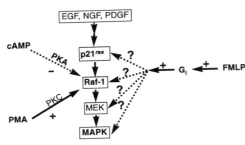

FIG. 1. The Raf-1, MAPK signaling cascade. Steps that are hypothetical or incompletely elucidated are indicated by dashed arrows and question marks. (See text for abbreviations.)

Activated MAPK translocates to the nucleus, where it acts directly to activate c-*jun* (13) and via p62^{TCF} to induce c-fos (14). Thus MAPK signaling probably plays a role in cell growth and division. However, neutrophils are terminally differentiated, post-mitotic cells with limited capacity for protein synthesis. They would therefore seem to be poor candidates in which to study the MAPK cascade. Nonetheless, human neutrophils contain MAPKs which respond to extracellular signals by undergoing phosphorylation and dephosphorylation (15). Several groups have recently demonstrated that, in cultured cells, EGF-induced MAPK activation may be inhibited by cAMP in a PKA-dependent manner (16,17). This observation has led us to hypothesize that, in neutrophils, the action of PGEs might be mediated by increments of [cAMP]$_i$ which would activate PKA and subsequently inhibit MAPK. We have studied both intact neutrophils and their granule-free cytoplasts, since these fragments permit analysis of neutrophil activation in the absence of nuclei, granules or intact microtubules (18,19).

METHODS

Human neutrophils were prepared according to the method of Boyum *et al.*. Blood from volunteer donors was collected into heparinized syringes and subjected to density centrifugation, dextran sedimentation and hypotonic lysis as previously described (20). This procedure yielded >98% neutrophils. Neutrophil superoxide anion (O$_2^-$)generation was assayed as previously described (21). Neutrophil carboxyl methyltransferase activity was assayed as previously described (22).

Neutrophil cytoplasts were prepared according to a modification of the method of Roos *et al.* (18). Briefly, neutrophils (0.5-4 x 10^8 cells) prepared as described above were pelleted (800 rpm x 10 min) and resuspended in 4 ml phosphate buffered saline (PBS) pH 7.4 containing 12.5% Ficoll 70 (Pharmacia) and 5 µg/ml cytochalasin B at 37°C and layered atop a discontinuous Ficoll gradient consisting of 16% and 25% Ficoll 70 layers, both in PBS pH 7.4 containing 5 µg/ml cytochalasin B and prewarmed to 37°C. Gradients were spun at 25,000 RPM in a Beckman SW27 centrifuge rotor for 30 min at 37°C. The cytoplasts were harvested from the 12.5%/16% interface, counted, washed twice and maintained until use in cell buffer containing 5 mM dextrose at 4°C.

Neutrophil MAPK activity was measured directly using an in-gel MAPK assay. Neutrophil cytoplasts (6.8x10^8/ml) in 45 µL cell buffer containing 5 mM dextrose were incubated in the absence or presence of FMLP or other agents for 1 to 20 min at 37°C. Reactions were stopped by the addition of 15 µL of 4X sample buffer. Alternatively, intact neutrophils were stimulated and prepared for analysis according to the method of

Torres *et al* (15). A portion of each sample (20 µl) was analyzed on 10% SDS-polyacry-lamide gel polymerized containing 0.25 mg/ml myelin basic protein (Sigma). After completion of electrophoresis, proteins in the gel were denatured and renatured according to a modification of the method of Kameshita and Fujisawa (23). Gels were subjected to a series of one hour baths consisting 50 mM tris pH 8.0, successively containing 20% isopropanol (2 baths), 0.035% ß-mercaptoethanol (ß-Me; 1 bath), and 0.035% ß-Me with 6 M guanidine (2 baths). Gels were then washed for 12-24 hr in a series of 5 baths containing 50 mM tris pH 8.0, 0.035% ß-Me, and 0.04% Tween-20, resulting in protein renaturation. To determine MAPK phosphorylation of the myelin basic protein intrinsic to the gel (i.e., in-gel MAPK activity), gels were incubated in phosphorylation buffer (20 mM Hepes, pH 7.4 containing 100 µM NaEGTA, 10 mM MgCl$_2$, 1 mM dithiothreitol, 250 µM ATP and 2.5 µCi/ml [^{32}P-γ]ATP) for 1 hr at 32°C. Reactions were stopped by transferring the gels into stop buffer containing 5% trichloroacetic acid and 1% sodium pyrophosphate. Gels were washed at least 5 times (30 min each) in stop buffer to remove unincorporated [^{32}P-γ]ATP. Gels were dried and myelin basic protein phosphorylation was visualized and quantitated by phosphorimaging (Molecular Dynamics, Sunnyvale, CA).

RESULTS

We first tested the effects of FMLP on neutrophil MAPK. Neutrophil cytoplasts were prepared as described, then stimulated with FMLP (100 nM) for 1 min prior to lysis with 4X sample buffer. We also tested the effects of 5 min stimulation with phorbol myristate acetate (PMA, 1µg/ml) on neutrophil MAPK activity. PMA, a potent activator of neutrophils that bypasses neutrophil G-protein linked seven-transmembrane-domain receptors by directly activating protein kinase C (PKC), has recently been shown to activate MAPK in cell culture through a PKC-dependent mechanism (24,25). Our data indicate that both FMLP and PMA activate MAPK in neutrophil cytoplasts (FIG.2).

Neutrophil responses to FMLP, including homotypic aggregation and superoxide anion generation, are generally rapid and transient. We therefore studied the kinetics of neutrophil MAPK activation from 1 to 20 min. Our data indicate that FMLP-induced MAPK activation peaks as early as 1 min after stimulation, with a rapid return to baseline (FIG. 3A). Thus the kinetics of the MAPK responses to FMLP (peak at 1 min) and PMA (persistent at 5 min) parallel those of other intracellular second messengers and neutrophil functions such as (O$_2^-$) generation (FIG.3B).

A

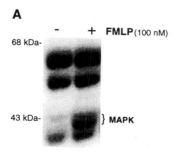

B

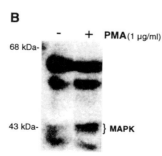

FIG. 2. Effects of **FMLP and PMA on MAPK.** Neutrophil cytoplasts, prepared as described, were incubated with or without FMLP for 1 min (panel A) or with or without PMA for 5 min (panel B). Reactions were stopped by the addition of sample buffer and analyzed for in-gel MAPK activity as described.

cAMP inhibits neutrophil responses including degranulation (5), chemotaxis (26), O_2^- generation (27), and bacterial killing (28). Prostaglandin E_1 inhibits neutrophil activation and elevates intracellular cAMP levels. In several cell lines, elevations of cAMP block MAPK activation in response to growth factors. We therefore tested the hypothesis

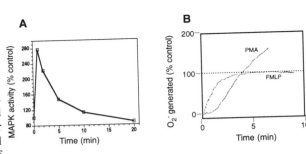

FIG. 3. Kinetics of MAPK activation by FMLP. A, Neutrophil cytoplasts, incubated in the presence of 100 nM FMLP for the times indicated, were lysed with sample buffer and analyzed for MAPK activity as described. B, Neutrophils were stimulated with 100 nM FMLP or 1μg/ml PMA and assayed for O_2^- generation as described.

that FMLP-induced MAPK activation in neutrophils would be inhibited by both PGE_1 and the cell-permeable cAMP analog dibutyryl cAMP (dbcAMP). Our data indicate that a 5 min preincubation with either dbcAMP or PGE_1 resulted in inhibition of both FMLP-induced neutrophil O_2^- generation (FIG. 4A) and FMLP-induced neutrophil MAPK activity (FIG. 4B).

N-acetyl-*S-all trans*-geranylgeranyl-L-cysteine (AGGC) is a potent and specific inhibitor of the prenylcysteine-directed carboxyl methylation of *ras*-related proteins. We have recently demonstrated that, in neutrophils, prenylcysteine-directed carboxyl methylation of *ras*-related proteins by a plasma membrane associated enzyme follows neutrophil activation, and that inhibition of *ras*-related protein carboxyl methylation markedly inhibits specific neutrophil functions such as superoxide anion generation and homotypic aggregation (22,29). The kinetics of FMLP-induced *ras*-related protein carboxyl methylation is identical to that of FMLP-induced MAPK activation (FIGS. 2A and 4C). Moreover, growth factors stimulate MAPK activation by a mechanism dependent on $p21^{ras}$ activation. We therefore tested the hypothesis that FMLP-induced neutrophil MAPK activation requires stimulated carboxyl methylation of $p21^{ras}$ and that inhibition of *ras*-protein carboxyl methylation would inhibit FMLP-induced MAPK activation. However, although preincubation with 20 μM AGGC markedly inhibited FMLP-induced O_2^- generation (FIG. 4A), it failed to inhibit FMLP-induced MAPK activation in intact neutrophils (Fig 4D).

DISCUSSION

Our data demonstrate that two agents that activate neutrophils via receptor-dependent and independent mechanisms also activate neutrophil MAPK. Neutrophil MAPK activation in response to both FMLP and PMA is rapid, but whereas the FMLP-induced response is transient, the PMA-induced response is more persistent. These observations are concordant with the physiologic effects of FMLP and PMA on neutrophils (e.g., kinetics of aggregation and O_2^- generation) and suggest that MAPK may indeed play a role in neutrophil activation. Whether other neutrophil agonists will be found to activate MAPK remains to be determined. It is possible that some, but not all neutrophil stimuli and some,

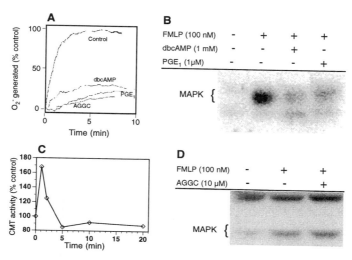

FIG. 4. dbcAMP and PGE₁ inhibit FMLP-induced MAPK. A, neutrophils were preincubated with or without dbcAMP (1mM), PGE₁ (1 µM) or AGGC (20µM) for 5 min prior to stimulation with 100 nM FMLP and measured for O₂⁻ as described. B, Neutrophil cytoplasts were preincubated with or without dbcAMP or PGE₁ for 5 min prior to 1 min stimulation with or without 100 nM FMLP and analyzed for in-gel MAPK activity. C, Neutrophils were stimulated with 100 nM FMLP and analyzed for carboxyl methyltransferase (CMT) activity as described. D, Neutrophils were preincubated with or without AGGC (20 µM) for 5 min prior to 1 min stimulation with 100 nM FMLP and analyzed for in-gel MAPK activity.

but not all neutrophil responses will be dependent on MAPK activation. In all other cell types studied to date MAPK activation acting over hours to days has been implicated in cell growth and division. The neutrophil response appears to be the first example of MAPK activation in excitable cells that become activated over seconds to minutes.

It has been recognized for many years that elevations of cytosolic cAMP inhibit neutrophil functions (5) and stimulate PKA activation in neutrophils (30). The observation that cAMP inhibits MAPK activation in cell cultures suggests a possible model for the effect of cAMP on neutrophils. cAMP-mediated inhibition of EGF-induced MAPK activation in cell culture appears to be PKA dependent: activation of PKA results in direct phosphorylation of Raf-1, apparently inhibiting its interaction with its upstream positive regulator, p21^{ras} (17). A similar mechanism may be involved in neutrophil MAPK inhibition. Indeed, our data suggests that neutrophil exposure to FMLP results in p21^{ras} and Raf-1 activation (manuscript in preparation). The failure of AGGC to block FMLP-induced MAPK activation is consistent with a model in which p21^{ras} activation, but not stimulated carboxyl methylation, is necessary for MAPK activation. Stimulated carboxyl methylation of *ras*-related proteins may be required for propagation of signals on pathways downstream of, or independent of, MAPK. Whether cAMP-induced inhibitory phosphorylation of Raf-1 will also block the ability of PMA to activate neutrophil MAPK through stimulatory PKC-dependent phosphorylation of Raf-1 remains to be determined.

Since multiple receptor classes for E prostaglandins have been defined (31), occupancy of various classes may explain the *in vivo* observation that PGEs have both inflammatory and anti-inflammatory effects (32,33). Nonetheless, both *in vivo* and *in vitro* the predominant effect of PGEs appears to be antiinflammatory. Engagement of the EP₂ receptor is associated with increases in intracellular cAMP (31). The human EP_2 receptor has recently been cloned, and its engagement in transfected cells increases $[cAMP]_i$ (34). Sequence analysis suggests a seven-transmembrane-domain receptor capable of interaction with a heterotrimeric G protein, presumably G_s. We have shown that PGE_1 is capable of inducing a greater than 300% increase in neutrophil intracellular cAMP within 2-5 min of exposure (5). We now demonstrate that PGE_1, most likely acting via EP_2 receptors and at concentrations as low as 1 µM, markedly inhibits neutrophil MAPK activity. It is probable that inhibition is due at least in part to the effect of PGE_1 on $[cAMP]_i$.

In summary, the kinetics of MAPK activation in neutrophils in response to FMLP and PMA are concordant with the kinetics of neutrophil activation, and both dbcAMP and PGE_1 inhibit both neutrophil and MAPK activation. We propose that the mechanism of PGE_1-induced global inhibition of neutrophil function may be via cAMP-induced, PKA-dependent inhibition of MAPK activation. The effect of PGE_1 on the FMLP response may thus represent a motif for crosstalk between seven-transmembrane-domain receptors linked to different classes of heterotrimeric G proteins (G_s and G_i, respectively). We are currently studying a variety of other eicosanoids to determine whether MAPK inhibition is a feature unique to the antiinflammatory prostaglandin classes.

REFERENCES

1. Zurier, RB. and Quagliata, F. (1971) *Nature* **234**, 304-306
2. Zurier, RB., Damjanov, I., Sayadoff, DM., and Rothfield, NF. (1977) *Arthritis Rheum.* **20**, 1449-1456
3. Kunkel, SL., Thrall, RS., Kunkel, RG., McCormick, JR., Ward, PA., and Zurier, RB. (1979) *J. Clin. Invest.* **64**, 1525-1527
4. Kitsis, E. A., Weissmann, G., and Abramson, S. B. (1991) *J. Rheum.* **18(10)**, 1461-1465
5. Zurier, R. B., Weissmann, G., Hoffstein, S., Kammerman, S., and Tai, H. H. (1974) *J. Clin. Invest.* **53**, 297-309
6. Warne, P. H., Viciana, P. R., and Downward, J. (1993) *Nature* **364**, 352-355
7. Zhang, X., *et al.* (1993) *Nature*   **364**, 308-313
8. Kyriakis, J. M., *et al.* (1992) *Nature* **358**, 417-421
9. Howe, L. R., Leevers, S. J., Gomez, N., Nakielny, S., Cohen, P., and Marshall, C. J. (1992) *Cell* **71**, 335-342
10. Dent, P., *et al.* (1992) *Science* **257**, 1404-1407
11. Ahn, N. G., *et al.* (1991) *J. Biol. Chem.* **266(7)**, 4220-4227
12. Gomez, N. and Cohen, P. (1991) *Nature* **353**, 170-173
13. Pulverer, B. J., Kyriakis, J. M., Avruch, J., Nikolakaki, E., and Woodgett, J. R. (1991) *Nature* **353**, 670-674
14. Gille, H., Sharrocks, A. D., and Shaw, P. E. (1992) *Nature* **358**, 414-417
15. Torres, M., Hall, F. L., and O'Neill, K. (1993) *J. Immunol.* **150**, 1563-1578
16. Cook, S. J. and McCormick, F. (1993) *Science* **262**, 1069-1072
17. Wu, J., Dent, P., Jelinek, T., Wolfman, A., Weber, M. J., and Sturgill, T. W. (1993) *Science* **262**, 1065-1068
18. Roos, D., Voetman, A. A., and Meerhof, C. J. (1983) *J. Cell Biol.* **97**, 368-377
19. Korchak, H. M., *et al.* (1983) *Proc. Natl. Acad. Sci. USA* **80**, 4968-4972
20. Boyum, A. (1968) *Scand. J. Clin. Lab. Invest.* **21 (Suppl 97)**, 77-78
21. Goldstein, I. M., Roos, D., Kaplan, H. B., and Weissmann, G. (1975) *J. Clin. Invest.* **56**, 1155-1163
22. Philips, M. R., *et al.* (1993) *Science* **259**, 977-980
23. Kameshita, I. and Fujisawa, H. (1989) *Anal. Biochem.* **183**, 139-143
24. Kolch, W., *et al.* (1993) *Nature* **364**, 249-252
25. Gause, K. C., *et al.* (1993) *J. Biol. Chem.* **268**, 16124-16129
26. Harvath, L., Robbins, J. D., Russell, A. A., and Seamon, K. B. (1991) *J. Immunol.* **146(1)**, 224-232
27. Ervens, J., Schultz, G., and Seifert, R. (1991) *Biochemical Society Transactions* **19**, 59-63
28. Bjornson, A. B., Knippenberg, R. W., and Bjornson, H. S. (1989) *J. Immunol.* **143(8)**, 2609-2616
29. Pillinger, M. H., *et al.* (1994) *J. Biol. Chem.* **269**, 1486-1492
30. Tsung, P-K., Sakamoto, T., and Weissmann, G. (1975) *Biochem. J.* **145**, 437-448
31. Davies, P. and MacIntyre, D. E. (1992) in *Inflammation: Basic Principles and Clinical Correlates* (Gallin, J. I., Goldstein, I. M., and Snyderman, R., eds) pp. 123-138, Raven Press, New York
32. Weissmann, G. (1993) in *Journal of Lipid Mediators* (Wolfe, L. S. and Ford-Hutchinson, A. W., eds) pp. 275-286, Elsevier Science Publishers
33. Reibman, J., Haines, K., and Weissmann, G. (1991) in *Mechanisms of Leukocyte Activation* (Grinstein, S. and Rotstein, O.D., eds) pp. 399-424, Academic Press
34. Bastien, L., *et al.* (1994) *J. Biol. Chem.* **269(16)**, 11873-11877

Advances in Prostaglandin, Thromboxane,
and Leukotriene Research, Vol. 23,
edited by B. Samuelsson et al.
Raven Press, Ltd., New York © 1995

INDUCIBLE PROSTAGLANDIN SYNTHASE
IN CELL INJURY

Nicolas G. Bazan, Victor L. Marcheselli, and Pranab K. Mukherjee

LSU Eye Center and Neuroscience Center
2020 Gravier Street, New Orleans, Louisiana, USA 70112

The activation of phospholipase A_2 and the resultant accumulation of free polyunsaturated fatty acids, notably arachidonic acid, is an early event in cell injury, cell activation, and in organ ischemia, such as cerebral ischemia.[1,2,3] Some of the accumulated second messengers may link ischemia-reperfusion injury with long-term cellular responses through the modulation of gene expression. One such second messenger is PAF (platelet-activating factor, 1-*O*-alkyl-2-acetyl-*sn*-glycero-3-phosphocholine), another phospholipase A_2 product (Fig. 1), that has been shown to induce the expression of the growth-related oncogenes c-*fos* and c-*jun* in SH SY5Y cells and in MOLT-4 T-lymphocytes.[4] Moreover, by inducing c-*fos* and c-*jun*, PAF leads to the expression of genes containing AP-1 responsive elements, and as a consequence, initiates gene cascades.[4,5] Since PAF antagonists inhibit brain gene expression in models of activity-dependent adaptive responses,[6,7] PAF-induced gene expression may be involved in plasticity responses and neuronal survival in stroke. During reperfusion after ischemia, there is a surge of oxygen as well as other effects not well understood that lead to enhanced lipid peroxidation. Mediators released from infiltrated polymorphonuclear leukocytes and microglia[7,8] may play a major role in limiting neuronal survival. Some of the free arachidonic acid released by phospholipase A_2 during brain ischemia is converted to prostaglandinsy and leukotrienes during the reperfusion phase. These second messengers elicit various actions at the microvasculature and on parenchymal neural cells. BN 52021, a PAF antagonist, elicits neuroprotection when administered to gerbils systemically after 10 min of ischemia produced by bilateral clamping of the carotid arteries.[9] These findings led to the search for the subcellular PAF binding site/s where the neuroprotective BN 52021 would compete for binding. It was found that, in cerebral cortex[10] and hippocampus (Marcheselli and Bazan, unpublished observations), there are PAF binding sites in microsomal and synaptic ending membranes. The site of PAF displacement by BN 52021 is on the presynaptic membranes.[5,10] Moreover, PAF enhances glutamate release when added to hippocampal neurons in culture and BN 52021 blocks this effect.[11] This suggests that excitatory amino acid neurotransmitter release and excitotoxic neuronal damage involve PAF as an agonist. The neuro-

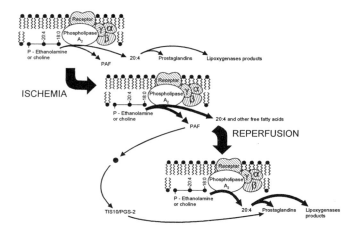

FIG. 1. Phospholipase A_2 and Arachidonic Acid Cascade
Activation mDuring Cerebral Ischemia and Subsequent Reperfusion

protective effect of BN 52021 in ischemia-reperfusion in gerbil brain[9] may be due partly to an inhibition of the PAF presynaptic binding site.[11,12]

The other PAF binding site is intracellular and was defined by a) using purified microsomal membranes and b) observing the displacement of [³H]PAF by different PAF antagonists.[10] This microsomal binding site displays the highest affinity for PAF thus far reported[5,10] and appear to mediate PAF's transcriptional activating properties.[4,5,13-16] The cell surface PAF receptor has been cloned[4,13-18]; however, the identity of the intracellular PAF receptor, as well as its possible relationships with the cell surface receptor, has not been defined. Here we summarize current studies on the role of a membrane lipid-derived second messenger, PAF, in cell injury and its activating effect on the inducible prostaglandin synthase gene. This gene seems to be regulated by activity-dependent plasticity and, by being turned on by PAF, leads to the synthesis of prostaglandins.

PAF and Transcriptional Activation

In the study of cell signaling, the identification of second messengers and intracellular sites that couple stimulation with gene transcription is a central issue. Many signals trigger the rapid and transient expression of immediate-early genes (primary genomic response genes, early response genes). In the nervous system, physiological and pathological events (such as long-term potentiation, ischemia, seizures, and NMDA receptor activation) initiate transcription of these genes. After the transcription takes place, and their mRNA is translated, in many instances other genes are activated, initiating gene cascades. Many of the immediate-early genes encode transcription factors. As a result of turning some of these genes on, long-term cellular responses such as neuronal plasticity occurs.

1-O-alkyl-2-acyl-sn-glycero-3-phosphocholine is the membrane lipid that gives rise to lyso-PAF and forms PAF in a subsequent step when catalyzed by an acetyl transferase (Fig. 1). Relatively little is known about the phospholipase(s) A$_2$ and other enzyme(s) or their trigger(s) involved in ischemia-reperfusion. However, PAF is accumulated in ischemia and during convulsions. It is also interesting to note that the phospholipid precursor of PAF is enriched in arachidonate and docosahexaenoate.[19] These polyunsaturated fatty acids are actively accumulated as free fatty acids during ischemia and convulsions.[1] PAF is a potential mediator of signal transcription coupling since a) it is undetectable in unstimulated neural tissue or in resting cells; b) seizures or ischemia trigger its production[20]; c) once generated it is often retained in cells[21] and neural cells,[22] and has been suggested to play a role as an intracellular messenger in several cells such as leukocytes and endothelial cells[23]; d) there are intracellular PAF binding sites in rat cerebral cortex[10] and hippocampus (Marcheselli and Bazan, unpublished observations); e) in transformed neural cells[4,5,13] as well as in other cells in culture[4,16] PAF rapidly and transiently augments c-*fos* and c-*jun* mRNA abundance; f) PAF's effect is at the transcriptional level[4]; g) phorbol esters and PAF synergistically stimulate c-*fos* expression indicating that the transcriptional effects of PAF are not mediated by protein kinase C[4]; h) 5′ deletion mutagenesis studies of the c-*fos* promoter indicate that the calcium-response element is necessary for the PAF-induced response[4]; i) in corneal organ culture, PAF activates the expression of c-*fos* and c-*jun*[24]; j) the hetrazepine BN 50730, a selective antagonist for the intracellular PAF binding site, inhibits c-*fos*, c-*jun* and *zif*-268 expression in several transformed[4,5,13-16] and primary cells[24] in culture; and k) c-*fos* and *zif*-268 expression triggered by electroconvulsive shock in hippocampus is inhibited by intraperitoneal or intracerebroventricular injection of the hetrazepine BN 50730,[25] the intracellular PAF antagonist.

PAF Enhances Expression of Inducible Prostaglandin Synthase

PAF stimulates transcription of the gene that encodes the inducible prostaglandin synthase.[26] The effect of PAF was studied using constructs of the promoter of the inducible prostaglandin synthase gene transfected to neural and non-neural cells.[26]

PAF's novel effect indicates that this mediator of cell injury and inflammation enhances gene expression and leads to the synthesis of other mediators of cell injury and inflammation. It is not yet known if this effect is part of the injury/inflammatory response, part of a pathway leading to cell death, or leads to repair.

Retinoic acid modulates gene expression through nuclear receptors that are members of a superfamily of ligand-dependent transcription factors. Since PAF may also affect gene expression through an intracellular site,[4,5] the effect of retinoic acid was studied. Retinoic acid induces the expression of constructs of the TIS10/PGS-2 promoter with a luciferase reporter transfected into neuroblastoma cells. Using the calcium phosphate co-precipitation transfection procedure in the presence of retinoic acid, there is a PAF-dependent (from 1 to 50 nM) activation of luciferase reporter constructs driven by regulatory regions of the TIS10/PGS-2 gene. BN 50730 inhibited this effect. The effect of PAF in the presence of retinoic acid is rapid, under the conditions of these experiments, indicating that a preexisting latent transcription factor(s) is engaged in the effect. Deletion studies of the TIS10/PGS-2 promoter/luciferase reporter constructs showed that deletion of sequences between -371 and -300 reduced the PAF inductive effect from 31-fold to 4.1-fold. BN 50730 inhibited the PAF inductive effect when incubated for 1 h with cultured cells before transfection. This indicates that a PAF receptor is involved in the expression of the inducible prostaglandin synthase and that a major PAF response site lies in this region. Further deletions showed no response to added PAF.

Membrane-Derived Lipid Second Messengers and Cell Injury

The membrane-derived second messengers accumulated during cell injury in brain or retina represents an overactivation of processes that regulate synaptic function.[27] Some of the membrane-derived lipid second messengers generated by injury may participate in the coupling of injury either with plasticity responses and repair/regenerative responses, or with cell death. PAF links injury response with transcriptional activation of immediate-early genes.[25,28] Several key mediators of nervous system function may also play roles in pathological conditions, depending upon the degree of impairment of neuronal activity. This duality is a feature of glutamate, an excitatory amino acid, that, by far, is the most abundant neurotransmitter of the mammalian brain. Glutamate plays a critical role in developmental plasticity, memory formation, etc. However, in stroke, seizures, neurotrauma and some neurodegenerative diseases, there is an abnormally high synaptic accumulation of glutamate, making it a critical effector of excitotoxic damage. Also, other mediators, such as interleukin-1 and, perhaps, amyloid peptide, coexist with neural cells under physiological conditions but may, when overproduced, be engaged in abnormal actions in diseases.

PAF also plays physiological roles and, when overproduced, may become an endogenous neurotoxin. Although PAF is most often referred to as a mediator of the inflammatory and immune responses as well as of cell injury, low PAF concentrations elicits sprouting in PC12 cells, whereas neuropathological changes occur when these cells are exposed to high PAF concentrations.[7,29] The presynaptic PAF binding site[29] linked to glutamate release[11] is a target through which PAF participates in excitotoxicity. However, the same presynaptic site involves PAF as a potential retrograde messenger in long-term potentiation.[29] The very high affinity binding site, localized intracellularly[10] and linked to immediate-early gene expression, may be a bridge between the initial response to ischemia and gene expression.[5] It is not yet known if two or more of these actions are interlinked or if there are different effects among the diverse cellular responses stimulated by PAF. The significance of the effect of PAF on gene expression may be related either to long-term adaptive responses or to nuclear events of apoptosis. PAF plays a role in ischemia-reperfusion damage in brain though several actions: its ability to increase intracellular Ca^{2+} [18,28] likely by activating a Ca^{2+} channel and by activating phospholipase C with resultant intracellular Ca^{2+} mobilization by inositol trisphosphate.

PAF stimulation of the inducible prostaglandin synthase gene[26] establishes a link between cell injury-generated PAF and the gene encoding the enzyme that catalyzes the cyclooxygenation of arachidonic acid. Arachidonic acid is readily available since cell injury such as cerebral ischemia promotes its accumulation.[1] The inducible prostaglandin synthase utilizes only a small proportion of the free arachidonic acid available under these conditions. PGE_2 synthesis under conditions of overstimulation (e.g., seizure) or ischemia-reperfusion, may require enhanced expression of inducible prostaglandin synthase. PGE_2 may comprise a feedback loop of the inflammatory response.

Knowledge about the prostaglandin synthase isoenzymes in the response of cells to stimulation and injury, as well as its physiological significance and pathological role, is just emerging. The inducible isoenzyme in brain has been reported to be predominantly expressed in neurons, mainly cortical and limbic.[30] No expression was detected in glia or vascular endothelium. The neuronal inducible prostaglandin synthase has been shown to be regulated by NMDA-dependent synaptic activity, implying a role of prostaglandins in activity-dependent neuronal plasticity.[30] Therefore, PAF, by turning on the inducible prostaglandin synthase in brain, may open up a pathway that may be involved in synaptic function. Prostaglandins are known to be cytoprotective against various forms of injury in the stomach,[31] and from ischemic injury in the kidney.[32] Moreover, prostaglandins are cytoprotective in embryonic retinal cells[33] as well as against glutamate-induced injury to cortical neurons in primary cultures.[34] Therefore prostaglandins being generated in the PAF-induced gene expression may limit damage to neurons and play a role in neuroprotection.

Acknowledgement: Supported by the National Institutes of Health, NINDS, NS 23002.

REFERENCES

1. Bazan NG. Effects of ischemia and electroconvulsive shock on free fatty acid pool in the brain. Biochim Biophys Acta. 1970;218:1-10.
2. Bazan NG. Arachidonic acid (AA) in the modulation of excitable membrane function and at the onset of brain damage. Ann N Y Acad Sci. 1989;559:1-16.
3. Bazan NG, Allan G, Rodriguez de Turco EB. Role of phospholipase A_2 and membrane-derived lipid second messengers in excitable membrane function and transcriptional activation of genes: Implications in cerebral ischemia and neuronal excitability. Progress in Brain Research. 1993;96:247-57.
4. Squinto SP, Block AL, Braquet P, Bazan NG. Platelet-activating factor stimulates a Fos/Jun/AP-1 transcriptional signaling system in human neuroblastoma cells. J Neurosci Res. 1981;24:558-66.
5. Bazan NG, Squinto SP, Braquet P, Panetta T, Marcheselli VL. Platelet-activation factor and polyunsaturated fatty acids in cerebral ischemia or convulsions: Intracellular PAF-binding sites and activation of a Fos/Jun/Ap-1 transcriptional signaling system. Lipids. 1991;26:1236-42.
6. Moises J, Allan G, Marcheselli VL, Mandahare V, Bazan NG. A PAF antagonist inhibits the expression of hippocampal immediate-early genes in a kindling model of epilepsy. Epilepsia. 1994;in press

7.　Siren A-L, McCarron RM, Liu Y, et al. Perivascular macrophage signaling of endothelium via cytokines: Mechanism by which stroke risk factors operate to increase stroke likelihood. In: Krieglstein J, Oberpichler-Schwenk H. eds. Pharmacology of Cerebral Ischemia. Stuttgart: Wissenschaftliche Verlagsgesellschaft, 1992:435-47.

8.　Giulian D, Vaca K. Inflammatory glia mediate delayed neuronal damage after ischemia in the central nervous system. Stroke. 1993;24 (Suppl):184-90.

9.　Panetta T, Marcheselli VL, Braquet P, Spinnewyn B, Bazan NG. Effects of a platelet-activating factor antagonist (BN 52021) on free fatty acids, diacylglycerols, polyphosphoinositides and blood flow in the gerbil brain: Inhibition of ischemia-reperfusion induced cerebral injury. Biochem Biophys Res Comm. 1987;149:580-7.

10.　Marcheselli VL, Rossowska M, Domingo MT, Braquet P, Bazan NG. Distinct platelet-activating factor binding sites in synaptic endings and in intracellular membranes of rat cerebral cortex. J Biol Chem. 1990;265:9140-5.

11.　Clark GD, Happel LT, Zorumski CF, Bazan NG. Enhancement of hippocampal excitatory synaptic transmission by platelet-activation factor. Neuron. 1992;9:1211-6.

12.　Bazan NG, Cluzel JM. Membrane-derived lipid second messengers as targets for neuroprotection: Platelet-activating factor. In: Marangos PJ, Lal H, eds.Emerging Strategies in Neuroprotection, Advances in Neuroprotection. Boston: Birkhauser, 1992:238-51.

13.　Squinto SP, Braquet P, Block AL, Bazan NG. Platelet-activation factor activates HIV promoter in transfected SH-SY5Y neuroblastoma cells and MOLT-4 T lymphocytes. J Mol Neurosci. 1990;2:79-84.

14.　Schulman PG, Kuruvilla A, Putcha G, Mangus L, F-Jonson J, Shearer WT. Platelet-activating factor induces phospholipid turnover calcium flux, and arachidonic acid liberation, eicosanoid generation, and oncogene expression in a human B cell line. J Immunol. 1991;146:1642

15.　Tripathy Y, Kandala J, Guntaka R, Lim R, Shukla S. Platelet-activating factor induces expression of early response genes c-*fos* and Tis-1 in human epidermoid carcinoma A-431 cells. Life Sci. 1991;49:1761-7.

16.　Mazer B, Domenico J, Sawami H, Gelfand EW. Platelet-activating factor induces an increase in intracellular calcium and expression of regularity genes in human B lymphoblastoma cells. J Immunol. 1991;146:1914-20.

17.　Nakamura M, Honda Z, Izumi T, et al. Molecular cloning and expression of platelet-activating factor receptor from human leukocytes. J Biol Chem. 1991;266:20400-5.

18.　Bito H, Nakamura M, Honda A, et al. Platelet-activating factor (PAF) receptor in rat brain: PAF mobilizes intracellular Ca^{2+} in hippocampal neurons. Neuron. 1992;9:1-10.

19.　Prescott SM, Zimmerman GA, McIntyre TM. Platelet-activating factor. J Biol Chem. 1990;265:17381-4.

20.　Kumar R, Harvey S, Kester N, Hanahan D, Olson M. Production and effects of platelet-activating factor in the rat brain. Biochim Biophys Acta. 1988;963:375-83.

21.　Yue TL, Lysko PG, Feuerstein G. Production of platelet-activating factor from rat cerebellar granule cells in culture. J Neurochem. 1990;54:1809-11.

22.　Bussolino F, Gremo F, Tetta C, Pescarmona G, Camussi G. Production of platelet-activating factor by chick retina. J Biol Chem. 1986;261:16502-8.

23. Henson P. Extracellular and intracellular activities of PAF. In: Snyder F, ed.Platelet-Activating Factor and Related Lipid Mediators. New York: Plenum Press, 1987:255-71.

24. Bazan HEP, Tao Y, Bazan NG. PAF induces collagenase expression in corneal epithelial cells, possibly through c-fos and c-jun activation. Proc Natl Acad Sci. 1993;90:8678-82.

25. Marcheselli VL, Bazan NG. Platelet-activating factor is a messenger in the electroconvulsive shock-induced transcriptional activation of c-fos and zif-268 in hippocampus. J Neurosci Res. 1994;37:54-61.

26. Bazan NG, Fletcher BS, Herschman HR, Mukherjee PK. Platelet-activating factor and retinoic acid synergistically activate the inducible prostaglandin synthase gene. Proc Natl Acad Sci. 1993;91:5252-6.

27. Bazan NG, Zorumski CF, Clark GD. The activation of phospholipase A_2 and release of arachidonic acid and other lipid mediators at the synapse: The role of platelet-activation factor. J Lipid Med. 1993;6:421-7.

28. Kornecki E, Ehrlich YH. Neuroregulatory and neuropathological actions of the ether phospholipid platelet-activating factor. Science. 1988;240:1792-4.

29. Kato K, Clark GD, Bazan NG, Zorumski CF. Platelet-activating factor as a potential retrograde messenger in CA1 hippocampal long-term potentiation. Nature. 1994;367:175-9.

30. Yamagata K, Andreasson KI, Kaufmann WE, Barnes CA, Worley PF. Expression of a mitogen-inducible cyclooxygenase in brain neurons: Regulation by synapic activity and glucocorticoids. Neuron. 1993;11:371-86.

31. Robert A, Nezamis JE, Lancaster C, Hanchar AJ. Cytoprotection by prostaglandins in rats. Prevention of gastric necrosis produced by alcohol, HCl, NaOH, hypertonic NaCl, and thermal injury. Gastroenterology. 1979;77:433-43.

32. Paller MS, Manivel JC. Prostaglandins protect kidneys against ischemic and toxic injury by a cellular effect. Kindey Int. 1992;42:1345-54.

33. Dymond JB, Kalmus GW. The cytoprotective properties of prostaglandin E_2 against the toxic effects of actinomycin C on embryonic neural retinal cells. Prostaglandins. 1992;44:129-34.

34. Cazevielle C, Muller A, Meynier G, Dutrait N, Bonne C. Protection by prostaglandins from glutamate toxicity in cortical neurons. Neurochem Int. 1994;24:395-8.

Advances in Prostaglandin, Thromboxane,
and Leukotriene Research, Vol. 23,
edited by B. Samuelsson et al.
Raven Press, Ltd., New York © 1995

Novel Mode of Monocyte 5-Lipoxygenase Stimulation

Ingo Weide and Thomas Simmet

Department of Pharmacology and Toxicology, Ruhr University,
D-44780 Bochum, Germany

Local contact activation is an important component of inflammatory reactions (1). In previous studies we have demonstrated that contact activation of human whole blood in vitro triggers not only generation of large amounts of platelet-derived TXB_2 but also induces release of both LTB_4 as well as cysteinyl-LT into the serum samples. In contrast to the TXB_2 formation, stimulation of LT biosynthesis in contact-activated blood was independent from endogenously generated thrombin (2).

Supplementation of human whole blood with either purified autologous mononuclear cells or monocytes but not with polymorphonuclear leukocytes led to an enhanced generation of LT upon contact activation. Since the polymorphonuclear leukocytes were shown to possess a functionally active 5-lipoxygenase pathway, these results indicated that the phenomenon of contact activation might selectively stimulate the 5-lipoxygenase pathway in peripheral monocytes (3).

By various pharmacological approaches we gained evidence that plasmin, presumably generated via the so-called contact-activated intrinsic fibrinolytic pathway, was responsible for the 5-lipoxygenase stimulation during contact activation. Thus, plasminogen activators, known as fibrinolytics, concentration-dependently stimulated the contact-mediated 5-lipoxygenase activation in monocytes. By contrast, various lysine analogues, known to inhibit binding of plasmin to plasmin binding sites, concentration-dependently inhibited the contact-mediated stimulation of the monocyte 5-lipoxygenase pathway. Moreover, plasmin inhibitors and a monoclonal antibody able to block plasminogen activation were potent inhibitors of the contact-mediated stimulation of the monocyte 5-lipoxygenase pathway (4).

In a more detailed study, we have now investigated the effect of purified plasmin on eicosanoid biosynthesis in human peripheral monocytes isolated on Percoll gradients.

METHODS

Blood collected from medication-free, apparently healthy, male volunteers was used for the isolation of peripheral monocytes by Percoll gradient centrifugation (4). The monocytes were finally resuspended in Hank's balanced salt solution (HBSS) containing essentially fatty acid-free bovine serum albumin 0.4% and were incubated at 37°C. LTB_4 was analysed radioimmunologically using the commercial radioimmunoassay from Amersham, UK. The determinations of prostanoids and reverse phase HPLC of LTB_4 were performed as described elsewhere (4). Plasmin, as well as plasminogen, after activation with streptokinase, were quantitated using the chromogenic substrate S-2251.

RESULTS

Incubation of human peripheral monocytes in HBSS did not induce any detectable release of LTB_4. However, when monocytes ($15x10^5$/ml) were incubated in the presence of low concentrations of human plasmin for 60 min, a concentration-dependent release of LTB_4 into the buffer samples could be detected (Fig. 1).

By contrast, plasmin in the concentrations used, did not significantly affect the release of the two major prostanoids formed by monocytes, namely TXB_2 and PGE_2 (data not shown).

Upon reverse phase HPLC profiling, immunoreactive LTB_4 was found to coelute in a single peak with the retention time of synthetic LTB_4 (data not shown).

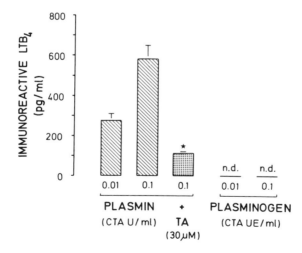

FIG. 1. Effects of human plasmin or plasminogen on the release of immunoreactive LTB_4 from human monocytes ($15x10^5$/ml) incubated in Hank's balanced salt solution for 60 min. Data represent means ± SEM of 4 experiments each. TA - tranexamic acid. n.d. - not detectable. * P<0.001 as compared to plasmin 0.1 CTA U/ml alone.

The stimulatory effect of plasmin (0.1 CTA U/ml) on the monocyte 5-lipoxygenase pathway was profoundly reduced by the lysine analogue tranexamic acid (30 μM)(Fig.1). Tranexamic acid (30 μM) did not reduce, however, the LTB_4 formation by monocytes stimulated with 1 μM ionophore A 23187 (data not shown).

In contrast to plasmin, plasminogen, in concentrations equivalent to those of plasmin, did not stimulate monocyte LTB_4 formation (Fig. 1).

DISCUSSION

Our results show that under the conditions used, human plasmin can stimulate the 5-lipoxygenase pathway in Percoll-isolated human monocytes leading to LTB_4 generation. The reason for the selective stimulation of the 5-lipoxygenase pathway as compared to the cyclooxygenase pathway remains unclear at present. However, it has previously been suggested that different sources of arachidonic acid might be liable for such an effect (5).

Tranexamic acid, as a lysine analogue, prevents binding of plasmin(ogen) to the appropriate binding sites on the monocyte membrane by interfering with the lysine binding sites located in kringle structure 1 to 4 of plasmin(ogen) molecules (6). The compound did not directly affect the 5-lipoxygenase pathway as shown by ionophore A 23187 stimulation, but inhibited only the plasmin-mediated stimulation. This indicates that association of plasmin via its lysine binding sites to the monocyte membrane might be required for the stimulatory activity (6). However, for transduction of the stimulatory effect, such association with the monocyte plasmin(ogen) binding sites alone is apparently not sufficient, since the zymogen plasminogen which carries the very same lysine binding sites as plasmin, but the catalytic center in a cryptic form only, was unable to stimulate the monocyte 5-lipoxygenase pathway. It appears, therefore, that similar to thrombin (7), the active catalytic center of plasmin might be essential for the stimulatory activity of the protease plasmin.

ACKNOWLEDGEMENTS

This work was supported by the Deutsche Forschungsgemeinschaft. The authors thank Mrs Bettina Tippler for expert technical assistance.

REFERENCES

1. Kozin F, Cochrane CG. In: Gallin JI, Goldstein IM, Snyderman R. *Inflammation.* New York: Raven Press; 1992:103-121.
2. Simmet Th, Weide I. *Thromb Res* 1991;62:249-261.
3. Weide I, Simmet Th. *Thromb Res* 1993;71:185-192.
4. Weide I, Römisch J, Simmet Th. *Blood* 1994;83:1941-1951.
5. Humes HL, Sadowski S, Galavage M et al. *J Biol Chem* 1982;257:1591-1594.
6. Miles LA, Dahlberg CM, Plescia J et al. *Biochemistry* 1991;30:1682-1691.
7. Vu TKH, Hung DT, Wheaton VI, Coughlin SR. *Cell* 1991;64:1057-1068.

Advances in Prostaglandin, Thromboxane,
and Leukotriene Research, Vol. 23,
edited by B. Samuelsson et al.
Raven Press, Ltd., New York © 1995

5-LIPOXYGENASE EXPRESSION IN CULTURED HUMAN KERATINOCYTES

Uwe Janßen-Timmen*, Philip Vickers†, Ulrike Beilecke*, Wolf Dieter Lehmann‡, Hans-Jürgen Stark¶, Norbert E. Fusenig¶, Thomas Rosenbach&, Matthias Goerig**, Olof Rådmark††, Bengt Samuelsson††, and Andreas J.R. Habenicht*

*University of Heidelberg, Medical School, Department of Internal Medicine, Division of Endocrinology, Bergheimerstr. 58, 69115-Heidelberg, F.R.G.; †Merck Frosst Center for Therapeutic Research, Quebec Canada; ‡Division of Spectroscopy, ¶Division of Differentiation and Carcinogenesis, German Cancer Center, Im Neuenheimer Feld 280, 69120-Heidelberg, F.R.G; & University of Berlin, Department of Dermatology, Augustenburger Str.1; **University of Erlangen-Nürnberg, Medical School, Department of Medicine, Division of Nephrology, Kontumazgarten 14-18, 90429-Nürnberg, F.R.G.; ††Karolinska Institutet, Department of Physiological Chemistry, Box 60400, S-10401 Stockholm, Sweden.

Until recently it was thought that expression of the gene encoding 5-lipoxygenase (arachidonate:oxygen 5-oxidoreductase, E.C. 1.13.11.12; 5-LO) is restricted to the hematopoietic system (4,12,13). However, attempts to identify the enzyme in other tissues yielded results that support the notion that it might be expressed in distinctive extrahematopoietic epithelia. Thus, Natsui et al. provided evidence that the 5-LO protein is present in the nuclear envelope of porcine pancreatic acinar cells (11) and the studies of Sjölander et al. and Dias et al. indicated the formation of 5-hydro(pero)xyeicosatetraenoic acid (5-H(P)ETE) and leukotriene (LT) B4 in human Henle intestine 407 cells and human colon CaCo-2 cells, respectively (3,14). The expression of the 5-LO pathway in the epithelium of the skin likewise remains a debatable issue (5,8,9,16). Several authors using primary and cultured skin keratinocytes reported the production of 5-HETE and LTB4 (8) but subsequent work challenged some of the earlier interpretations (reviewed in 6).

We have used a human keratinocyte cell line, HaCaT, and primary normal human foreskin and adult trunk skin keratinocytes as models to study the expression of the 5-LO pathway in extrahematopoietic epithelia. Since HaCaT keratinocytes maintain a high differentiation potential in vitro and in vivo (1), most experiments were performed with these cells. In the report detailed below and in unpublished studies we show that the 5-LO gene is expressed in HaCaT keratinocytes and in normal skin keratinocytes under culture conditions that favour their differentiation.

HaCaT keratinocytes were maintained in Dulbecco´s minimal essential medium supplemented with 10% fetal calf serum (1,7,15) under nondifferentiating conditions at low cell density or under differentiation conditions as confluent monolayers. Under nondifferentiation conditions the expression of the late keratinocyte differentiation marker, involucrin, is low. However, after the cells had been maintained as confluent monolayers for prolonged periods of time in medium supplemented with fetal calf serum and > 1 mM Ca++, involucrin levels increased by a factor of approximately 10. This keratinocyte differentiation system was used to study the expression of the 5-LO gene during prokeratinocyte-keratinocyte transformation. When 5-LO enzyme activity was assayed in homogenates prepared from both types of cells, we found a major upregulation of 5-HETE- and LTB4-producing activities in the differentiating cells (Table 1). 5-LO enzyme induction was most pronounced between days 4 and 13 corresponding to the time period when the cells approached confluency and showed increased involucrin formation.

Table 1. 5-H(P)ETE and LTB4 formation in HaCaT keratinocytes. Fresh HaCaT homogenates were incubated with 40 μM AA for 30 minutes as described by Denis et al. (2). After addition of 18-O-labeled internal standards, extraction, and derivatization, 5-HETE and LTB4 were quantitated by gas chromatography negative ion chemical ionization mass spectrometry as described by Lehmann et al. (10).

Days After Seeding	5-HETE	LTB4
	(nmoles/mg protein)	
4d sample 1	0.084	0.008
4d sample 2	0.061	0.017
4d boiled	0.035	0.001
50d sample 1	15.388	0.709
50d sample 2	13.631	0.688
50d boiled	0.035	0.001

We next studied the possibility that the increase in apparent 5-LO enzyme activity levels in differentiating HaCaT keratinocytes is associated with increased levels of 5-LO mRNA, 5-LO protein, and with the ability of intact keratinocytes to produce LTs. Northern blots, quantitative reverse transcription-polymerase chain reaction analyses of 5-LO mRNA, Western blots, and determination of the stereochemistry of 5-HETE as the S enantiomer established that functional 5-LO is present in differentiating HaCaT keratinocytes whereas it is low in their undifferentiated counterparts. Moreover, experiments performed in intact monolayer cultures of differentiated HaCaT keratinocytes revealed the formation of both LTB4 and LTC4 in response to Ca++ ionophore A23187. Although significantly lower expression levels of 5-LO mRNA, 5-LO protein, and cell-free 5-LO enzyme activity were found in primary human skin keratinocytes when compared to HaCaT keratinocytes, these results indicate that skin keratinocytes possess an inherent capability to express the 5-LO gene. Thus, it will be a challenge for future studies to identify the 5-LO gene-inducing factor(s) present in the differentiation medium (17). When taken together our results demonstrate that cultured HaCaT keratinocytes and primary keratinocytes express the bona fide 5-LO gene (12) if the prokeratinocytes are maintained under differentiation conditions for prolonged time periods.

Several inflammatory skin diseases are characterized by epidermal infiltration by leukocytes of various lineages some of which are producers of LTs (5). The majority of investigators have therefore assumed that epidermal LTs are derived from leukocytes that have been recruited into the skin, or that have been produced following export of leukocyte-derived LTA4 and subsequent metabolism by keratinocytes (6, 9, 16). While these assumptions remain viable, the ability of cultured keratinocytes to express the 5-LO gene raises the possibility that the 5-LO pathway plays a primary role in skin biology.

ACKNOWLEDGEMENTS

This work was supported by grants of the DFG Bonn, the European Community (Biomed 1 program) Brussels, the Stiftung Verum für Verhalten und Umwelt Munich, and the Swedish Medical Research Council (03X-217 and 03X-7464)

REFERENCES

1. Boukamp, P., Chen, J., Gonzales, F., Jones, P.A., and Fusenig, N.E. J. Cell Biol. 1992;116:1257-71.
2. Denis, D., Falgueyret, J.-P., Riendeau, D., and Abramovitz, M. J. Biol. Chem. 1991;266:5072-9.
3. Dias, V.C., Wallace, J.L., and Parsons, H.G. Gut 1992;33:622-7.
4. Dixon, R.A.F., Diehl, R.E., Opas, E. et al. Nature 1990;343:282-4.
5. Fauler, J., Neumann, C., Tsikas, D., and Frölich, J. J. Invest. Dermatol. 1992;99:8-11.
6. Ford-Hutchinson, A.W. Skin Pharmacol 1993;6:292-7.
7. Fusenig, N.E. In Keratinocyte Handbook (Leigh, I., Watt, F., Lane, B. eds.) Cambridge University Press 1994; in press.
8. Grabbe, J., Rosenbach, T., Czarnetzki, B.M. J. Invest. Dermatol 1985;85:527-30.
9. Iversen, L., Fogh, K., Ziboh, V.A., Kristensen, P., Schmedes, A., and Kragballe, K. J. Invest. Dermatol 1993;100:293-8.
10. Lehmann, W.D., Metzger, K., Stephan, M., Beilecke, U., Zalán, I., Habenicht, A.J.R., and Fürstenberger, G. Anal. Biochem 1994, submitted.
11. Natsui, K., Ueda, N., Yamamoto, S., Komatsu, N., and Watanabe, K. Biochim. Biophys. Acta 1991;1085:241-7.
12. Samuelsson, B., and Funk, C.D. J. Biol. Chem 1989;264:19469-72.
13. Samuelsson, B., Dahlén, S.-E., Lindgren, J.A., Rouzer, C.A., and Serhan, C.N. Science 1987;237:1171-6.
14. Sjölander, A., Schippert, A., and Hammarström, S. Prostaglandins 1993;45:85-96.
15. Smola, H., Thiekötter, G., and Fusenig, N.E. J. Cell Biol. 1993;122:417-29.
16. Solá, J., Godessart, N., Vila, L., Puig, L., and de Moragas, J.M.J. Invest. Dermatol. 1992;98:333-9.
17. Steinhilber, D., Rådmark, O., and Samuelsson, B. Proc. Natl. Acad. Sci. USA 1993;90:5984-8.

Advances in Prostaglandin, Thromboxane,
and Leukotriene Research, Vol. 23,
edited by B. Samuelsson et al.
Raven Press, Ltd., New York © 1995

Regulation of leukotriene C_4 synthase in human platelets via receptor-mediated mechanisms

Charlotte Edenius, Susanne Tornhamre, Barbro Näsman-Glaser,
Inger Eriksson, Susanne Björkholm and Jan Åke Lindgren.

Department of Medical Biochemistry and Biophysics, Division of Physiological Chemistry,
Karolinska Institutet, S-171 77 Stockholm, SWEDEN

Arachidonic acid is transformed by the 5-lipoxygenase to leukotriene (LT) A_4. This unstable epoxide is a key intermediate in the biosynthesis of leukotrienes and lipoxins (1). Platelets are devoid of 5-lipoxygenase activity, but convert LTA_4 to LTC_4 and may therefore participate in the production of this compound via transcellular mechanisms (1,2). This may be of importance under inflammatory conditions, such as asthma, since activation and accumulation of platelets in the lung have been demonstrated during bronchoconstriction. In addition, platelets transform LTA_4 to lipoxins (1). Platelet activation leads to altered metabolism of LTA_4, with increased formation of lipoxins and decreased LTC_4 biosynthesis (3). In the present study the regulation of platelet LTC_4 production has been further investigated.

METHODS

Preparations of human platelet suspensions (400×10^6 platelets/ml) from peripheral blood, determination of platelet aggregation, incubation procedures, sample purification and HPLC determination of LTC_4 were performed as described (4).

RESULTS AND DISCUSSION

Receptor-mediated platelet activation is induced via G protein-coupled phospholipase C activation and subsequent stimulation of protein kinase (PK) C (5). This process is initiated via ligand binding to distinct receptors for thrombin, thromboxane (TX) A_2 or platelet activating factor. In the present investigation thrombin and the TXA_2 analogue U-46619 suppressed platelet LTC_4 synthase activity, as demonstrated by decreased conversion of exogenous LTA_4 to LTC_4 (table 1). The degree of inhibition was dependent on the substrate concentration

Table 1 *Effect of platelet activating agents on LTC$_4$ synthase activity*

Pretreatment :	LTC$_4$ (% of control)			
	-	IM	13-APA	carbacyclin
Thrombin	45 ± 12	49 ± 9	53 ± 8	92[1] ± 3[2]
U-46619	49 ± 14	49 ± 10	88 ± 13	96 ± 12
Collagen	57 ± 10	88 ± 12	80 ± 10	n.d.
AA	45 ± 8	102 ± 14	107 ± 4	n.d.
PMA	55 ± 5	56 ± 5	63 ± 8	n.d.

Platelets were preincubated at 37°C in the presence or absence of indomethacin (IM; 10 μM; 5 min), 13-azaprostanoic acid (13-APA; 50 μM; 5 min) or carbacyclin (4 nM; 1 min) and incubated with or without thrombin (0.2 U/ml), U-46619 (1 μM), collagen (200 μg/ml), arachidonic acid (AA; 8 μM) or PMA (80 nM) for another 5 min. Thereafter LTC$_4$ synthase activity was assayed by incubation with 10 μM LTA$_4$ for 5 min. Values are expressed as % of basal LTC$_4$ synthase activity (mean±SD) in the absence of stimulatory agent (control). n.d: not determined; [1]40 nM carbacyclin; [2] range

used to determine LTC$_4$ synthase activity. Consequently, maximal thrombin-induced platelet activation provoked 78% suppression of LTC$_4$ synthesis at 0.3 μM LTA$_4$, as compared to only 35% inhibition at a substrate concentration of 30 μM. Unstimulated control platelets produced 1165 ± 609 pmol LTC$_4$/ml (mean ± SD; n=44) after incubation with 10 μM LTA$_4$ for 5 min. Stimulation of endogenous TXA$_2$ formation with collagen or arachidonic acid also attenuated the capacity of platelets to transform LTA$_4$ to LTC$_4$ (table 1). These effects were counteracted by indomethacin. As expected, the inhibition of LTC$_4$ synthase activity induced by collagen, arachidonic acid or U-46619 was also blocked by 13-azaprostanoic acid, a thromboxane receptor antagonist (table 1).

Direct activation of PKC with phorbol ester mimicked receptor-mediated inhibition of LTC$_4$ synthase activity (table 1). In agreement, preincubation with the PKC inhibitor staurosporine totally abolished the inhibitory effects on LTC$_4$ formation induced by receptor-mediated platelet activation or PMA (results not shown). Interestingly, the stable prostacyclin analogue carbacyclin counteracted the decreased LTC$_4$ synthase activity observed after receptor-mediated platelet activation (table 1). Stimulation of the prostacyclin receptor triggers the cyclic AMP system, which inhibits platelet activation mainly by suppression of phospholipase C activity, thereby abolishing phosphoinositide hydrolysis and the subsequent activation of PKC.

The onset and progress of the inhibitory effects on LTC$_4$ synthase activity provoked by thrombin (fig 1A) and U-46619 (results not shown) closely followed the aggregatory response induced by these agonists. Similarly, attenuation of LTC$_4$ formation paralleled platelet aggregation in concentration-response experiments (fig 1B). However, the inhibition of LTC$_4$ synthase activity could be distinguished from the aggregatory response. Thus, decreased LTC$_4$ synthesis after platelet activation with thrombin (fig 1C) or PMA (results not shown) was elicited also in platelets that were prevented from aggregation by incubation in the absence of magnetic stirring. This crucial finding excludes the possibility that the attenuated LTC$_4$ formation was a secondary phenomenon due to decreased LTA$_4$ availability in aggregated platelets.

In summary, the present findings indicate that the LTC$_4$ synthase in human platelets is regulated via receptor-mediated, PKC-dependent transduction pathways. The possible involvement of thromboxane A$_2$ and prostacyclin in the regulation of platelet LTC$_4$ synthase activity indicate a link between cyclooxygenase

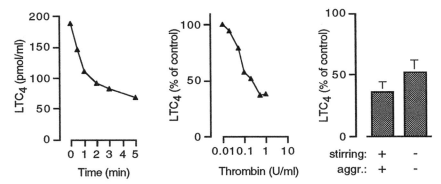

Fig 1: *Effect of thrombin on platelet LTC₄ synthase activity.* Platelet suspensions (400 x 10⁶/ml) were preincubated for 5 min at 37°C prior to stimulation with thrombin. LTC₄ synthase activity was assayed A) after various times of exposure to thrombin (0.2 U/ml) B) after exposure to various concentrations of thrombin (0.01-1-U/ml) for 5 min and C) after exposure to thrombin (0.2 U/ml) for 5 min in the presence or absence of magnetic stirring. Enzyme activity was assayed by incubation with 10 μM LTA₄ for 30 sec (A) or 5 min (B and C) and LTC₄ formation was determined by HPLC. aggr.: aggregation

products and formation of cysteinyl leukotrienes. The finding that inhibition of TXA₂ production can lead to increased LTC₄ formation may be of particular interest for the understanding of the mechanisms behind aspirin-induced asthma. Further investigations of the regulation of LTC₄ synthesis in platelets and other cells are in progress.

ACKNOWLEDGEMENTS

This project was supported by the Swedish Medical Research Council (proj. no. 03X-6805), Berth von Kantzows Foundation, King Gustaf V:s 80-years Fund, the Royal Swedish Academy of Science, Lars Hierta´s Memorial Foundation and Karolinska Institutet.

REFERENCES

1. Lindgren, J. Å. and Edenius, C.. Transcellular biosynthesis of leukotrienes and lipoxins via leukotriene A₄ transfer. *Trends Pharmacol. Sci.* 1993; 14:351-354.
2. Edenius, C., Heidvall, K. and Lindgren, J. Å. Novel transcellular interaction: Conversion of granulocyte-derived leukotriene A₄ to cysteinyl-containing leukotrienes by human platelets. *Eur. J. Biochem.* 1988; 178:81-86.
3. Edenius, C., I. Forsberg, Stenke, L. and Lindgren, J. Å. Lipoxin formation in human platelets. In: Samuelsson, B, Ramwell, P., Folco, G. and Granström, E. *Advances in Prostaglandin Thromboxane and Leukotriene Research, vol 21,* 1990, pp 97-100.
4. Tornhamre, S., Edenius, C. and Lindgren, J. Å. Receptor-mediated inhibition of leukotriene C₄ synthase activity in human platelets - evidence for protein kinase C-dependent signal transduction. *J Exp Med.* 1994. Submitted.
5. Brass, L. F., Hoxie, J. A. and Manning, D. R.. Signaling through G proteins and G protein-coupled receptors during platelet activation. *Thromb. Haemostas.* 1993; 70:217-223.

Advances in Prostaglandin, Thromboxane,
and Leukotriene Research, Vol. 23,
edited by B. Samuelsson et al.
Raven Press, Ltd., New York © 1995

Antibodies to ICAM-1 ameliorate inflammation in acetic acid induced inflammatory bowel disease

Patrick Y-K Wong[1], Gang Yue[1], Kingsley Yin[1], Masayuki Miyasaka[2], Caryl L. Lane[3], Anthony M. Manning[3], Donald C. Anderson[3] and Frank F. Sun[4].

[1]*Dept. of Cell Biology, University of Medicine and Dentistry New Jersey, Stratford, NJ 08084;* [2]*Dept. of Immunology, The Tokyo Metropolitan Institute of Medical Sciences, Tokyo, Japan;* [3]*Dept. of Adhesion Biology and* [4]*Hypersensitivity Diseases Research, The Upjohn Labs., Kalamazoo, MI 49001*

Recently, immunohistochemical localization of a number of adhesion molecules was characterized from tissues of patients with inflammatory bowel disease (IBD) and compared with the profile in normal colon tissues (1). The results demonstrated that there was a marked increase in the expression of the integrins, LFA-1, macrophage antigen-1 (Mac-1) and their counter-receptor, ICAM-1.

Although there have been studies using monoclonal antibodies (mAbs) against human CD18 (the common β-subunit of the heterodimer integrins) in a rabbit model of IBD (2), no information on the role of ICAM-1 in the inflammatory response of rat IBD has been reported. Importantly, the above-mentioned study administered the antibody before the inflammatory insult. In other models of inflammation, ICAM-1 mAb inhibited the development of adjuvant arthritis (3) and renal ischemic-reperfusion injury (4). In these studies, either high levels of mAb were given on multiple occasions during the course of the study (5 mg/kg; arthritis) or as a single high dose (1 mg/rat) in a model of acute inflammation (ischemic-reperfusion injury). We have examined for the first time the effects of a single, relatively low dose of specific murine mAb against rat ICAM-1 in an acetic acid-induced chronic model of rat IBD.

Male Sprague Dawley rats were divided equally into 2 groups. One group received acetic acid (HOAc) intraanally to induce IBD while the other received saline as control. After 24h, each of the 2 groups was subdivided into three groups which received ICAM-1 antibody (1A29), murine IgG1 control, (non-blocking antibody to human E-selectin CL37) or no treatment. Seven days after acetic acid or vehicle treatment, rats were sacrificed and the colon examined. The whole colon was slit longitudinally and any visible damage was scored on a 0-5 scale of increasing tissue damage. Eight cm of colonic tissue containing the major gross pathologic area (if any) was weighed to determine the ratio of distal colon weight to body weight as index of edema. A 4 cm segment containing the area(s) of major gross pathologies was cut. This segment was then longitudinally sectioned into 3 strips for measurement of (i) myeloperoxidase (MPO) activity, (ii) superoxide and (iii) nitric oxide (NO) production (measured as nitrite levels).

Table 1 shows that HOAc treatment caused a marked increase in damage score. Treatment with ICAM-1 antibody reduced the damage score by 50%. There were no signs of inflammation in any rats without HOAc treatment. MPO activity of colonic tissue was measured as a specific index of neutrophil infiltration. MPO activity decreased by more than two-fold in IBD rats treated with ICAM-1 mAb compared with the two groups of positive controls but the MPO activity was still higher than rats not treated with HOAc.

Exp. I.P.	1A29 + HOAc	1A29 + saline	CL37 + HOAc	CL37 + saline	HOAc	Saline
Damage score	2.5 ± 0.4	0	5 ± 0	0	4.6 ± 0.3	0
MPO (U/5mg)	1.4 ± 0.3	$0.3\pm.004$ **	4.3 ± 0.3 **	$0.4\pm.01$ **	4.6 ± 0.4 **	$0.4\pm.006$ **
O^{2-} (cps/g) x 10^{-4}	2.2 ± 0.3	0.7 ± 0.1 **	16.2 ± 0.8 **	$0.4\pm.04$ **	14.9 ± 2.2 **	0.9 ± 0.2 **
O^{2-} (cps/g) x 10^{-4} (+fMLP)	3.6 ± 0.7	1.2 ± 0.6 *	23.8 ± 1.8 **	$0.8\pm.003$ **	42.2 ± 1.7 **	4.1 ± 3 **
nitrite (nmoles/g)	23.5 ± 1.2	20.6 ± 2.7	35.3 ± 5.1	19.7 ± 1.8	38.7 ± 6.9	31.8 ± 4.6

Table 1: Effects of different treatments on various inflammatory parameters. * $P < 0.05$ when compared to 1A29 + HOAc. ** $P < 0.01$ when compared to 1A29. I.P. = inflammatory parameters. Exp. = experimental procedures. 1A29 is the ICAM-1 mAb. CL37 is the non-blocking mAb.

Superoxide formation was measured as an indication of the formation of reactive oxygen species by infiltrating leukocytes. Tissue from rats given HOAc alone or HOAc with non-blocking mAb generated substantially more superoxide as compared with rats treated with saline only. Treatment with ICAM-1 mAb reduced superoxide generation by approximately 85%. To ensure that the increased superoxide levels was due to an increased infiltration of leukocytes a high dose of fMLP was added to the tissue medium for 10 mins before superoxide generation was measured again. A similar pattern emerged where HOAc treated rats had a greater capacity to generate superoxide than IBD rats treated with ICAM-1 mAb or rats which did not have IBD.

Formation of NO has been implicated as a mediator in the development and the pathogenesis of chronic IBD (5). Nitrite, a stable metabolic product of the NO reaction with O_2 and water was used as an indicator for the generation of NO. HOAc administration modestly increased tissue nitrite levels. Treatment with anti-ICAM-1 decreased the formation of nitrite similar to the trends seen with other inflammatory parameters.

The ratio of distal colonic weight to body weight was measured as an index of edema. Tissues taken from rats given HOAc or HOAc and non-blocking mAb had an increased ratio compared to rats treatment with ICAM-1 mAb. The body weights of all rats treated with HOAc were not significantly different between groups.

Although the exact mechanism is not well understood, there is little doubt that the cardinal signs of this inflammation are due to the rapid and prolonged infiltration of leukocytes together with the release of inflammatory mediators such as cytokines, arachidonic acid metabolites and reactive oxygen species. These inflammatory mediators can either increase vascular permeability and/or damage cells directly or indirectly through a mechanism secondary to increased leukocyte adhesion and infiltration. Central to this pathology of infiltrating leukocytes, is the role of adhesion molecules such as ICAM-1. In this study, we provide evidence that ICAM-1 plays a critical role in the development of IBD. Our results support the hypothesis that the prevention of infiltration of leukocytes and the prevention of release of their respiratory products can substantially reduce inflammation in IBD.

REFERENCES

1. Nakamura, S., Ohtani, H., Watanabe, Y. et al., In situ expression of the cell adhesion molecules in inflammatory bowel disease. *Lab. Invest.* (1993); 69(1), 77-85.
2. Wallace, J.L., Higa, A., McKnight, G.W and MacIntyre, D.E. Prevention and reversal of experimental colitis by a monoclonal antibody which inhibits leukocyte adherence. *Inflammation,* (1992); 16(4), 343-354.
3. Iigo Y., Takahashi, T., Tamatani, T. et al., ICAM-1-dependent pathway is critically involved in the pathogenesis of adjuvant arthritis in rats. *J. Immunol.,* (1991); 147(12), 4167-4171.
4. Kelly, K.J., Williams, W.W. Jr., Colvin, R.B. and Bonventre, J.V. Antibody to ICAM-1 protects the kidney against ischemic injury. *Proc. Natl. Acad. Sci., USA,* (1994); 91, 812-816.
5. Miller, M.J.S., Sadowska-Krowicka, H., Choinaruemol, S., Kakkis, J.L. and Clark, D.A. Amelioration of chronic ileitis by nitric oxide synthase inhibition. *J. Pharm. Exp. Ther.,* (1993); 264(1), 11-16.

Advances in Prostaglandin, Thromboxane, and Leukotriene Research, Vol. 23,
edited by B. Samuelsson et al.
Raven Press, Ltd., New York © 1995

SYNERGISTIC PREVENTION OF ENDOTOXIN INDUCED MORTALITY IN RATS BY PGE1 AND PARTICLES

David F. Eierman, Machiko Yagami, Scott M. Erme, Sharma R. Minchey, Paul A. Harmon and Andrew S. Janoff

The Liposome Company, Inc., Princeton, NJ, 08540, USA

Opinion concerning the role of prostaglandins in the inflammatory cascade is divided. Pro-inflammatory prostaglandin activities such as vasodilation and hyperalgesia have been used to explain the mechanism by which non-steroidal anti-inflammatory drugs exert their effects while numerous anti-inflammatory prostaglandin activities have been identified including the inhibition of leukocyte activation and subsequent inhibitions of O_{2-} release and cytokine production[1,2]. These anti-inflammatory effects are mediated by increased intracellular cAMP which is dramatically augmented by phagocytic stimuli [3,4]. This suggests a role for surface adhesive proteins and their receptors in the systemic prostaglandin response.

The synergistic effect of PGE1 and particles on neutrophil cAMP elevation and the direct effect of PGE1 itself on preventing neutrophil adhesion to capillary endothelium[5] led us to investigate whether large unilamellar liposome vesicles, i.e., biodegradable 100 nm egg phosphatidyl choline particles, plus PGE1 might be effective in lethal models of experimental endotoxemia. We found that liposomes labelled with 2 mole% of the fluorescent probe rhodamine PE and opsonized with purified human fibronectin, fibrinogen or sera targeted to human leukocytes and primary cultures of human arterial and venous endothelial cells only if these cells were activated by exposure to endotoxin or cytokines. Targeting was blocked by antibodies to the opsonins or to cellular $\alpha5\beta1$ and $\alpha V\beta3$ integrin receptors.

We therefore assessed the efficacy of PGE1 and liposomes in a rat model of endotoxemia. As shown in Figure 1, PGE1 when administered alone was pro-inflammatory. It increased both the rate and extent of the LPS induced mortality. In contrast, liposomes reduced mortality. Remarkably, PGE1 administered in combination with liposomes became anti-inflammatory and afforded complete protection against endotoxin induced death. The protective effect of PGE1 + liposomes was confined to survival. All animals receiving endotoxin exhibited non-purulent conjunctivitis, profuse watery diarrhea and profound lethargy. Dying animals exhibited syncope and shock. Surviving animals recovered completely.

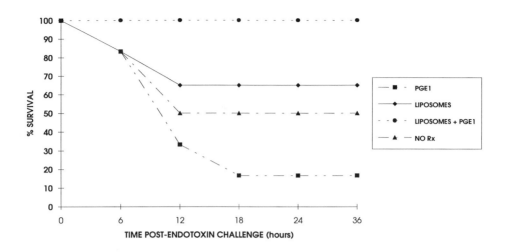

FIGURE 1: Liposomes + PGE1 attenuate LPS induced mortality while PGE1 alone leads to increased mortality. Male Sprague-Dawley rats were injected i.v. with 50 mg/kg LPS at time 0. Free PGE1 or liposomal PGE1 (at 40 ug/kg) were simultaneously injected i.v. Survival was assessed at the indicated times. For each group n=12.

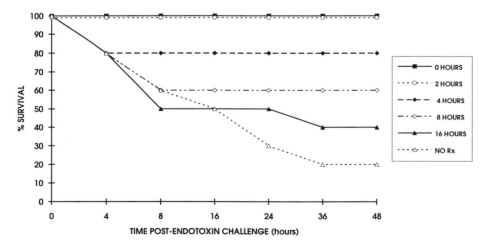

FIGURE 2: PGE1 + liposome dosing post-LPS "rescues" animals from endotoxic shock and subsequent mortality. Male Sprague-Dawley rats were injected i.v. with 75 mg/kg LPS at time 0. Liposomal PGE1

(at 40 ug/kg) was administered as a single i.v. bolus to groups of animals beginning at either 0, 2, 4, 8, or 16 hour post-LPS. Survival was assessed at the indicated times. For each group n=10.

The extraordinary protection afforded to animals in our model by PGE1 + liposomes led us to further assess this treatment modality. We induced endotoxemia and administered single bolus i.v. injections of PGE1 + liposomes at various times post-challenge. As shown above in Figure 2, "rescue" of animals from lethal endotoxic shock was achieved even when treatment was with-held for significant periods of times after endotoxin challenge. While some mortality occurred prior to treatment, all animals alive at up to 8 hours post-challenge survived. Even animals treated up to 16 hours post-challenge showed a significantly increased survival as compared to controls. We are unaware of any experimental or clinical data that suggests successful intervention is possible in the later stages of systemic inflammatory disease.

These data demonstrate that, in rats, the lethal consequences of high dose endotoxin challenge are exacerbated by the i.v. administration of exogenous PGE1, but attenuated by the i.v. administration of endocytosable particles. Moreover we show that particles can act in concert with PGE1 to completely rescue animals from the lethal late stage sequelae of experimental endotoxemia. These data illustrate that the endocytosis of particles can transform the overall systemic response to prostaglandin E1 from pro- to anti-inflammatory and suggest a rationale for new therapeutic modalities.

References

1. Vane JR. Prostaglandins a mediators of inflammation. In: Samuelsson B and Paoletti R. *Adv Prost Thromb Res*, Vol2. New York: Raven Press; 1976:791-801.

2. Abramson SB and Weissmann G. The mechanisms of actions of antiinflammatory drugs. *Arth Rheum* 1989;32:1-9.

3. Weissmann G, Zurier RB, Spieler PJ, and Goldstein IM. Mechanisms of lysosomal enzyme release from leukocytes exposed to immune complexes and other particles. *J Exp Med* 1971;134:149s-165s.

4. Zurier RB, Weissmann G, Hoffstein S, Kammerman S, and Tai HS. Mechanisms of lysosomal enzyme release from human leukocytes. *J Clin Invest* 1974;53:297-309.

5. Grant, MM, Burnett CM and Fein AM. Effect of prostaglandin E1 infusion on leukocyte traffic and fibrosis in acute lung injury induced by bleomycin in hamsters. *Crit Care Med.* 1991;19:211-217.

Advances in Prostaglandin, Thromboxane,
and Leukotriene Research, Vol. 23,
edited by B. Samuelsson et al.
Raven Press, Ltd., New York © 1995

INDUCTION OF PROSTAGLANDIN H SYNTHASE-2 IN RAT CARRAGEENIN-INDUCED PLEURISY AND EFFECT OF A SELECTIVE COX-2 INHIBITOR

Makoto Katori, Yoshiteru Harada, Ko Hatanaka, Masataka Majima
Michiko Kawamura, Takashi Ohno[1], Akira Aizawa[2] and
Shozo Yamamoto[3]

[1]*Department of Pharmacology,* [2] *Department of Molecular Biology, Kitasato University
School of Medicine, Sagamihara, Kanagawa, 228 and* [3] *Department of Biochemistry, Tokushima
University School of Medicine, Tokushima 770, Japan*

Recently, inducible prostaglandin H synthase (PGHS)-2 or cyclooxygenase (COX)-2, besides constitutive COX-1, was identified[1] in cells in vitro. Messenger RNA of COX-2 was expressed in many isolated or cultured cells in vitro by PMA, LPS, inflammatory mediators and cytokines. This new COX-2 shows 60 % homology in the amino acid sequence with that of constitutive COX-1. The expression of this COX-2 was reported to be inhibited by glucocorticosteroids. However, still we have very few evidence that COX-2 is expressed in cells of inflammatory sites of animal models. Thus we tested whether COX-2 is really expressed in inflammatory sites and demonstrated that COX-2 was induced in the inflammation site of carrageenin-induced rat pleurisy [2].

MATERIALS AND METHODS

Carrageenin pleurisy was induced in male Sprague-Dawley rats (9-10 weeks old) by intrapleural injection of 0.2 ml of 2% λ-carrageenin[3]. Dexamethasone (0.3-30 mg/kg, i.p.) was injected 2 hrs before carrageenin injection. Aspirin (100 mg/kg, i.p.) or NS-398 (N-[2-cyclohexyloxy-4-nitrophenyl] methane-sulfonamide, Taisho Pharmaceutical Co., Tokyo, 3 mg/kg, i.p.) was injected 1 hr before carrageenin. Rats were exsanguinated under ether anesthesia at given times. Cells in the pleural exudate were harvested and mononuclear cells and polymorphonuclear leukocytes were separated by elutriation using LymphoprepTM. Rat peritoneal cells were collected 19 hr after intraperitoneal injection of casein (0.4

mg/40 ml). Microsomal fractions of lung, stomach and kidney from normal and pleurisy rats were prepared. The pleural cells, the peritoneal cells and the microsomal fractions were submitted to Western blot and Northern hybridization analyses. Anti-sera used for Western blot analysis were rabbit anti-bovine PGHS-1 antiserum[4] and rabbit anti-murine PGHS-2 antiserum (Cayman Chemical, Ann Arbor). Probes used for Northern hybridization were murine PGHS-1 cDNA and murine PGHS-2 cDNA (Cayman Chemical). The prostanoid levels in the pleural exudate were measured using enzyme-immunoassay kits. ^{3}H-arachidonic acid were incubated in the presence of 5 mM tryptophan and 1μM of hemoglobin with PGHS-1 (sheep seminal vesicles) or PGHS-2 (sheep placenta, Cayman Chemical) for assay of selective inhibitors.

RESULTS AND DISCUSSION

In the rat carrageenin pleurisy, the pleural exudate started to be accumulated from 1 hr and reached a plateau at 19 hr after carrageenin injection. The plasma exudation for 20 min into the pleural cavity, assessed by exudation of pontamine sky blue after intravenous injection, was rapidly increased up to 5 hr and declined gradually thereafter. The level of 6-keto-PGF$_{1\alpha}$, PGE$_2$ and TXB$_2$ in the pleural exudate were increased between 1 and 7 hr after carrageenin injection. PGE$_2$, which showed a peak at 3-5 hr, was mainly contributed to the plasma exudation among these prostanoids, as reported before (3). The plasma exudation and the exudate volume at 1-5 hr were inhibited by aspirin. Using Western blot analysis, COX-2 was detected neither in white cells in peripheral blood and in the pleural cells before carrageenin, but was detected in the cells of the pleural exudate from 1 hr. The level was at maximum at 5 hr (Figure 1 A), being reduced thereafter, and was hardly detected at 19 hr. This agreed well with the results of our previous paper (2). COX-2 was induced mainly by mononuclear cells, not by polymorpho-nuclear leukocytes, in the pleural exudate. COX-1 was present at the same level in the peripheral white blood cells and in the cells before and after carrageenin injection. Messenger RNA of COX-2 was also expressed in the cells of the exudate at 5 hr, as detected by an Northern hybridization analysis (Figure 1 B). Dexamethasone suppressed the induction of COX-2 at the doses larger than 3 mg/kg. The prostanoid levels in the pleural exudate were suppressed by dexamethasone. A new anti-inflammatory drug, NS-398 inhibited COX-2 at smaller doses (IC$_{50}$=10 μM) than those for inhibition of COX-1 from sheep vesicular gland (IC$_{50}$=200 μM) in vitro, whereas indomethacin showed 10 times higher inhibition on COX-1 than COX-2. The plasma exudation and the exudate volume at 5 hr in the carrageenin-induced pleurisy was markedly suppressed by NS-398 (3 mg/kg, i.p.) at the same degree to that by aspirin (100 mg/kg, i.p.). Only COX-1, not COX-2, was detected in the microsomal fraction of lung, stomach and kidney of the pleurisy rats and the non-pleurisy rats. Selective COX-2 inhibitors may exert their anti-inflammatory actions without side effects on stomach and kidney.

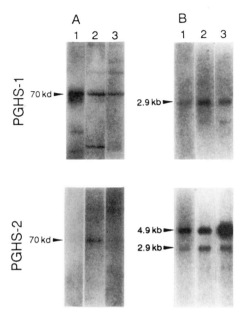

Figure 1. Western blot analysis of PGHS-1 and PGHS-2 (A) and Northern hybridization analysis of their mRNA (B). [A], lane 1, 2 & 3: cells in the pleural lavage from normal rats, cells in the pleural exudate at 5 hr of the pleurisy and at 19 hr of the pleurisy, respectively. The position of 70-kDa molecular marker protein is indicated. [B], lane 1: cells in the pleural exudate at 5 hr of the pleurisy; lane 2 &3: casein-induced peritoneal cells incubated for 4 hr at 37°C with (lane 3) or without (lane 2) PMA (30 nM). The position of 4.9- and 2.9 kb size markers are indicated.

REFERENCES

1. DeWitt DL, Meade EA, Smith WL. PGH synthase isoenzyme selectivity: The potential for safer nonsteroidal antiinflammatory drugs. *Amer J Med* 1993: 95; Suppl. 2A: 40S-46S.
2. Harada Y, Hatanaka K, Saito M et al. Detection of inducible prostaglandin H synthase-2 in cells in the exudate of rat carrageenin-induced pleurisy. *Biomed Res* 1994; 15: 127-130.
3. Harada Y, Tanaka K, Uchida Y et al. Changes in the levels of prostaglandins and thromboxane and their roles in the accumulation of exudate in rat carrageenin-induced pleurisy--A profile analysis using gas chromatography-mass spectrometry. *Prostaglandins* 1982; 23: 881-895.
4. Ishimura K, Suzuki T, Fukui K et al. Immunocytochemical localization of prostaglandin endoperoxide synthase in the bovine intestine. *Histochemistry* 1993; 99: 485-490.

Advances in Prostaglandin, Thromboxane,
and Leukotriene Research, Vol. 23,
edited by B. Samuelsson et al.
Raven Press, Ltd., New York © 1995

Cyclooxygenase in Rat Pleural Hypersensitivity Reactions

Adrian R. Moore, Dean Willis, Derek Gilroy, Annette Tomlinson, Ian
Appleton and Derek A. Willoughby

*Department of Experimental Pathology, St. Bartholomew's Hospital Medical College,
London EC1M 6BQ, Great Britain.*

Cyclooxygenase (COX) converts arachadonic acid to prostaglandins (PGs) which
in acute inflammation are proinflammatory because of a combination of
vasodilatation and hyperalgesia. The inhibition of COX therefore results in
antiinflammatory effects and is the basis for the pharmacological actions of non-
steroidal antiinflammatory drugs[1]. COX exists as two known isoforms, a
constitutive form (COX1) and a more recently identified inducible form (COX2).
The inducible isoform can be expressed in a variety of cells following exposure to
cytokines that are generated as part of the inflammatory response[2]. The aim of
this study was to measure the activity of COX and determine a role for COX2 in
an Arthus reaction and a model of delayed hypersensitivity.

MATERIALS AND METHODS

Male Wistar rats (150 ± 10g) were sensitised by intradermal injection at the
base of the tail with 0.1ml 50:50 incomplete Freund's adjuvant and saline
containing bovine serum albumin (BSA, 10mg/ml) or whole cell pertussis vaccine
(2×10^9 organisms/ml). Twelve days after sensitisation the animals were challenged
intrapleurally with 0.1ml saline containing 10mg/ml BSA (Arthus reaction) or 2×10^9
organisms/ml pertussis vaccine (delayed hypersensitivity reaction). Groups of
animals (n=7) were killed at various time intervals after challenge and exudates
were collected by pleural lavage[3]. Exudate volumes, total and differential cell
counts were recorded. Cell pellets were prepared by centrifugation.

COX activity was measured by radioimmunoassay of PGE_2 in the presence
of excess arachidonic acid[3].

COX2 protein levels of exudate cells were determined by Western blot
analysis or immunocytochemistry[3].

Results are expressed as the mean ± s.e.m.

RESULTS

Intrapleural injection of either BSA or pertussis into non-sensitised animals resulted in no recoverable exudates at any of the time points (data not shown). The BSA reaction resulted in exudate volumes that were measurable at 2 hours, peaked at 6 hours and greatly reduced at 24 hours (Table 1). Inflammatory cell influx showed a similar pattern with the neutrophil being the dominant cell. The pertussis reaction resulted in exudate volumes that were measurable at 2 hours but greatly increased at both 24 and 48 hours (Table 2). Inflammatory cell influx showed a similar pattern. Neutrophils were dominant at 2 hours and mononuclear cells dominant at 48 hours.

Biochemical determinations showed COX activity at all time points in both models. In the Arthus reaction, activity was greatest at 6 hours. In the pertussis reaction there appeared to be raised activity at 2 hours and at 48 hours.

In the Arthus reaction, Western blot showed COX2 to be present at all time points. Qualitatively, the intensity of the bands appeared greatest at 2 hours. In the pertussis model, COX2 protein was barely detectable at 2 hours but was present as intense bands at 24 and 48 hours. Immunocytochemistry showed COX2 staining to be present in a proportion of neutrophils in both models and a proportion of mononuclear cells in the pertussis reaction at 24 and 48 hours.

	2 hours	6 hours	24 hours
Exudate vol. ml	0.83 ± 0.19	1.16 ± 0.23	0.11 ± 0.01
Total cells x10^6	11.2 ± 1.3	16.8 ± 2.8	8.6 ± 0.7
Total PMN x10^6	7.9 ± 0.9	10.9 ± 1.8	4.6 ± 0.4
Total Mϕ x10^6	3.3 ± 0.4	5.9 ± 1.0	4.0 ± 0.3
ngPGE$_2$/pellet/min	9.9 ± 3.0	11.3 ± 2.0	9.1 ± 1.9

Table 1   Characterisation of inflammation resulting from an active Arthus reaction to BSA in the rat pleural cavity.

	2 hours	24 hours	48 hours
Exudate vol. ml	0.41 ± 0.07	2.95 ± 0.55	3.01 ± 0.83
Total cells x10^6	15 ± 3	31 ± 2	99 ± 27
Total PMN x10^6	11.6 ± 2.3	19.2 ± 1.2	25.0 ± 6.8
Total Mϕ x10^6	3.4 ± 0.7	11.8 ± 0.8	74 ± 20.2
ngPGE$_2$/pellet/min	11.5 ± 1.4	7.0 ± 1.5	14.9 ± 2.5

Table 2   Characterisation of inflammation resulting from intrapleural challenge with pertussis vaccine into sensitised rats.

DISCUSSION

It has previously been shown that COX2 is present in complement-dependent acute inflammation (rat carrageenan pleurisy[3]) and in murine chronic granulomatous inflammation[4]. The current study extends these observations and shows COX2 to be present in an Arthus reaction and a model of delayed hypersensitivity. In both models, COX2 was present at or before the peak of fluid and cell accumulation, and coincident with highest COX activity measurements. In the Arthus reaction, the neutrophil would appear to be the major source of COX2 whereas in the pertussis model, mononuclear cells also appear to be making a contribution. These results support the concept that COX2 derived mediators have a role to play in these reactions although a contribution from COX1 cannot be ruled out. Selective COX2 inhibitors are likely to prove effective antiinflammatory compounds which by sparing COX1 should result in compounds with fewer side effects than current NSAIDs.

ACKNOWLEDGEMENTS

A.R.M. is supported by ONO Pharmaceutical Company Ltd, D.W. is supported by Laboratoires OM, A.T. is supported by Servier and I.A. is in receipt of a Royal Society Smith & Nephew Fellowship .

REFERENCES

1.   Vane JR. Inhibition of prostaglandin synthesis as a possible mechanism of action for the aspirin-like drugs. *Nature* 1971;231:232-5.

2.   Xie W., Robertson DL. & Simmons DL. Mitogen inducible prostaglandin G/H synthase: a new target for non-steroidal antiinflammatory drugs. *Drug Dev. Res.* 1992;25:249-65.

3.   Tomlinson A., Appleton I, Moore AR., et al. Cyclooxygenase and nitric oxide synthase isoforms in rat carrageenan-induced pleurisy. *Br. J. Pharmacol.* 1994 In press.

4.   Vane JR., Mitchell JA., Appleton I., et al. Inducible isoforms of cyclooxygenase and nitric oxide synthase in inflammation. *Proc. Natl. Acad. Sci. USA* 1994;91:2046-50.

Advances in Prostaglandin, Thromboxane, and Leukotriene Research, Vol. 23,
edited by B. Samuelsson et al.
Raven Press, Ltd., New York © 1995

Leukotrienes and Other Mediators of the Schultz-Dale Reaction in Guinea-Pig Lung Parenchyma

Eva Wikström Jonsson and Sven-Erik Dahlén

*Asthma Research Group, Division of Physiology I, Department of Physiology & Pharmacology
and Institute of Environmental Medicine,
Karolinska Institutet, S-171 77 Stockholm, Sweden*

It has recently been established that leukotrienes are major mediators of antigen-dependent contractions in human airways (1). There is however a need for experimental models of leukotriene mediated responses in preparations other than human bronchi. The aim of this study was to evaluate whether the mediators of the contraction evoked by antigen-challenge in strips of guinea-pig lung parenchyma (GPLP) were similar to those of human airways.

MATERIALS AND METHODS

Male guinea-pigs were sensitised by i.p. and s.c. injections of ovalbumin (OA), 10 mg dissolved in 400 µl saline respectively. After a minimum of four weeks, the animals were sacrificed by cervical dislocation and exsanguination. Following perfusion with ice cold Tyrode's solution (20 ml) via the pulmonary artery, the lungs were excised and strips of guinea-pig lung parenchyma were prepared and mounted in organ-baths as previously described (2). The preparations were challenged with cumulatively rising concentrations of antigen (OA 0.001-10 µg/ml). Enzyme Immuno Assay of cysteinyl-leukotriene release (3) was performed with reagents from Cayman Chemical Company, Ann Arbor, MI. Thromboxane analysis was performed with Radio Immuno Assay as described (4).

RESULTS AND CONCLUSIONS

Challenge with ovalbumin yielded a concentration-dependent, biphasic contractile response, which consisted of a sharp initial peak-phase and a sustained plateau-phase. The response to OA was not affected by histamine antagonism alone (mepyramine, H_1, 1μM, and metiamide, H_2, 1μM). Thus, histamine did not seem to be involved in the response. The contractile response was associated with release of thromboxane A_2 (net increase of TXB_2 in bath fluid 3.2 ± 1.7 nM, mean $\pm$ SD, n=8). Challenge with OA in the presence of indomethacin resulted in TXB_2-levels below the detection limit (0.3 nM; n=7), but the OA-induced contraction was not affected by cyclooxygenase inhibition (indomethacin or diclofenac 10μM). Neither did combined TP-antagonism (BAY u3405 3μM) and thromboxane synthase inhibition (CS-518 3μM) block the contraction. Therefore, important contributions by contractile cyclooxygenase products were excluded. In contrast, 5-lipoxygenase inhibition (BAY x1005 30μM, MK-886 100μM or BW A4C 10μM) inhibited the peak-phase substantially, indicating that 5-lipoxygenase products were involved (shown for BAY x1005 in fig.1).

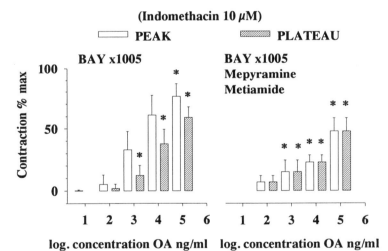

FIG. 1. Leukotriene biosynthesis inhibition (BAY x1005 30μM) significantly inhibited the plateau-phase of the contractile response to antigen, whereas the peak contraction was unaffected. When histamine antagonists (mepyramine 1μM and metiamide 1μM) were combined with BAY x1005, both the peak and the plateau were substantially depressed. Star denotes significant difference vs controls.

Since the time-course of the remaining OA-contraction was histamine-like, the effect of histamine-antagonism in combination with lipoxygenase inhibition was assessed in another series of experiments. Addition of antihistamines substantially depressed also the peak-phase, whereas the plateau-phase was not further inhibited (fig. 1). These results were reproduced using the cysteinyl-leukotriene receptor antagonist ICI 198,615 (3μM), confirming that cysteinyl-leukotrienes and histamine synergistically mediate the peak-phase, whereas cysteinyl-leukotrienes alone contribute to the peak-phase. The results also imply that cysteinyl-leukotrienes released during the anaphylactic contraction act at conventional Cys-LT$_1$ receptors in GPLP.

The remaining anti-histamine- and anti-leukotriene-resistant component of the OA-induced contraction could not be attenuated by pretreatment with the Platelet Activating Factor (PAF) antagonist WEB 2086 10μM or by NO-synthesis inhibition (L-NAME 0.1mM). The NK$_2$-receptor antagonist SR 48968 (500nM) could not reverse the residual contractile response, when administered on the plateau-phase.

In summary, as shown for IgE-dependent contractions of human bronchi (1), the Schultz-Dale response in GPLP is mediated by histamine and cysteinyl-leukotrienes. At the highest antigen-dose, there is however a residual response in GPLP, which is not sensitive to PAF- or NK$_2$-antagonism.

ACKNOWLEDGEMENTS

Supported by the Swedish Medical Research Council (14X-9071), the Swedish Association Against Chest and Heart Diseases, the Swedish Association Against Asthma and Allergy (RmA), the Swedish Society for Medical Research, the Institute of Environmental Medicine and Karolinska Institutet.

REFERENCES

1. Björck T, Dahlén S-E. Leukotrienes and Histamine Mediate IgE-Dependent Contractions of Human Bronchi: Pharmacological Evidence Obtained with Tissue from Asthmatic and Non-Asthmatic Subjects. *Pulm. Pharmacol.* 1993;6:87-96.

2. Wikström E, Westlund P, Nicolaou KC, Dahlén S-E. Lipoxin A$_4$-Induced Release of Thromboxane in the Guinea-Pig Lung: Studies of Its Characteristics Using Lipoxin A$_4$-Methyl Ester. *J. Lipid Mediators* 1992;5:205-217.

3. Pradelles P, Antoine C, Lellouche J-P, Maclouf J. Enzyme Immunoassays for Leukotrienes C$_4$ and E$_4$ Using Acetylcholinesterase. *Methods Enzymol.* 1990;187:82-89.

4. Granström E, Kindahl H, Samuelsson B. Radioimmunoassay for Thromboxane. *Anal. Lett.* 1976;9:611-627.

Advances in Prostaglandin, Thromboxane,
and Leukotriene Research, Vol. 23,
edited by B. Samuelsson et al.
Raven Press, Ltd., New York © 1995

Arachidonic Acid Liberation from Rat Tracheal Epithelial Cells by Alveolar Macrophages

Andreas Reimann, Gernot Brunn, Claudia Hey, Ignaz Wessler[*] and Kurt Racké[#]

Department of Pharmacology, J.W. Goethe-University, Theodor-Stern-Kai 7,
*D-60590 Frankfurt; * Department of Pharmacology, University of Mainz,*
Obere Zahlbacher Str. 67, D-55101 Mainz.

In the airways arachidonic acid (AA) derived mediators can exert a large variety of effects. The different eicosanoids can either stimulate or inhibit airway smooth muscles, ion transport and mucus secretion (see 6) and inhibit neurotransmission (5). The airway epithelium is a major source of prostaglandins (6), whereas macrophages, which are present in the airway epithelium of asthmatic patients in large numbers, can in addition release thromboxane A_2 and leukotrienes (2,4). Macrophages by releasing numerous other chemotoxins appear to play a key role in airway inflammatory reactions (4). Macrophages and macrophages derived mediators, such as GM-CSF, can stimulate the generation of leukotrienes in eosinophils and neutrophils (see 4). The present experiments should test whether alveolar macrophages (AM) may also affect AA metabolism in tracheal epithelial cells in primary culture.

METHODS

Tracheae of newborn rats, cut into small pieces, were explanted onto 55 mm diameter culture dishes (3) and cultured in RPMI-1640 medium with 15 % fetal bovine serum, supplemented with epidermal growth factor and few other growth hormones and with reduced calcium concentration (60-80 μM). These conditions allow selective proliferation of epithelial cells (1). Confluent epithelial layers were obtained after about 4 weeks and all cells showed a positive staining with a pan-cytokeratin-antibody. Confluent cell layers were incubated with ^{3}H-AA (370 kBq) for 16 h. After intensive washing, the cells were incubated for 3 consecutive 1 h periods in Krebs-HEPES medium and the outflow of ^{3}H-compounds was determined. ^{3}H-Compounds were separated by gra-

author for correspondence

dient reverse phase HPLC allowing the identification of TxB_2, PGE_2/D_2, $PGF_{2\alpha}$ LTB_4, 15-, 12- and 5-HETE and AA (7).

AM were freshly prepared by broncho-alveolar lavage of isolated rat lungs. They were either added to the epithel cells (10^6 AM per dish) or incubated for 1 h in Krebs medium to obtain AM-conditioned medium which was then added to the epithel cells (see Table 1). In some experiments AM were also labelled with ^3H-AA and the outflow of ^3H-compounds determined.

RESULTS

In medium of unstimulated epithelial cells, the fraction coeluting with ^3H-PGE_2/D_2 represented the main fraction (2130 ± 339 DPM, mean $\pm$ SEM, n=25) compared to ^3H-LTB_4 (250 ± 42 DPM) and ^3H-AA (450 ± 52 DPM) or other metabolites (< 150 DPM). Table 1 summarizes the acute effects of the calcium ionophore A 23187 and phorbol 12-myristate 13-acetate (PMA) on the outflow of AA metabolites. Both drugs caused, compared to the controls, a slight increase in the outflow of ^3H-AA, but only A 23187 enhanced the outflow of ^3H-prostaglandins without affecting that of ^3H-LTB_4.

AM showed only a very low rate of spontaneous outflow of ^3H-AA and ^3H-AA-metabolites. As shown in Table 2, in AM, PMA and A 23187 caused an 3-4fold increase in the ^3H-AA outflow, but PMA selectively stimulated the outflow of cyclooxygenase products without enhancing the outflow of ^3H-LTB_4, whereas A 23187 caused a marked increase in the outflow of cyclooxygenase products and an enormous stimulation of ^3H-LTB_4 outflow.

Addition of unlabelled AM to epithelial cells, labelled with ^3H-AA, caused a marked rise in release of ^3H-AA and of several lipophilic AA metabolites and an about 7fold increase in release of ^3H-prostaglandins and of an unidentified metabolite (HPLC retention time of 52 min). AM-conditioned medium caused a substantial liberation of only ^3H-AA without significant effects on the outflow of ^3H-prostanoids or other ^3H-AA metabolites (Table 1).

TABLE 1: Effects of the ionophore A 23187 (10 μM), phorbol 12-myristate 13-acetate (PMA, 100 nM), alveolar macrophages (AM) or AM-conditioned medium (AM-CM) on the release of AA metabolites from rat tracheal epithelial cells in primary culture labelled with ^3H-AA.

	PGs	LTB_4	52 min	L-M	AA	
Ctr.	75 ± 15	155 ± 74	85 ± 15	110 ± 35	50 ± 7	%
A 23187	273 ± 39	137 ± 51	189 ± 53	240 ± 83	104 ± 11	%
PMA	55 ± 8	43 ± 2	57 ± 13	125 ± 45	185 ± 26	%
AM	489 ± 30	76 ± 14	744 ± 129	1893 ± 505	3782 ± 1316	%
AM-CM	164 ± 49	93 ± 9	158 ± 48	146 ± 55	1553 ± 677	%

Epithelial cells, labelled with ^3H-AA were incubated for 3 consecutive 1 h periods with Krebs-HEPES solution. Test stimuli were present during the 2nd incubation period. Given are means $\pm$ SEM (n=3-4) of the outflow of HPLC-separated ^3H-compounds during the 2nd incubation period expressed as % of the respective value of the first period. PGs: PGE_2/D_2; 52 min: unidentified peak with HPLC retention time of 52 min; L-M: sum of lipophilic metabolites (HPLC retention time between 65-80 min).

TABLE 2: Effects of the ionophore A 23187 (10 μM) and phorbol 12-myristate 13-acetate (PMA, 100 nM) on the release of AA metabolites from rat alveolar macrophages (AM) labelled with ^{3}H-AA.

	TxB$_2$	Pgs	LTB$_4$	L-M	AA	
Ctr.	63 ± 10	116 ± 48	195 ± 53	79 ± 26	106 ± 48	%
A 23187	1.040 ± 351	1.170 ± 340	41.000 ± 11.000	2.690 ± 857	394 ± 54	%
PMA	434 ± 137	727 ± 233	97 ± 17	605 ± 98	289 ± 80	%

AM, labelled with ^{3}H-AA were incubated for 3 consecutive 1 h periods. Test stimuli were present during the 2nd incubation period. Given are means$\pm$SEM (n=3-4) of the outflow of HPLC separated ^{3}H-compounds during the 2nd incubation period expressed as % of the respective value of the first period. PGs: sum of PGE$_2$/D$_2$ and PGF$_{2\alpha}$; L-M: sum of lipophilic metabolites (HPLC retention time between 65-80 min)

CONCLUSIONS

In AM and tracheal epithelial cells protein kinase C and intracellular free calcium differentially activate cyclo-oxygenase and lipoxygenase pathways of AA metabolism in a cell-specific manner.

AM can cause marked liberation of AA from tracheal epithelial cells, and this is accompanied by an enhanced formation of prostaglandins and different other AA metabolites. Humoral factors as well as cell to cell interactions appear to be involved in the described effects of AM.

ACKNOWLEDGMENTS

Supported by the Deutsche Forschungsgemeinschaft (Ra 400/3-2).

REFERENCES

1 Emura, M., Riebe M, Ochiai M, Aufderheide M, Germann P, Mohr U. New functional cell-culture approach to pulmonary carcinogenesis and toxicology. *Cancer Res Clin Oncol* 1990;116:557-62.

2 Fels A A S, Cohn ZA. The alveolar macrophage. *J Appl Physiol* 1986; 60:353-369.

3 Lechner JF, LaVeck MA. A serum-free method for culturing normal bronchial epithelial cells. *J Tissue Cult Methods* 1985;9:43-8.

4 Lee TH, Lane SJ. The role of macrophages in the mechanisms of airway inflammation in asthma. *Am Rev Resp Dis* 1992; 145:S27-S30.

5 Racké K, Bähring J, Langer C, Bräutigam M, Wessler I. Prostanoids inhibit release of endogenous norepinephrine from rat isolated trachea. *Am Rev Resp Dis* 1992;146:1182-86.

6 Raeburn D. Eicosanoids, epithelium and airway reactivity. *Gen Pharmac* 1990; 21:11-16.

7 van Scott MR, McIntire MR, Henke DC. Arachidonic acid metabolism and regulation of ion transport in rabbit Clara cells. *Am J Physiol* 1990; 259:L213-L221.

Advances in Prostaglandin, Thromboxane,
and Leukotriene Research, Vol. 23,
edited by B. Samuelsson et al.
Raven Press, Ltd., New York © 1995

Airway hyperresponsiveness induced by 13-hydroxyoctadecadienoic acid (13-HODE) is mediated by sensory neuropeptides

Ferdi Engels, Anneke H. van Houwelingen
Theresa L. Buckley, Marco J. van de Velde
Paul A.J. Henricks and Frans P. Nijkamp

*Department of Pharmacology, Utrecht Institute for Pharmaceutical Sciences
Utrecht University, P.O. Box 80082, 3508 TB Utrecht, The Netherlands*

Asthma is a multifactorial disease and is characterized by direct airway narrowing due to smooth muscle spasm, thickening of the submucosa and airway plugging with mucus. Many asthmatics also suffer from airway hyperresponsiveness, i.e. they display an exaggerated airway narrowing after inhaling contractile stimuli. Indeed, the acute and long-term effect of antiasthma drugs in reducing airway hyperresponsiveness is considered an important factor with respect to their clinical effectiveness. Both neural mechanisms and humoral factors are involved in the regulation of normal airway calibre. Dysregulation of these systems may be responsible for airway hyperresponsiveness. Thus, the hypothesis of an imbalance between excitatory and inhibitory autonomic nervous pathways has been the subject of much research over the years [1]. Current thinking, however, suggests that these abnormalities are likely to be secondary to the disease, rather than primary defects. It is possible that airway inflammation may interfere with autonomic control by the action of several inflammatory and immune cell types and their mediators [1]. Indeed, airway hyperresponsiveness is often associated with local inflammatory reactions. Lipid mediators originating from inflammatory and immune cells, including arachidonic acid-derived products like prostaglandins, thromboxanes, and leukotrienes, but also platelet-activating-factor (PAF), have been clearly shown to be able to induce airway hyperresponsiveness [2]. Surprisingly, lipid mediators derived from the unsaturated fatty acid linoleic acid, e.g. 13-hydroxyoctadecadienoic acid (13-HODE), have not been the subject of much research in relation to airway reactivity, notwithstanding the fact that these mediators are formed by several cell types within the respiratory tract [3,4]. We have recently shown that 13-HODE, when administered via an aerosol, is able to induce airway hyperresponsiveness to histamine in guinea pigs *in vivo* [5]. The goal of the present experiments was to gain insight into the mechanisms by which 13-HODE can induce hyperresponsiveness in isolated guinea pig tracheal tissues. Our results suggest that 13-HODE- induced hyperresponsiveness is mediated/modulated by the release of neuropeptides from sensory nerve endings.

MATERIAL AND METHODS

Tracheas from male Dunkin-Hartley guinea pigs were cut into pieces containing two cartilage rings. From each trachea, three preparations were obtained from both the proximal and the distal part. The tracheal preparations were mounted in organ baths containing Krebs solution and the development of tension by the tracheal preparations was measured by an isometric smooth muscle transducer. The experimental protocol included (1) a 15 min equilibration period, during which 2000 mg tension was applied to the tracheal preparation, (2) a 15 min period during which 4000 mg tension was applied in order to increase the stability of the preparation, and (3) a 45 min equilibration period during which 2000 mg tension was applied to the tracheal preparation again. Subsequently, the tracheal preparations were incubated for 30 min with 1 μM 13-HODE or vehicle. Finally, a concentration-response curve for histamine was constructed. The contractile responses to histamine were analyzed by a computerized iterative non-linear curve fitting routine based on the 4-parameter logistic equation.

RESULTS AND DISCUSSION

Incubation of tracheal preparations with 13-HODE for 30 min resulted in a small but reproducable decrease of the smooth muscle tension. Subsequent applications of increasing concentrations of histamine indicated that 13-HODE did not have an effect on the tracheal sensitivity to histamine (no changes in EC_{50} values), but significantly enhanced the maximal development of tension in response to histamine. The enhancement was only seen with tracheal preparations that were taken from the distal part of the tissue (see table I). These results indicate that 13-HODE not only can induce airway hyperresponsiveness to histamine *in vivo* [5], but also is able to increase histamine responsiveness *in vitro*. The finding that 13-HODE only affects the distal part of the trachea might point to the involvement of sensory nerve endings which contain neuropeptides like the tachykinins substance P and neurokinin A. Indeed, it has been shown that the release of substance P-like immunoreactivity from sensory nerve endings was particularly abundant in the lower tracheal and bronchial tissues [6]. To substantiate the involvement of neuropeptides from sensory nerve endings in the 13-HODE-induced hyperresponsiveness, two different approaches were followed: (1) tracheal preparations were depleted of neuropeptides by *in vitro* treatment with capsaicin, and (2) an antagonist of NK_1/NK_2 tachykinin receptors, FK224 [7] (generous gift of Fujisawa Pharmaceutical Co., Osaka, Japan), was used to prevent the activity of tachykinins after their release. We observed that 13-HODE-induced hyperresponsiveness was completely abolished both by capsaicin treatment and by FK224. These findings confirm our hypothesis that neuropeptides from sensory nerve endings play a role in 13-HODE-induced airway hyperresponsiveness. Interestingly, peptidergic neural pathways have also been implicated in some pulmonary actions of other lipid mediators such as eicosanoids and PAF [8].

Table I.   The effect of 13-HODE on the maximal development of tension of guinea pig tracheal preparations in response to histamine.

| | maximal tension (mgf) | |
	proximal	distal
control	1647 ± 80	1539 ± 115
13-HODE	1853 ± 114	2061 ± 151*

* $p < 0.05$ with Student's unpaired t-test, n=6-7

REFERENCES

1.   Barnes PJ. Modulation of neurotransmission in airways. *Physiol Rev* 1992;72:699-729.
2.   Arm JP. Lipoxygenase derivatives in asthma. In: Tarayre JP, Vargaftig B, Carilla E *New Concepts in Asthma.* London: The Macmillan Press Ltd., 1993:114-36.
3.   Oosthuizen MJ, Engels F, van Esch B, Henricks PAJ, Nijkamp FP. Production of arachidonic acid and linoleic acid metabolites by guinea pig tracheal epithelial cells. *Inflammation* 1990;14:401-8.
4.   Engels F, Kessels GCR, Schreurs AJM, Nijkamp FP. Production of arachidonic acid and linoleic acid metabolites by human bronchoalveolar lavage cells. *Prostaglandins* 1991;42:441-50.
5.   Henricks PAJ, Engels F, Van der Linde HJ, Nijkamp FP. 13-Hydroxy-linoleic acid induces airway hyperreactivity to histamine in guinea-pigs. *Eur J Pharmacol* 1991;197:233-4.
6.   Manzini S, Conti S, Maggi CA, Abelli L, Somma V, Del Bianco E, Geppetti P. Regional differences in the motor and inflammatory responses to capsaicin in guinea pig airways. *Am Rev Respir Dis* 1989;140:936-41.
7.   Hirayama Y, Lei Y-H, Barnes PJ, Rogers DF. Effects of two novel tachykinin antagonists, FK224 and FK888, on neurogenic airway plasma exudation, bronchoconstriction and systemic hypotension in guinea-pigs *in vivo. Br J Pharmacol* 1993;108:844-51.
8.   Manzini S, Perretti F, Meini S. Interactions between sensory neuropeptides and lipid mediators in the airways. *J Lipid Mediators* 1993;8:67-79.

Advances in Prostaglandin, Thromboxane, and Leukotriene Research, Vol. 23,
edited by B. Samuelsson et al.
Raven Press, Ltd., New York © 1995

Furosemide Attenuates Bronchial Responsiveness To Antigen Challenge "In Vitro"

Giancarlo Folco, Manlio Bolla, Elena Santinelli, Sebastiano Bianco*, Piersante Sestini**, Maurizio Mezzetti° and Angelo Sala.

*Center for Cardiopulmonary Pharmacology, Inst. of Pharmacological Sciences, Univ. of Milan, 20133 Milan, *S. Raffaele Hospital, Milan, **Inst. of Respir. Dis., Univ. of Siena, °Division of Thoracic Surgery, Policlinico di Milano, Italy*

Sulfidopeptide leukotrienes (LT) are synthesized by numerous cell types and exert potent biological effects in the immediate surrounding of their site of synthesis. Substantial evidence is available on the potential role of LT in various lung diseases such as asthma; in fact LT have been detected in bronchoalveolar lavages from atopic patients following local challenge with specific antigen (1).

The search for new therapies to asthma has remarkably increased over the last two decades in line with our deeper understanding of the pathophysiology of the disease. Recently novel perspectives in the treatment of allergic asthma have attracted interest; inhaled furosemide (F), a loop diuretic that can interfere with ion and water transport across airway epithelium, has been proved to exert protective effects on allergen-induced early and late asthmatic reactions (2), as well as on bronchoconstriction induced by exercise (3).

In the present paper we report that furosemide significantly attenuate the LT-dependent maximal contraction obtained with antigen challenge in isolated, human bronchial strips; this effect was partially reversed by indomethacin.

METHODS

Bronchi (internal caliber of 2-3 mm) were isolated following surgery for bronchial carcinoma or bronchiectasis and spiralized to obtain a strip 2-3 mm wide and of varying length (2-3 cm). Strips were suspended under isometric tension of 500 mg, at 37°, in a Krebs-Henseleit solution and, whenever necessary, medicated with indomethacin (10 µM) and pyrilamine (1 µM). After a resting period of 1 hour, tissue contractilitya was tested using cumulative concentrations of acetylcholine (Ach, 10-300 µM) . After washing and recovery of basal tension, strips were treated with F or blank solution for 30' and challenged with a specific anti-human IgE antibody (0.01-1.0 µg/ml).

RESULTS

Immunological challenge of isolated human bronchial strips, evoked a

contraction which was slow in onset and sustained. F (0.1-1.0 mM), antagonized
the increase in bronchial tone caused by the anti-human IgE antibody (Fig. 1A).
Reference contractions of bronchial strips induced by Ach were also

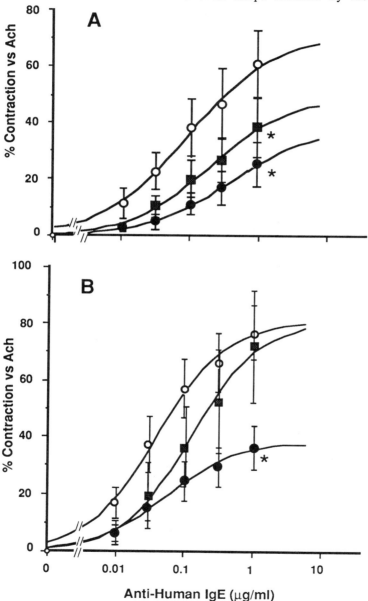

Fig 1: Effect of F, 0.1 mM (solid squares) and 1.0 mM (solid circles), on the
contraction of isolated, human bronchial strips, induced by immunological
challenge (open circles). * p<0.05   Panel **A**: untreated human bronchial strips.
Panel **B**: human bronchial strips pretreated with pyrilamine (1µM) and
indomethacin (10µM).

non-competitively antagonized by 0.1 mM F only, while the maximal contraction observed with a non receptor-mediated agonist, ($BaCl_2$, 30 mM), was unaffected.

Pretreatment of bronchial specimens with antihistamine and indomethacin, made the anti-IgE-induced bronchial contraction specifically LT-dependent, since the contractile tone was fully reverted by specific, LTD_4 receptor antagonists, compound LY171883 (10 µM) and SKF 104353 (1 µM). F (0.1 mM) did not alter the basal tone of the preparations and caused a non significant shift to the right of the dose response curve obtained with antigen challenge (Fig.1B) without affecting maximal contractile response. F, at 1 mM only, caused a slight drop of the basal tone of the preparation and decreased significantly the anti-IgE-induced contraction of human bronchial tissue (Fig. 1B).

DISCUSSION

The present results indicate that F, at 0.1 mM, attenuates the immunologic contraction of human, isolated bronchi; a possible involvement of bronchodilatory prostaglandins is likely, in light of the reversal of this effect with indomethacin, according with data recently reported by Pavor et al. (4). However, at 1 mM, a direct effect of F on bronchial contractility is plausible, since F was able to affect non-competitively the tissue response to Ach, in agreement with data showing direct airway smooth muscle relaxation by F. Moreover aerosolized F has been reported to increase the PD_{20} values for methacoline in healthy volunteers, although this was not observed in asthmatic patients.

F, at 0.1 mM, causes a non-significant rightward shift of the LT-dependent contractile response of human bronchial strips to antigen challenge, while, at 1.0 mM, a significant inhibition of the maximal bronchial contraction is observed.

The concentration of F utilized in these experiments is within the range attainable in the epithelial lining fluid *in vivo*. Knowles and coll. (5), after aerosol administration of amiloride, estimated a drug concentration on airway surfaces which was diluted approximately 50 folds when compared to the solution delivered. This would result, in our case, in a concentration of 0.6 mM of F.

Taken together our results suggest that:
- a direct effect of F on human bronchial smooth muscle contractility takes place
- an involvement of bronchodilatory prostanoids is likely.

REFERENCES

1. Miadonna A, Tedeschi A, Brasca C, Folco GC, Sala A, Murphy RC. Mediator release after endobronchial antigen challenge in patients with respiratory allergy. *J Allergy Clin Immunol* 1990; 85(5): 906-913.
2. Bianco S, Pieroni MG, Refini RM, Rottoli L, Sestini P. Protective effect of inhaled furosemide on allergen induced early and late asthmatic reactions. *N Eng J Med* 1989; 321:1069-1073
3. Bianco S, Vaghi A, Robuschi M, and Pasargiklian M. Prevention of exercise-induced bronchoconstriction by inhaled frusemide. *The Lancet* 1988; II:252-5.
4. Pavord I, Holland D, Baldwin A, Tattersfield A, Knox A. The effects of diuretics on allergen-induced contractions of passively sensitized human bronchi in vitro. *Am. Rev. Resp. Dis.* 1993; 147(4): A839.
5. Knowles MR, Church NL, Waltner WE, et al. A pilot study of aerosolized amiloride for the treatment of lung disease in cystic fibrosis. *N Engl J Med* 1990; 322: 1189-94.

Advances in Prostaglandin, Thromboxane,
and Leukotriene Research, Vol. 23,
edited by B. Samuelsson et al.
Raven Press, Ltd., New York © 1995

THROMBOXANE BIOSYNTHESIS AND PULMONARY FUNCTION IN CYSTIC FIBROSIS

Giovanni Davì, Luciana Iapichino, Vincenzo Balsamo, Antonina Ganci, Carlo Giammarresi, Paola Patrignani and Carlo Patrono.

Departments of Medicine and Pharmacology, University of Chieti and the Cystic Fibrosis Center, Di Cristina Hospital, Palermo, Italy.

Cystic fibrosis (CF) is the most common autosomal recessive genetic disorder occurring in the caucasian population[1]. The disease is characterized by an exocrine dysfunction, impairment of electrolyte transport and abnormal mucus secretion[2]. Its pulmonary manifestations include airway obstruction by thick, tenacious secretions and recurrent respiratory infections eventually perpetuating airway and pulmonary parenchimal injury[2].

The defective gene responsible for cystic fibrosis[3] encodes for a protein of 1480 amino-acids called the cystic fibrosis transmembrane conductance regulator. This protein is likely to represent a dysregulated chloride channel, but may also be involved in the control of arachidonic acid release through its annexin-like sequence[4].

The majority of patients with cystic fibrosis die in early adulthood from respiratory failure associated with pulmonary hypertension and cor pulmonale. Patients with a forced expiratory volume in one second (FEV_1) less than 30 percent of the predicted value have a 50 percent chance of dying within two years[5].

An increase in the excretion of 11-dehydro-thromboxane B_2, a major enzymatic metabolite of the vasoconstrictor and bronchoconstrictor thromboxane A_2, occurs in both primary and secondary forms of pulmonary hypertension[6]. Whether enhanced thromboxane biosynthesis is a cause or a result of pulmonary hypertension is unknown, but it may play a part in the development and maintenance of both forms of the disorder[6]. Previous studies in patients with cystic fibrosis have suggested altered platelet behavior, as reflected by ex-vivo measurements of platelet aggregation and eicosanoid production[7]. Platelet-derived thromboxane A_2 might exert local contractile effects on pulmonary blood vessels and bronchial smooth muscle, possibly contributing to the pathophysiology of CF.

In the present study, we sought to determine whether the formation of thromboxane is altered in vivo through measurements of a major enzymatic metabolite of thromboxane B_2 in the urine of patients with cystic fibrosis. Moreover, we attempted to correlate these biochemical measurements with the degree of pulmonary dysfunction.

DESIGN OF THE STUDIES

We studied 19 patients with cystic fibrosis (8 women and 11 men, 6 to 23 years of age), attending the Cystic Fibrosis Center of Di Cristina Children's Hospital. The diagnosis of cystic fibrosis was based on typical clinical findings or a family history of cystic fibrosis together with an abnormal sweat chloride value[1]. Genotyping was performed in 15 of the 19 patients. All were undergoing frequent, routine assessment of their pancreatic and pulmonary function. The FEV_1, and SaO_2 were measured in order to evaluate the degree of decline in pulmonary function. Patients were followed-up on average for 35 months after measurement of thromboxane metabolite excretion. Seven died during follow-up and one underwent lung transplantation. Nineteen healthy subjects (8 women and 11 men) with a similar age distribution (range 7-20 years of age) were also studied as controls. Patients and controls were asked to abstain from taking aspirin-like drugs during 10 days prior to urine sampling.

In the first phase of the study, a comparison of 11-dehydro-thromboxane B_2 excretion and in vitro platelet function was performed in 15 cystic fibrosis patients and 15 controls. Immunoreactive 11-dehydro-TXB_2 was extracted and measured as previously described[8].

To characterize the enhanced biosynthesis of thromboxane in patients with cystic fibrosis as being primarily of platelet or non-platelet origin, we evaluated the short-term effects of a relatively platelet-selective regimen of aspirin therapy (50 mg per day for seven days) on the degree of suppression and the recovery of 11-dehydro-thromboxane B_2 excretion in three cystic fibrosis patients (2 M, 1 F; aged 7 to 20 years).

RESULTS AND DISCUSSION

Results from the first phase of the study indicated an abnormally high 11-dehydro-thromboxane B_2 excretion and normal platelet function in cystic fibrosis patients. In fact, urinary immunoreactive 11-dehydro-thromboxane B_2 averaged 56.1±31.7 ng/hr (mean±SD) in cystic fibrosis patients and 16.8±5.0 ng/hr in controls ($p<0.001$). The urinary excretion of 11-dehydro-thromboxane B_2 was inversely related to both $FEV1$ and SaO_2 to a statistically significant extent ($r = -0.777$, $P=0.0001$ and $r = -0.462$, $P=0.046$, respectively).

All pts with FEV_1 less than 50 percent of the predicted value had metabolite excretion in excess of 2SD above the normal mean.

At variance with the in vivo evidence of enhanced thromboxane biosynthesis, ex vivo capacity measurements of platelet function did not reveal any abnormality in cystic fibrosis. Thus, the threshold aggregating concentrations of arachidonate, ADP, collagen and epinephrine as well as collagen- and arachidonate-induced thromboxane B_2 production in platelet-rich plasma were not significantly different in patients and controls.

Before aspirin administration, the rate of metabolite excretion averaged 75.3±21.2 ng/hr. At the end of one week of aspirin administration, 11-dehydro-thromboxane B_2 excretion was significantly reduced to 15.5±5.8 ng/hr ($P<0.01$) and the recovery of metabolite excretion was slow upon aspirin withdrawal (49 percent and 77 percent of the baseline excretion rate at 4 and 8 days, respectively). This finding is consistent with the time-dependent return of unacetylated platelet cyclooxygenase and the capacity for synthesis of thromboxane B_2 to the systemic circulation on withdrawal of aspirin administration[9].

At least two distinct mechanisms might account for enhanced thromboxane biosynthesis in this setting. Firstly, a persistent activation of platelets has been suggested to occur in association with a sustained elevation of pulmonary artery pressure, regardless of the cause[6]. This in turn may reflect the endothelial dysfunction described in patients with chronic obstructive lung disease, including patients with end-stage cystic fibrosis[10]. Impairment of the synthesis and release of endothelium-derived relaxing factor and prostacyclin from pulmonary endothelial cells might contribute to local platelet activation. Secondly, infection and the ensuing inflammatory response, that are considered to be the proximate cause of lung destruction in cystic fibrosis, are self-sustaining because of defective clearance of pseudomonas and other organisms from the lung[11].

The results of the low-dose aspirin study are consistent with the hypothesis that enhanced thromboxane metabolite excretion reflects to a large extent platelet thromboxane biosynthesis because of the profound suppression by aspirin as well as the time-dependent pattern of recovery of 11-dehydro-thromboxane B$_2$ excretion upon drug withdrawal.

The potential functional consequences of enhanced synthesis and release of thromboxane A$_2$ are related to its being a potent inducer of irreversible platelet aggregation, vasoconstriction and broncho-constriction as well as having a promitogenic effect on airway smooth muscle cells. Whether any of these effects play a role in the functional and structural changes characteristic of cystic fibrosis remains to be determined.

REFERENCES

1. Rosenstein BJ. The spectrum of cystic fibrosis mutations. Lancet 1994; 343: 746-7.

2. Weinberger SE. Recent advances in pulmonary medicine. N Engl J Med 1993; 928: 1389-97.

3. Rommens JM, Iannuzzi MC, Kerem B et al. Identification of the cystic fibrosis gene: chromosome walking and jumping. Science 1989; 245: 1059-65.

4. Levistre R, Lemnaouar ML, Rybkine T, Biriziat G, Masliah J. Increase of bradykinin-stimulated arachidonic acid release in a DF508 cystic fibrosis epithelial cell line. Biochim Biophys Acta 1993; 1181: 233-9.

5. Kerem E, Reisman J, Corey M, Canny GJ, Levison H. Prediction of mortality in patients with cystic fibrosis. N Engl J Med 1992; 326: 1187-91.

6. Christman BW, McPherson CD, Newman JH, et al. An imbalance between the excretion of thromboxane and prostacyclin metabolites in pulmonary hypertension. N Engl J Med 1992, 327: 70-5.

7. Stead RJ, Barradas MA, Mikhailidis DP et al. Platelet hyperaggregability in cystic fibrosis. Prostaglandins Leukotrienes and Medicine 1987; 26: 91-103.

8. Davì G, Catalano I, Averna M, et al. Thromboxane biosynthesis and platelet function in type-II diabetes mellitus. N Engl J Med 1990; 322:1769-74.

9. Patrignani P, Filabozzi P, Patrono C. Selective cumulative inhibition of platelet thromboxane production by low-dose aspirin in healthy subjects. J Clin Invest 1982; 69: 1366-72.

10. Dinh-Xuan AT, Higenbottam TW, Clelland CA, et al. Impairment of endothelium-dependent pulmonary-artery relaxation in chronic obstructive lung disease. N Engl J Med 1991; 324: 1539-47.

11. Davis PB. Cystic fibrosis from bench to bedside. N Engl J Med 1991; 325: 575-6.

Advances in Prostaglandin, Thromboxane,
and Leukotriene Research, Vol. 23,
edited by B. Samuelsson et al.
Raven Press, Ltd., New York © 1995

Lupus Anticoagulant IgGs do not depend on serum for the induction of Cyclooxygenase-2 by Human Endothelial Cells

Aïda Habib[1], Marta Martinuzzo[2], Marilyne Lebret[1], Sylviane Lévy-Toledano[1], Luis O. Carreras[2] and Jacques Maclouf[1]

[1]*U 348 INSERM, Hôpital Lariboisière, 75475 Paris cedex 10 France and* [2]*University Institute of Biomedical Sciences, Fundación Favaloro, 1078 Buenos Aires, Argentina*

Antiphospholipid (aPL) antibodies have been characterized by their reactivity with negatively charged phospholipids *in vitro*. The association of these antibodies with clinical problems such as thrombosis or fetal loss in patients with the aPL syndrome is still not elucidated. However, their capacity to affect the generation of eicosanoids such as thromboxane (TX) or prostacyclin, deriving respectively from platelets and vascular cells seemed to provide a reasonable basis to explain some of the clinical manifestations of this syndrome. An increased formation of TXA_2 could reflect the thrombotic tendency and contribute to the thromboembolic complications of these patients. Asumptions concerning the role of prostacyclin and TXA_2 during pregnancy and fetal life also explained the obstetric complications in patients with lupus anticoagulant (LA) (1). In a recent study we found a significant increase in urinary excretion of platelet-derived metabolites, with a smaller increase in the vascular cell metabolite 2,3-dinor-6-keto-$PGF_{1\alpha}$, suggesting an imbalance of the TXA_2/PGI_2 equilibrium without inhibition of vascular PGI_2 (2). The *ex vivo* evaluation of sera or purified IgGs from these patients on defined *in vitro* systems such as platelets or vascular cells has also been evaluated. Contradictory findings have been published on the effect of sera or immunoglobulin fractions containing LA or aPL antibodies on prostacyclin production from vascular cells (3). Clearly, the heterogeneity of the syndrome and/or criteria for diagnosis and the diversity of the methodology may affect the outcome of the final response. We have shown recently in normal donors an increase of thrombin-induced platelet aggregation, serotonin release and TX synthesis by $F(ab')_2$ from IgGs of six patients with LA (4) suggesting that these antibodies may promote the thrombotic tendency of affected patients.

Recent data on the regulation of cyclooxygenases (Cox) by nucleated cells have expanded the possibilities of the rate-limiting steps participating in the formation of PGs (5). In addition to constitutive Cox-1, endothelial cells also contain an inducible form of the enzyme which is the product of a primary response gene: Cox-2 (6). This novel Cox allows the cell to modify rapidly its capacity to generate PGs with a nearly total absence of variation of Cox-1 (7). Novel data support the concept that aPL antibodies may also recognize a variety of protein-phospholipid complexes as recently demonstrated for ß-2-glycoprotein I (8). Such findings may indicate that subgroups of patients' IgGs recognizing other epitopes, could account for the heterogeneity of the syndrome. We have shown elsewhere that in a series of 9 patients presenting the aPL syndrome, most of the patients IgGs can promote the synthesis of Cox-2 in human endothelial cells (Habib et al. submitted). We undertook this study to evaluate the influence of serum impact on the induction of Cox-2 by patients' IgGs in endothelial cells.

Incubation of a patient's IgGs with HUVEC was performed in the presence of 5% serum (usual conditions) or 0.7% bovine serum albumin (compatible with the cell viability for short times of incubation, i.e. less than 6 h). Although serum alone induces the expression of Cox-2 (7), the patients' IgGs stimulated the induction of Cox-2 (see figure 1, lanes 1 and 2) compared to controls, irrespective of the incubation medium.

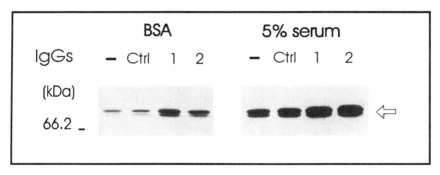

FIG.1 Effect of serum on the induction of Cox-2 in HUVEC by aPL IgGs. HUVEC were incubated in the absence or presence of IgGs in either 0.7% BSA or 5% human serum. After 6-h incubation, cell monolayers were washed, lyzed, run on a SDS-PAGE; transfer and visualization of the immune complexes was done as described previously (7). *(-)*, no addition; ***Ctrl***, pool of normal IgGs; ***1 and 2***, patients' IgGs.

When albumin was used rather than serum, the responses varied very little, suggesting that removal of serum factors did not affect the reactivity of the patients

IgGs. However, residual ß-2-glycoprotein I could still be present on the surface of endothelial cells at a sufficient concentration and this interaction may account for this effect. We also possess substantial support for recognition of the phospholipid epitope based on the important neutralization of the effect of the antibodies by preincubation with phospholipids using either micelles or liposomes (9).

ACKNOWLEDGMENTS

This work was performed as part of an exchange program between INSERM, France and CONICET, Argentina; it was supported in part by grants from the Association pour la Recherche sur le Cancer (ARC) (grant 2076). A.H. is supported by a scholarship from Association Sanofi Thrombose pour la Recherche (Sanofi, Paris).

REFERENCES

1. Carreras LO and Vermylen J. "Lupus" anticoagulant and thrombosis. Possible role of inhibition of prostacyclin formation. *Thromb Haemostas.* 1982;48:38-40.
2. Lellouche F, Martinuzzo ME, Said P, Maclouf J, and Carreras LO. Imbalance of thromboxane/prostacyclin biosynthesis in patients with lupus anticoagulant. *Blood* 1991;78:2894-2899.
3. Carreras LO and Maclouf J. The lupus anticoagulant and eicosanoids. *Prostaglandins, Leukotrienes and Essential Fatty Acids* 1993;49:483-488.
4. Martinuzzo ME, Maclouf J, Carreras LO and Lévy-Toledano S. Antiphospholipid antibodies enhance thrombin-induced platelet activation and thromboxane formation. *Thromb. Haemostas.* 1993;70: 667-6711.
5. Smith WL. Prostanoid biosynthesis and mechanisms of action. *Am. J. Physiol.* 1992;263:F181-F191.
6. Jones DA, Carlton DP, McIntyre TM, Zimmerman GA and Prescott SM. Molecular cloning of human prostaglandin endoperoxide synthase Type II and demonstration of expression in response to cytokines. *J. Biol. Chem.* 1993;268:9049-9054.
7. Habib A, Creminon C, Frobert Y, Grassi J, Pradelles P, and Maclouf J. Demonstration of an inducible cyclooxygenase in human endothelial cells using antibodies raised against the C-terminal region of the cyclooxygenase-2. *J. Biol. Chem.* 1993;268:23448-23454.
8. Galli M, Comfurius P, Maassen C et al. Anticardiolipin antibodies (ACA) directed not to cardiolipin but to a plasma protein cofactor. *Lancet* 1990;335: 1544-1547.
9. Pierangeli SS, Harris EN, Gharavi AE, Goldsmith G, Branch DW, and Dean WL. Are immunoglobulins with lupus anticoagulant activity specific for phospholipids? *Br. J. Haematol.* 1993;85: 124-132

Advances in Prostaglandin, Thromboxane, and Leukotriene Research, Vol. 23,
edited by B. Samuelsson et al.
Raven Press, Ltd., New York © 1995

RESTORATION OF PROSTACYCLIN SYNTHESIS BY TRANSFER OF PROSTAGLANDIN H SYNTHASE cDNA.

K.K. Wu, P. Zoldhelyi, J.T. Willerson, R. Meidell, J. McNatt and X-M Xu

Department of Internal Medicine, Division of Hematology, The University of Texas Health Science Center at Houston Medical School, Houston, Texas 77030

Endothelium is endowed with a number of molecules which play important roles in protecting blood vessels and maintaining blood fluidity (1). Among these molecules, prostacyclin is a potent inhibitor of platelet aggregation and activation, vasoconstriction and smooth muscle cell proliferation (1,2). Its continuous synthesis is probably responsible for maintaining vascular wall integrity. Endothelial dysfunction and/or depletion due to injury may result in a comprised production of PGI_2 leading to uncontrolled platelet aggregation and vascular lesions. Because of its potent biological action and physiological importance, PGI_2 and its analogs have been administered systematically for treatment of vascular diseases. The therapeutic efficacy has been marginal because PGI_2 acts as an autacoid with extremely short half-life (3,4). To achieve therapeutic efficacy, a large dose of PGI_2 or stable analogs is required which is accompanied by undesirable side effects. A reasonable strategy is to deliver PGI_2 locally or to augment its synthesis in situ at the vascular lesion.

Availability of viral vectors has rendered the approach of augmenting PGI_2 synthesis in situ possible. As biosynthesis of PGI_2 is catalyzed serially by 3 enzymes, selection of the rate-limiting enzyme for gene transfer is critical for maximal formation of PGI_2. Prostaglandin H synthase (PGHS) undergoes inactivation during catalysis and is considered to be the key rate limiting step. There are two isoforms of PGHS. PGHS-1 is constitutively expressed and physiologically important whereas PGHS-2 is inducible and is thought to be involved in pathophysiological processes such as inflammation.

As PGHS-1 is the constitutive PGHS in vascular endothelial cells, it is, a candidate for gene transfer. To test this hypothesis, we transferred PGHS-1 cDNA into an endothelial cell line, EA.hy926 by a retroviral vector, BAG (5).

The PGHS-1 expression in this cell line was increased by 20-30 fold accompanied by a marked increase in the PGI_2 synthesis in response to physiologic agonists. To determine whether an increased basal level of PGHS-1 prolonged the duration of PGHS catalytic activity and therefore increased not only the extent but also the duration of PGI_2 synthesis, we challenged the transfected cells repeatedly with AA or ionophore hourly and measured the ability of the cells to continue to respond to these stimuli. This PGHS-1 augmented cell line showed only partial (30%) inactivation of the enzyme for each catalysis. Therefore, the duration of PGI_2 synthesis is closely related to the enzyme mass. These results confirm the notion that enhanced PGHS-1 expression is not only associated with a higher extent but also a more prolonged synthesis of PGI_2. These data give credence for transferring PGHS-1 to augment PGI_2 synthesis.

Although earlier studies showed promising ß-galactosidase transfer data with autologous endothelial cell transfer by retrovirus (6-8), its low transfecting efficiency renders its use in direct in vivo vascular gene transfer unsatisfactory (9,10). We, therefore, evaluated the transfer of PGHS-1 by an adenoviral vector which was prepared by homologous recombination described previously (11). Treatment of cultured endothelial cells with adenovirus carrying PGHS-1 cDNA (Ad-CMV-PGHS-1) for 48 h resulted in a large increase in PGI_2 synthesis when the transfected cells were stimulated with ionophore or AA. Analysis of eicosanoids by reverse-phase HPLC shows concomitant increases in PGE_2 and $PGF_{2\alpha}$. Increase in the enzyme activity was accompanied by an increase in PGHS-1 mRNA.

To determine whether Ad-CMV-PGHS-1 transfers PGHS-1 cDNA into the vascular cells at the damaged vessel wall and restores PGI_2 synthesis effectively, we administered Ad-CMV-PGHS-1 to the porcine carotid arterial segments damaged by crush injury via a perforated catheter for 30 min. Animals were sacrificed on day 3, injured carotid arterial segments were dissected and PGI_2 synthesis by these segments in response to AA or ionophore was measured. PGI_2 productions were increased by 3-fold in Ad-CMV-PGHS-1 infected vessel when compared to those of control arteries. These results suggest that a 30-min administration of Ad-CMV-PGHS-1 may be sufficient to achieve a significant augmentation of PGI_2 synthesis by damaged vessel wall.

We have begun to determine whether restoration of PGI_2 by Ad-CMV-PGHS-1 is effective in preventing thrombus formation in a porcine carotid balloon-catheter angioplasty model. Balloon catheters were introduced into carotid arteries via transfemoral catheterization. Flow changes were monitored by Doppler continuously for 10 days. Ad-CMV-PGHS-1 or control were instilled into the damaged vessel wall for 30 min. Animals were sacrificed on day 10. The damaged vascular segments were dissected and their response to AA or ionophore was determined. There was a 5-fold increase in PGI_2 production in vessels infected with Ad-CMV-PGHS-1. Based on cyclic flow changes and histological examinations on day 10, there was a significant reduction in thrombosis in Ad-CMV-PGHS-1 treated pigs and the antithrombotic efficacy was related to Ad-CMV-PGHS-1 viral titers.

In summary, our findings indicate that overexpression of PGHS-1 leads to a significant increase in the extent and duration of PGI_2 production.

Adenoviral-mediated transfer of PGHS-1 to damaged vessel wall may prevent thrombosis in vivo. Gene transfer of PGHS-1 to the damaged vessel wall represents a new modality for treating arterial and microvascular thrombosis.

ACKNOWLEDGEMENTS

The authors thank Scott Biedermann and Nena Aleksic for technical assistance, Teri Trevino and Beverly Curbello for secretarial assistance. This work was supported by grants from U.S. National Institutes of Health (P50 NS-23327 to K.K. Wu, HL-50179 to J.T. Willerson, and HL-50675 to K.K. Wu).

REFERENCES

1. Wu KK. Endothelial cells in hemostasis, thrombosis and inflammation. Hospital Prac 1992;April 15:145-166.
2. Pomerantz KB, Hajjar DP. Eicosanoids in regulation of arterial smooth muscle cell phenotype, proliferative capacity and cholesterol metabolism. Arteriol 1989;9:413-29.
3. Szczeklik A, Grygleewski. Actions of prostacyclin in man. In:Vane JR, Bergström. *Prostacyclin*. New York: Raven Press; 1979:393-407.
4. Fressinger JN, Schäfer M. Trial of iloprost versus aspirin treatment for critical limb ischemia of thromboangiitis obliterans. Lancet 1990;335:555-7.
5. Xu X-M, Ohashi K, Sanduja SK, Ruan K-H, Wang L-H, Wu KK. Enhanced prostacyclin synthesis in endothelial cells by retrovirus-mediated transfer of Prostaglandin H synthase cDNA. J Clin Invest 1993;91:1843-49.
6. Nabel EG, Plantz G, Boyce FM, Stanley JC, Nabel GJ. Recombinant gene expression in vivo within endothelial cells of arterial wall. Science 1989;244:1342-44.
7. Zwiebel JA, Freeman SM, Kantoff PW, Cornetta K, Ryan US, Anderson WF. High-level recombinant gene expression in rabbit endothelial cells transduced by retroviral vectors. Science 1989;243:220-22.
8. Wilson JM, Birinyi LK, Salomon RN, Libby P, Callow AD, Mulligan RC. Implantation of vascular grafts lined with genetically modified endothelial cells. Science 1989;244:1344-46.
9. Flugelman MY, Jaklitsch MT, Newman KD, Casscells W, Bratthauer GL, Dichek DA. Low level in vivo gene transfer into the arterial wall through a perforated balloon catheter. Circulation 1992;85:1110-17.
10. Lim CS, Chapman GD, Gammon RS, Muhlestein JB, Bauman RP, Stack RS, Swain JL. Direct in vivo gene transfer into the coronary and peripheral vasulatures of the intact dog. Circulation 1991;83:2007-11.
11. Willard JE, Landau C, Glamann DB, Burns D, Jessen ME, Pirwitz MJ, Gerard RD, Meidell RS. Genetic modification of the vessel wall: comparison of surgical and catheter-based techniques for delivery of recombinant adenovirus. Circulation: in press.

*Advances in Prostaglandin, Thromboxane,
and Leukotriene Research, Vol. 23,*
edited by B. Samuelsson et al.
Raven Press, Ltd., New York © 1995

Expression of 15-lipoxygenase in Transplant Coronary Artery Disease

Stefano Ravalli, Charles C. Marboe, Vivette D. D'Agati, Elliott
Sigal, Robert E. Michler, Paul J. Cannon

*Departments of Medicine, Division of Cardiology (SR, PJC), Cardiothoracic Surgery
(REM) and Pathology (CCM, VDD), Columbia University College of Physicians and
Surgeons, New York, New York and Syntex Discovery Research (ES), Palo Alto,
California*

Coronary artery disease in the transplanted heart (TCAD) is currently the leading cause of death after the first post-transplant year and the most frequent cause of long-term cardiac allograft failure (1). The pathogenesis of TCAD is unclear. Established risk factors include: multiple episodes of rejection, cytomegalovirus infection and the development of serum antibodies directed against donor HLA alloantigens. The possible contribution of lipid peroxidation has not been extensively studied. In atherosclerosis, 15-lipoxygenase (15-LO), which catalyzes the oxygenation of arachidonic and linoleic acids, has been implicated in the oxidative modification of low density lipoprotein (LDL) (2). Recently, 15-LO mRNA and protein have been localized to macrophages in atherosclerotic lesions in humans and experimental animal models (3). The mechanisms of regulation of 15-LO expression are yet to be defined, but it appears that the enzyme is stimulated by the cytokine IL-4 and inhibited by γ-interferon (4). IL-4 levels have been reported to be higher in the coronary sinus blood than in arterial blood in patients following transplantation, despite adequate immunosuppression (5). Whether IL-4 induces 15-LO expression in the coronary arteries of transplanted hearts is unknown. Accordingly, the objective of this study was to determine whether 15-LO is present in the vascular lesions of TCAD.

METHODS

Coronary arteries were obtained from the explanted cardiac grafts of 8 patients undergoing retransplantation for TCAD and from the native hearts of 5 patients with ischemic heart disease (3), hypertrophic cardiomyopathy (1) and valvular heart disease (1). Immunohistochemistry was performed using the avidin-biotinylated horseradish peroxidase complex. A rabbit polyclonal antibody against human recombinant 15-LO was utilized in all cases. Macrophages, endothelial and smooth muscle cells were identified with specific monoclonal antibodies.

RESULTS

Normal coronary and pulmonary arteries had no detectable 15-LO expression. Two different types of TCAD were observed. The first one consisted of concentric proliferation of myointimal cells overlying an intact internal elastic lamina. Intra- or extracellular lipids or calcifications were not present in these lesions. There was no 15-LO immunoreactivity in this type of graft arteriosclerosis. The second form of TCAD consisted of lesions characteristic of complex atheromatous plaques, with lipid-filled foam cells, a fragmented internal elastic lamina, extracellular lipid deposits and patchy calcifications. Immunostaining for 15-LO was uniformly apparent in these "atheromatous" lesions. The 15-LO staining was prominent in spindle-shaped cells present throughout the intima, which were recognized by a monoclonal antibody to α-actin, establishing their origin from smooth muscle cells. Macrophages and foam cells also exhibited prominent 15-LO immunoreactivity. Surprisingly, the majority of 15-LO positive foam cells were of smooth muscle cell origin, while the remainder were macrophages. In the atheromatous form of TCAD, 15-LO immunostaining was also present in endothelial cells, although the intensity of staining varied significantly from one arterial region to another.

DISCUSSION

The present study demonstrates the expression of 15-LO in the lipid-rich, atheromatous form of TCAD. Using specific antibodies, 15-LO was localized to the cytoplasm of smooth muscle cells and macrophages. 15-LO staining of foam cells, the majority of which was of smooth muscle cell origin, was very prominent. Endothelial cells also stained positively for 15-LO in this type of lesion. No immunohistochemical evidence for 15-LO was found, on the other hand, in coronary arteries showing only myointimal hyperplasia.

The causes of TCAD are not well understood. Current theories suggest that chronic rejection to foreign HLA antigens expressed on graft vascular endothelial cells is associated with the release of cytokines. This in turn promotes the expression of growth factors which initiate intimal smooth muscle cell migration and proliferation (6). The absence of 15-LO staining in myointimal hyperplastic lesions suggests that the enzyme does not participate in their pathogenesis. In contrast, the intense immunostaining observed in the lipid-rich, atheromatous lesions indicates a possible role of 15-LO and lipid peroxidation. Since endothelial cells of normal vessels, medial smooth muscle cells and monocytes did not manifest 15-LO immunostaining, the data suggest that 15-LO expression is induced in the atheromatous lesions of TCAD. The nature of the signal for 15-LO expression in this context is unknown. Conceivably, it could be the cytokine IL-4, a product of the T_H2 subset of helper T lymphocytes, which is present in increased amounts in coronary sinus blood from cardiac allografts, even in adequately immunosuppressed patients (5). In conclusion, the present study suggests that 15-LO and lipid peroxidation may play a role in the development of the lipid-rich form of TCAD.

REFERENCES

1. Hosenpud JD, Shipley GD, Wagner CR. Cardiac allograft vasculopathy: current concepts, recent developments, and future directions. *J Heart Lung Transplant* 1992;11:9-23.
2. Witztum JL. Role of oxidized low density lipoprotein in atherogenesis. *Br Heart J* 1993; 69 (Supp):S12-S18.
3. Yla-Herttuala S, Rosenfeld ME, Parthasarathy S, et al. Gene expression in macrophage-rich human atherosclerotic lesions. 15-lipoxygenase and acetyl low density lipoprotein receptor messenger RNA colocalize with oxidation specific lipid-protein adducts. *J Clin Invest* 1991;87:1146-1152.
4. Conrad DJ, Kuhn H, Mulkins M, Highland E, Sigal E. Specific inflammatory cytokines regulate the expression of human monocyte 15-lipoxygenase. *Proc Natl Acad Sci USA* 1992;89:217-221.
5. Fyfe A, Daly P, Galligan L, Pirc L, Feindel C, Cardella C. Coronary sinus sampling of cytokines after heart transplantation: evidence for macrophage activation and interleukin-4 production within the graft. *J Am Coll Cardiol* 1993;21:171-176.
6. Salomon RN, Hughes CCW, Schoen FJ, Payne DD, Pober JS, Libby P. Human coronary transplantation-associated arteriosclerosis. Evidence for a chronic immune reaction to activated graft endothelial cells. *Am J Pathol* 1991;138:791-798.

Advances in Prostaglandin, Thromboxane, and Leukotriene Research, Vol. 23,
edited by B. Samuelsson et al.
Raven Press, Ltd., New York © 1995

Blood Cell-Vascular Wall Interactions And The Production Of Coronary Contracting Sulfidopeptide Leukotrienes in Isolated, Cell- Perfused, Rabbit Heart

Angelo Sala, Giuseppe Rossoni, Carola Buccellati, Tullio Testa, Ferruccio Berti, Jacques Maclouf[*] and Giancarlo Folco

Center for Cardiopulmonary Pharmacology, Inst. of Pharmacological Sciences, University of Milan, Milan 20133 Italy and [*]U-348 INSERM, Hopital Lariboisiere, Paris CEDEX 10, France

Leukotriene (LTs) formation may involve the participation of different cell types whereby donor cells (i.e. polymorphonuclear leukocytes, PMNL) synthesize and donate the unstable intermediate LTA_4 to acceptor cells (i.e. platelets, P; endothelial cells, EC) for further metabolism into LTC_4 (1). This process suggests that the cellular environment (i.e. cell-cell interactions) is an important control in the production of eicosanoids. Evidence obtained in our laboratory (2) suggests that challenge of PMNL present within the coronary vasculature, causes a LTD_4-dependent coronary vasoconstriction, favoured by uptake of PMNL-derived LTA_4 by endothelial cells. Peptide LTs appear to be released during episodes of myocardial ischemia, as indicated by enhanced urinary LTE_4 excretion (3) and might contribute to the extension of ischemic damage and to post-ischemic ventricular disfunction during reperfusion (4).

In light of the further contribution provided by platelets to the final production of sulfidopeptide leukotrienes, we have studied the effects on cardiac functions of reperfusion with mixed PMNL-platelet preparations, in isolated normal rabbit heart, following challenge with A-23187.

METHODS

Rabbit hearts were isolated and perfused retrogradely through the aorta as previously described (2). Coronary perfusion pressure (CPP), left ventricular pressure (LVP) and left ventricular end-diastolic pressure (LVEDP) were monitored continuously. Blood cells were prepared as described (5). PMNL (5×10^6 cells) and/or platelets (2×10^8 cells) were supplied with Ca^{++} (2 mM) and Mg^{++} (0.5 mM) and infused into the perfusing medium (50 ml) of recirculating hearts At the end of the experiment, the entire heart reservoir (approx. 45 ml) was collected, spiked with 50,000 dpm ^3H-LTD_4 as well as 25 ng of PGB_2, and stored at -20°C until HPLC analysis (2).

RESULTS

Challenge with A23187, 0.5 µM, of rabbit hearts perfused under recirculating conditions with human PMNL resulted in a marked increase in coronary perfusion pressure, associated with a slight rise in LVEDP (mm Hg, basal 11 ± 0.8, 30' after A-23187, 19 ± 5 n=9). The increase in CPP was slow in onset and very persistent, reaching about 250% of basal values at 30' after A23187 challenge (Fig. 1A).

When human P $(2\times10^8$ cells/ml), were added to the perfusing buffer and challenged, negligible changes in CPP and LVEDP occurred. Combined perfusion with PMNL and P resulted, after A-23187 challenge only, in an earlier and steeper rise in CPP (Fig. 1A). The presence of P seemed to be responsible for the more prompt increase in CPP taking place around 10'; however at 30', CPP attained values similar to those achieved in presence of challenged PMNL alone. This phenomenon seemed to correlate well with the changes in LVEDP, where the combination of PMNL and P triggered a more severe derangement of cardiac contractility (30' after A-23187, LVEDP mm Hg 58 ± 20) than that observed with challenged PMNL alone. Pretreatment of the heart with the LTD_4 receptor antagonist LY171883 caused a marked protection against the effect of cell activation on the heart (Fig. 1A)

The increase in CPP observed in presence of PMNL was accompanied by elevated levels of sulfidopeptide LTs. The additional presence of platelets did not change significantly the levels of sulfidopeptide leukotrienes (fig. 1B).

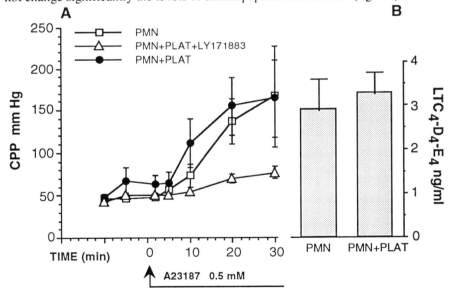

Fig. 1 A. Coronary perfusion pressure (CPP) of isolated rabbit hearts perfused with human blood cells (closed circles: PMNL+platelets; closed squares: PMNL; closed triangles: PMNL+platelets+LY171883 10 µM), and challenged with calcium ionophore A23187 (0.5 µM). B. LT concentrations as measured by RP-HPLC. Mean ± SD.

DISCUSSION

These results show that challenge of blood cells that are recirculating in a spontaneously beating, perfused rabbit heart, causes a marked and progressive increase in CPP. Addition of P to the PMNL preparations, does not change the maximal increase in coronary tone, but the time course profile of this event shows an earlier rise than with PMNL alone.

Analytical evidence proofs unequivocally presence of sulfidopeptide LT in the recirculating medium, with preferential formation of LTD_4. The changes in heart mechanics, observed in presence of PMNL, i.e. increase in LVEDP, suggest onset of an ischemic process. This event is aggravated by combined presence of PMNL and P and is associated with stiffness of the heart. These alterations were fully prevented by the LT-receptor antagonist LY171883.

The functional modifications observed, likely reflect local formation of sulfidopeptide LTs as probable consequence of tight interactions between PMNL, P and coronary EC. It is likely that in our experimental model an efficient uptake of LTA_4 by EC (and/or P) takes place, favouring final conversion of the epoxide intermediate into LTC_4-LTD_4. In spite of a faster onset of the vascular response, addition of aspirinized P to the recirculating PMNL, expected to result into augmented transcellular biosynthesis of LTs, did not change the maximal increase in CPP at 30'. This could be explained by the fact that a high rate of transcellular biosynthesis was already taking place. Moreover, uptake of PMNL-derived LTA_4 by P could result in LTC_4 formation predominantly at luminal sites and therefore not in favourable conditions to reach vascular smooth muscle layers.

Taken together, our results underline the importance of transcellular metabolism, particularly those steps involved in the transfer of PMNL-derived LTA_4 and its conversion by vascular or perivascular acceptor cells to cysteinyl LT. The activation of the 5-LO biosynthetic pathway in the context of a tight interaction between circulating blood cells and coronary vasculature, has an important outcome in the alteration of coronary flow and cardiac contractility. This event may become critical in those pathological conditions associated with presence of oxLDL, where leukocytes adhesion is enhanced.

REFERENCES

1. Maclouf J, Murphy RC and Henson P. Transcellular sulfidopeptide LT biosynthetic capacity of vascular cells. *Blood* 1989, 74:703-707.
2. Sala A, Rossoni G, Buccellati C, Berti F, Folco GC and Maclouf J. Formation of sulfidopeptide-leukotrienes by cell-cell interaction causes coronary vasoconstriction in isolated, cell-perfused heart of the rabbit. *Br. J. Pharmacol.* 1993 , 110:1206-1212.
3. Carry, M., Korley, V., Willerson, J.T., Weigelt, L., Ford-Hutchinson, A.W. & Tagari, P. Incresed urinary excretion in patients with cardiac ischemia. In vivo evidence for 5-lipoxygenase activation. *Circulation* 1992, 85:230-236.
4. Hock CE, Beck LD, Papa LA. Peptide LT receptor antagonism in myocardial ischemia and reperfusion. *Cardiovascular Research* 1992, 26:1206-1211.
5. Haslett C, Guthrie LA, Kopaniac MM, Johnston RB, Henson PM, Modulation of multiple neutrophil functions by preparative methods for trace concentrations of bacterial LPS. *Am. J. Pathol.* 1985, 119:101-110.

Advances in Prostaglandin, Thromboxane,
and Leukotriene Research, Vol. 23,
edited by B. Samuelsson et al.
Raven Press, Ltd., New York © 1995

Urinary Thromboxane has Diagnostic Value in Myocardial Infarction

M.L. Foegh, Y. Zhao, L. Madren, M. Rolnick[1],
T.O. Stair[2], and P.W. Ramwell[3]

*Departments of Surgery, Emergency Medicine[2] and Physiology and Biophysics[3],
Georgetown University Medical Center, Washington DC 20007; Emergency Medical Department[1],
Fairfax Hospital, Fairfax Virginia, 22046.*

Thromboxane A_2 metabolizes rapidly into numerous urinary metabolites, eleven-dehydro-thromboxane B_2 (11-dehydro-TXB_2), 2,3-dinor-thromboxane B_2 (2,3-dinor-TXB_2) and thromboxane B_2 (TXB_2) and appears to be associated with thrombotic events. They could form the basis for a rapid and accurate differential diagnosis of patients presenting in the emergency room with chest pain which can contain the substantial costs associated with admission to an intensive care unit.

Patients (247 men and 122 women, 30 to 94 years) presenting to the emergency room of two local hospitals with chest pain were studied. Information was obtained on current medication, aspirin or other anti-inflammatory drugs during the preceding days. The times of chest pain onset and of arrival in the emergency room were noted. A urine sample was taken in the emergency room and daily for up to five days, for those patients admitted. Urine was stored at -70°C for i-TXB_2, i-2,3-dinor-TXB_2 and i-11-dehydro-TXB_2 analysis. Myocardial infarction (MI) was defined as an increase in the myocardial band fraction of plasma creatinine and changes in the ECG. The MI group was sub-classified as either Q-wave or non Q-wave infarctions. Unstable angina was defined as chest pain occurring at rest for >15 minutes with no increase in the myocardial band fraction of creatinine phosphokinase. The results of the 11-dehydro-TXB_2 and 2,3-dinor TXB_2 measurements are published elsewhere[1].

Patients were diagnosed as follows: MI (n=103), unstable angina, (n=137), cardiovascular disease but no MI or unstable angina, (n=70), of which half had congestive heart failure, (n=38). Other diagnoses numbered 59. All three urine

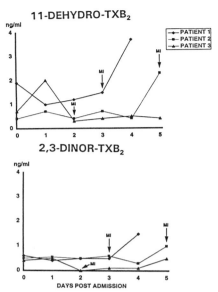

Fig.1 Daily levels metabolites in patients developing MI after admission and all on aspirin

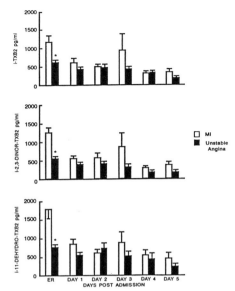

Fig. 2 Metabolite levels in patients with MI compared to unstable angina i-TXB$_2$ includes 60% 2,3 dinor TXB$_2$

metabolites increased. Intake of aspirin did not prevent an increase in urine thromboxane in patients with MI, as 11-dehydro-TXB$_2$ levels were not affected. This was particularly seen in three patients who developed myocardial infarction after admission (Figure 1). All patients received aspirin upon admission, and an increase was seen in 11-dehydro-TXB$_2$ only.

Urine thromboxane metabolites were all significantly higher in the patients with MI compared to those with unstable angina. (Figure 2). On the day of admission the i-TXB$_2$ is significantly lower in those patients with unstable angina. I-TXB$_2$ declines rapidly on the following day when levels overlap with those of patients with unstable angina.

Discussion

Urine metabolites increase during MI, but are not significantly elevated on the second day[2]. This rapid fall may be due to treatment with aspirin or, more likely, the high thromboxane level is a phenomenon related to the acute occlusion of the coronary artery. Urine thromboxane metabolites do not increase to the same extent in patients with unstable angina thus allowing for use of urinary thromboxane as a diagnostic tool in an emergency room setting. Fitzgerald et al.[3] described increased levels in both patients with unstable angina and in MI cases allowing no discrimination between the two diagnoses. However, in the current study, urine samples were obtained more rapidly following MI, which may have accounted for the significant difference between the two groups.

Currently most patients with cardiovascular problems take aspirin daily. Thus it is encouraging that previous intake of aspirin affects only the 2,3-dinor-TXB_2 but not 11-dehydro-TXB_2. This allows use of the rapid ELISA test for 11-dehydro-TXB_2 as a diagnostic tool in the emergency room. Other studies have shown increased levels of thromboxane metabolites in patients with either MI or unstable angina[2,3]. This is the first report to show statistical differences between MI patients and other patients presenting with chest pains. An earlier study involving 166 patients[4] showed that although the majority of patients diagnosed with MI had greater levels of TXB_2 in their urine than did a control group, the differences overall were not statistically significant. Furthermore some patients with confirmed MI had low levels of thromboxane excretion similar to that of the other groups. Although there are differences between our study and the one reported by Lorenz et al.[4] such as the nature of the thromboxane immuno-assay, the basis for MI diagnosis, and different control groups, some patients undergoing MI in the present study also had low levels of thromboxane metabolites. This may result from these patients undergoing a non Q-wave MI which we and others[4,5] have shown to be associated with lower levels of urine thromboxane metabolites. The timing of the urine sampling in relation to the onset of the MI appears to be critical.

To conclude, patients with acute MI have higher urinary i-TXB_2, i-11-dehydro-TXB_2 and i-2,3-dinor-TXB_2 than patients with unstable angina or undergoing a cardiac event. The same results are obtained whether the thromboxane A_2 metabolites are expressed in pg/ml urine or pg/mg creatinine. In patients taking aspirin i-11-dehydro-TXB_2 still increases during MI. Thromboxane measurement provides a rapid means of diagnosing MI in patients presenting with chest pain.

Acknowledgement. This work was supported by Grant NIH-HL40069.

REFERENCES

1. Foegh ML, Zhao Y, Madren L et al. Urinary thromboxane A_2 metabolites in patients presenting in the emergency room with acute chest pain. *J Intern Med* 1994;235:153-61.
2. Foegh ML, Eliasen K, Johansen S, Helfrich GB and Ramwell PW. Coronary artery thrombosis and elevated urine immunoreactive thromboxane B_2. *Prostaglandins* 1986;32:781-8.
3. Fitzgerald DJ, Roy L, Castela F, Fitzgerald GA. Platelet activation in unstable coronary disease. *N Engl J Med* 1986;315:983-9.
4. Lorenz RL, Hamm CW, Riesner H, Bleifeld W. A prospective study of the diagnostic value of urinary thromboxane in patients presenting with acute chest pain. *J Intern Med* 1990;227:429-34.
5. Djurup R, Chiabrando C, Jörres A et al. Rapid direct enzyme immunoassay of 11-keto-thromboxane B_2 in urine, validated by immunoaffinity/gas chromatography-mass spectrometry. *Clin Chem* 1993;39:2470-7.

Advances in Prostaglandin, Thromboxane,
and Leukotriene Research, Vol. 23,
edited by B. Samuelsson et al.
Raven Press, Ltd., New York © 1995

Serum Lipids and Fatty Acids in Populations on a Lake-fish Diet or on a Vegetarian Diet, in Tanzania

Claudio Galli[1], M.T. Angeli[1], M. Puato[2], G. Caroli[2], and P. Pauletto[2].

[1] Institute of Pharmacological Sciences, University of Milan, Italy
[2] Institute of Clinical Medicine, University of Padua, Italy

Dietary fatty acids (FA) modulate variables (serum cholesterol and blood pressure) that are risk factors for coronary heart disease (CHD), as shown by comparative studies in populations from countries on different diets, and by feeding-studies in groups of subjects fed different types of fats. The widespread use of manufactured foods in economically advanced countries, however, progressively minimizes dietary differences among large population groups, whereas comparisons among populations from different countries are limited by confounding (e.g. genetic) factors in dietary responses. Studies in genetically homogeneous populations living in defined areas, where distribution of processed food is minimal and the diet strictly reflects the local availability of food items, allow comparisons among groups of identical ethnic origin but on sharply different and yet totally natural diets.

THE LUGARAWA STUDY

The attention of the World Health Organization (WHO), has been recently focussed on regional differences in risk factors for CHD among population groups living in areas with distinctly different dietary patterns. The Lugarawa Study, supported by WHO, was coordinated by the Istitute of Clinical Medicine, University of Padua, Italy, in order to investigate on the observed differences in blood pressure (BP) values between population groups living in the Lugarawa area in Tanzania, in two villages, one (Lupingu) on the shores of lake Nyasa, and the other (Madilu), at the distance of about 120 kilometers from the Lake. The diet in the coastal village is mainly based on fish from the lake, whereas in the rural area grains, potatoes and vegetables are the main components of the diet. Based on these observations, the project was aimed to investigate the relations between serum FA profiles, reflecting the fat intake with the diet, and BP and serum total cholesterol (TC) and triglyceride (TG) levels. This report is focussed on the differences in serum TC and TG, and in serum FA between the two groups.

STUDY DESIGN

654 subjects (368 men and 286 women) in Madilu, and 622 (370 men and 252 women) in Lupingu, aged 15 to over 80 years, were recruited. Dietary surveys indicate that daily average intakes are as follows. Madilu village (Vegetarian Diet, VD) : 2200 total calories, 900 from maize (250 g), 680 from beans (300 g), 80 from potatoes (100 g), 140 from bananas (200 g), and 400 from low alcohol beverages (1 L); Lupingu village (Fish Diet, FD) : 2040 total calories, 600 from fish (500 g), 990 from tapioca, a starch obtained from the root of the cassava (300 g), 150 from beans (50 g) and 300 from low alcohol beverages (0.75 L). BP were measured in all subjects, whereas representative serum samples (total of 61, 26 M and 35 W in the FD group, and 55, 24 M and 31 W, in the VD group) were collected, frozen and shipped as such to Italy for routine biochemical tests, serum lipid (Institute of Clinical Medicine, Padua) and serum FA (Institute of Pharmacological Sciences, Milan) analyses. In addition, samples of typical lake fish were included for FA analysis. Measurements were carried out by conventional methods for serum lipids (cholesterol and triglycerides) and by gas chromatography for FA methyl ester analyses.

RESULTS AND DISCUSSION

The values for serum total cholesterol and triglycerides are markedly lower in the FD group than in VD. It is of interest that serum cholesterol is lower in the FD group, an effect which is not consistently occurring in subjects fed fish-derived n-3 FA. Analyses of serum FA profiles in the two groups reveal marked, partly unexpected, differences in the major polyunsaturated FA (PUFA), also in comparisons with values in Italian subjects, as shown in Table I. Compared to VD, levels of linoleic acid (18:2 n-6) are lower and those of EPA, 22:5 and DHA, higher in FD, as expected. However, in FD, arachidonic acid (20:4 n-6) is not reduced, being even higher than in VD, in spite of the elevated levels of n-3 FA. Among the n-3 FA, DHA is more elevated than EPA. The two groups differ also from the Italian subjects, since, in these, 18:2 is higher and 20:4 lower than in the Tanzanian subjects, and n-3 FA are lower even than in VD. In order to correlate the somewhat unexpected serum FA profile in the FD group with dietary FA, we analyzed the FA patterns of four types of lake fish and compared the values with those reported for a tropical fish and for mackerel, a North Atlantic fish (Table II). In the four lake fish, DHA is the predominant n-3 FA, whereas EPA is generally lower than in cold-water fish. 20:4 n-6 is present in appreciable concentrations, quite higher than those of EPA. The FA profiles resemble those of the tropical halibut (1) and of other fishes from tropical waters, reported in the literature (2). The FA patterns of the lake fishes are thus reflected in serum FA of the FD group (high 20:4 and DHA, and EPA lower than in populations eating cold-water fish (3). Similar influences of diets rich in tropical Australian fish fed to volunteers have been reported (4). It can be calculated that the daily intakes of 20:4 in the FD group are in the order of 0.5-0.8 g, and thus the fish from lake Nyasa is a good dietary source of this FA, as reported for Northern Australian coastal fish (2).

Major FA n-6	Bantu Population VD (n=55)	Italian Normal FD (n=61)	Subjects (n=16)
18:2	23.97±0.59	14.85±0.55	34.55±1.99
20:3	1.75±0.06	1.15±0.05	1.87±0.15
20:4	8.30±0.26	9.85±0.34	7.00±0.30
22:4	0.51±0.03	0.48±0.04	0.16±0.01
22:5	0.34±0.02	0.68±0.03	0.12±0.01
n-3			
20:5	0.72±0.03	2.48±0.17	0.64±0.08
22:5	0.62±0.04	1.11±0.06	0.31±0.04
22:6	1.49±0.14	5.93±0.23	1.39±0.09

Table 1. Fatty Acid Composition of Serum Total Lipids

	Nyasa Lake Fish (local name)					
	Kambale	Mfui	Njenu	Mbelele	Eq. Indian halibut [a]	N. Atl. mackerel (Oil)
Fat (g%)	1.8	1.1	4.9	10.3	1.7	
n-6 FA						
20:4	5.9	8.0	5.8	4.3	6.3	0.4
n-3 FA						
20:5	2.1	3.1	1.8	4.2	5.9	7.6
22:5	5.2	3.7	5.0	1.8		
22:6	13.3	19.1	7.8	8.6	10.4	7.7

a. Viswanathan Nair PG and Gopakumar K. (1978)

Table 2. Lipid content and PUFA levels in four major types of fish consumed in coastal villages on Nyasa Lake

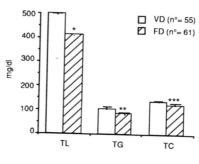

* p< 0.001 ** p< 0.01 *** p< 0.05

Fig. 1. TL, Total Lipids; TG, Triglycerides; TC, Total Cholesterol (mg/dl) levels in the two population groups. VD Vegetarian Diet (Madilu) and FD, Fish Diet (Lupingu).

The differences in serum lipids between the two groups can be ascribed to the high serum n-3 FA, reflecting the diet. It is interesting, however, that lower lipids are associated with relatively high levels of serum 20:4. In conclusion, our data indicate that populations on distinctly different unprocessed diets and with major differences in the intake and proportions of n-3 and n-6 PUFA show profound differences in some risk factors for CHD such as serum cholesterol and tryglycerides. These differences do not appear to be dependent upon modifications of the n-6 FA levels in serum lipids, induced by the high n-3 FA intake.

REFERENCES

1. Knapp HR and FitzGerald, GA. The antihypertensive effects of fish oil. A controlled study of polyunsaturated fatty acids supplements in essential hypertension. N Engl J Med. 1989; 320:1037-43
2. Viswanathan Nair PG and Gopakumar K. Fatty acid compositions of 15 speciesJof fish from tropical waters; Food Sci 1978, 43:1162
3. Sinclair AJ, O'Dea K and Naughton JM. Elevated levels of arachidonic acid in fish from Northern Australian coastal waters. Lipids 1983, 18:877-881
4. Bang HO, Dyerberg J and Brøndum Nielsen A. Plasma lipid and lipoprotein pattern in Greenlandic west-coast Eskimos. Lancet 1971, 11:1143-6
5. Sinclair AJ, O'Dea K, Dunstan G, Ireland PD and Niall M. Effects on plasma lipids and fatty acid composition of very low fatty diets enriched with fish or kangaroo meat. Lipids 1987, 22:523-29

Advances in Prostaglandin, Thromboxane, and Leukotriene Research, Vol. 23, edited by B. Samuelsson et al. Raven Press, Ltd., New York © 1995

Inhibition of Cyclooxygenase activity in human Endothelial Cells by Homocysteine

Isabelle Quéré, Aïda Habib, Gérard Tobelem and Jacques Maclouf

U 348 INSERM, Hôpital Lariboisière, 75475 Paris cedex, 10 France

In humans, various reports have now ascertained homocysteine (HC) as an independent risk factor in atherosclerosis also associated with arterial thrombotic events (1). Indeed platelet activation *in vivo* in homozygous homocystinuria has been demonstrated by measuring an increased excretion of the urinary metabolite of the platelet-derived thromboxane A_2 (2). Interference of HC with various aspects of the endothelial cell functions *in vitro* has been demonstrated such as reduction in cellular binding sites for t-PA (3) or of an inhibitor of protein C activation (4). The synthesis of the potent antiagregant prostacyclin (PGI_2) by vascular cells also constitutes an important pathway by which an efficient homeostasis is maintained between the vessel wall and circulating elements of blood such as platelets. In vitro studies have shown that low concentrations (<100 µmol/L) of HC stimulated the biosynthesis of prostacyclin by rat aorta whereas higher concentrations (>1 mmol/L) inhibited this production (5). In contrast, in a recent report, Wang and colleagues (6) failed to observe any variation of prostacyclin production by cultured human vascular endothelial cells (HUVEC). In this study, we evaluated the influence of HC as modulator of prostacyclin production by HUVEC.

RESULTS:

HC at concentrations from 0.3 to 6 mM, showed a reduction of 6-keto-$PGF_{1\alpha}$ from HUVEC (figure 1A, open circles); this effect was similar when cyclooxygenase (Cox) activity was tested by adding exogenous arachidonic acid (figure 1 B, open circles). Cells were stimulated with IL-1α, a cytokine known to promote the formation of 6-keto-$PGF_{1\alpha}$ as well as to induce Cox synthesis in HUVEC (7) (figure 1A and B, closed circles). HC induced a reduction of the stimulatory effects of IL-1 reflected on Cox activity. In both conditions, the effect of HC reached a plateau at 3 mM. After 4 hours in the presence of 3 mM HC, there was a significant reduction in the formation of 6-keto-PGF$_{1\alpha}$ in the supernatant of IL-1-treated HUVEC which persisted up to 24h (figure 1C). Although at 0.3 mM HC a reduction of 6-keto-PGF$_{1\alpha}$ was observed, it never reached significance. When Cox contents was tested by incubating excess amount of exogenous substrate, HC exerts a strong reduction in enzyme activity (figure 1D).

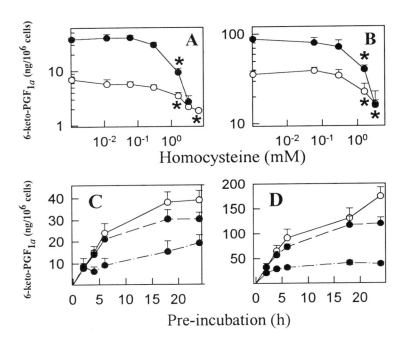

Figure 1. Effect of HC on prostacyclin metabolism by HUVEC. Upper panels: Panel A, dose-response of HC on 6-keto-PGF$_{1\alpha}$ production by HUVEC incubated for 4 h with HC in the absence (O——O), or presence of IL-1 (25 U/ml, 6h) (●——●). Panel B. Cox activity was evaluated after replacement of supernatant with Hanks' buffer containing 1 mg/ml albumin and incubation with arachidonic acid (10 μM) for 30 min at 37°C. 6-keto-PGF$_{1\alpha}$ was analyzed by EIA (8). *, $p < 0.05$ Kruskal-Wallis test. Lower panels: Time-dependence effect of HC on 6-keto-PGF$_{1\alpha}$ production after 6h-incubation with IL-1 (25 U/ml). Panel C, PG in supernatant of control cells (O), and in the presence of 0.3 mM (●- - -●) or 3 mM (●- • - •●) HC. Panel D. Cox activity measured as described above. IL-1 was subsequently added for 6h to the cells. Data are plotted as mean ± S.D. of 4-5 experiments in duplicate.

When 1 μM PGH_2 was added to HUVEC that had been incubated in the presence of 3 mM HC for more than 4 hours, the concentrations of 6-keto-$PGF_{1\alpha}$ did not vary suggesting that prostacyclin synthase was not modified by HC.

In summary, HC exerted a strong inhibition of prostacyclin liberation in the supernatant of controls and activated cells but also from exogenously added arachidonic acid which reflects a change in activity. In other experiments western blot analysis showed that HC inhibits the expression of Cox-2 in a dose-dependent fashion, in agreement with the change in Cox activity observed at the cellular level.

ACKNOWLEDGMENTS

This work was supported in part by grants from Institut National de la Santé et de la Recherche Médicale, from Action Paroi Vasculaire and from the Association pour la Recherche sur le Cancer (ARC) (grant 2076) I. Q. was supported by Fondation de la Recherche Médicale; A.H. is supported by a scholarship from Association Sanofi Thrombose pour la Recherche (Sanofi, Paris).

REFERENCES

1.   Graham I.A. Homocysteine as a risk factor for cardiovascular disease. Trends Cardiovasc. Med. 1991;6:244-49.

2.   Di Minno G., Davi G., Margaglione et al. Abnormally high thromboxane biosynthesis in homozygous homocystinuria. Evidence for platelet involvement and Probucol-sensitive mechanism. J. Clin. Invest. 1993;92:1400-06.

3.   Hajjar K.A. Homocysteine-induced modulation of tissue plasminogen activator binding to its endothelial cell membrane receptor. J. Clin. Invest. 1993;91:2873-79.

4.   Rodgers, G.M. and Conn M.T. Homocysteine, an atherogenic stimulus, reduces protein C activation by arterial and venous endothelial cells. Blood.1993; 75:895-901.

5.   Panganamala R.V., Karpen C.W., and Merola A.J. Peroxide-mediated effects of homocysteine on arterial prostacyclin synthesis. Prosta Leuko Med. 1986;22:349-56.

6.   Wang J.W., Dudman N.P.B. and Wilcken E.L. Effects of homocysteine and related compounds on prostacyclin production by cultured human vascular endothelial cells. Thromb. Haemostas. 1993;70:1047-52.

7.   Jones D.A., Carlton, D.P. McIntyre T.M., Zimmerman G.A. and Prescott S.M. Molecular cloning of human prostaglandin endoperoxide synthase Type II and demonstration of expression in response to cytokines. J. Biol. Chem. 1993;268:9049-54.

8.   Pradelles P., Grassi J. and Maclouf J. Enzyme immunoassay of eicosanoids using acetylcholine esterase as label: an alternative to radioimmunoassay. Anal. Chem. 1985;57:1170-73.

Advances in Prostaglandin, Thromboxane,
and Leukotriene Research, Vol. 23,
edited by B. Samuelsson et al.
Raven Press, Ltd., New York © 1995

ONO-AP-500-02: A non prostanoid prostaglandin I2 mimetic with inhibitory activity against thromboxane synthase

Kigen Kondo, Koji Machii, Masami Narita, Akihiko Kawamoto, Shinichi Yamasaki and Nobuyuki Hamanaka

Minase Research Institute, Ono Pharmaceutical Co., LTD.
3-1-1 Sakurai, Shimamoto-cho, Mishima-gun, Osaka 618, Japan

During research to develop an orally and long lasting prostaglandin (PG) I2 analog, we found a novel compound, {7,8-Dihydro-5-[(E)-2-[(a-(3-pyridyl)-benzylidene aminooxy]ethyl]-1-naphtyl-oxy} acetic acid : ONO-AP-500-02. Although ONO-AP-500-02 possesses a non-prostanoid structure, it shows potent PGI2 activity and inhibitory activity against thromboxane(TX) A2 in vitro and in vivo. Here we describe biochemical and pharmacological properties of ONO-AP-500-02.

MATERIALS AND METHODS

BINDING ASSAYS OF PROSTANOID RECEPTORS

Assays of binding to IP and TP receptors were carried out using human platelets (1,2). Assays of binding to EP and FP receptors were conducted using membrane fractions from rat uterus, guinea pig ileum or rat ovary (3).

EFFECTS ON HUMAN TX SYNTHASE IN VITRO

TX synthase activity was measured by the reaction of membrane fractions of human platelet (30 μg/ml) with 50 μM PGH2 at 22°C for 3 min. and formed TXB2, a stable metabolite of TXA2, was measured by the enzyme immuno assay kit (EIA, Cayman). Test compounds were incubated for 2 min. with membrane fractions before addition of PGH2.

PLATELET AGGREGATION OF DIFFERENT SPECIES IN VITRO

Citrated platelet rich plasma (PRP) was prepared by centrifugation at 180 x g (for dog and human), 200 x g (for rabbit) for 10 min.. Test compounds were added to PRP 2 min. before the addition of ADP (4 μM, 10-20 μM and 10 μM for human, dogs and rabbit, respectively) and platelet aggregation was monitored as changes in light transmission.

SIMULTANEOUS MEASUREMENT OF INHIBITORY ACTIVITY AGAINST PLATELET AGGREGATION AND THE FORMATION OF TXB2 IN RATS

Male SD rats weighing 250-300 g were anesthetized with pentobarbital (30 mg/kg, i.p.) and cannula was inserted into the duodenum. One hr after administration of ONO-AP-500-02 dissolved in M/15 phosphate buffer (pH7.4) through cannula, heparinized and citrated blood samples were prepared. For measurement of effects on platelet aggregation, citrated PRP prepared by centrifugation (1,200 x g for 10 min.) was stimulated by the addition of 10 μM ADP. To heparinized whole blood, 10 μM Ca^{2+} ionophore (A-23187) was added to stimulat TX formation in vitro. The reaction was continued at 37°C for 10 min. and plasma was prepared by centrifugation at 12,000 x g for 30 seconds. The concentrations of TXB2 were determined by EIA after purification with Sepack C-8 .

RESULTS AND DISCUSSIONS

BINDING OF ONO-AP-500-02 TO PROSTANOID RECEPTORS

As shown in the Table human platelets contained one binding site of iloprost and ONO-AP-500-02 inhibited the specific binding of [^{3}H]-iloprost with a Ki value of 89 nM. Guinea pig ileum and rat uterus contained high and low affinity binding sites. However, ONO-AP-500-02 showed no inhibition against specific binding to a EP receptor in guinea pig ileum, to a TP receptor in human platelets and to a FP receptor in rat ovary at doses up to 10,000 nM. These results suggest that ONO-AP-500-02 has a specific interaction with IP receptor.

Binding studies on various subtypes of prostanoid receptors

Subtype	Source	Ligand	Kd (nM)	Bmax (fmol/mg)	Ki values (nM) of ONO-AP-500-02
IP	Human platelet	^{3}H-Iloprost	9.9	2,000	89
EP	Guinea pig ileum	^{3}H-PGE2	2.5 (high) 33 (low)	95 490	>10,000
TP	Human platelet	^{3}H-SQ29548	12	780	>10,000
FP	Rat ovary	^{3}H-PGF2α	3.0 (high) 33 (low)	200	>10,000

EFFECTS OF ONO-AP-500-02 ON PLATELET AGGREGATION IN DIFFERENT SPECIES IN VITRO

Since prostacyclin has been known to inhibit platelet aggregation in different species, we studied the effects of ONO-AP-500-02 on human, dog and rabbit platelet aggregation induced by ADP. Though concentrations required to cause 50% inhibition (IC_{50}) of platelet aggregation were different among these tissues, ONO-AP-500-02 could inhibit platelet aggregation in a dose dependent manner. Species differences were estimated by calculating IC_{50} values and human platelets were the most sensitive to ONO-AP-500-02 (IC_{50} value was 1.5×10^{-7} M) followed by dog platelets (IC_{50} value was 1.2×10^{-6} M) and rabbit platelets (IC_{50} value was 1×10^{-5} M).

EFFECTS OF ONO-AP-500-02 ON HUMAN TX SYNTHASE

ONO-AP-500-02 contains the pyridine function that often inhibits TX synthase. Therefore, we studied effects of ONO-AP-500-02 on human TX synthase in platelets. Under the same conditions that a specific TX synthase inhibitor, OKY-046, inhibited the enzyme with IC_{50} value of 3 nM, ONO-AP-500-02 did inhibit the enzyme with an IC_{50} value of 10 nM .

EFFECTS OF INTRADUODENAL ONO-AP-500-02 ON PLATELET AGGREGATION AND THE FORMATION OF TX IN RATS

We examined if ONO-AP-500-02 could inhibit platelet aggregation and TX synthase after intraduodenal administration in anesthetized rats. ONO-AP-500-02 at doses from 3 to 30 mg/kg inhibited platelet aggregation and the formation of thromboxane B2 . Further, the doses causing 50 % inhibitions of platelet aggregation and TXB2 formation were 11 mg/kg and 8.5 mg/kg . These results indicate that even in in vivo systems ONO-AP-500-02 exerted both activities at similar doses in rats.

We here demonstrate that ONO-AP-500-02 is a novel PGI2 mimetic with a non-prostanoid structure. ONO-AP-500-02 inhibited platelet aggregation and TX synthase in in vitro and in vivo systems. PGI2 and TX synthase inhibitors could prevent platelet aggregation through different mechanisms. PGI2 increases the intracellular cAMP levels not only in platelets but also in smooth muscle. PGI2 sometimes caused adverse effects mainly due to effects on vascular smooth muscle (headache, facial flushing or hypotension). However, inhibitors of TX synthase have little effect on the cardiovascular system at doses that inhibit platelet aggregation. ONO-AP-500-02 stimulates PGI2 receptors and inhibits TX synthase in vitro and in vivo and may be useful as an anti-platelet agent with less adverse effects than PGI2 and/or its mimetics.

REFERENCES

1. Andrew I. Schafer, Barry Cooper, Donald O'Hara and Robert I. Handin. Identification of platelet receptor for prostaglandin I2 and D2. The Journal of Biological chemistry 1979; 254: 2914-2917.

2. Anders Hedberg, Steven E. Hall, Ogletree, Don N. Harris and Eddie C.-K. Liu. Characterization of [5,6-3H]SQ 29,548 as a high affinity radioligand, binding to thromboxane A2/Prostaglandin H2-receptors in human platelets. The Journal of Pharmacology and Experimental Therapeutics 1988; 245: 786-792.

3. Andrew C. Karaplis and William S. Powell. Specific binding of prostaglandin E1 and E2 adrenal Medulla. The Journal of Biological Chemistry 1981; 256: 2414-2419.

Advances in Prostaglandin, Thromboxane,
and Leukotriene Research, Vol. 23,
edited by B. Samuelsson et al.
Raven Press, Ltd., New York © 1995

A Double-Blind, Multi-Center, Dose Comparison Study of TTC-909 for the Treatment of Peripheral Vascular Disorders

Kensuke Esato

First Department of Surgery
Yamaguchi University School of Medicine
Ube City, Yamaguchi Prefecture, Japan

INTRODUCTION

Prostaglandins are known to feature strong platelet aggregation inhibition and vasodilatation, but there are problems such as instability and adverse reactions such as headache due to the strong vasodilatation.

The novel TTC-909 used in this trial is a lipid emulsion of clinprost, a stable derivative of prostacyclin (figure 1), which was jointly developed by Teijin Ltd. and Taisho Pharmaceutical Co., Ltd.

The drug was developed by utilizing the tendency of lipid microsphere's good distribution to arteriosclerotic lesions in vascular walls [1], so that clinically small amounts of clinprost could effectively work at the lesion sites of vascular, thus reducing systemic adverse reactions.

In the present study we investigated the optimal dose of TTC-909 for peripheral vascular disorders (PVD) with the double-blind method, and the results are reported below. This study was performed in Japan from October 1991 till December 1992.

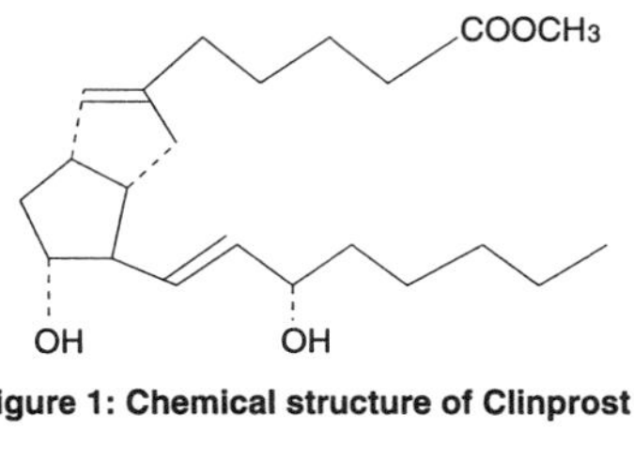

Figure 1: Chemical structure of Clinprost

SUBJECTS AND METHOD

The subjects were PVD of Fontaine IV, who had given their informed consent. Patients who underwent surgery to improve hemodynamics within one month before the start of administration were excluded as subjects.

TTC-909 was infused at the dose of 1, 2, or 4µg of clinprost in bolus infusion, once a day, 7 days a week, for 4 weeks.

The total number of patients enrolled in the study was 157, but 20 patients were excluded from analysis because of administration method violation, incomplete administration period, etc. In consequence, 47 cases was enrolled in the 1µg group, 45 in the 2µg group and 45 in the 4µg group. There was no significant difference in the backgrounds of three groups.

RESULTS

Global Improvement rates of moderately improved or better were 61.7% in the 1 µg group, 66.7% in the 2µg group, and 44.4% in the 4µg group (Table 1).

Ulcer size was measured and expressed as the square root of the long diameter multiplied by the short diameter (mm). Taking the ulcer size at the start of administration as 100, the time-course changes also indicate the highest improvement for the 2µg group (Figure 2).

The severity rating of pain at rest was evaluated on a 4-point rating scale as [1] -: no pain at all, [2] ±: rarely feeling pain, [3] +: ingestion of analgesics needed, and [4] ++: unable to sleep at night because of pain. The improvement rates of moderately improved or better were 56.8% in the 1µg group, 60.0% in the 2µg group, and 41.5% in the 4µg group.

The overall incidence of adverse reactions was low, involving mainly symptoms due to vasodilatation such as dizziness, headache, and fever, and digestive symptoms such as vomiting, diarrhea, and soft stools. But all symptoms were temporary, involving no serious episodes. There was no significant difference in incidence between the dose groups.

DISCUSSION

The improvements in ulcer size and in pain at rest suggest that 2 µg/day is the optimal dose of this drug. These results can be compared with references in the literature [2, 3], and in comparison with other similar PGs, TTC-909 recorded high improvement and safety rates, suggesting its usefulness in treating PVD.

Work is now in progress to investigate the reason for the low improvement rate in the 4µg group with the transcutaneous oxygen tension method.

	Markedly improved	Moderately improved	Slightly improved	No change	Aggravated	Total
1μg group	10 (21.3%)	19 (40.4%)	8 (17.0%)	3 (6.4%)	7 (14.9%)	47
2μg group	16 (35.6%)	14 (31.1%)	7 (15.6%)	3 (6.7%)	5 (11.1%)	45
4μg group	8 (17.8%)	12 (26.7%)	14 (31.1%)	4 (8.9%)	7 (15.6%)	45

Table 1: Global Improvement Ratings

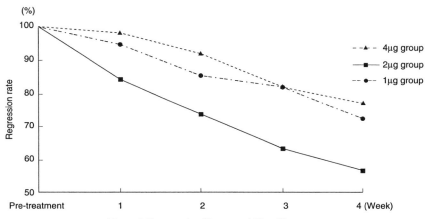

Figure 2. Progressive Changes of Ulser Size

REFERENCES

1. Mizushima Y et al. Tissue distribution and anti-inflammatory activity of corticosteroids incorporated in lipid emulsion. *Ann Rheum Dis* 1982;41:263-267.
2. Katsumura T. et al. Investigation of the clinical usefulness of Lipo-PGE$_1$ against chronic arterial occlusion - A double-blind, intergroup, comparative trial. *Cardioangiology* 1986; 20(4):331-350.
3. Ishitobi K. et al. Therapeutic results of the prosta- cyclin derivative iloprost against chronic arterial occlusion. *Jpn J of Clinical and Experimental Med* 1991; 68(6):246-260

Advances in Prostaglandin, Thromboxane,
and Leukotriene Research, Vol. 23,
edited by B. Samuelsson et al.
Raven Press, Ltd., New York © 1995

Influence of Prostaglandin E₁ on In Vitro Oxidation of Human Low Density Lipoproteins

Helmut Sinzinger, Norbert Leitinger, Anthony Oguogho, and Waltraud Rogatti

*University of Nuclear Medicine, University of Vienna, Wilheim Auerswald
Atheroschlerosis Research Group (ASF), Vienna, Austria*

There are a number of reports that the oxidative modification of low density lipoproteins (LDL) is an important initial event in the pathogenesis of atherosclerosis (1,2). It is well known that the oxidatively modified LDL is taken up via a scavenger receptor of monocyte derived macrophages (3). By the subsequent accumulation of cholesterol the macrophages develop into foam cells. The finding that massive accumulation of foam cells is observed in early atherosclerotic lesions supports the hypothesis that unlimited uptake of the oxidatively modified LDL by macrophages is involved in the development of atherosclerosis in vivo.

During the last few years a variety of mechanisms have been proposed by which prostaglandins might influence the progression of atherosclerosis. Among others, the influence on in vivo platelet function, mitotic activity, activation and proliferation of smooth muscle cells, intracellular cholesterol synthesis and degradation as well as on fibrinogen synthesis has been well discussed.

This study was designed to further characterize the activity of prostaglandins on atherosclerosis.

Materials and Methods

Human LDL (d = 1,019 - 1,063 kg/l) were isolated by ultracentrifugation from the plasma of normolipidemic healthy subjects using an established protocol (4). EDTA and KBr were separated from the isolated LDL by column chromatography (Econo-Pac, 10DG, Bio-Rad, California, USA). LDL were adjusted to a concentration of 0,25 mg/ml and oxidation was initiated by addition of 5 μM Cu^{2+}. The influence of PGE_1 and its metabolites 13,14-dihydro-PGE_1, 13,14-dihydro-15-keto-PGE_1 and 15-keto-PGE_1 was tested at concentrations of 0,001 ng/ml, 1 ng/ml, 200 ng/ml, 800 ng/ml, 1000 ng/ml, 1600 ng/ml in phosphate buffered saline, pH 7,2. Oxidation of LDL was monitored continuously at 234 nm for 3 hrs in a Hitachi U-2000 spectrophotometer (Hitachi, Japan) for the development of conjugated dienes (5).

Results

Influence of PGE₁ and its metabolites 13,14-dihydro-PGE₁, 13,14-dihydro-15-keto-PGE₁ and 15-keto-PGE₁ on in-vitro oxidation of LDL

The parameter assessed from kinetic studies of LDL oxidation in the study was the lag-phase defined by the intercept of the tangent to the curve and the time axis.

PGE₁ showed a concentration-dependent acceleration of the oxidation process, expressed by a shortening of the lag-phase by 18%, 42%, 60%, 84% using concentrations of 200, 400, 800 and 1600 ng/ml, respectively, compared to the control (Fig. 1). However, the degree of acceleration varied using LDL isolated from different patients plasma.

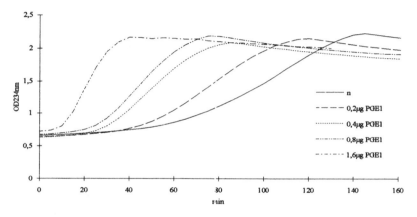

Fig. 1. Influence of PGE₁ on the kinetics of LDL oxidation. LDL (0,25 µg/ml) was incubated with various concentrations of PGE₁. Oxidation was induced by the addition of 5µM coppersulfate and the development of conjugated dienes was monitored by measuring the absorption at 234 nm.

Prostavasin (Schwarz Pharma AG, Monheim, Germany) also showed a shortening of the lag-phase. However, this effect was attenuated by increasing concentrations of Prostavasin. Therefore we tested the stabilizing agent α-cyclodextrin and we observed an attenuation of the oxidation process. The biologically inactive metabolite of PGE₁, 13,14-dihydro-15-keto-PGE₁ also caused an acceleration of the oxidation of LDL similar to PGE₁. The metabolite 13,14-dihydro-PGE₁ showed an attenuation of the oxidation process, whereas 15-keto-PGE₁ caused an acceleration.

Discussion

Our results demonstrated a concentration-dependent effect of prostaglandins on copper-induced in-vitro oxidation of LDL. We observed a marked shortening of the lag-phase by increasing concentrations of PGE_1.

Previous in-vivo studies showed an increased blood clearence of LDL after treatment with PGE_1. An influence of PGE_1 on LDL-receptor expression was discussed as the underlying mechanism. The data presented suggest that PGE_1 accelerates the LDL-oxidation process, at least at therapeutical concentrations. In consequence, oxidized LDL particles would be taken up by the scavenger receptor which resulted in a faster clearence from the blood.

The half-life of PGE_1 is very short. PGE_1 is metabolised to 15-keto-PGE_1, which was shown to be biologically inactive. The intermediate product 13,14-dihydro-PGE_1 again, however, is biologically active.

Normally, PGE_1 and 13,14-dihydro-PGE_1 have similar biological capacities. As to our knowledge, beside the effect on smooth muscle, this is the first mechanism where these two compounds show a different behaviour.

The presented findings suggest an additional effect of prostaglandins on atherogenesis via their influence on the oxidative modification of the LDL particles.

References

1. Steinberg D., Parthasarathy S., Carew TE., Khoo JC., Witztum JL. Beyond cholesterol. Modifications of low density lipoprotein that increase its atherogenicity. *N Engl J Med* 1989;320:915-24.

2. Esterbauer H., Gebicki J., Puhl H., Jurgens G. The role of lipid peroxidation and antioxidants in oxidative modification of LDL. *Free Rad Biol Med* 1992;13:341-90.

3. Steinbrecher UP., Witztum JL., Parthasarathy S., Steinberg D. Decrease in reactive amino groups during oxidation or endothelial cell modification of LDL. *Arteriosclerosis* 1987;7:135-43.

4. Havel RJ., Eder HA., Bragdon JH. The distribution and chemical composition of ultracentrifugally seperated lipoproteins in human serum. *J Clin Invest* 1955;34:1345-53.

5. Esterbauer H., Striegl G., Puhl H., Rotheneder M. Continuous monitoring of in vitro oxidation of human low density lipoprotein. *Free Rad Res Comm* 1989;6:67-75.

*Advances in Prostaglandin, Thromboxane,
and Leukotriene Research, Vol. 23,*
edited by B. Samuelsson et al.
Raven Press, Ltd., New York © 1995

PRINCIPLES OF THROMBOREGULATION: CONTROL OF PLATELET REACTIVITY IN VASCULAR DISEASE

AJ Marcus, LB Safier, WE Kaminski, N Islam, KA Hajjar, E Jendraschak,
RL Silverstein, MJ Broekman, C von Schacky, and JH Fliessbach

Departments of Medicine and Pathology, New York VA Medical Center and
Cornell University Medical College, New York, New York 10010

The initial modality of host defense following vessel injury is the blood platelet. Platelets adhere to subendothelium, aggregate and produce a releasate which recruits additional platelets, culminating in formation of the hemostatic platelet plug. The latter is accompanied by thrombin-induced consolidation and fibrin deposition between cohesive platelets. This process is multicellular in origin because erythrocytes promote and neutrophils inhibit formation of the platelet thrombus. Endothelial cells in the microenvironment are endowed with three protective mechanisms (thromboregulators) which limit the size of the hemostatic plug or thrombus. These include an ectoADPase on the endothelial cell surface, the eicosanoids, and the endothelium-dependent relaxing factor or nitric oxide. In blood vessels afflicted with advanced atherosclerosis such as coronary or cerebral arteries, an ulcer or fissure in the fibrous cap of the atheroma is a strong stimulus which can transform the platelet into a major prothrombotic moiety. Induction of excessive platelet activation cannot be contained by normal thromboregulation. Thus, erythrocytes further activate platelets in an aspirin-insensitive manner and neutrophil blockade of platelet reactivity is not sufficient for prevention of vascular occlusion. Recent appreciation that additional cell types and metabolic pathways are involved in control of platelet reactivity in occlusive vascular disease has given rise to development of new hypotheses for prevention. Novel strategies aimed at restoration of defense systems such as thromboregulation are needed in order to improve our therapeutic approach to thrombosis - which, at present, is far from satisfactory.

Primary Hemostasis: Relationship to Thrombosis

Interruption of continuity of a normal blood vessel evokes an initial response to the injury known as primary hemostasis (1). An intense vasoconstriction occurs which is accompanied by the process of platelet activation.   Immediate adherence of platelets to collagen in the subendothelium which has been exposed to the injury occurs.   Collagen is one of the strongest platelet agonists known and it instantly produces platelet activation, leading to secretion of additional fluid-phase agonists.   Among these are adenosine diphosphate (ADP), thromboxane A_2 (TXA_2), and serotonin (5-HT).   The secretory products recruit other platelets which will aggregate and cohere to the initial layer of platelets on the subendothelium. In this manner, a hemostatic plug is formed (2,3).   Activation induces a change in platelet shape from a disk to a spiny sphere.   During this process, the platelet membrane phospholipoprotein surface rearranges itself so that a catalytic procoagulant surface is formed.   Activated coagulation factor X is bound to this platelet surface in the presence of activated factor V.   Factor VII, which belongs to the extrinsic coagulation system is also activated at the platelet surface (1).   These interactions rapidly culminate in formation of thrombin which is a highly potent platelet agonist and also induces contraction and consolidation of the platelet plug.   Furthermore, thrombin is the catalyst for transformation of fibrinogen to fibrin.   Fibrin strands interlace the interstices of the platelet plug and render it difficult to reverse therapeutically (4).

Secondary Hemostasis

Thrombin mediates reinduction of platelet activation and recruitment as well as promoting further fibrin deposition.   These events are defined as secondary hemostasis.   At this point, the hemostatic platelet plug is tightly consolidated and impermeable.   The break in continuity of the blood vessel is completely sealed.   Platelets have actually formed a nidus which can withstand the back pressure of the circulation and cannot be dislodged. Superimposed upon this is participation of other cells which promote platelet reactivity such as erythrocytes, and neutrophils which serve to limit the size of the platelet thrombus and metabolize lipoxygenase products released from activated platelets (5-7).

In sharp contrast to normal hemostasis occurring in traumatized, but otherwise healthy vessels, arterial thrombosis in atherosclerotic vessels can be interpreted as a misdirected or abnormal consequence of normal hemostasis (2,8-10).   Although thrombi resemble hemostatic plugs morphologically (11), their development is quite different from that of hemostatic plugs.   An arterial thrombus almost always occurs at sites of pathologic vascular damage.   The deeply fissured or ulcerated advanced atherosclerotic plaque in the vessel wall is the major offender.   The plaque may contain an eroded fibrous cap with lipid-rich necrotic tissue and inflammatory cells (12-16).   These lesions have marked agonistic potential (16).   They promote far more adhesion, activation, secretion, recruitment, and consolidation than the injured healthy vessel surface initially described. Furthermore, lipid-overloaded arterial plaques serve as a focus for intermittent thrombus formation as a consequence of recurrent fissuring, as well as slow release of incorporated thrombin (4,9,13,17).   The size of pathologic thrombi and the extent of associated damage to normal tissues frequently surpass the capacity of normal control systems.   Thus, a pathologic thrombus can extend or embolize, thereby producing a totally stenotic vessel, leading to ischemic necrosis and death.   The multiple factors involved in development of arterial thrombosis and the associated myofibrotic response allows one to appreciate how difficult clinical management of these occlusive events can be (3,15,16).

We now know that several additional cell types modulate the growth of platelet thrombi (5,18). Time-course studies of evolving thrombi as viewed by electron microscopy initially demonstrate platelets adhering to subendothelium. With the passage of time, the platelet thrombus becomes admixed with erythrocytes, neutrophils, and later, occasional monocytes. Superimposed upon this are normal, metabolically viable endothelial cells adjacent to and in the vicinity of the lesion (11,19). The presence of multiple cells in a thrombus is not passive or random. Biochemical and functional interactions between platelets and other cells in proximity to the thrombus have been demonstrated *in vitro* (18,20,21) and there is strong evidence for their presence *in vivo*.

Many of the above interactions are thromboregulatory, in that they culminate in enhancement or inhibition of platelet reactivity. Thus, intact erythrocytes in close proximity to activated platelets strongly enhance platelet reactivity, arachidonate release, and thromboxane formation (22,23). In sharp contrast, neutrophils (24) and endothelial cells (25-27) down-regulate platelet activation and recruitment, both of which serve to limit thrombus size. The aforementioned interactions occur in the setting of cell proximity, cell motion and/or direct contact. Inhibitory or prothrombotic effects can be due to secretory products of one or more cell types after activation by a specific agonist(s) or to surface-connected modulators (2). In some instances, the phenomenon of transcellular metabolism occurs in which a metabolic product of one cell is transformed by another into a biologically active compound (5,18). Transcellular metabolism can also result in formation of a metabolite that cannot be synthesized by either cell alone. Examples of transcellular metabolism have been demonstrated *in vitro* between platelets and endothelial cells, as well as neutrophils, erythrocytes and smooth muscle cells (21). These studies from our own and several other laboratories indicate that development and reversibility of thrombosis represents an integrated group of multicellular biochemical events (1). This will eventually guide therapeutic design.

Control of Platelet Reactivity by Endothelial Cells

As long as the endothelium remains biochemically and physically intact, platelets in the circulation are not activated (there is no shape change which would verify it) (6,28). Also, circulating viable platelets produce a substance(s) that maintains vascular integrity and prevents spontaneous hemorrhage (1). As a consequence of vascular injury, platelets do become activated, whereupon endothelial cells respond in a manner that is directed toward limitation or reversal of the consequences of platelet reactivity. We define this response as endothelial thromboregulation.

Thromboregulation can be studied *in vitro* (3). This is carried out with combined suspensions of cultured human umbilical cord endothelial cells and human platelets at high density and in motion. The procedure can be carried out in aggregometer cuvettes or over monolayers in culture (25,27). Under these conditions, both functional and biochemical parameters can be measured simultaneously. In point of fact, platelets become unresponsive to all agonists when in proximity to endothelial cell suspensions. This unresponsiveness is due to at least three separate endothelial cell thromboregulatory systems. They include the eicosanoids, the endothelium-dependent relaxing factor or nitric oxide (EDRF/NO), and the ectonucleotidase, ATP-diphosphohydrolase which is capable of hydrolyzing ADP and ATP (27,29,30).

Table 1 summarizes the biologic activities of thromboregulators.

TABLE 1. *Inhibitory thromboregulators associated with endothelial cells*

Class	Type	Aspirin sensitivity	Mode of action
Eicosanoids	PGI_2, PGD_2	Inhibited	⬆ cAMP
Nitrovasodilators	EDRF/NO	Insensitive	⬆ cGMP
Ecto-nucleotidases	ATPDase	Insensitive	⬇ ADP

We have been studying the human endothelial cell ectoADPase in detail. The enzyme belongs to a family of immunoglobulin-like genes on human chromosome 19. This includes a subgroup of sequences related to the carcinoembryonic antigen. The polypeptides are strongly conserved in sequence. They may function as receptors, adhesion molecules, and in recognition and signal transduction. We have solubilized the ectoADPase from endothelial cell membranes and believe that a single band on an AMP affinity column represents the enzyme at a molecular weight of 72,000. A cloning strategy was developed which utilizes putative homology to a rat liver plasma membrane ectoADPase of known cDNA sequence. We utilized degenerate oligonucleotide primers which are homologous to the rat ectoADPase for PCR amplification of homologous segments from the human endothelial cell cDNA.

The ectoADPase completely blocks platelet reactivity in the absence of prostacyclin and nitric oxide. We currently believe that this cell-associated, aspirin insensitive enzyme is the prime regulator of platelet reactivity.

REFERENCES

1. Marcus AJ. Platelets and their Disorders. In: Ratnoff OD, Forbes CD, eds. *Disorders of Hemostasis*. 3rd ed. Philadelphia: W. B. Saunders, 1994;

2. Marcus AJ. Cellular interactions of platelets in thrombosis. In: Loscalzo J, Schafer AI, eds. *Thrombosis and Hemorrhage*. ed. Boston, MA: Blackwell Scientific Publications, 1994;279-289.

3. Marcus AJ, Safier LB. Thromboregulation: Multicellular modulation of platelet reactivity in hemostasis and thrombosis. *FASEB J* 1993;7:516-522.

4. Szczeklik A, Dropinski J, Radwan J, et al. Persistent generation of thrombin after acute myocardial infarction. *Arterioscler Thromb* 1992;12:548-553.

5. Marcus AJ. Thrombosis and inflammation as multicellular processes. Pathophysiological significance of transcellular metabolism. *Blood* 1990;76:1903-1907.

6. Kroll MH, Schafer AI. Biochemical mechanisms of platelet activation. *Blood* 1989;74:1181-1195.

7. Kroll MH. Mechanisms of platelet activation. In: Loscalzo J, Schafer AI, eds. *Thrombosis and Hemorrhage*. ed. Boston, MA: Blackwell Scientific Publications, 1994;247-277.

8. Bick RL, Pegram M. Syndromes of hypercoagulability and thrombosis: A review. *Semin Thromb Hemost* 1994;20:109

9. DiCorleto PE. Cellular mechanisms of atherogenesis. *Am J Hypertens* 1993;6 Suppl.314S-318S.

10. Harker LA. Platelets and vascular thrombosis. *N Engl J Med* 1994;330:1006-1007.

11. Woolf N. Thrombosis. In: McGee JO, Isaacson PG, Wright NA, eds. *Oxford Textbook of Pathology*. ed. New York: Oxford University Press, 1992;509-519.

12. Stary HC, Chandler AB, Glagov S, et al. A definition of initial, fatty streak, and intermediate lesions of atherosclerosis. A report from the committee on vascular lesions of the Council on arteriosclerosis, American Heart Association. *Circulation* 1992;89:2462-2478.

13. Fuster V, Badimon L, Badimon JJ, et al. The pathogenesis of coronary artery disease and the acute coronary syndromes. *N Engl J Med* 1992;326:242-250-310-318.

14. Ross R. The pathogenesis of atherosclerosis: a perspective for the 1990s. *Nature* 1993;362:801-809.

15. Myler RK, Frink RJ, Shaw RE, et al. The unstable plaque: Pathophysiology and therapeutic implications. *J Invas Cardiol* 1990;2:117-128.

16. MacIsaac AI, Thomas JD, Topol EJ. Toward the quiescent coronary plaque. *J Am Coll Cardiol* 1993;22:1228-1241.

17. Davies MJ. A macro and micro view of coronary vascular insult in ischemic heart disease. *Circulation* 1990;82:II-38-II-46.

18. Maclouf J. Transcellular biosynthesis of arachidonic acid metabolites: from in vitro investigations to in vivo reality. *Bail Clin Haem* 1993;6:593-608.

19. Ross R. Atherosclerosis: A defense mechanism gone awry. *Am J Pathol* 1993;143:987-1002.

20. Brezinski DA, Nesto RW, Serhan CN. Angioplasty triggers intracoronary leukotrienes and lipoxin A_4. Impact of aspirin therapy. *Circulation* 1992;86:56-63.

21. Maclouf J, Fitzpatrick FA, Murphy RC. Transcellular biosynthesis of eicosanoids. *Pharmacol Res* 1989;21:1-7.

22. Santos MT, Valles J, Marcus AJ, et al. Enhancement of platelet reactivity and modulation of eicosanoid production by intact erythrocytes. *J Clin Invest* 1991;87:571-580.

23. Valles J, Santos MT, Aznar J, et al. Erythrocytes metabolically enhance collagen-induced platelet responsiveness via increased thromboxane production, ADP release, and recruitment. *Blood* 1991;78:154-162.

24. Valles J, Santos MT, Marcus AJ, et al. Down-regulation of human platelet reactivity by neutrophils. Participation of lipoxygenase derivatives and adhesive proteins. *J Clin Invest* 1993;92:1357-1365.

25. Marcus AJ, Weksler BB, Jaffe EA, et al. Synthesis of prostacyclin from platelet-derived endoperoxides by cultured human endothelial cells. *J Clin Invest* 1980;66:979-986.

26. Broekman MJ, Eiroa AM, Marcus AJ. Inhibition of human platelet reactivity by endothelium-derived relaxing factor from human umbilical vein endothelial cells in suspension. Blockade of aggregation and secretion by an aspirin-insensitive mechanism. *Blood* 1991;78:1033-1040.

27. Marcus AJ, Safier LB, Hajjar KA, et al. Inhibition of platelet function by an aspirin-insensitive endothelial cell ADPase. Thromboregulation by endothelial cells. *J Clin Invest* 1991;88:1690-1696.

28. Brass LF, Hoxie JA, Kieber-Emmons T, et al. Agonist receptors and G proteins as mediators of platelet activation. *Adv Exp Med Biol* 1993;344:17-36.

29. Côté YP, Filep JG, Battistini B, et al. Characterization of ATP-diphosphohydrolase activities in the intima and media of the bovine aorta: Evidence for a regulatory role in platelet activation in vitro. *Biochim Biophys Acta Mol Basis Dis* 1992;1139:133-142.

30. Yagi K, Shinbo M, Hashizume M, et al. ATP diphosphohydrolase is responsible for ecto-ATPase and ecto-ADPase activities in bovine aorta endothelial and smooth muscle cells. *Biochem Biophys Res Commun* 1991;180:1200-1206.

Advances in Prostaglandin, Thromboxane,
and Leukotriene Research, Vol. 23,
edited by B. Samuelsson et al.
Raven Press, Ltd., New York © 1995

Mechanisms for Lipoxin A4 Induced Neutrophil Dependent Cytotoxicity for Human Endothelial Cells

Johan Bratt,* Richard Lerner, Bo Ringertz, and Jan Palmblad

Departments of Rheumatology and Medicine, The Karolinska Institute at Stockholm Söder Hospital, S-118 83 Stockholm, Sweden

Neutrophil polymorphonuclear (PMN) granulocytes adhere rapidly to the vascular endothelium in response to inflammatory agents (1,2). During this adhesion and the subsequent transendothelial migration activated PMN may mediate an injury to endothelial cells. This is an important event in the pathogenesis of the vasculitis that characterizes rheumatic diseases and reperfusion situations and may be an early event in atherosclerosis (3-7).

In an in vitro model of vasculitis we have evaluated mechanisms for how neutrophil granulocytes kill cultured human umbilical vein endothelial cells (HUVEC) in response to the double dioxygenation product of arachidonic acid, lipoxin A4 (LXA4) and to formyl-methionyl-leucyl-phenylalanine (fMLP). We also evaluated this effect of leukotriene B4 (LTB4), platelet activating factor (PAF) and phorbol myristate acetate (PMA).

Methods

HUVEC were grown to confluence and labeled with ^{51}Cr. PMN and stimuli were added and the release of ^{51}Cr to supernatants were assessed after 4 hours (8).

Results

LXA4 as well as fMLP caused neutrophils to damage the HUVEC. The cytolysis induced by LXA4 and fMLP was dose dependent, with maxima at 100 nM (which caused 2.7- and 2.3-fold increases of ^{51}Cr release, respectively, relative to buffer treated controls). LXA4 also conferred a peak of cytotoxicity at 0.1 nM (which caused 2.2-fold increase of ^{51}Cr release). Leukotriene B4, platelet activating factor (PAF) and zymosan activated serum were inefficient. Phorbol myristate acetate (PMA) caused the most prominent cytotoxicity, but evident first at $1\mu M$ (fig.1).

We then assessed the role of toxic oxygen metabolites for the cytolysis process. The LXA4 (as well as the fMLP) effect was abrogated by superoxide dismutase (fig.2) and catalase but not by mannitol. Neutrophils from a patient with chronic granulomatous disease were incapable of mediating any cytotoxicity. Next, we analysed whether release of proteases from PMN were of significance. α-2-macroglobulin, α-1-antitrypsin inhibited the LXA4 effect (fig.3).

The role of adhesion molecules was addressed. Addition of a mAb to CD18 inhibited neutrophil dependent cytotoxicity to LXA4 and fMLP. MAbs to intercellular adhesion molecule-1 (ICAM-1) or P-selectin blocked 100% and 52%, respectively, of the LXA4 induced cytotoxicity (fig.4).

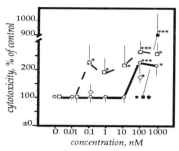

Fig. 1. Dose-response curves for various stimuli. HUVEC were exposed for 4 hours to PMN alone (controls) or PMN stimulated by fMLP, LXA4, LXB4, PAF, LTB4 and PMA in various concentrations. ZAS was also tested (0.5% resp. 1%) and gave no cytotoxicity above that of the controls. The FCS concentration was 1%. Mean and SE values for 3-48 experiments, run in duplicates. o = fMLP, □ = LXA4, ◇ = LXB4, ● = PAF, ◆ = LTB4,

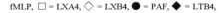

■ = PMA.

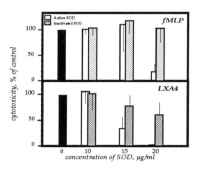

Fig. 2. The effect of active or H_2O_2- inactivated SOD on the cytotoxicity induced by 100 nM fMLP or LXA4. Mean and SE values for 3-5 experiments, run in duplicates.

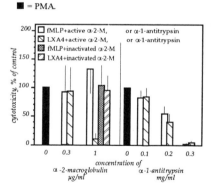

Fig. 3. The effect of active, inactive α-2-macroglobulin (α-2-M) or α-1-antitrypsin on the cytotoxicity induced by 100 nM fMLP or LXA4. Mean and SE values for 3 experiments, run in duplicates.

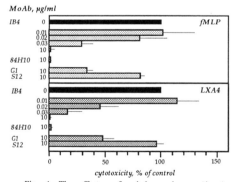

Fig. 4. The effect conferred by various mAbs (as described under Results) on the cytotoxicity induced by 100 nM of fMLP or LXA4. A control mAb, D3/9 directed against CD45, was also used and conferred no inhibitory effect on the cytotoxic reaction. Mean and SE values for 3 experiments, run in duplicates.

Since previous results have indicated that LXA4 might cause PAF expression on HUVEC we used the PAF receptor antagonist WEB-2086 in order to block cytolysis. The LXA4 effect was inhibited by WEB-2086 (Table 1).

Likewise, treating neutrophils with pertussis toxin impaired PMN cytolysis in response to LXA4 (Table 1).

Table 1. The effect of WEB-2086 or pertussis toxin on the fMLP or LXA4 induced endothelial cytolysis

	WEB (10 μM)	n	Pertussis toxin (750 ng/ml)	n
fMLP, 100 nM	73.9±15.1	4	100.0±0	2
LXA4, 100 nM	77.1±22.9	4	77.3±1.1	2

This table shows the inhibition (expressed as percent of untreated controls) conferred by the PAF receptor antagonist WEB-2086 and by pertussis toxin on the fMLP or LXA4 induced cytotoxicity. PMN were treated with pertussis toxin for 2 hours at 37°C prior to addition to the HUVEC monolayers, and subsequently stimulated by fMLP or LXA4, while WEB 2086 were added to the HUVEC simultaneously with the PMN. Mean and SE values for the number (n) of separate experiments, run in duplicates.

Discussion.

This novel effect of LXA4, as a potent promoter of neutrophil mediated cytotoxicity for HUVEC, is a process dependent on PMN adhesion proteins, oxygen radicals, proteases, and apparently associated with endogenous PAF expression and requiring pertussis sensitive G proteins. It occurs at LXA4 concentrations that has been noted in vivo after angioplasty (9). Thus, LXA4 might be of significance for vasculitides that accompanies rheumatic and autoimmune diseases.

This study was supported by grants from the Swedish Medical Research Council (19X-05991, 19P-8884), The Swedish Association against Rheumatism, King Gustaf V's 80-year Fund, the Funds of the Karolinska Institute, Södersjukhuset and The Swedish Medical Society.

References.

1. Zimmerman GA, Prescott SM, Mcintyre TM: Endothelial cell interactions with granulocytes: tethering and signaling molecules. *Immunol. Today* 1992;13:93-100.
2. Springer T: Adhesion receptors of the immune system. *Nature* 1990;346:425-34.
3. Fauci AS, Leavitt RY: Vasculitis. In:*Artritis and alied conditions.* Eleventh edition. Edited by DJ Mccarty. Philadelphia, Lea & Febiger, 1989.
4. Weiss SJ: Tissue destruction by neutrophils. *N. Engl. J. Med.* 1989;320:365-76.
5. Ricevuti GA, Mazzone A, Pasotti D, de Servi S, Specchia G: Role of granulocytes in endothelial injury in coronary heart disease in humans. *Atherosclerosis.* 1991;91:1-14.
6. Mehta JL, Nichols WW, Mehta P: Neutrophils as potential participants in acute myocardial ischemia: Relevance to reperfusion. *J. Am. Coll. Cardiol.* 1988;11:1309-16.
7. Cybulsky MI, Gimbrone MA: Endothelial expression of a mononuclear leukocyte adhesion molecule during atherogenesis. *Science* 1991;251:788-91.
8. Bratt J, Lerner R, Ringertz B, Palmblad J: Lipoxin A4 induces neutrophil dependent cytotoxicity for human endothelial cells. *Scand. J. Immunol.* 1994;39:351-4.
9. Brezinski DA, Nesto RW, Serhan CN: Angioplasty triggers intracoronary leukotrienes and lipoxin A4. *Circulation* 1992;86:56-63.

*Advances in Prostaglandin, Thromboxane,
and Leukotriene Research, Vol. 23,*
edited by B. Samuelsson et al.
Raven Press, Ltd., New York © 1995

Thromboxane A_2 synthase inhibitor, DP-1904, decreases TNFα secretion from monocytes and inhibits E-selectin and ICAM-1 expression on the endothelial cell surfaces.

H.Kameda[1], T.Yoshida[1], Y.Ichikawa[2] and M.Homma[1]

*1)Department of Internal Medicine, Keio University School of Medicine, Shinjuku-ku, Tokyo 160, Japan
2)Division of Internal Medicine, Institute of Medical Science, St.Marianna University School of Medicine, Kanagawa 216, Japan*

TXA_2 is an important modulator of hemodynamics and microcirculation. In lupus nephritis, enhanced urinary excretion of TXB_2 and decreased excretion of $6\text{-keto-}PGF_2\alpha$ were observed(1). After that, TXA_2 receptor antagonists improved renal function in lupus patients(2), and increased GFR and decreased proteinuria in murine model(3). Moreover, DP-1904, a thromboxane synthase inhibitor, was shown to improve renal function in rat renal ischemia model(4). These authors suggested the possibility that TXA_2 played an important role in lupus nephritis and they attributed their results mainly to the hemodynamic effects of TXA_2 inhibitors. In the present paper, We clarified the significant role of TXA_2 in leukocyte extravasation in lupus nephritis.

METHODS

Isolation and culture of human monocytes and measurement of TXA_2, PGE_2 and TNFα
The purified mononuclear cells from venous blood were seeded onto dishes and adherent cells were collected as monocytes. Monocytes were incubated with or without lipopolysaccharide, and DP-1904 was added ten minutes before LPS treatment. The supernatants were subjected to radioimmunoassay for TXA_2 and PGE_2, or ELISA for TNFα.
Culture of HL60 cells and adhesion assay
Promyelocytic cell line HL60 cells were differentiated with vitamin D_3 into macrophage-like cells, radiolabeled with ^{51}Cr, distributed over the HUVEC. HUVEC monolayers were washed to remove non-adherent cells, and remaining cells were lysed and counted for radioactivity.
Indirect immunofluorescence
The endothelial surface expression of the adhesion monocules were analysed with indirect immunofluorescence. Briefly, HUVEC monolayers were fixed with 1% paraformaldehyde and incubated with anti-ICAM-1 or E-selectin monoclonal antibodies, and then with FITC-conjugated anti-mouse IgG antibodies. The fluorescence intensity was measured with confocal laser cytometer ACAS570.

RESULTS AND DISCUSSION

DP-1904, a TXA_2 synthase inhibitor, decreased TXB_2 production, metabolite of TXA_2, from human monocytes in dose-dependent manners. On the other hand, PGE_2 production was remarkably increased with DP-1904.

PGE_2 was reported to suppress LPS-induced TNFα secretion from murine peritoneal macrophages[5] and human monocytes[6]. So we examined the effect of DP-1904 pretreatment on LPS-induced TNFα secretion from human monocytes. DP-1904 decreased TNFα secretion in dose-dependent manners(Fig.1a). U-46619, a TXA_2 receptor agonist, induced significant increase in TNFα secretion, but this increase was not comparable to the reduction of TNFα secretion with DP-1904. These data suggested that those suppression by DP-1904 pretreatment was chiefly attributed to the increased endogeneous PGE_2 production by monocytes.

TNFα has been shown to induce augmented leukocyte-endothelial adhesion[7]. So we investigated the effect of DP-1904 on the HL60 cell adhesion to endothelial monolayers. Only 4% of HL60 cells were adhered to resting endothelial cells, and the adherence was increased to 28% with TNFα treatment(Fig.1b). The supernatants of monocytes induced similar increase in the adherence of HL60 cells, and this increment was significantly reduced when monocytes were cultured in the presense of DP-1904 10^{-5} M. The supernatants of LPS-activated monocytes increased the adherence of HL60 cells, and DP-1904 did not show a significant reduction of the adherence of HL60 cells under these conditions. These results suggested that DP-1904 reduced TNFα production by monocytes and decreased the augmentative effect of monocyte-supernatants on the adhesion of HL60 cells to endothelial monolayers.

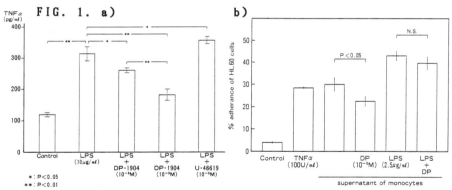

FIG. 1. a) Effect of DP-1904 and U-46619 on TNFα production by human monocytes.

b) Effect of DP-1904 on HL60 cell adherence to HUVEC monolayers.

In order to determine the molecular mechanisms of those increased adhesion of leukocytes to endothelial cells induced by culture supernatants of monocytes, we examined the endothelial surface expression of adhesion molecules, ICAM-1 and E-selectin, induced by conditioned media of HL60 cells differentiated into macrophage-like cells with Vit.D_3 . Both ICAM-1 and E-selectin expression was increased with TNFα treatment, and also with the conditioned media of macrophage-like cells(Fig.2). Those increased expression was reduced when macrophage-like cells were

cultured in the presense of DP-1904. The culture supernatants of
LPS-activated macrophage-like cells induced higher expression of
ICAM-1 and E-selectin. Those increased expression was also reduced by the treatment of macrophage-like cells with DP-1904 as
for ICAM-1, but not for E-selectin under those conditions.

FIG.2.

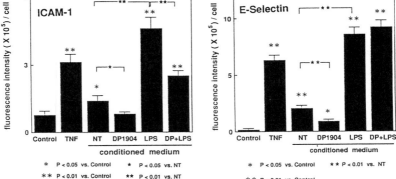

FIG.2. Effect of DP-1904 on ICAM-1 and E-selectin expression
on the endothelial cell surfaces induced by culture
supernatants of macrophage-like cells.

In conclusion, TXA₂ synthase inhibitor, DP-1904, inhibits
leukocyte adhesion to endothelial cells, which may be involved in
the mechanisms of the reduced renal injury by DP-1904 other than
its hemodynamic effects.

REFERENCES

1. Patrono C, Ciabattoni G, Remuzzi G, Gotti E, Bombardieri S, Di Munno O. et al. Functional significance of renal prostacyclin and thromboxane A_2 production in patients with systemic lupus erythematosus. *J Clin Invest* 1985;76:1011-8.

2. Pierucci A, Simonetti BM, Pecci G, Mavrikakis G, Feriozzi S, Cinotti GA et al. Improvement of renal function with selective thromboxane antagonism in lupus nephritis. *N Engl J Med* 1989;320:421-5.

3. Spurney RF, Fan P-Y, Ruiz P, Sanfilippo F, Pisetskey DS and Coffman TM. Thromboxane receptor blockade reduces renal injury in murine lupus nephritis. *Kidney Int*1992;41:973-82.

4. Masumura H, Kunitada S, Irie K, Ashida S and Abe Y. A thromboxane A_2 synthase inhibitor, DP-1904, prevents rat renal injury. *Eur J Pharmacol* 1991;193:321-7.

5. Kunkel SL, Wiggins RC, Chensue SW and Larrick J. Regulation of macrophage tumor necrosis factor production by prostaglandin E_2. *Biochem Biophys Res Comm* 1986;137:404-10.

6. Hart PH, Whitty GA, Piccoli DS and Hamilton JA. Control by IFN-γ and PGE₂ of TNFα and IL-1 production by human monocytes. *Immunology* 1989;66:376-83.

7. Gamble JR, Harlan JM, Klebanoff SJ and Vadas MA. Stimulation of the adherence of neutrophils to umbilical vein endothelium by human recombinant tumor necrosis factor. *Proc Natl Acad Sci* 1985;82:8667-71.

Advances in Prostaglandin, Thromboxane,
and Leukotriene Research, Vol. 23,
edited by B. Samuelsson et al.
Raven Press, Ltd., New York © 1995

Augmented Platelet - Endothelial Adhesion Induced by PGI₂ Receptor Desensitization

Harald Darius, Christiane Binz, Kerstin Veit, and Andreas Fisch

Department of Medicine II, J.Gutenberg - Univ., 55101 Mainz, Germany

Acute myocardial ischemia and unstable angina are pathophysiologic situations with an increased body prostacyclin (PGI_2) synthesis and a decreased number of PGI_2 binding sites on platelets. The role of platelet PGI_2 receptor desensitization in platelet-endothelial cell adhesion was studied. In the presence of thrombin washed human platelets adhered to cultured human umbilical vein endothelial cells. Adhesion was markedly augmented if platelet PGI_2 receptors were desensitized or if endothelial cell PGI_2 synthesis was inhibited by aspirin. Thus, increased PGI_2 synthesis in vivo may result in platelet PGI_2 receptor desensitization with platelet hyperresponsiveness and augmented adhesion to the vascular endothelium in the presence of thombin.

Materials & Methods

Endothelial cells from human umbilical veins (HUVECs) were harvested and cultured according to standard techniques (1) and identified by light microscopy and indirect immunofluorescence staining for vWF antigen.

Blood was drawn from volunteers, anticoagulated with ACD and platelet rich plasma obtained. Platelets were radiolabeled by incubation with ^{14}C-arachidonic acid (55 mCi/mmol; 0.9 μmol/l for 3 hrs at 37°C).

Platelet PGI_2 receptors were desensitized by incubation of PRP with iloprost (1-100 nmol/l) for 3 h at 37°C. Platelet PGI_2 receptor desensitization was determined in binding experiments using ^3H-iloprost (5 nmol/l). Non-specific binding was measured with iloprost (10 μmol/l) for 10 min at 30°C. Then ^3H-iloprost was added at a concentration adapted from the predetermined K_D-value (7.1 nmol/l) and incubated for 10 min at 30°C. Reaction was terminated by centrifugation (12.000xg for 12s) and radioactivity of the platelet homogenate was measured (LKB-Wallac 1410).

Platelet - endothelial cell adhesion was investigated using confluent HUVECs in 24-well plates and labeled washed human platelets suspended in tyrode buffer. Platelet count was adjusted to 2.5 x 10^8 cells/ml. All adhesion experiments were performed in duplicate with HUVECs of the first or second passage. The endothelial cell monolayer with adhering platelets was gently washed three times with HBSS under standardized conditions to remove non-adhering platelets. Platelet adherence (%) was calculated as the level of radioactivity of the solubilized sample divided by the total radioactivity of the platelets added to each well, times100.

Results

Platelet PGI_2 receptors were desensitized by incubation with iloprost at concentrations of 1, 10, or 100 nmol/l for 3 h. This caused a dose-dependent decrease in PGI_2 binding sites from a control value of 361±17 to 352±29 (P > 0.05), 220±15 (P < 0.01) and 181±19 (P < 0.001) fmol/10^9 platelets with 1, 10, and 100 nmol/l iloprost (n=6), respectively.

Coincubation of washed platelets (10^8 platelets/well) and confluent HUVECs for 15 min resulted in platelet adhesion of 0.7±0.1% to the endothelial cells. Addition of thrombin in concentrations ranging from 0.04 to 0.2 U/ml caused a dose-dependent increase in platelet adhesion to a maximum of 3.2±0.6% with 0.2U/ml thrombin (n=6).

When platelets were desensitized by preincubation with iloprost 10, 30 or 100 nmol/l the number of binding sites decreased by 23.3±2.8, 40.5±3.1 and 58.8±2.7%, respectively. This dose-dependent receptor desensitization resulted in a desensitization-dependent increase in platelet adhesion amounting to 21.7±0.7% adhesion with iloprost 100nmol/l and thrombin 0.2U/ml (Fig.1). When the data for the iloprost-induced receptor desensitization and increased platelet - endothelial cell adhesion were plotted a strong positive correlation was disclosed with a correlation coefficient of 0.96 for iloprost concentrations between 10 and 100 nmol/l.

Fig1: Significant augmentation of thrombin-stimulated platelet adhesion to human endothelial cells following platelet PGI_2 receptor desensitization by preincubation with iloprost (10-100 nmol/l for 3hrs). The data represent mean ± SEM of 6 independent experiments performed in duplicate.
* : P<0.01, ** : P<0.001

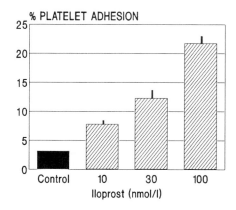

Discussion

In our experiments iloprost caused a dose-dependent diminuition of PGI_2 binding sites on human platelets being significantly lower than control already following incubation with 10 nmol/l for 3 hrs.

If PGI_2 receptor desensitization occurrs in vivo in humans two questions arise. First, are there physiologic or pathophysiologic situations in which a receptor desensitization is provoked and becomes detectable ex vivo and second, is the observed receptor desensitization of any physiologic importance. FitzGerald (2) reported in 1984 that PGI_2 metabolites in urine were markedly elevated in patients with severe atherosclerosis. A decreased number of platelet binding sites for PGI_2 in patients with spontaneous angina or acute myocardial ischemia has been reported (3,4,5). Although it has not yet conclusively demonstrated that prostacyclin receptors are diminished in those patients who exert an elevated prostacyclin metabolite excretion in urine, the evidence for this hypothesis is still increasing.

In case of prostacyclin receptor desensitization either during infusion therapy with PGI_2 or its analogs (4) or in pathophysiologic situations (3-5) the question of its physiologic importance is still unresolved. The main purpose of this study was to investigate the effect of prostacyclin receptor desensitization on the adhesion of human platelets to human endothelial cells in culture. Platelet preincubation with iloprost caused a dose-dependent PGI_2 receptor desensitization and in accordance with the decreased number of binding sites a marked increase in platelet adhesion to endothelial cells was observed (Fig.1). The augmented platelet adhesion of receptor desensitized platelets was comparable to the enhanced adhesion following ASA pretreatment (data not shown). The data for the decrease in PGI_2 binding sites and the increase in platelet adhesion were correlated with a coefficient of correlation of 0.96. Thus, the antiadhesive effect of endogenous PGI_2 in our model was completely lossed if the platelet PGI_2 receptor were desensitized.

These findings may have implications for the treatment of patients with vascular disease with PGI_2, PGE_1 or their analogs, since duration and dose of treatment are important factors for induction of PGI_2 receptor desensitization.

References

1. Curwen K, Kim H, Vazquez M, et al. J Lab Clin Med 1982;100:425-431.
2. FitzGerald G, Smith B, Pedersen A. N Engl J Med 1984;310:1065-1068.
3. Neri-Serneri GG, Modesti PA, Fortini A, et al. Lancet 1984; 2: 838-841.
4. Jaschonek K, Faul C, Renn W. Eur J Pharmacol 1988; 147: 187-196.
5. Kahn NN, Mueller H, Sinha AK. Circ Res 1991; 66: 932-940.
6. Modesti PA, Fortini A, Poggesi L, et al. Thromb Res 1987; 48: 663-669.

Advances in Prostaglandin, Thromboxane,
and Leukotriene Research, Vol. 23,
edited by B. Samuelsson et al.
Raven Press, Ltd., New York © 1995

Effects of 5-oxo-ETE on Neutrophils, Eosinophils, and Intestinal Epithelial Cells

William S. Powell, Sylvie Gravel, P. Stamatiou, and R. John MacLeod

Meakins-Christie Labs, McGill University, 3626 St. Urbain St., Montreal, Quebec, Canada, H2X 2P2

Human neutrophils contain a highly specific dehydrogenase which converts 5S-hydroxy-6,8,11,14-eicosatetraenoic acid (5S-HETE) to 5-oxo-ETE (Fig. 1). This enzyme is present in the microsomal fraction and requires $NADP^+$ as a cofactor. Only relatively small amounts of 5-oxo-ETE are formed from 5-HETE by resting cells, but its synthesis is strongly stimulated by phorbol myristate acetate (PMA), which appears to act by stimulating NADPH oxidase (1).

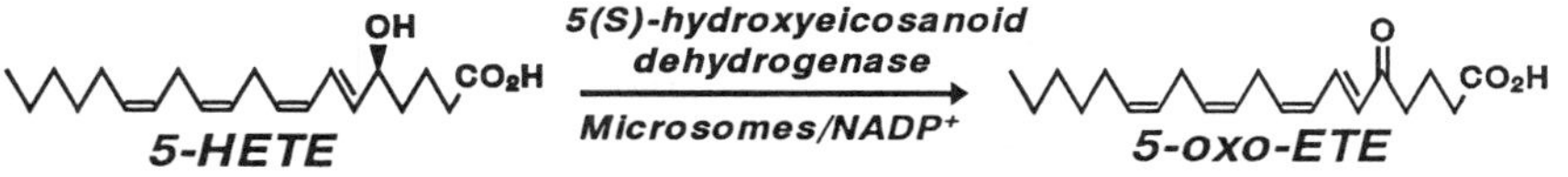

FIG. 1. Formation of 5-oxo-ETE from 5-HETE

5-Oxo-ETE is a potent agonist of human neutrophils, causing chemotaxis, increased cytosolic calcium levels, and degranulation (2,3). Although it is about one-tenth as potent as leukotriene B_4 (LTB_4), it clearly acts by a mechanism independent of the LTB_4 receptor, since its actions are not prevented by an LTB_4 antagonist or by prior desensitization of cells to LTB_4 (2,3). Cross-desensitization experiments suggest that 5-oxo-ETE interacts with a receptor with affinities for eicosanoids in the order 5-oxo-ETE > 5-oxo-15-hydroxy-ETE > 5S-HETE > LTB_4 (2). Although 5-oxo-ETE has similar actions to LTB_4 on human neutrophils, the fact that it acts by an independent mechanism raises the possibility that it could have a different spectrum of biological actions on other cells.

RESULTS AND DISCUSSION

5-Oxo-ETE stimulates adhesion of neutrophils to endothelial cells

Incubation of 5-oxo-ETE with a mixture of human neutrophils and human umbilical vein endothelial cells (HUVEC) lead to a marked increase in the numbers of neutrophils adhering to the HUVEC. The magnitude of this response was about the same as that for LTB_4 whereas the potency of 5-oxo-ETE (EC_{50}, ca. 2 nM) was about one-half that of LTB_4 (EC_{50}, 1 nM). Interestingly, the response to 5-oxo-ETE (maximum at 30 min) was slower than that to LTB_4 (maximum at 15 min) and was much more prolonged. Preincubation of 5-oxo-ETE with HUVEC, followed by washing and addition of neutrophils also resulted in enhanced adherence of neutrophils, the magnitude of this effect being about 3 times greater than that observed for LTB_4.

5-Oxo-ETE is a potent chemotactic agent for human eosinophils

The chemotactic effects of 5-oxo-ETE and other lipid mediators on eosinophils from healthy human subjects were evaluated. Eosinophils were purified by immunomagnetic removal of neutrophils. Chemotaxis was measured by direct counting of cells after staining with hematoxylin and chromotrope 2R and is expressed as the number of cells per high power field calculated as a percentage of the maximum response to 5-oxo-ETE. At a concentration of 1 nM (Fig. 2, left), 5-oxo-ETE had a slightly greater effect than platelet-activating factor (PAF) in stimulating chemotaxis. The effects of these two agonists were additive at this concentration. At higher concentrations (1 μM), the response to 5-oxo-ETE was about 3 times greater than that to PAF (Fig. 2, right). Addition of 1 nM 5-oxo-ETE to 1 μM PAF resulted in a more than additive increase in chemotaxis.

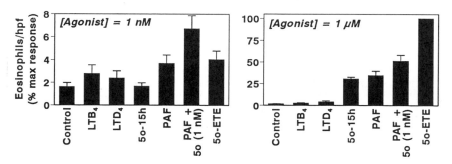

FIG. 2. Chemotactic effects of lipid mediators (1 nM, left; 1 μM, right) for human eosinophils. Responses to PAF in the presence of 1 nM 5-oxo-ETE are also shown (second bars from right in each panel).

5-Oxo-ETE induces volume reduction of intestinal epithelial cells

Incubation of jejunal crypt epithelial cells from guinea pigs with 5-oxo-ETE resulted in a reduction in cell volume. This response could be blocked by blockers of both Cl⁻ (anthracene 9-carboxylate) and K^+ (barium) channels as well as by staurosporine, an inhibitor of protein kinase C and other protein kinases. These experiments would suggest that the volume reduction induced by 5-oxo-ETE was caused by a protein kinase C-mediated increase in K^+ and Cl⁻ efflux from the epithelial cells. Of the substances investigated (LTD_4, bradykinin, and 5-HETE) 5-oxo-ETE was by far the most potent, with an EC_{50} of about 40 pM. In contrast, LTB_4 had no detectable effect on cell volume.

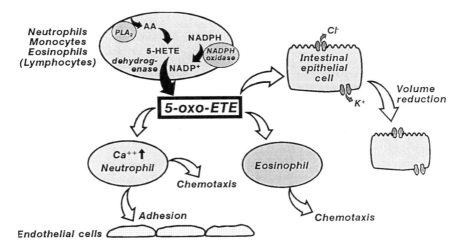

FIG. 3. Synthesis and biological activities of 5-oxo-ETE

5-Oxo-ETE is a potent stimulus of neutrophils, eosinophils, and epithelial cells (Fig. 3). In some cases it has actions similar to those of LTB_4, but in others it clearly has a different spectrum of activities. Because it is synthesized by inflammatory cells, 5-oxo-ETE may be an important mediator of inflammation.

REFERENCES

1. Powell WS, Zhang Y, Gravel S. Effects of phorbol myristate acetate on the synthesis of 5-oxo-6,8,11,14-eicosatetraenoic acid by human polymorphonuclear leukocytes. Biochemistry. 1994;33:3927-33.
2. Powell WS, Gravel S, MacLeod RJ, Mills E, Hashefi M. Stimulation of human neutrophils by 5-oxo-6,8,11,14-eicosatetraenoic acid by a mechanism independent of the leukotriene B₄ receptor. J Biol Chem. 1993;268:9280-6.
3. O'Flaherty JT, Cordes J, Redman J, Thomas MJ. 5-Oxoeicosatetraenoate, a potent neutrophil stimulus. Biochem Biophys Res Commun. 1993;192:129-34.

Advances in Prostaglandin, Thromboxane,
and Leukotriene Research, Vol. 23,
edited by B. Samuelsson et al.
Raven Press, Ltd., New York © 1995

Regulation of 12-Lipoxygenase by Platelet-Derived Growth Factor in Vascular Smooth Muscle Cells.

R. Natarajan, W. Bai, J. Gu, V. Rangarajan, and J. Nadler.

Department of Diabetes, City of Hope National Medical Center, Duarte, California 91010, U.S.A.

Platelet-derived growth factor-BB (PDGF) is a potent mitogen and chemotactic agent for vascular smooth muscle cells (VSMC) (1,2). PDGF also plays an important role *in vivo* in restenosis and formation of the neointimal lesion after balloon injury (3) and therefore has a key role in the pathogenesis of atherosclerosis. The binding of PDGF to its cell surface receptor leads to the stimulation of the receptor tyrosine kinase (1,4) followed by the activation of several signal transducing proteins. PDGF has also been shown to cause the release of arachidonic acid from membrane phospholipids (5). Arachidonic acid can itself serve as a substrate for several enzymes including the lipoxygenase (LO) and the cyclooxygenase. The signalling mechanisms of PDGF bear some resemblance to that of another VSMC growth factor, angiotensin II (AII). We have recently shown that the AII can increase the activity and expression of the 12-LO in porcine VSMC (PVSMC) (6). Furthermore, the LO pathway seems to play an important role in the growth-promoting effects of AII in PVSMC (7). In the present study we have examined whether PDGF can increase 12-LO activity and also expression of the 12-LO protein and mRNA.

METHODS

Recombinant human PDGF-BB was obtained from GIBCO-BRL. PVSMC were cultured as described (6). For studies of 12-LO activity, serum-starved cells were treated for 2 hr. with PDGF followed by measurement of immunoreactive 12-LO product, 12-hydroxyeicosatetraenoic acid (12-HETE) or intracellular 12-LO activity as described (6). For studies of the regulation of

12-LO protein or RNA expression, serum-starved cells were treated with PDGF-BB for 24 hr. followed by Western immunoblotting or RNA extraction (for reverse transcriptase polymerase chain reaction, RT-PCR) as described (6).

RESULTS AND DISCUSSION

PDGF treatment for 2 hr. did not alter the levels of released 12-HETE. However, it caused a significant dose-dependent increase in the levels of the cell-associated 12-HETE as seen in Table 1. This PDGF treatment also caused a marked increase in intracellular 12-LO activity (conversion of arachidonate to 12-HETE as measured by HPLC), which was blocked by the LO inhibitor baicalein and potentiated by the cyclooxygenase blocker, ibuprofen. These results suggest that PDGF can increase 12-LO activity in PVSMC.

TABLE 1. *Effect of PDGF treatment for 2 hr on immunoreactive cell-associated 12-HETE levels in PVSMC*

Treatment	12-HETE (pg/10^6 cells)
Basal	824±83
PDGF(2×10^{-11}M)	1205±191[*]
PDGF(2×10^{-10}M)	1571±140[**]
PDGF(2×10^{-9}M)	1769±102[**]

Results are expressed as mean±SE. *,p<0.05 vs basal; **,p<0.01 vs basal.

In order to determine whether PDGF-induced increase in 12-HETE formation is via increased transcriptional (mRNA) or translational (protein) expression of the 12-LO enzyme, we examined the effect of PDGF on leukocyte-type 12-LO mRNA and protein expression. We have previously shown the presence and AII-induced regulation of the leukocyte-type 12-LO in PVSMC (6). We now observed that PDGF could also up-regulate the levels of 12-LO mRNA transcripts (4-fold over control) at 24 hr as identified by RT-PCR. In addition, immunoblotting using a specific 12-LO peptide antibody, showed that PDGF caused a dose-dependent increase in levels of leukocyte-type 12-LO protein (72kD) at 24 hr with even a dose as low as 10^{-12}M causing a marked increase (fold increase over control by densitometry: PDGF 10^{-12}M, 2.3 fold; PDGF 10^{-11}M, 4.7 fold; PDGF 10^{-10}M, 3.5 fold).

LO products have several cardiovascular and growth promoting effects. 12-HETE is a potent inducer of smooth muscle migration (8) and the HETEs have direct hypertrophic effects and also mediate AII effects in VSMC (7). The present studies indicate that PDGF is a potent inducer of 12-LO activity and expression. Earlier studies have indicated that the chemotactic effects of PDGF in VSMC could be attenuated by a LO inhibitor such as caffeic acid but not by a cyclooxygenase inhibitor (9). Our results suggest that PDGF-induced 12-LO activity and expression may be a novel mechanism for the mitogenic and chemotactic effects of PDGF observed in the atherosclerotic process.

ACKNOWLEDGEMENTS

The authors thank N. Gonzales and L. Lanting for their excellent technical assistance and Drs. T. Yoshimoto and S. Yamamoto (Tokushima University, Japan) for the porcine 12-LO cDNA. This work was supported by grants from National Institutes of Health, R29 HL48920 and RO1 DK39721 to RN and JN.

REFERENCES

1. Ross R, Raines WE, Bowen-Pope DF. The biology of platelet-derived growth factor. *Cell* 1986;46:155-169.
2. Grotendorst G, Sepp HEJ, Kleinman HK, Martin GR. Attachment of smooth muscle cells to collagen and their migration towards platelet-derived growth factor. *Proc Natl Acad Sci USA* 1982;71:3669-3672.
3. Jawien A, Bowen-Pope DF, Schwartz SM, Clowes AW. Platelet-derived growth factor promotes smooth muscle migration and intimal thickening in a rat model of balloon angioplasty. *J Clin Invest* 1992;89:507-511.
4. Williams LT. Signal transduction by the platelet-derived growth factor. *Science* 1989;243:1564-1570.
5. Domin J, Rozengurt E. Platelet-derived growth factor stimulates a biphasic mobilization arachidonic acid in Swiss 3T3 cells. *J Biol Chem* 1993;268:8927-8934.
6. Natarajan R, Gu JL, Rossi J, Gonzales N, et al. Elevated glucose and angiotensin II increase 12-lipoxygenase activity and expression in porcine aortic smooth muscle cells. *Proc Natl Acad Sci USA* 1993;90:4947-4951.
7. Natarajan R, Gonzales N, Lanting L, Nadler J. Role of the lipoxygenase pathway in angiotensin II-induced vascular smooth muscle cell hypertrophy. *Hypertension* 1994;23[suppl I]:I-142-I-147.
8. Nakao J, Ooyama T, Ito H, Chang W, Murota S. Comparative effect of lipoxygenase products of arachidonic acid on rat aortic smooth muscle migration. *Atherosclerosis* 1982; 44:339-342.
9. Nakao J, Ito H, Chang WC et.al. Aortic smooth muscle cell migration caused by PDGF is mediated by lipoxygenase products of arachidonic acid. *Biochem Biophys Res Commun* 1983;112:866-871.

Advances in Prostaglandin, Thromboxane,
and Leukotriene Research, Vol. 23,
edited by B. Samuelsson et al.
Raven Press, Ltd., New York © 1995

Biological Properties of 12(S)-HETE in Cancer Metastasis

Xiang Gao [a] and Kenneth V. Honn [a, b, c]

Departments of [a] Radiation Oncology, [b] Chemistry, and [c] Pathology, Wayne State University, Detroit, Michigan 48202, USA

Metastasis is a cascade of linked and sequential steps involving multiple host cell-tumor cell interactions (1). To successfully create a metastatic colony, a cell or group of tumor cells must be able to complete all of the steps in the metastatic cascade, including detachment, intravasation, arrest (on endothelium), extravasation and proliferation. Multiple cell-host interactions, such as tumor cell-platelet, tumor cell-endothelial cell and tumor cell-matrix protein interactions, are influenced by positive and negative regulatory factors. Eicosanoids and other bioactive lipids have been shown to be involved in various aspects of neoplasia including cell transformation, proliferation, invasion and metastasis. Platelets and endothelial cells with which tumor cells interact during hematogenous metastasis are capable of producing a vast array of lipid mediators by either direct or transcellular metabolism of precursors. Platelets and some tumor cells are capable of converting arachidonic acid (AA) through the 12-lipoxygenase (12-LOX) pathway into 12(S)-hydroxyeicosatetraenoic acid [12(S)-HETE]. The generation of 12(S)-HETE and other fatty acids occurs in response to cell activation by various cytokines and growth factors. The production of these fatty acids [i.e. 12(S)-HETE] in response to cell activation, may suggest their role in as yet unidentified cell signaling pathway(s).

12-Lipoxygenase and its regulation in tumor cells. Lipoxygenases insert molecular oxygen into *cis, cis*-pentadiene-containing lipid molecules generating various hydroperoxides. So far three animal lipoxygenases have been identified; they are 5-, 12-, and 15-lipoxygenases named after the positions where oxygen is inserted to the AA moiety. 5-lipoxygenase metabolizes AA to hydroperoxyeicosatetraenoic acid (5-HPETE) which is further converted to 5-HETE and leukotrienes. 12-lipoxygenase (EC 1.13.11.31) metabolizes AA to 12-HPETE which is subsequently transformed to 12-HETE and hepoxilins. Similarly, 15-lipoxygenase catalyzes the reaction that generates 15-HPETE and subsequently 15-HETE and lipoxins. Three types of 12-lipoxygenases have been reported. The first is human platelet-type 12-lipoxygenase expressed normally in platelets, HEL (human erythroleukemia) cells, and umbilical vein endothelial cells. Platelet-type 12-lipoxygenase metabolizes only AA (but not C-18 fatty acids such as linoleic acid) to form exclusively 12(S)-HETE. The second is porcine leukocyte-type 12-lipoxygenase which metabolizes both arachidonic acid and linoleic acid thus generating 12(S)-HETE as well as small amounts of 15(S)-HETE. The third type of 12-lipoxygenase (sometimes termed epithelial 12-lipoxygenase) has been isolated from bovine tracheal epithelial cells and rat brain, which shares more homology with 15-lipoxygenase and leukocyte-type 12-lipoxygenase than with platelet-type 12-lipoxygenase. This type of 12-

lipoxygenase, like reticulocyte 15-lipoxygenase and leukocyte-type 12-lipoxygenase, catalyzes the formation of both 12(S)-HETE and 15(S)-HETE. Recently, mouse homologues of both platelet-type and leukocyte-type 12-lipoxygenases have been reported (see 1 and references therein for a review).

Although six 12-lipoxygenase cDNAs have been cloned from five species, its genomic structure has only been characterized from human, pig, and mouse. All 12-lipoxygenase genes isolated have 14 exons and the size of the exons, but not introns, are highly conserved among different species. The human, porcine, and mouse promoter sequences of 12-lipoxygenase genes have been identified by different groups, yet little is known about their regulation. Multiple GC boxes were found in the 5' region, raising the possibility of 12-lipoxygenase as a housekeeping gene. However, this is not very likely since 12-lipoxygenase activity is inducible. All 12-lipoxygenase promoters, except the mouse platelet-type 12-lipoxygenase promoter, contains no typical TATA box. The human platelet-type 12-lipoxygenase promoter contains 4 putative GC boxes, 2 CACCC boxes, 3 AP-2 sites, and 1 glucocorticoid-responsive element (GRE) (see 1 and references therein for a review). The porcine 12-lipoxygenase promoter possesses 9 GC boxes and 2 AP-2 sites. In mouse, platelet-type 12-lipoxygenase promoter has 3 GC boxes, 1 TATA site, 1 TATA-like site, and 1 AP-2 site, whereas leukocyte-type 12-lipoxygenase promoter contains 1 GC box, 1 TATA-like site, and 1 AP-1 site. We have isolated the 12-lipoxygenase promoter from a human colon carcinoma cell line (Clone A) and the sequence is nearly identical to the published human platelet-type 12-lipoxygenase promoter sequence with a point mutation affecting one of the four GC boxes (X. Gao and K. V. Honn, unpublished data). The GRE is activated by glucocorticoid, androgen, mineralococrticoid and progesterone. The AP-2 site is inducible by TPA, cAMP and retinoic acid. The AP-1 site could be induced by TPA and other protein kinase C (PKC) activators. Indeed, it has been shown that treatment of HEL cells with TPA increases 12-lipoxygenase mRNA and activity. Furthermore, EGF, glucose, and angiotensin II have been demonstrated to increase 12-lipoxygenase mRNA expression, stimulate 12-lipoxygenase activity and therefore the production of HETE and HODE (i.e., hydroxyoctadecaenoic acids). Recently, we and others identified authentic platelet-type 12-lipoxygenase mRNA in Clone A (human colon adenocarcinoma) cells (2) and DU 145 (human prostatic adenocarcinoma) cells (3) and observed that 12-lipoxygenase mRNA and protein were upregulated by 12-(S)-HETE treatment in Clone A cells (4).

12(S)-HETE as a signaling molecule. 12(S)-HETE is the major arachidonic acid (AA) metabolite of 12-LOX. Many different types of normal cells including platelets, neutrophils, macrophages, endothelial cells, and smooth muscle cells can generate 12(S)-HETE (5-7). However, the level of 12(S)-HETE generated by normal cells under resting physiological conditions is minimal. The physiological functions of this eicosanoid are not fully characterized, but accumulated data indicate that it is involved in a wide-spectrum of biological activities such as stimulating insulin secretion by pancreatic tissue, chemoattracting leukocytes, and facilitating the attachment of macrophages to rat glomeruli during inflammation (5). 12(S)-HETE also has been observed to reduce prostacyclin biosynthesis by vascular endothelial cells (8) and play a vital role in platelet activation and aggregation (9, 10). More recently, 12(S)-HETE is found to be the most prominent AA metabolite in menstrual blood (11) and in intrauterine tissues (12). However, the biological significance of these findings is not yet clear. A growing body of recent evidence suggests that 12(S)-HETE may act as a second messenger in stimulus-response coupling in some cells (13-16). For example, angiotensin II stimulates 12-HETE biosynthesis and aldosterone secretion by adrenal cortical cells. Pharmacologic inhibitors of 12-HETE biosynthesis suppress angiotensin II-induced aldosterone secretion, and exogenous 12-HETE increases aldosterone secretion (14). A similar series of observations suggest the participation of 12-HETE or its precursor in neurotransmitter peptide-induced hyperpolarization by Aplysia neuronal cells (13). 12(S)-HETE, like LTB4, has been shown to promote epidermal proliferation (15). On the other hand, treatment of rat renal cortical slices with 12-HPETE or 12-HETE, but not LTB4 or 5-HPETE, blocked the PGI_2- or iloprost-induced renin secretion (17). In addition, 12-HETE has been shown to significantly increase intracellular levels of cyclic AMP (cAMP) in human arterial smooth muscle cells (18).

We investigated a possible role of 12(S)-HETE on regulating expression of the 12-LOX gene, integrin genes (α_{IIb} and $\beta3$), tumor suppressor genes (deleted in colon carcinoma [DCC], p53, retinoblastoma [Rb], adenomatous polyposis coli [APC], mutated in colon carcinoma [MCC]), and oncogene MDM-2 in human colon carcinoma (Clone A) cells (for background information, see 1, 4, 19-22). It was found that 12(S)-HETE upregulated 12-LOX, α_{IIb}, $\beta3$ and MDM-2, but downregulated DCC mRNA levels (4). Preliminary results indicated that 12(S)-HETE also increased 12-LOX and MDM-2 at the protein level. The effects of 12(S)-HETE were antagonized by the PKC inhibitor, Calphostin C. No alteration was observed for p53, Rb, APC, and MCC genes. The mechanism of mRNA regulation by 12(S)-HETE may be transcriptional, since actinomycin D could abolish the 12(S)-HETE effect on gene expression (4). Interestingly, when Clone A cells were treated with BHPP, a 12-LOX selective inhibitor, stimulation of the DCC gene and suppression of the 12-LOX, MDM-2, α_{IIb}, and $\beta3$ gene expression were observed (4). This suggests that endogenous 12(S)-HETE in the Clone A cells may also be functioning in terms of regulating gene expression. The ability of 12(S)-HETE to upregulate 12-LOX, integrins, oncogene and downregulate tumor suppressor gene might contribute to its ability to increase tumor cell metastasis.

Our laboratory has performed comprehensive studies on the molecular mechanisms underlying the versatile 12(S)-HETE effects on various tumor cells (see 1 for a review). In tumor cells, external 12(S)-HETE, through binding to the cell surface receptor, activates a pertussis toxin-sensitive G protein (23, KVH, unpublished observations), which in turn activates PLC. Stimulation of PLC activates the phosphoinositide metabolism generating from PIP_2 both DAG and IP_3, which together activate PKC. Functionally activated PKC mediates protein (e.g., cytoskeletal elements) phosphorylation resulting in a modulation of a variety of phenotypic properties of metastasizing tumor cells such as adhesion, spreading, and motility (24-28). Tumor cell adhesion to endothelial cells activates the 12-lipoxygenase, leading to arachidonic acid metabolism to 12(S)-HETE. 12(S)-HETE, by unknown mechanisms, activates PKC and translocates PKC to the plasma membrane. PKC subsequently phosphorylates and reorganizes the cytoskeletal elements which mobilize $\alpha_{IIb}\beta3$ integrin-containing vesicles to the plasma membrane. Cytoskeletal rearrangements induced by 12(S)-HETE also are involved in modulation of tumor cell spreading on matrix and tumor cell motility. Tumor cell-derived 12(S)-HETE likewise acts on endothelial cells, resulting in enhanced $\alpha v\beta3$ integrin surface expression and tumor cell adhesion, and PKC-dependent phosphorylation and reorganization of cytoskeleton and endothelial cell retraction. In addition, 12(S)-HETE may promote tumor cell release of cathepsin B to degrade the subendothelial matrix. In vivo, tumor cell interactions with platelets (through $\alpha_{IIb}\beta3$ integrins and many other receptors) will lead to platelet aggregation, activation and release reactions. Platelet-derived 12(S)-HETE, which can be released to the foci of tumor cell-platelet-endothelial cell interactions, can similarly act on endothelial cells to initiate the diverse biological responses described above, thus contributing to tumor cell metastasis.

12(S)-HETE effects on modulating tumor invasion and metastasis. 12(S)-HETE can enhance the invasive and metastatic potentials of tumor cells via modulating several steps of this complex process (1). 12(S)-HETE has been shown to promote tumor cell motility, enhance tumor cell release of proteolytic enzyme cathepsin B, reorganize tumor cell cytoskeleton, modulate tumor cell interactions with matrix, and induce endothelial cell retraction (see 1 for a review). Several lines of experimental evidence suggest that the ability of tumor cells to generate 12(S)-HETE is correlated with their metastatic potential. First, subpopulations of murine B16 amelanotic melanoma (B16a) have been isolated by centrifugal elutriation that demonstrate differential metastatic capabilities. The high metastatic subpopulation of B16a cells (HM340) synthesized 4 times more 12(S)-HETE than the low metastatic subpopulation of B16a (LM180) cells when equal amounts of substrates were supplied (29). The generation of higher amount of 12(S)-HETE in HM340 cells appears to result from the presence of a higher level of 12-lipoxygenase mRNA in these cells (30). Second, the correlation of 12(S)-HETE production and metastatic potential also was evaluated in several other tumor cell systems, i.e., Dunning rat prostate carcinoma (AT2.1 and GP 9F3, low metastatic cell lines; MAT Lu and MLL, high metastatic lines) (31), murine B16 melanoma (F1, low metastatic; F10, high metastatic) (29, 30), and murine K-1735 melanoma (C1-11, low metastatic clone; M1, high metastatic clone). In all these experiments it was observed that the high metastatic tumor cell lines generate a significantly higher level of 12(S)-HETE than low metastatic counterparts (1). Third, tumor cell adhesion to fibronectin provokes a spike of 12(S)-HETE generation within 10 min indicating a late-type signaling activation of tumor cell 12-lipoxygenase (26). Morphological studies demonstrated that tumor cell spreading on fibronectin is followed by 12-lipoxygenase translocation to the cell surface (26.). Fourth, adhesion of tumor cells to vascular endothelium is accompanied or immediately followed by a surge of 12(S)-HETE biosynthesis by tumor cells, which was correlated with tumor cell-induced endothelial cell retraction (32). Low metastatic B16a cells generated little 12(S)-HETE upon adhesion and did not induce endothelial cell retraction. In contrast, high metastatic B16a cells adhering to endothelium biosynthesized large amounts of 12(S)-HETE and induced prominent retraction of endothelial cell monolayers (32). Fifth, pretreatment of tumor cells with a selective platelet-type 12-lipoxygenase inhibitor, BHPP (N-benzyl-N-hydroxy-5-phenylpentanamide; 2) dose-dependently inhibited adhesion-induced tumor cell biosynthesis of 12(S)-HETE and endothelial cell retraction (32), platelet-enhanced tumor cell-induced endothelial cell retraction (33), tumor cell (i.e., HM340 B16a cells) adhesion to endothelium and matrix (2, 29), and lung colonization by high metastatic B16a cells (29). Sixth, in rat Dunning R3327 model, 12(S)-HETE was found to increase the motility (determined by the colloidal gold phagokinetic track assay) and invasion (measured as their ability to invade through basement membrane Matrigel-coated filters) of low metastatic AT2.1 cells (31). Finally, 12(S)-HETE has recently been shown to stimulate PKC-mediated release of cathepsin B from tumor cells (34). Interestingly, 12(S)-HETE induced release of native and latent cathepsin B activity in the high metastatic murine B16a cells, but did not induce the release of cathepsin B from low metastatic B16-F1 cells. This suggested that there may be an enhanced response to 12(S)-HETE in more malignant cells. Similar results also were obtained in immortalized and ras-transfected MCF-10 human breast epithelial cells, in which 12(S)-HETE induced cathepsin B release from the ras-trancfected, but not the immortalized cells (34). Taken together, these data implicate 12-lipoxygenase and 12(S)-HETE production as an important determinant of tumor cell invasion and metastasis.

12-Lipoxygenase as a prognostic marker in human prostate cancer. Since 12(S)-HETE has aforementioned global effects on tumor cell invasion and metastasis and tumor cells possess the 12(S)-HETE-generating enzyme (12-LOX), we tested for the potential use of 12-lipoxygenase as a predictor for the aggressiveness of human prostate cancer (3). The 12-lipoxygenase mRNA expression levels in matching prostate normal and cancerous tissues were measured by in situ hybridization (ISH) and quantitative reverse transcription-polymerase chain reaction (RT-PCR). A statistically significantly greater number of cases were found to have an elevated level of 12-lipoxygenase among T3, high grade, and surgical margin positive than T2, intermediate grade, and surgical margin negative prostatic adenocarcinomas. Therefore, our data suggest 12-lipoxygenase may serve as an indicator for progression and prognosis of prostate cancer (3). This enzyme also may be a novel potential target for the development of anti-invasive and anti-metastatic agents.

REFERENCES

1. Honn KV, Tang DG, Gao X, et al. 12-lipoxygenases and cancer metastasis. *Cancer Metastasis Rev.*, (In press)
2. Chen YQ, Dunies ZM, Liu B, et al. Endogenous 12(S)-HETE production by tumor cells and its role in metastasis. *Cancer Res.* 1994; 54:1574-1579.
3. Gao X, Gringnon D, Honn KV, et al. Elevated 12-lipoxygenase mRNA expression: a novel marker for poor prognosis in human prostate cancer. *J Natl Cancer Inst* (Submitted).
4. Gao X, Hagmann W, Zacharek A, et al. Eicosanoids, cancer metastasis, and gene regulation. In:Honn KV, Nigam S, Marnett LJ. *Eicosanoid and other bioactive lipid in cancer, inflammation, and radiation injury.* Norwell, MA: Kluwer Academic Publishers; 1994: 537-547.
5. Spector AA, Gordon JA, Moore SA. Hydroxyeicosatetraenoic acids (HETEs). *Prog Lipid Res* 1988; 27:271-323.
6. Natarajan R, Gu J-L, Rossi J, et al. Elevated glucose and angiotensin II increase 12-lipoxygenase activity and expression in porcine aortic smooth muscle cells. *Proc Natl Acad Sci USA* 1993; 90:4947-4951.
7. Kim JA, Gu J, Natarajian R, et al. Evidence that a leukocyte type of 12-lipoxygenase is expressed in normal human vascular and mononuclear cells. *Clin Res* 1993; 41:148A.
8. Hadjiagapiou C, Spector AA. 12-hydroxyeicosatetraenoic acid reduces prostacyclin production by endothelial cells. *Prostaglandins* 1986; 31:1135-1144.
9. Sekiya F, Takagi J, Usui T, et al. 12S-hydroxyeicosatetraenoic acid plays a central role in the regulation of platelet activation. *Biochem Biophys Res Commun* 1991; 179:345-351.
10. Scheider MR, Tang DG, Schirner M, et al. Prostacyclin and its analogues: antimetastatic effects and mechanisms of action. *Cancer Metastasis Rev.* Inpress, 1994
11. Hofer G, Bieglmayer CH, Kopp B, et al. Measurement of eicosanoids in menstrual fluid by the combined use of high pressure chromatography and radioimmunoassay. *Prostaglandins* 1993; 45:413-426.
12. Wetzka B, Schafer W, Scheibel M. Eicosanoid production by intrauterine tissues before and after labor in short-term tissue culture. *Prostaglandins* 1993;45:571-581.
13. Piomelli D, Volterra A, Dale N, et al. Lipoxygenase metabolites of arachidonic acid as second messengers for presynaptic inhibition of Aplysia sensory cells. *Nature* 1987; 328:38-43.
14. Nadler JL, Natarajian R, Stern N. Specific action of the lipoxygenase pathway in mediating angiotensin II-induced aldosterone synthesis in isolated adrenal glomerula cells. *J Clin Invest* 1987; 80:1763-1769.
15. Chan CC, Duhamel L, Ford-Hutchison A. Leukotriene B4 and 12-hydroxyeicosatetraenoic acid stimulate epidermal proliferation in vivo in the guinea pig. *J Invest Dermatol* 1985; 85:333-334.
16. Glasgow WC, Afshari CA, et al. Modulation of the epidermal growth factor mitogenic response by metabolites of linoleic and arachidonic acid in Syrian hamster embryo fibroblasts. Differential effects in tumor suppressor (+) and (-) phenotypes. *J Biol Chem* 1992; 267:10771-10779

17. Antonipillai I. 12-lipoxygenase products are potent inhibitors of prostacyclin-induced renin release. *Proc Soc Exp Biol Med* 1990; 194:224-230.
18. Etingin OR, Hajjar DP. Evidence for cytokine regulation of cholesterol metabolism in herpes virus-infected arterial cells by the lipoxygenase pathway. *J Lipid Res* 1990; 31:299-305.
19. Chen YQ, Gao X, Timar J, et al. Identification of the $\alpha_{IIb}\beta_3$ integrin in murine tumor cells. *J. Biol. Chem.* 1992; 267:17314-17320.
20. Gao X, Honn, KV, Grigonn D, et al. Frequent loss of expression and loss of heterozygosity of the putative tumor suppressor gene DCC in prostatic carcinomas. *Cancer Res.* 1993; 53:2723-2727.
21. Gao X, Wu N, Grignon D, et al. High frequency of mutator phenotype in human prostatic adenocarcinoma. *Oncogene* 1994; 9: 2999-3003.
22. Gao X, Wu N, Grignon D, et al. Allelic deletion of microsatellite loci on chromosome 6p in a subset of human prostate cancer. *Cancer Mol. Biol. J.* (In press)
23. Liu B, Khan WA, Hannun YA, et al. 12(S)-HETE and 13(S)-HODE regulation of protein kinase C alpha in melanoma cells: Role of receptor mediated hydrolysis of inositol phospholipids. (Submitted)
24. Chopra H, Timar J, Chen YQ, et al. The lipoxygenase metabolite 12(S)-HETE induces a cytoskeleton-dependent increase in surface expression of integrin $\alpha_{IIb}\beta_3$ on melanoma cells. *Int J Cancer* 1991; 49:774-786.
25. Chopra H, Timar J, Rong X, et al. Is there a role for the tumor cell integrin aIIbb3 and cytoskeleton in tumor cell-platelet interaction? *Clin Expl Metastasis* 1992; 10:125-138.
26. Timar J, Chen YQ, Liu B, et al. The lipoxygenase metabolite 12(S)-HETE promotes $\alpha_{IIb}\beta_3$ integrin-mediated tumor cell spreading on fibronectin. *Int J Cancer* 1992; 52: 594-603.
27. Timar J, Silletti S, Bazaz R, et al. Regulation of melanoma-cell motility by the lipoxygenase metabolite 12(S)-HETE. *Int J Cancer* 1993; 55:1003-1010.
28. Timar J, Tang D, Bazaz R, et al. PKC mediates 12(S)-HETE-induced cytoskeletal rearrangement in B16a melanoma cells. *Cell Motil Cytoskel* 1993; 26:49-65.
29. Liu B, Mamett LJ, Chaudhary A, et al. Biosynthesis of 12(S)-hydroxyeicosatetraenoic acid by B16 amelanotic melanoma cells is a determinant of their metastic potential. *Lab Invest.* 1994; 20:314-323.
30. Tang DG, Honn KV. 12-Lipoxygenase, 12(S)-HETE, and Cancer Metastasis. *Annals New York Acad Sci* (in press)
31. Liu B, Maher RJ, Hannun YA, et al. 12(S)-HETE enhancement of prostate tumor cell invasion: Seledctive role of PKCα. *J Natl Cancer Inst* 1994; 86:1145-1151.
32. Honn KV, Tang D, Grossi I, et al. Tumor cell-derived 12(S)-Hydroxyeicosatetraenoic acid induces microvascular endothelial cell retraction. *Cancer Res.* 1994; 54: 565-574.
33. Honn KV, Tang DG, Grossi IM, et al. Enhanced endothelial cell retraction mediated by 12(S)-HETE: A proposed mechanism for the role of platelets in tumor cell metastasis. *Exp Cell Res* 1994; 210:1-9.
34. Honn KV, Timar J, Rozhin J, et al. A lipoxygenase metabolite, 12-(S)-HETE, stimulates protein kinase C-mediated release of cathepsin B from malignant cells. *Exp Cell Res* (in press)

Advances in Prostaglandin, Thromboxane,
and Leukotriene Research, Vol. 23,
edited by B. Samuelsson et al.
Raven Press, Ltd., New York © 1995

INVOLVEMENT OF CYCLOOXYGENASE-2 IN BONE LOSS INDUCED BY INTERLEUKIN-1β

Takahiro Sato, Ikuo Morita, Kouji Sakaguchi,
Kenichi Nakahama and Sei-itsu Murota

*Department of Physiological Chemistry, Graduate School,
Tokyo Medical and Dental University, 1-5-45,
Yushima, Bunkyo-ku, Tokyo, Japan,*

Osteoclast has been know to be derived from hematopoietic stem cell (1). In the course of the development of osteoclast from stem cell, stroma cell is known to play some important roles by providing various kinds of associated factors with the osteoclast formation (2). On the other hand, a mouse bone marrow cell culture provides an ideal experimental system in vitro capable of examining the processes of the osteoclast development from stem cell (3). By using this assay system, we examined the mechanism of IL-1β induced osteoclast formation. After 8 days, the cultures received some factors that could stimulate osteoclast development, showed some typical osteoclasts formed which can easily be distinguished from other types of cells by their specific feature of multinuclear giant size and positive staining with tartrate-resistant acid phosphatase. The effects of IL-1β on the osteoclast formation and PGE_2 production in the mouse bone marrow cell cultures were examined. IL-1β caused a remarkable increase in the number of osteoclast in a dose dependent fashion, which was accompanied by PGE_2 production in the culture. To know the relationship between PGE_2 production and osteoclast formation in the IL-1β treatment, we examined the effect of indomethacin on the IL-1β effects. There was a good correlation between PGE_2 production and osteoclast formation. PGE_2 production declined with increasing doses of indomethacin, in proportion to that, osteoclast formation also declined. The stimulatory effect of IL-1β on the osteoclast formation was blocked by indomethacin completely, while the effect of PGE$_2$ exogenously added to the culture was not blocked by indomethacin at all. Concomitant addition of IL-1β caused an additional increase in the osteoclast formation, and only the additional increase was blocked by indomethacin. These results suggest that the endogenous PGE$_2$ induced by IL-1β plays an important role in the osteoclast formation. To know whether the enhanced PGE$_2$ production due to the IL-1β treatment was accompanied by protein synthesis or not, next we examined the effect of cycloheximide on the PGE$_2$ production. The increased PGE$_2$ production due to the IL-1β treatment was blocked by cycloheximide in a dose dependent fashion, suggesting that induction of some new enzyme was involved in the PGE$_2$ production. Therefore, next we examined, whether IL-1β could induce cyclooxygenase (COX) or not. The time course of the Northern blot analysis of COX-2 mRNA during the IL-1β treatment showed that the IL-1β treatment caused a time dependent increase in the expression of COX-2 mRNA. The amount of the mRNA started to increase 30min after the IL-1β treatment and reached the maximum level 2h after the IL-1β treatment. On the other hand, concomitant treatment with cycloheximide caused super-induction of COX-2 mRNA, suggesting that some degradation enzyme of COX-2 mRNA was involved in this process. The stimulatory effect of IL-1β on the induction of COX-2 mRNA was dose dependent. Since dexamethasone (DEX) has been known to inhibit COX-2 induction in various kinds of cells, next we examined the effect of DEX on the IL-1β effects. The data on the Northern blot analysis of COX-2 mRNA expression under the DEX treatment showed that, DEX blocked COX-2 mRNA accumulation almost completely. However, DEX block the cycloheximide induced super induction of COX-2 mRNA only slightly. As we expected, DEX inhibited the IL-1β induced osteoclast formation in a dose dependent fashion. These data strongly suggest that COX-2 induction plays a key role in the IL-1β induced osteoclast formation. To know whether protein kinase C (PKC) is involved in the IL-1β induced osteoclast formation, next we examined the effect of Calphostin C, a specific inhibitor of PKC, on the IL-1β induced osteoclast formation. Calphostin C (CAL) caused significant inhibition of IL-1β induced osteoclast formation. The data on the Northern blot analysis of COX-2 mRNA under the CAL treatment showed that CAL abolished the IL-1β induced COX-2 mRNA expression, suggesting that PKC is deeply involved in the COX-2 mRNA induction by IL-1β.

EXPERIMENTAL PROCEDURES

Bone marrow mononuclear cells were isolated from 7 weeks old male ddy mice (Sankyo Laboratory, Japan) and were cultured as described previously (3). After being cultured for 8 day, aliquots of conditioned medium were assayed for the levels of PGE$_2$ using an enzyme immunoassay system (Amersham, USA) and the cell layers were stained with tartrate-resistant acid phosphatase, a marker enzyme of osteoclast as described (4). The total cellular

RNA was isolated as described previously (5). The purified RNA was then denatured with glyoxal and dimethyl sulfoxide, electrophoresed on a 1.0% agarose gel, and transferred to a nylon membrane filters (Amersham, USA). The RNA was hybridized to ^{32}P-labeled COX-2 and glyceraldehyde-3-phosphate dehydrogenase (GAPDH) cDNA probes.

CONCLUSIONS

1.   The mechanism in which IL-1β enhances osteoclast formation was investigated in relation to PGE_2.

2.   In the mouse bone marrow cell cultures, IL-1β caused a dose-dependent increase in the number of osteoclast via endogenous PGE_2 production.

3.   Northern blot analysis showed that IL-1β induced COX-2 mRNA.

4.   When COX-2 mRNA induced by IL-1β was blocked by DEX, the increased osteoclast formation by IL-1β was also suppressed.

5. PGE_2 production through the COX-2 mRNA induction was exclusively involved in the IL-1β induced osteoclast formation, which was regulated by PKC.

ACKNOWLEDGMENT

The COX-2 cDNA probe used in the series of experiments was kindly provided by Dr. David L. DeWitt and Dr. William L. Smith (Department of Biochemistry, Michigan State University), to whom the authors thanks are due.

REFERENCES

1.   Udagawa N, Takahashi N, Akatsu T. Tanaka H, Sasaki T, Nishihara T, Koga T, Martin TJ and Suda T *Proc. Natl. Acad. Sci. USA* 1990; 87: 7260-4.
2.   Suda T, Takahashi N and Martin TJ *Endocrine Rev.* 1992; 13: 66-80.
3.   Takahashi N, Yamana H, Yoshiki S, Roodman GD, Mundy GR, Jones SJ, Boyde A and Suda T *Endocrinology* 1988; 122: 13703-82.
4.   Burstone MS *J. Natl. Cancer Inst.* 1958; 21: 523-39.
5.   Chomczynski P and Sacchi N *Anal. Biochem.* 1987; 162: 156-9.

Advances in Prostaglandin, Thromboxane,
and Leukotriene Research, Vol. 23,
edited by B. Samuelsson et al.
Raven Press, Ltd., New York © 1995

TRANSFORMING GROWTH FACTOR-BETA AND 1,25-DIHYDROXYVITAMIN D_3 INDUCE 5-LIPOXYGENASE ACTIVITY DURING MYELOID CELL MATURATION

D. Steinhilber[§], M. Brungs[§], O. Rådmark[¶] and B. Samuelsson[¶]

[¶]*Dept. of Medical Biochemistry and Biophysics, Karolinska Institutet, Box 60400, S-10401 Stockholm, Sweden and* [§]*Pharmaceutical Institute, University of Tübingen, Auf der Morgenstelle 8, D-72076 Tübingen, F.R.G.*

1. INTRODUCTION

Leukotrienes are important mediators of inflammation and are released from leukocytes after stimulation [1]. The capability of leukocytes to release leukotrienes is upregulated during myeloid cell maturation. Using DMSO differentiation of HL-60 cells as a model for myeloid cell maturation we observed that a protein factor in serum was required for upregulation of 5-lipoxygenase (5-LO) activity [2]. TGFß was identified as an inducer of cellular 5-LO activity [3]. TGFß1 (2 ng/ml) and a combination of TGFß1 and GM-CSF (1 ng/ml) lead to a 10- and 32-fold induction of cellular 5-LO activity, respectively. 5-LO activity in cell homogenates (3- and 6-fold induction, respectively) and 5-LO protein levels (2- or 5-fold induction, respectively) were less affected. No appreciable effects were observed on 5-LO and FLAP mRNA levels as determined by RT-PCR analysis.

During purification of the 5-LO stimulatory activity from serum, protein and lipid fractions were separated and it was found that serum lipids markedly enhanced the effect of the serum factor [3]. Cellular 5-LO activity of DMSO differentiated HL-60 cells correlated with CD14 expression [2]. Recently, it was reported that CD14 expression in HL-60 cells is strongly induced by 1,25-dihydroxyvitamin D_3 (VD3) plus TGFß [4] and that VD3 mediated differentiation of monocytes to macrophages enhances 5-LO activity [5].

In the present study we investigated the effects of TGFß, VD3 and related differentiation inducers on 5-LO activity, 5-LO protein and mRNA expression in HL-60 cells.

2. METHODS

Cell culture, preparation of lipid and protein fractions of serum, determination of 5-LO activity, Western blot and RT-PCR analysis were performed as described [2,3].

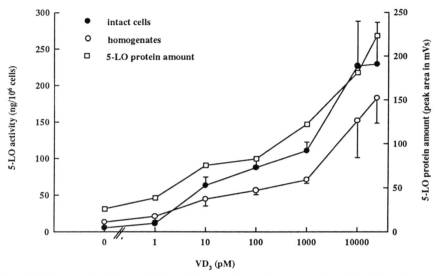

Fig. 1. Effects of VD3 on 5-LO activity and protein expression. HL-60 cells were differentiated for 4 days in serum free medium with 1.5 % DMSO, 1% serum protein fraction and the indicated concentrations of VD3.

3. RESULTS AND DISCUSSION

5-LO activity of intact HL-60 cells was rather low when they were differentiated in the absence of lipid fraction or VD3. Addition of lipid fraction increased 5-LO activity from 5.4±2.7 to 20.3±13.3 ng 5-LO products/10^6 cells (n=3). When the lipid fraction was replaced by VD3, there was a concentration dependent induction of 5-LO activity and 5-LO protein expression (fig. 1). Induction of 5-LO activity and protein expression was detectable at very low concentrations of VD3 (10pM). VD3 (24 nM) increased cellular 5-LO activity from 5.4 to 229.2±57.2 ng/10^6 cells (n=3) and lead to an about 14-fold induction of 5-LO protein amount and 5-LO activity in cell homogenates. This difference in protein expression corresponded to 4-fold differences in 5-LO mRNA expression as determined by reverse transcription and competitive PCR analysis (data not shown).

Next, induction of 5-LO activity and protein expression by VD3, TGFß, DMSO and retinoic acid (RA) alone and combinations of TGFß or VD3 with other compounds was investigated (fig. 2). No 5-LO expression was detectable in undifferentiated cells. TGFß alone was a poor inducer of 5-LO expression. DMSO increased 5-LO protein expression and 5-LO activity in cell homogenates but failed to induce 5-LO activity in intact cells. However, VD3 alone and especially the combination of TGFß and VD3 induced high levels of 5-LO expression and activity. Other combinations were less active. Similar results were

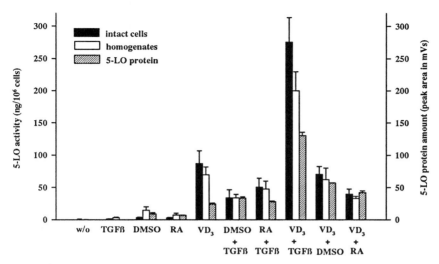

Fig. 2. Effects of differentiation inducers on 5-LO activity and protein expression. HL-60 cells were differentiated in serum free medium for 4 days in the presence of the TGFß (1 ng/ml), DMSO (1.5%), retinoic acid (RA, 1 μM), VD3 (24 nM) or combinations of these compounds.

obtained when 5-LO mRNA expression was determined by RT-PCR (data not shown).

It is concluded that VD3 and TGFß are potent inducers of 5-LO activity and protein expression in HL-60 cells. Also, in contrast to DMSO, combination of both compounds seems to affect the expression of cellular components which are important for 5-LO activity in the intact cell.

4. REFERENCES

1. Samuelsson, B., Dahlén, S.-E., Lindgren, J.-Å., Rouzer, C.A. and Serhan, C.N. Leukotrienes and lipoxins: Structures, biosynthesis, and biological effects. *Science* 1987;237:1171-1176.
2. Steinhilber, D., Hoshiko, S., Grunewald, J., Rådmark, O. and Samuelsson, B. Serum factors regulate 5-lipoxygenase activity in maturating HL-60 cells. *Biochim Biophys Acta* 1993;1178:1-8.
3. Steinhilber, D., Rådmark, O. and Samuelsson, B. Transforming growth factor beta upregulates 5-lipoxygenase activity during myeloid cell maturation. *Proc Natl Acad Sci USA* 1993;90:5984-5988.
4. Morikawa, M., Harada, N., Soma, G. and Yoshida, T. Transforming growth factor-beta1 modulates the effect of 1-alpha,25-dihydroxyvitamin D3 on leukemic cells. *In Vitro Cell Dev Biol* 1990;26:682-690.
5. Coffey, M.J., Gyetko, M. and Peters-Golden, M. 1,25-Dihydroxyvitamin D3 upregulates 5-lipoxygenase metabolism and 5-lipoxygenase activating protein in peripheral blood monocytes as they differentiate into mature macrophages. *J Lipid Med* 1993;6:43-51.

Advances in Prostaglandin, Thromboxane,
and Leukotriene Research, Vol. 23,
edited by B. Samuelsson et al.
Raven Press, Ltd., New York © 1995

MODULATION OF EGF CELL SIGNALING TYROSINE PHOSPHORYLATION BY LINOLEIC ACID METABOLITES

Thomas E. Eling, Angela L.Everhart and Wayne C. Glasgow

Laboratory of Molecular Biophysics,NIEHS,NIH
Research Triangle Park,NC 27709,USA

This laboratory is investigating arachidonic acid and linoleic acid metabolites formed by prostaglandin H synthase and lipoxygenase as modulators of growth factor signaling pathways that lead to cellular proliferation (1,2). We have chosen to focus on epidermal growth factor (EGF) and employ Syrian hamster embryo (SHE) fibroblasts in these studies (2). SHE cells are an immortalized preneoplastic cell line established by treatment of primary fibroblasts with a carcinogen. The cells were selected for two variants. The supB+ variant inhibits tumorigenicity of tumor cells in cell-cell hybrids while supB- does not inhibit tumorigenicity. Epidermal growth factor (EGF) stimulates mitogenesis which is attenuated by lipoxygenase but not prostaglandin H synthase (PHS) inhibitors. Arachidonic acid is metabolized to PGE_2 by SHE cells to a limited extent and no lipoxygenase-derived arachidonic acid metabolites were observed. EGF does not stimulate the expression of PHS-2 in these cells. EGF stimulates the production of lipoxygenase-derived metabolites of linoleic acid. We characterized 13-hydroxyoctadecadienoic acid (13-HODE) as the major metabolite with 9-hydroxyoctadecadienoic (9-HODE) as a minor product (2). Subsequent chiral analysis determined that 13(S)-HODE was the only enantiomer formed, while 9(S,R)-HODE were observed (4) Figure 1.

The metabolism of linoleic acid by SHE cells is regulated by the tyrosine kinase activity of the EGF receptor (EGFR). The tyrosine kinase inhibitor, methyl 2,5-dihydroxycinnamate inhibits not only EGF-dependent mitogenesis but also the formation of 13(S)-HODE from endogenous and exogenous linoleic

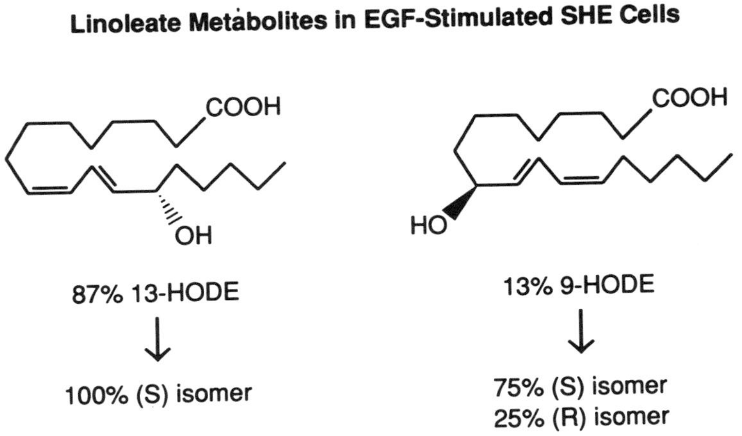

Linoleate Metabolites in EGF-Stimulated SHE Cells

87% 13-HODE

13% 9-HODE

↓

↓

100% (S) isomer

75% (S) isomer
25% (R) isomer

Fig. 1. EGF-dependent metabolism of linoleic acid by SHE cells.

acid(2). Furthermore, the addition of linoleic acid metabolites potently augmented EGF-dependent mitogenesis in the supB+ variant but not in the supB- variant of SHE cells. The metabolites by themselves were not mitogenic. In contrast,the addition of PGE_2 potently inhibited EGF-dependent mitogenesis (5). We have recently defined the structural requirements of analogous lipid metabolites necessary for stimulation of EGF-dependent mitogenesis. A high specificity was observed for the (S)-isomer of 13-HODE. Corresponding metabolites of arachidonic acid and linolenic acid were weakly active (4). 13(S)-HpODE was more potent than 13(S)-HODE and effective at nanomolar concentration. These results suggest a specific interaction between 13(S)-HpODE with intercellular components of the EGF signaling pathway.

EGF binds to its receptor (EGFR) and activates the intrinsic tyrosine kinase activity which is a critical activity that leads to cellular proliferation. EGFR kinase activity auto-phosphorylates the cytoplasmic portion of the receptor and phosphorylates a family of signaling proteins which include GAP (GTPase activating protein). These events initiate a kinase cascade, a series of enzymes in which each member phosphorylates the subsequent protein and thereby activates the next member of the series. The stimulation of EGF-dependent mitogenesis by the linoleic acid metabolites could occur by modulation of the EGF signaling pathway.

Tyrosine phosphorylation initiated by the tyrosine kinase activity of the EGFR can be examined by Western analysis of whole cell lysates using specific antibodies against signaling proteins and phosphorylated tyrosine moieties. We examined the auto-phosphorylation of the EGFR (170 Kd) and tyrosine phosphorylation of the GTPase activting protein, GAP (120Kd) most likely as a RAS-GAP complex. EGF produced both a concentration and time dependent tyrosine phosphorylation of the EGFR and GAP proteins as measured with anti-phosphorylated tyrosine antibody. At 37° C, the tyrosine phosphorylation of the EGFR and RAS-GAP complex proteins peaked at approximately 1-2 minutes and then rapidly declined. The decay of the tyrosine phoshporylated EGFR and GAP proteins was faster in the SupB+ cells than in the supB- cells. Pre-incubation of SHE cells with 13(S)-HpODE or 13(S)-HODE at 10^{-9} to 10^{-6} M increased the half-lives of the tyrosine phosphorylated EGFR and GAP proteins in the supB+ but was not effective with the supB- variant.   With EGF alone the phosphorylated EGFR was not detectable after 2 minutes, but with EGF and 13-HpODE, the phosphorylated receptor was still detectable at 5 minutes. This finding is in agreement with the observation that linoleic acid metabolites stimulated EGF-dependent mitogenesis in the supB+ but not the supB- variant. EGFR and GAP protein levels measured by Western analysis with specific antibodies were not altered by the treatments.   Other arachidonic acid and linoleic acid metabolites were not effective. These findings suggest that 13(S)-HpODE and 13(S)-HODE stimulate EGF-dependent mitogenesis and up-regulate the EGF signaling pathway by prolonging tyrosine phosphorylation dependent on the EGFR tyrosine kinase. The mechanism(s) by which the linoleic acid metabolites modulates the EGF tyrosine phosphorylation signaling cascade remains to be elucidated.

REFERENCES

1.   Nolan RD, Danilowicz RM, Eling TE.   Role of arachidonic acid metabolism in the mitogenic response of BALB/c 3T3 fibroblasts to epidermal growth factor. *Mol Pharmacol* 1988;**33**:650-6.
2.   Glasgow WC, Eling TE.   Epidermal growth factor stimulates linoleic acid metabolism in BALB/c 3T3 fibroblasts. *Mol Pharmacol* 1990;**38**:503-10.
3.   Glasgow WC, Afshari CA, Barrett JC, Eling TE. Modulation of the epidermal growth factor mitogenic response by metabolites of linoleic and arachidonic acid in Syrian hamster embryo fibroblasts: Differential effects in tumor suppressor gene (+) and (-) phenotypes. *J Biol Chem* 1992;**267**:10771-9.
4.   Glasgow WG and Eling TE.   Structure-activity relationship for potentiation of EGF-dependent mitogenesis by oxygenated metabolites of linoleic acid. *Arch Biochem Biophys* 1994 (accepted).
5.   Cowlen MS and Eling TE.   Effects of prostaglandins and hydroxyoctadecadienoic acid on epidermal growth factor-dependent DNA synthesis and c-*myc* proto-oncogene expression in Syrian hamster embryo cells. *Biochim Biophys Acta* 1993;**1174**:234-40.

*Advances in Prostaglandin, Thromboxane,
and Leukotriene Research, Vol. 23,*
edited by B. Samuelsson et al.
Raven Press, Ltd., New York © 1995

Effect of PGE$_2$ on c-Myc and Bcl-2 Production and Programmed Cell Death in Human Lymphocytes.

F. Pica *, O. Franzese, C. D'Onofrio, L. Paganini,
C. Favalli, E. Bonmassar and E. Garaci.

*Department of Experimental Medicine and Biochemical Sciences, University of Rome "Tor
Vergata", and * Institute of Experimental Medicine, CNR, Rome, Italy.*

Prostaglandins of the E series (PGE) play a role in the control of the immune response in normal and pathological conditions. In particular, PGE$_2$ is known to down regulate selected immune functions among which T cell mitogenesis, IL-2 production and IgM production, though enhancing the synthesis of certain antibody isotypes in B cells (1, 2).

The administration of a synthetic analog of PGE$_2$ in mice induces thymocyte apoptosis (3). Like PGE$_2$, other intracellular cAMP elevating agents induce thymocyte apoptosis *in vitro* (4). In addition, a possible role of PGE$_2$-induced apoptosis in the immunosuppression occurring during HIV infection has been suggested by our very recent experiments (5).

Programmed cell death (PCD) is a biological phenomenon, typically accompanied by the morphological features of apoptosis (6), naturally occurring in different tissues, but which can also be induced by a number of external signals (i.e. glucocorticoids, irradiation, withdrowal of growth factors, etc.). Recent work has made clear that induction of PCD is a response mediated by multiple and interacting intracellular pathways regulated by gene expression. Oncogenes and oncosuppressor genes are involved in this regulation. At present, there are convincing data relating apoptosis to c-myc, bcl-2, p53 and APO-1/fas. In this work we present our preliminary results on the effects of PGE$_2$ on c-Myc and Bcl-2 protein expression and in relation to PCD in immature and mature human lymphocytes.

c-Myc and Bcl-2 production in human lymhocytes after *in vitro* PGE$_2$ treatment.

Resting human peripheral blood lymphocytes (PBL) or cord blood lymphocytes (CBL) were cultured up to one week in RPMI 1640 medium plus 20% foetal calf serum and treated, at the onset of the culture, with concentrations of PGE$_2$ ranging from 0.1 to 10 μM. At various times, equal amount (100 μg/ml) of proteins per sample were separated on SDS-PAGE gels and electroblotted onto nitrocellulose membranes as previously described (7). For specific immune staining of c-Myc

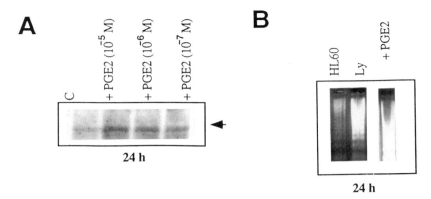

Fig. 1. c-Myc protein levels (**A**) and DNA fragmentation (**B**) in untreated and PGE₂-treated CBL. (In **B**, UV-irradiated HL60 cells were used as positive control).

and Bcl-2 protein, a mouse anti-human monoclonal antibody (Santa Cruz Biotech., Inc., Santa Cruz, CA) and a polyclonal antisera (Pharmingen, San Diego, CA) were respectively used.

Under these experimental conditions PGE₂ increased, dose and time-dependently, the levels of c-Myc protein with different kinetics depending on the maturation stage of lymphocytes. In fact, the more immature lymphocyte population, represented by CBL, responded to the PGE₂ treatment with an enhanced production of c-Myc protein in the first 24 h of culture (Fig. 1A), whereas in PBL, which are mature cells, the same phenomenon occurred generally later (data not shown). Unlike the effects on c-Myc production, equivalent concentrations of PGE₂ apparently did not modify the levels of Bcl-2 protein in both cell populations, at all the culture time points we tested (data not shown). These observations have been repeatedly confirmed in different blood donors.

Programmed cell death in human lymhocytes after *in vitro* PGE₂ treatment.

Nuclear DNA fragmentation into 200-bp fragments, indicative of PCD, was observed both in CBL and PBL populations after treatment with various concentrations of PGE₂. To evaluate DNA fragmentation, DNA was extracted sequentially with phenol, phenol/chloroform, precipitated in ethanol and electrophoresed on 1.5% agarose gel (8).

PGE₂ treatment induced DNA fragmentation that was clearly detectable in CBL after 24 h of culture, while in the untreated controls no sign of this phenomenon was found (Figure 1B). DNA fragmentation was also observed in PBL, though considerably later, i. e. from 72 h to 5 days after the onset of the culture (data not shown), suggesting a different sensitivity to PGE₂ action by immature and mature human lymphocytes.

Conclusions.

Our experiments show that PGE₂ treatment *in vitro* can increase the intracellular levels of c-Myc protein in human lymphocytes, whereas the constitutive Bcl-2 levels were not affected. At the same time PGE$_2$ induced PCD, as evaluated by nuclear DNA fragmentation in treated lymphocytes versus untreated controls. Both c-Myc overproduction and PCD were dose-dependent and occurred concomitantly in PGE$_2$-treated cultures. Lymphocytes at lower differentiation/maturation stage responded with higher sensitivity to PGE$_2$, as shown by earlier occurrence of both c-Myc induction and PCD in CBL than in PBL. Great variability in the response to PGE$_2$ was found in lymphocytes isolated from different donors; therefore larger number of donors needs to be examined. It has to be underlined that the extremely short half life of c-Myc protein (9) makes it difficult to detect this protein, especially in freshly isolated lymphocytes grown in the absence of mitogens or specific growth factors. However our preliminary results clearly indicate a possible role of c-Myc in the PGE$_2$-induced PCD in human lymphocytes. The fact that without a second survival signal, such as that provided by growth-factor receptor interaction, c-Myc is able to induce apoptosis whereas in the presence of this additional signal it can lead to progression through the cell cycle, has been recently suggested (8). Interestingly, in our experiments, Bcl-2 protein, whose expression in lymphoid tissue is restricted to long-lived cells and which can inhibit apoptosis induced by several other stimuli in addition to cytokine deprivation (9), was apparently not modified by PGE$_2$ at the same time points when c-Myc levels increased. Studies are in progress to contribute to a better understanding of the interplay between PGE$_2$ and c-Myc in human lymphocyte commitment towards proliferation or death.

AKNOWLEDGEMENTS
Supported in part by Ministero della Sanità, VI AIDS Research Project (E.G.) and in part by CNR, PF Biotecnologie e Biostrumentazione (C.D'O), Rome, Italy.

REFERENCES
1. Phipps R.P., Stein S.H. and Roper R.L. A new view of prostaglandin E regulation of the immune response. *Immunol Today* 1991; 12: 349-52.
2. Favalli C., Garaci E., Etheredge E., Santoro M.G., and Jaffe B.M. Influence of PGE on the immune response in melanoma bearing mice. *J Immunol* 1980; 125: 897-901.
3. Mastino A., Piacentini M., Grelli S. et al. Induction of apoptosis in thymocytes by prostaglandin E$_2$ in vivo. *Develop Immunol* 1992; 2:263-71.
4. Mc Conkey D.J., Orrenius S. and Jondal M. Agents that elevate cAMP stimulate DNA fragmentation in thymocytes. *J Immunol* 1990; 145: 1227-30.
5. Mastino A., Grelli S., Piacentini M. et al. Correlation between induction of lymphocyte apoptosis and prostaglandin E 2 production by macrophages infected with HIV. *Cell Immunol* 1993; 152:120-30.
6. Wyllie A.H. Apoptosis (The 1992 Frank Rose Memorial Lecture). *Br J Cancer* 1993; 67:205-8.
7. D'Onofrio C., Franzese O., De Marco A., Bonmassar E. and Amici C. Antiproliferative activity of cyclopentenone prostaglandins in early HTLV-1 infection is independent of IL-2 and is associated with HSP70 induction. *Leukemia* 1994; (in press).
8. Bissonnette R.P., Echeverri F., Mahboubi A. and Green D.R. Apoptotic cell death induced by c-myc is inhibited by bcl-2. *Nature* 1992; 359:552-4.
9. Shi Y., Glynn J.M., Guilbert L.J., Cotter T.G., Bissonnette R.P., Green D.R. Role for c-myc in activation-induced apoptotic cell death in T cell hybridomas. *Science* 1992; 257:212-4.

Advances in Prostaglandin, Thromboxane,
and Leukotriene Research, Vol. 23,
edited by B. Samuelsson et al.
Raven Press, Ltd., New York © 1995

Regulation and Signal Transduction of PAF Receptor

Takashi Izumi, Zen-ichiro Honda, Hiroyuki Mutoh,
Kazuhiko Kume, and Takao Shimizu

Department of Biochemistry, Faculty of Medicine, The University of Tokyo,
Tokyo 113, Japan

Platelet-activating factor (1-*O*-alkyl-2-acetyl-*sn*-glycero-3-phosphocholine; PAF) is a potent proinflammatory mediator, causing microvascular leakage, vasodilatation, contraction of smooth muscle, and activation of neutrophils, macrophages, and eosinophils (1-4). PAF is thought to play important roles in allergic disorders, inflammation, and endotoxin shock. Specific PAF receptors on the plasma membrane of target cells mediate these versatile processes. Our group isolated a cDNA clone for guinea pig PAF receptor using Xenopus Oocyte expression system (5). Subsequently, human and rat homologues were isolated (6-9). The analysis of PAF receptor cDNAs indicated that they have 341 or 342 amino acids with the molecular mass of about 39 kDa. Hydropathy profiles suggested the seven transmembrane segments characteristic to a G-protein coupled receptor superfamily. In the cytoplasmic tails, serine/threonine residues as possible phosphorylation sites are conserved among species.

In this study, we will discuss about genomic structure and transcriptional regulation for PAF receptor, and also the signal transduction in Chinese hamster ovary (CHO) cells expressing transfected PAF receptor cDNA.

STRUCTURE AND REGULATION OF PAF RECEPTOR GENE

Structure of Human PAF Receptor Gene

Human PAF-R cDNAs have been cloned from leukocytes (6), HL-60 cells (7), and from heart (8). All of them contained an identical coding region sequences. However, the upstream of the initial ATG codon of the heart cDNA was different from that of leukocyte type. Only -1 to -38 of the 5'-untranslated region was common to both leukocyte and heart cDNAs. Three exons were isolated from a genomic library using DNA probes corresponding to these specific sequences (10). Two 5'-noncoding exons are alternatively ligated to the third exon which contains the total open reading frame. As a result, two species of mRNA are yielded; named as Transcript 1 and 2 (Fig. 1). Exon specific primers for polymerase chain reaction revealed that Transcript 1 is distributed ubiquitously while Transcript 2 is not detected in peripheral leukocytes, EoL-1 cells (an eosinophilic cell line), and the brain (10). By primer extension analysis, a single RNA start site (-327) was identified for Transcript 1, and two sites (-259, -249) for Transcript 2.

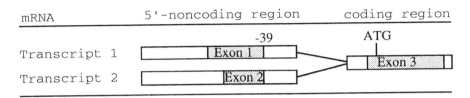

Fig. 1 The structure of the human PAF receptor gene.

Properties of the Promoter Regions

Sequence analysis of the upstream region of the RNA start site of exon 1 revealed that the putative promoter region has neither TATA nor CCAAT box, but contains consensus sequences for NF-κB and Sp-1. The sequence for NF-κB repeats three times. The other characteristic feature is that it contains a homologous sequence to the "*Initiator*" sequence, which was found in the murine terminal deoxynucleotidyltransferase (TdT) gene (11). The RNA start site is surrounded by a pyrimidine-rich sequence shown in Fig. 2.

```
PAF  receptor        5'-CCTCTTTCT-3'
TdT                  5'-CCTCATTCT-3'
         (underlined: RNA start site)
```

Fig. 2 The "*Initiator*" sequence in Exon 1 of PAF receptor and murine terminal deoxynucleotidyltransferase (TdT) gene.

The murine TdT gene contains *Initiator* and is tightly regulated during differentiation of B and T lymphocytes. These sequences may act as a functional promoter related to cell differentiation. When EoL-1 cells which have only Transcript 1 were stimulated by sodium butyrate, they were differentiated to eosionophilic phenotypes. And the expression of PAF receptor was closely associated with cell differentiation (Izumi, T., unpublished observation). In this case, *Initiator* may act as a promoter related the differentiation.

The upstream region of the RNA start site of exon 2 contained neither TATA nor CCAAT box as that of exon 1. The promoter region for Transcript 2 contains consensus sequences for AP-2, TGF-ß inhibitory element, SP-1, and AP-1.

Thus, the transcription of the two distinct mRNAs for the human PAF receptor is regulated in different manners. Existence of these two distinct promoters may play roles in the regulatory control of PAF-R gene expression in different cells and under different conditions (12).

PAF RECEPTOR-MEDIATED SIGNAL TRANSDUCTION

Previous studies have indicated that PAF receptor-induced signals involve guanine nucleotide regulatory proteins (G-proteins) (13-15). Although it is clear that the PAF receptor is coupled to various effector systems through G-proteins, the identities of the involved G-protein have not been characterized yet.

Many groups have shown that PAF mediates inositol phospholipid turnover in a variety of cells through the activation of PI-specific phospholipase C (PLC). PLC hydrolyzes PIP_2 to produce IP_3 and DG. IP_3 initiates the release of Ca^{2+} from intracellular stores, while DG activates protein kinase C.

It has been known that PAF stimulates phosphorylation of several proteins in many cells. The activation of protein kinases through PAF receptor is thought to be involved in the mitogenic and differentiating actions of PAF.

Signal Transduction in the CHO Cells Expressing Guinea Pig PAF Receptor

To study the signal transduction mechanisms through PAF receptor, we isolated a CHO cell line which stably expressed the transfected guinea pig PAF receptor cDNA and analyzed the signal transduction in the CHO cells (16).

In the CHO cells, PAF induced inositolphosphate turnover, arachidonic acid release, and inhibition of forskolin-stimulated cAMP accumulation, in dose-dependent manners. PAF also stimulated mitogen-activated protein (MAP) kinase and MAP kinase kinase activities. The EC_{50} values were about 1 nM for each signal. However, in the parent CHO cells, these signals were below the detectable limits.

The MAP kinase is considered to play a key role in the kinase cascade during differentiation, proliferation, and the cell-cycle transition (17). PAF also stimulates proliferative and differentiating signals in neuroblastoma cells, pheochromocytoma cells, and lymphocytes. Such effects produced by PAF may be explained by the activation of MAP kinase through the PAF receptor. The MAP kinase also activates cytosolic phospholipase A_2 (18). This might be a possible mechanism of PAF-induced arachidonic acid release.

Effects of Pertussis Toxin (PTX) on the PAF-induced Signals

The effects of PTX on the PAF-induced signals in the CHO cells were examined. PTX completely abolished the inhibitory effects of PAF on forskolin-stimulated cAMP accumulation. In contrast, inositol phosphates production was not changed. MAP kinase cascade and arachidonic acid release were inhibited by 40-60%. These results indicate that PAF appears to transduce signals through PTX-sensitive and -insensitive G-proteins.

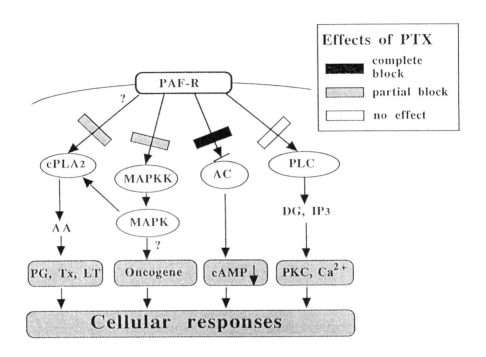

Fig. 3 Signal transduction through PAF receptor expressed in CHO cells and the effects of pertussis toxin (PTX).

cPLA2, cytosolic phospholipase A2; MAPK, mitogen-activated protein kinase; MAPKK, MAPK kinase; AC, adenylate cyclase; PLC, phospholipase C.

Fig. 3 summarizes the signal transduction induced by PAF in the CHO cells. A single receptor mediate various effects through multiple G-proteins. It is coupled to PLC through PTX-insensitive G-protein, possibly Gq, and to adenylate cyclase through Gi. The precise pathways for the activation of PLA2 and MAP kinase have not been elucidated yet.

However, these observation were obtained from the studies in an artificial CHO cell system with overexpression of PAF Receptor. It is important to study the signal transduction mechanisms in the native target cells for PAF such as leukocytes and macrophages, and also to study the relationship between PAF-induced signals and cell-specific functions. Furthermore, the signal transduction in PAF target cells should be studied to understand the role of PAF in physiological and pathological conditions.

ACKNOWLEDGMENTS

This work was supported in part by a grant-in-aid from the Ministry of Education, Science and Culture, and the Ministry of Health and Welfare of Japan, and by grants from the Uehara Memorial Foundation, the Yamada Science Foundation, and the Ono Medical Research Foundation.

REFERENCES

1.   Hanahan DJ. Platelet activating factor: a biologically active phosphoglyceride. *Annu Rev Biochem* 1986;55:483-509.

2.   Braquet P, Touqui L, Shen TY, Vargaftig BB. Perspectives in platelet-activating factor reseach. *Pharmacol Rev* 1987;39:97-145.

3.   Snyder F. Biochemistry of platelet-activating factor: a unique class of biologically active phospholipids. *Proc Soc Exp Biol Med* 1989;190:125-35.

4.   Prescott SM, Zimmerman GA, McIntyre TM. Platelet-activating factor. *J Biol Chem* 1990;265:17381-4.

5.   Honda Z, Nakamura M, Miki I, et al. Cloning by functional expression of platelet-activating factor receptor from guinea-pig lung. *Nature* 1991;349:342-6.

6.   Nakamura M, Honda Z, Izumi T, et al. Molecular cloning and expression of platelet-activating factor receptor from human leukocytes. *J Biol Chem* 1991;266:20400-5.

7.   Ye RD, Prossnitz ER, Zou AH, Cochrane CG. Characterization of a human cDNA that encodes a functional receptor for platelet activating factor. *Biochem Biophys Res Commun* 1991;180:105-11.

8.   Sugimoto T, Tsuchimochi H, McGregor CGA, Mutoh H, Shimizu T, Kurachi Y. Molecular cloning and characterization of the platelet-activating factor receptor gene expressed in the human heart. *Biochem Biophys Res Commun* 1992;189:617-24.

9.   Bito H, Honda Z, Nakamura M, Shimizu T. Cloning, expression and tissue distribution of rat platelet-activating-factor-receptor cDNA. *Eur J Biochem* 1994;221:211-8.

10.   Mutoh H, Bito H, Minami M, et al. Two different promoters direct expression of the two distinct forms of mRNAs of human platelet-activating factor receptor. *FEBS Lett* 1993;322:129-34.

11.   Smale ST, Baltimore D. The "initiator" as a transcription control element. *Cell* 1989;57:103-13.

12. Müller E, Dupuis G, Turcotte S, Rola-Pleszczynski M. Human PAF receptor gene expression: Induction during HL-60 cell differentiation. *Biochem Biophys Res Commun* 1991;181:1580-6.

13. Shimizu T, Honda Z, Nakamura M, Bito H, Izumi T. Platelet-activating factor receptor and signal transduction. *Biochem Pharmacol* 1992;44:1001-1008.

14. Shukla SD, Thurston J A. W., Zhu CY, Dhar A. Platelet activating factor receptor functions via phosphoinositide turnover and tyrosin kinase. In: Shukla SD, ed. Platelet activating factor receptor: Signal mechanisms and molecular biology. Boca Raton: CRC Press, 1992: 41-59.

15. Chao W, Olson MS. Platelet-activating factor: receptors and signal transduction. *Biochem J* 1993;292:617-29.

16. Honda Z, Takano T, Gotoh Y, Nishida E, Itoh K, Shimizu T. Transfected platelet-activating factor receptor activates mitogen-activated (MAP) kinase and MAP kinase kinase in Chinese hamster overy cells. *J Biol Chem* 1994;269:2307-15.

17. Davis RJ. The mitogen-activated protein kinase signal transduction pathway. *J Biol Chem* 1993;268:14553-6.

18. Lin LL, Wartmann M, Lin AY, Knopf JL, Seth A, Davis RJ. cPLA2 is phosphorylated and activated by MAP kinase. *Cell* 1993;72:269-78.

Advances in Prostaglandin, Thromboxane, and Leukotriene Research, Vol. 23,
edited by B. Samuelsson et al.
Raven Press, Ltd., New York © 1995

Platelet Activating Factor Induces Transformation of Human Fibroblasts

S.A.L. Bennett and H.C. Birnboim

Department of Biochemistry, University of Ottawa and Ottawa Regional Cancer Centre, Ottawa, Ont, Canada K1H 8L6

The correlation between chronic inflammation and an increased predisposition to development of human cancers (1) suggests that pro-inflammatory agents synthesized and released by activated phagocytes at sites of injury may play a role in tumour progression. One such agent, platelet activating factor (PAF:1-*O*-alkyl-2 -acetyl-glycero-3-phosphocholine) has been shown to phenotypically transform murine cells *in vitro* (2). PAF is a family of potent pro-inflammatory and hypertensive ether lipids. Its diverse biological activities are mediated by interaction with specific cell-surface receptors and intracellular binding sites and are dependent upon activation of a wide variety of second messengers, including arachidonic acid metabolites, protein tyrosine kinases and protein kinase C (3,4). In the present study, the possibility that PAF may play a role in human cancers through specific signal transduction pathways was investigated by evaluating PAF-induced changes in human fibroblast (HF) phenotype *in vitro*.

MATERIALS AND METHODS

Normal diploid HF cultures, prepared from neonatal foreskins, were grown in DMEM plus 10% fetal calf serum (FCS, Gibco). 1×10^5 cells were treated for 1 hr with vehicle (Fisher), PAF (Avanti Biochem), lyso-PAF (Sigma), or PAF plus CV3988 (Calbiochem), indomethacin (Sigma), staurosporine (LC Services), or genestein (UBI) at the concentrations noted in the text. Treatments were carried out in DMEM plus 0.2% bovine serum albumin at 37°C. Where co-incubations are indicated, agents were added 15 min prior to PAF. Following treatment, HFs were assayed for changes in (i) saturation density, (ii) growth in low serum, and (iii) anchorage independent (AI) growth. Saturation density and growth in low serum were established by incubating cells in DMEM+10% FCS or DMEM+0.5% FCS respectively for 25 days. Cell number was determined at various time intervals by cell counts using a Coulter counter. AI growth was assayed by suspending cells in 0.3% agarose over a layer of 0.6% agarose containing DMEM+10% FCS. AI colonies (>80 μm in dia.) were scored 50 days after treatment. In each assay, cells received twice weekly feedings with appropriate medium.

RESULTS AND DISCUSSION

Although a correlation between chronic inflammation and predisposition to cancer in humans has been recognized for many years, causal mechanisms have yet to be determined. Our results suggest that PAF, a known endogenous inflammatory agent at physiologically relevant concentrations, may contribute to the multi-step process of malignant transformation. As depicted in Fig. 1 (Panel A and B),

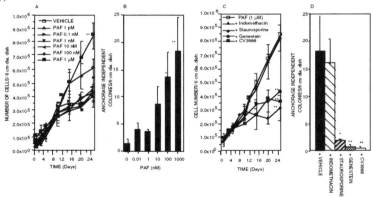

FIG.1. PAF treatment induces growth in low serum (Panel A) and AI growth (Panel B) in HFs. PAF (1μM)-induced growth in low serum (Panel C) and AI growth (Panel D) is attenuated by CV3988 (10μM), staurosporine (50nM), and genestein (1μg/ml) but not by indomethacin (200nM). Each data point represents the mean ± SEM of a minimum of 5 plates. ANOVA and Dunnetts tests were performed on the final day of testing to determine statistically significant differences from vehicle treated cells. *p<0.05, **p<0.01.

treatment of HFs with PAF induced a long-term, dose-dependent increase in the ability of cells to (i) proliferate with limiting amounts of exogenous growth factors (autonomous cell growth in low serum medium) and (ii) clonally expand in a non-permissive environment (AI growth); characteristics commonly associated with tumour cells cultured *in vitro*. Lyso-PAF (0.1nM-1μM), PAF's immediate metabolite, had no effect on HF phenotype (data not shown). It is important to note that phenotypic transformation was observed only when cells were cultured under sub-optimal growth conditions. PAF had no effect on HF saturation density when cells were grown in DMEM+ 10 % FCS (data not shown).

In an attempt to identify some of the mechanism(s) underlying PAF-mediated transformation of HFs, cells were pretreated with either a PAF antagonist, CV3988, a cyclooxygenase metabolism inhibitor, indomethacin, a putative protein kinase C inhibitor, staurosporine, or a putative tyrosine kinase inhibitor, genestein (Fig 1, Panel C and D). None of these agents were found to affect vehicle (0.1% DMSO)-treated HF phenotype at the concentrations employed (data not shown). CV3988, staurosporine, and genestein effectively blocked PAF-induced growth in low serum and AI growth. Inhibition of the cyclooxygenase pathway of arachidonic acid metabolism had no effect on PAF-induced transformation. These results provide the first evidence that PAF can induce phenotypic transformation of human cells *in vitro* and that this effect is PAF-specific, receptor-mediated, and dependent upon protein tyrosine kinase and protein kinase C activity.

(This research was funded by the a grant from the Medical Research Council (MRC) of Canada to HCB and a MRC studentship to SALB. The authors thank Cai-Ying Zhou for her skilful assistance.)

REFERENCES

1. Templeton AC. Acquired diseases. In:Fraumeni JF, *Persons at high risk of cancer: an approach to cancer etiology and control*. New York: Academic Press; 1975:84.
2. Bennett SAL, Leite LCC, Birnboim HC. Platelet activating factor, an endogenous mediator of inflammation, induces phenotypic transformation of rat embryo cells. *Carcinogenesis* 1993;14:1289-6.
3. Chao W, Olson MS. Platelet-activating factor: Receptors and signal transduction. *Biochem J* 1993;292:617-9.
4. Gerard C, Gerard NP. The pro-inflammatory seven-transmembrane segment receptors of the leukocyte. *Curr Opin Immunol* 1994;6:140-5.

Advances in Prostaglandin, Thromboxane,
and Leukotriene Research, Vol. 23,
edited by B. Samuelsson et al.
Raven Press, Ltd., New York © 1995

Evidence for the predominant role of intracellular PAF Binding Sites in the Regulation of Phospholipase A_2 in Human Neutrophils

Santosh Nigam*, Saeed Eskafi, Stefan Müller, Hong Zhang

Eicosanoid Research Div., Department of Gynecology, University Medical Center Steglitz, Free University Berlin, D-12200 Berlin, Germany.

The receptor-mediated activation of human polymorph neutrophils (PMN) by ligands such as chemotactic peptide N-formyl-methionine-leucine-phenylalanine (fMLP) is coupled with the activation of phospholipases C and A_2 (1). Phospholipase A_2 (PLA_2) hydrolyzes arachidonic acid (AA) and lysophospholipid from the *sn*-2 position of 1-alkyl-2-arachidonoyl-*sn*-3-glycerophosphocholine of the membrane (2). Currently, it is accepted that the cytosolic PLA_2 ($cPLA_2$) and not the secretory PLA_2 ($sPLA_2$) is primarily responsible for the release of AA (3) in most of the cell systems. The reasons for this assumption are based on the observations, such as low requirements of Ca^{++} concentrations (μM for $cPLA_2$ vs mM for $sPLA_2$), fatty acid preference of $cPLA_2$ at the *sn*-2 position (3), resistance of $cPLA_2$ to disulfide-reducing agents (3) and increased concentrations of cytosolic Ca^{++} (4). In addition, it is stimulated by phosphorylation via protein kinase C (PKC) , but inhibited by staurosporine, an inhibitor of PKC (5). Conversely, previous studies from our laboratory have shown that the inhibition of PKC by staurosporine potentiated the activation of PLC and PLA_2 in fMLP-challenged human PMN (6,7).

In the present study, we describe a novel mechanism for the regulation of PLA_2 in human PMN, which involves the activation of recently identified intracellular platelet-activating factor (PAF) binding sites (8). We believe, that the release of AA and lyso-PAF via intracellular PAF binding sites in human PMN constitutes the major pathway as compared with the $cPLA_2$ pathway.

RESULTS AND DISCUSSION

Fig. 1 shows the potentiating effect of 1 μM staurosporine (3-fold) on the formation of 20-carboxy-LTB_4, a metabolite of leukotriene B_4 (LTB_4) in fMLP-activated human neutrophils. This observation is, however, in contradiction to the currently reported mechanism for the release of AA and PAF in different cell systems, in which the inhibition of PKC has been shown to decrease the AA release (7).Thus, it is evident that the $cPLA_2$ pathway does not describe alone the mechanism for eicosanoid and PAF formation in human neutrophils.

Author for correspondence

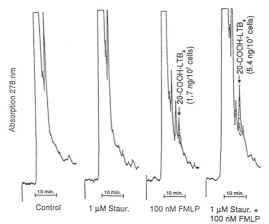

Figure 1: *Effect of staurosporine on the formation of 20-COOH-LTB$_4$ in fMLP-challenged human neutrophils*

Since 5-lipoxygenase products and PAF are potent stimuli of human neutrophils, it was of interest to know if these agonists, which are formed intracellularly, participated in the enhanced release of AA and PAF formation in presence of staurosporine. While MK 886 (a kind gift from Dr. A. Ford-Hutchinson, Canada), a potent inhibitor of 5-lipoxygenase was ineffective, a dose-dependent inhibition was observed by WEB 2086, a specific PAF receptor antagonist (Fig.2). WEB 2086 at a concentration of 3.0 μM caused a maximal inhibition of 80 % of staurosporine-potentiated PAF formation and 71% of AA release. This suggested that a regulatory process dealing with the endogenously produced PAF, which is strictly retained in the cell (9), is involved in the release of AA and formation of PAF.

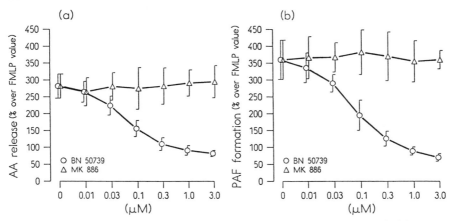

Figure 2: *Effect of MK 886 and WEB 2086 on AA release and PAF formation in fMLP-challenged human neutrophils pretreated with staurosporine*

Recently, our laboratory has presented evidence for the presence of specific high affinity cytosolic binding sites for PAF in human neutrophils (K$_d$ = 4.29 nM), the estimated number of binding sites (B$_{max}$) being 219 fmol/100 μg protein. The [^{3}H]PAF binding studies in fMLP-challenged human neutrophils demonstrated a significant decrease of the affinity of [^{3}H]PAF binding sites (K_d = 7.6 nM) with a concomitant increase of B_{max} to 312 fmol/100 µg protein. Upon pretreatment of cells with 1 µM staurosporine, the decrease in the affinity of [^{3}H]PAF binding sites was almost completely restored(K_d = 4.68 nM; B_{max} =272 fmol/100 µg protein). Thus, it can be implicated that the activation of PKC by diacylglycerol in fMLP-challenged human neutrophils might represent the down regulation with respect to the action of intracellular PAF binding sites, which can be reversed by staurosporine.

The present data and the previous studies from others (3-5) and our laboratory (2,6,7) led us to suggest a novel mechanism for the regulation of cPLA$_2$ in human neutrophils. Increased intracellular Ca^{++} and the stimulation of PKC translocate the cPLA$_2$ from cytosol to the membrane where AA and lysophospholipid are released from the phospholipid pool. PKC also phosphorylates at the same time the cytosolic PAF binding sites and decreases their affinity towards the endogenously synthesized PAF. The use of staurosporine inhibits the PKC and thus the activation of cPLA$_2$, but increases the affinity of cytosolic PAF binding sites by dephosphorylation. Together with PAF as an agonist the intracellular PAF binding sites apparently translocate to the membrane and stimulate the PLC, leading to hydrolysis of PIP$_2$ to IP$_3$ and DG. Whereas the so released IP$_3$ causes elevation of intracellular Ca^{++} (6), which is predominantly responsible for the activation of cPLA$_2$, DG is no longer capable of activating PKC in presence of excess staurosporine. Thus, we conclude, that the activation of cPLA$_2$ in human neutrophils occurs via three different pathways: (a) PKC, (b) cytosolic PAF binding sites, and / or (c) elevation of intracellular Ca^{++}.

ACKNOWLEDGEMENT:

This study was supported by a grant from the DFG, Bonn, F.R.G. (Ni 242/9-1).

REFERENCES:

1. Abdel-Latif AA. Calcium-mobilizing receptors, polyphosphoinositides, and the generation of second messengers. Pharmacol. Rev. 1986; 38: 227-72.
2. Müller S & Nigam S. Arachidonic acid release and platelet-activating factor formation by staurosporine in human neutrophils challenged with n-formyl peptide. Eur. J. Pharmacol. 1992; 218: 251-58.
3. Lin LL, Wartman M, Lin AY, Knopf JL, Seth A, Davis RJ. cPLA$_2$ is phosphorylated and activated by MAP kinase. Cell 1993; 72: 269-78.
4. Clark JD, Lin LL, Kriz RW, Ramesha CS, Sultzman LA, Lin AY, Milona N, Knopf JL. A novel arachidonic acid-selective cytosolic PLA$_2$ contains a calcium-dependent translocation domain with homology to PKC and GAP. Cell 1991; 65: 1043-51.
5. Lin LL, Lin AY, Knopf JL. Cytosolic phospholipase A$_2$ is coupled to the hormonally regulated release of arachidonic acid. P.N.A.S. USA 1992; 89: 6147-51.
6. Nigam S, Müller S, Walzog B. Effect of staurosporine on fMet-Leu-Phe-stimulated human neutrophils: dissociated release of of inositol 1,4,5 triphosphate, diacylglycerol and intracellular calcium. Biochim. Biophys. Acta 1992; 1135: 301-08.
7. Svetlov S & Nigam S. Calphostin C, a specific protein kinase C inhibitor, activates human neutrophils: effect on phospholipase A$_2$ and aggregation. Biochem. Biophys. Res. Comm. 1992; 190: 162-66.

Advances in Prostaglandin, Thromboxane, and Leukotriene Research, Vol. 23,
edited by B. Samuelsson et al.
Raven Press, Ltd., New York © 1995

ABT-299, A Potent Antagonist of Platelet Activating Factor

James B. Summers, Daniel H. Albert, Steven K. Davidsen,
Richard G. Conway, James H. Holms, Terrance J. Magoc,
Gongjin Luo, Paul Tapang, David A. Rhein, and George W. Carter

*Immunoscience Research Area, D47J AP10,
Abbott Laboratories, Abbott Park, IL 60064*

Platelet Activating Factor (PAF) is a phospholipid mediator which acts through specific cellular receptors to induce a wide range of biological effects. It has been implicated as an important mediator in several disorders including septic shock, asthma, and ischemia/reperfusion injury (1, 2). In view of the potent pathophysiologic effects of PAF and the broad scope of diseases in which it may play a role, there appears to be therapeutic potential for agents which antagonize the action of PAF at its receptor.

We wish to report the discovery of ABT-299, a novel prodrug that is rapidly converted *in vivo* to A-85783.0, a highly potent, specific antagonist of PAF (FIG. 1). ABT-299 shares the pharmacologic properties of A-85783, but has much greater aqueous solubility rendering it useful for parenteral administration.

RESULTS AND DISCUSSION

Solubility of ABT-299 and Conversion to A-85783.0

ABT-299 is rapidly converted to A-85783.0 in the presence of plasma esterases. The prodrug displayed a half life of 3.8 min in human plasma at 37 °C. This conversion was substantially inhibited by the addition of the esterase inhibitor diisopropyl fluorophosphate. The prodrug is also rapidly converted *in vivo*. Following a 1 mg/kg intravenous dose to rat, ABT-299 had an half life of

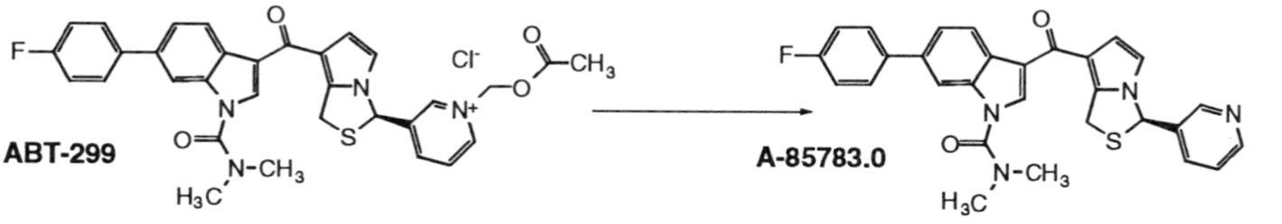

FIG 1. Conversion of ABT-299 to A-85783.0.

about 3 min and was no longer detectable in plasma (<10 nM) 20 min after administration. In contrast, A-85783.0 was detectable immediately after dosing where it exhibited an extended duration (*vide supra*).

ABT-299 is considerably more stable in the absence of plasma esterases, particularly in acidic buffer. At pH 3 only about 10% conversion was noted after one week at 25 °C. In this aqueous medium ABT-299 is also much more soluble than A-85783.0. Solubilities of greater than 25 mg/mL and less than 0.001 mg/mL, respectively, were observed.

In Vitro Inhibitory Activity

A-85783 is a potent inhibitor of $[^3H]$–PAF binding to receptors on rabbit platelet membranes ($K_i = 3.8$ nM). This inhibition is competitive, reversible, and stereoselective (enantiomer $K_i = 760$ nM). Interactions of A-85783 with the PAF receptor are highly specific. A survey of more than three dozen other receptors showed no inhibitory activity from the compound at concentrations up to 10 μM.

A-85783 also inhibits PAF induced cellular responses. For example, it blocks PAF induced elastase release from human neutrophils ($A_2 = 0.5$ nM) and PAF induced serotonin release from rabbit platelets ($K_b = 1.1$ nM). Selectivity was also demonstrated in the latter assay. A-85783 failed to inhibit thrombin or calcium ionophore induced serotonin release.

Inhibition of the Effects of Exogenous PAF *In Vivo*

Intradermal administration of PAF induces localized cutaneous vascular permeability as evidenced by an edematous wheal (3). ABT-299 given 1 h prior to PAF challenge (50 ng) was highly effective at inhibiting this response in rats following either intravenous or oral administration ($ED_{50} = 0.006$ mg/kg and 0.08 mg/kg, respectively). Virtually identical activities were observed whether the prodrug or its active form were administered. A-85783.0 displayed ED_{50} values of 0.007 mg/kg and 0.06 mg/kg following intravenous and oral dosing in this assay.

This paradigm was also used to demonstrate the selectivity of ABT-299 *in vivo*. The compound had no effect on the vascular permeability produced by intradermal injection of serotonin or histamine in the rat.

When PAF (50 ng) is injected into a mouse paw, a robust edema is induced that increases the size of the paw by 50% within one hour (4). ABT-299 inhibited this response with an ED_{50} of 0.01 mg/kg, intravenously. Following oral administration A-85783.0 displayed an ED_{50} of 0.09 mg/kg.

Intravenous administration of PAF results in transient but profound hypotensive episode (5). Following a 10 nmole/kg dose of PAF, mean arterial pressure in the rat fell by 60% around 5 min then returned to within 70% of baseline by 30 min. Administration of ABT-299 15 min prior to PAF challenge inhibited PAF induced hypotension ($ED_{50} = 0.005$ mg/kg iv). In the dog, a dose of 0.1 mg/kg, iv, completely inhibited the nearly lethal hypotension induced by 1 nmole/kg of PAF.

Assays involving exogenously administered PAF were also used to assess the duration of anti-PAF effects in animals. For example, in the PAF induced cutaneous vascular permeability assay described above, a dose of 0.1 mg/kg, iv, of ABT-299 produced about 90% inhibition at one hour after administration and inhibition was still greater than 50% inhibition after 15 h. Similarly, a dose 0.1 mg/kg, iv of ABT-299 inhibited 50% of PAF induced hypotension in the rat for more than 16 h.

Activity in models of endotoxic shock

Administration of lipopolysaccharide (LPS) to rats produces many of the hallmarks of septic shock including systemic hypotension, vascular leak, disseminated intravascular coagulation (DIC), organ damage/failure and high mortality. ABT-299 has been shown to be highly effective in blocking each of these characteristics.

LPS (25 mg/kg) given intraarterially to rats produces a transient fall in mean arterial pressure followed by a partial recovery and then a sustained period of hypotension which reaches a maximum of about 60% baseline levels 1 h after challenge. ABT-299 when administered 15 min prior to challenge produced a dose related inhibition of the second phase hypotensive response (ED_{50} = 0.01 mg/kg, iv). A dose of 0.1 mg/kg completely blocked this effect of LPS.

ABT-299 was also highly effective when administered after LPS challenge. When given intraarterially 20, 40, or 60 min after LPS, the compound (0.1 mg/kg, iv) rapidly reversed the hypotension and restored blood pressure to baseline.

ABT-299 has also been demonstrated to inhibit LPS induced DIC, intestinal damage, vascular permeability, lethality and other characteristics of septic shock in animals. Results of these and other studies will be reported in full elsewhere.

CONCLUSIONS

ABT-299 is a prodrug which is rapidly converted to A-85783 *in vivo* or in incubations with plasma. ABT-299 and A-85783 have been shown to be potent inhibitors of PAF mediated effects in a variety of *in vitro* and *in vivo* assays. They have also been shown to be highly effective in modulating the signs and symptoms of endotoxic shock in animal models.

REFERENCES

1. Koltai M, Hosford D, Guinot P, Esanu A, Braquet P. Platelet activating factor. A review of its effects, antagonists and possible future clinical implications. *Drugs* 1991;42:9-29, 174-204.
2. Summers J, Albert D. Platelet Activating Factor Antagonists. *Adv Pharmacol* 1994; in press.
3. Hwang SB, Li CL, Lam MH, Shen TY. Characterization of cutaneous vascular permeability induced by PAF in guinea pigs and rats and its inhibition by PAF receptor antagonists. *Lab Invest* 1985;52:617-630.
4. Goldenberg M, Meurer R. A pharmacologic analysis of the action of platelet-activating factor in the induction of hindpaw edema in the rat. *Prostaglandins* 1984;28:271-278.
5. Terashita Z-I, Tsushima S, Yoshioka Y, Nomura H, Inada Y, Nishikawa K. CV-3988 - a specific antagonist of platelet activating factor (PAF). *Life Scie* 1983;32:1975-1982.

Advances in Prostaglandin, Thromboxane,
and Leukotriene Research, Vol. 23,
edited by B. Samuelsson et al.
Raven Press, Ltd., New York © 1995

Streptokinase - Prostacyclin - Nitric Oxide: *In Vivo* Interactions

Ryszard J. Gryglewski and Józef Święs

Chair of Pharmacology, Medical College of Jagiellonian University
31-531 Cracow, 16 Grzegórzecka, Poland

Prostacyclin (PGI_2), nitric oxide (NO) and tissue plasminogen activator (t-PA) constitute the most prominent triad among all endotelial products. PGI_2 and NO are interlinked in many ways. They show platelet-suppressant, fibrinolytic, vasodilator and cytoprotective properties which are mediated by cyclic nucleotides, i.e. cyclic-AMP and cyclic-GMP, respectively (5). On the other hand t-PA along with plasminogen activator inhibitor (PAI) are likely to be involved in thrombolytic action of PGI_2 (11), and NO (4,10), PGI_2 and NO are released in coupled manner (3,9), and therefore their interactions are highly feasible. *In vitro* there is an ample evidence for a synergism between PGI_2 and NO in their platelet-suppressant action (8,14) and vasorelaxant additive interaction (8). In patients with peripheral vascular disease PGI_2 and molsidomine (a NO-donor) synergize in their fibrinolytic actions (2). Little is known about interactions between PGI_2 or NO with t-PA.

In light of the above we decided to explore whether or not the *in vitro* outlined interactions between endothelial mediators occur also *in vivo*, first, between endogenous PGI_2 and NO, and second, between PGI_2 analogues and NO-donors. For this purpose we implemented our original method (2) for simultaneous assaying of extracorporal thrombolysis and thrombogenesis along with pressor effects of drugs administered intravenously.

METHODS

In vivo cat model

Our method of simultaneous monitoring of thrombolysis or thrombogenesis and mean arterial blood pressure in anaesthetized cats (7) was extended by integrating of heart rate from tripolar ECG, recording of *dp/dt* and radioimmunoassay of c-GMP, TXB_2 or 6-keto-$PGF1\alpha$ (Amersham kits) in plasma from arterial blood samples.

Mongrel cats body weight 1.5-2.5 kg were anaesthetized with pentobarbital (30 mg/kg i.p.) and heparinized (2500 units/kg i.v.). Mean arterial blood pressure was recorded from the right carotid artery by a Stadham transducer while thrombolysis or thrombogenesis were assayed in an extracorporal circulation. This consisted of the arterial blood (from the left carotid artery) superfusing (37°C, 3 ml/min) a collagen strip (Achilles tendon of a rabbit). After superfusion blood was returned to the venous system of the animal. The weight of collagen strip was continuously monitored through an auxotonic spring-balanced lever connected to a Harvard 386 transducer. During superfusion the collagen strip gained in weight (300 - 500 mg) owing to the deposition of thrombi composed of platelet aggregates, a few patches of fibrin and blood cells trapped in between them. This gain in weight reached a stable plateau after the first 15 -20 min of superfusion. In our *in vivo* system PGI_2 or iloprost (0.3 - 3.0 µg/kg, i.v.) had a dose dependent thrombolytic effect which appeared as a short lasting (10-20 min) loss in weight of the detector strip. This thrombolytic action is not unique for exogenous PGI_2 and its analogues (7). Endogenous PGI_2 has the same thrombolytic action when it is released into circulation by activating muscarinic (17) or kinin (16) receptors. The thrombolytic action of the above releasers of PGI_2 is blocked by the pretreatment with a megadose of aspirin (50 mg/kg i.v.). Incidentally, in our *in vivo* system aspirin and other anti-platelet drugs have no thrombolytic action of their own.

Drugs

The following drugs were administered as bolus injections or infused intravenously: prostacyclin sodium salt (PGI_2, Wellcome U.K., 0.3 µg/kg,i.v.), iloprost (IL, Schering, Germany, 0.3 µg/kg, i.v.), metacholine hydrochloride (Sigma, U.S.A., 3 µg/kg,i.v.), 3-morpholinesydnonimine (SIN-1, GEA, Denmark, 30 µg/kg, i.v. or 5 µg/kg/min, i.v.), streptokinase (Sigma, U.S.A. 3000 U/kg, i.v. or 100 U/kg/min, i.v.), ε-aminocaproic acid (Epsicapron, Polfa, Poland, 100 mg/kg, i.v.), heparin sulphate (Sigma, U.S.A., 2500 U/kg, i.v.) , acetylsalicylic acid (ASA, Polfa, Poland, 50 mg/kg, i.v.) camonagrel (a TXA_2 synthase inhibitor of Ferrero Group, Spain, 10 mg/kg, iv.), N^G-nitro-L-arginine (L-NNA, Sigma U.S.A. 300 µg/ kg/ min, i.v.) and methylene blue (MB, Sigma U.S.A., 10 mg/kg, iv.).

Statistics

Unpaired Student's t test was used for comparison of means ± standart deviation (S.D.) out of n experiments at a level of statistical significance $p < 0.05$.

RESULTS

Metacholine (Mch, n = 10) produced both a fall in blood pressure (BP, by 46.2 ± 8.3%) and thrombolysis (THL, by 34.0 ± 6.2%). The pretreatment with L-NNA significantlly diminished the hypotensive response to Mch (BP dropped by 21.3 ± 3.4 %) and did not influence THL (37.1 ± 5.8%). The superimposed bolus injection of ASA over the infusion of L-NNA hardly changed the BP response to Mch (18.4 ± 4.5 %), however, ASA abolished THL response to Mch. PGI_2 or IL at a range of doses 0.3 - 1.0 µg/kg i.v.,n = 22) produced no hypotension. Their THL response ranged from 25 - 47 % and was not influenced by pretreatment with either ASA or L-NNA. The basal plasma levels of 6-keto-$PGF_{1\alpha}$ were 147 ± 38 pg/ml (n = 4), and increased after Mch to 375 ± 53 pg/ml. The pretreatment with ASA blunted this Mch-induced rise in 6-keto-$PGF_{1\alpha}$ down to 182 ± 37 pg/ml. Mch induced also a rise in plasma c-GMP level from 1.1 ± 0.3 pmol/ml to 4.3 ± 0.6 pmol/ml This rise in c-GMP was not diminished by the ASA pretreatment (4.8 ± 0.7 pmol/ml).

Camonagrel induced THL (by 38.4 ± 7.3 %, n=7) associated with a drop of TXB_2 plasma level from 261 ± 66 to 176 ± 53 pg/ml and a rise of 6-keto-$PGF_{1\alpha}$ from 217 ± 57 to 350 ± 91 pg/ml. At the same time c-GMP plasma levels did not change significantly (from 1.7 ± 0.3 to 1.5 ± 0.3 pmole/ml).

Intravenous injections of SIN-1 produced hypotension and thrombolysis. Only this last was reduced by the pretreatment with ASA or with MB from $28.5 \pm 5.2\%$ (n =6) to $4.4 \pm 2.0\%$ and $10.3 \pm 3.0\%$, respectively.

Infusions or injections of streptokinase (SK) produced a biphasic response; first, thrombogenesis (THG) during first 30 -90 min and then a long lasting thrombolysis (THL). Maximum THG mounted up to $+ 21.6 \pm 8.2\%$ (SK injection) or $+ 43.2 \pm 7.5\%$ (SK infusion) of increase in the thrombi weight, whereas maximum THL were $- 28.1 \pm 7.7\%$ (n=9, SK injection) or $- 58.7\%$ (n=5, SK infusion). The THG and THL phases of the SK action were not influenced by pretreatment with ASA, L-NNA and SIN-1 (5 μg/kg/min i.v. infusion). Both phases were abolished by the pretreatment with ε-aminocaproic acid. The SK-induced THG did not occur during the infusion of IL (5ng/kg/min i.v., n=5) or after the pretratment with camonagrel (n =4). In these experiments the SK-induced THL phase was augmented by IL from -28.1 $\pm$ 7.7% to -72.0 $\pm$ 10.8% and by camonagrel to -75.6 $\pm$ 6.4%.

DISCUSSION

No matter how disappointing it seems, in our *in vivo* model endogenous PGI_2 and NO did not interact with each other. Stimulation of muscarinic receptors resulted in a coupled release of PGI_2 - the one responsible for thrombolysis and NO which alone mediated a fall in blood pressure. The most likely explanation for lack of interaction betwen endogenous PGI2 and NO is that these mediators do not see each other since PGI_2 is released intraluminally and NO abluminally (5,6). Selective inhibition of NO-synthase by L-NNA did not change the thrombolytic action of metacholine that was abolished by a megadose of aspirin. Inhibition of TXA_2 synthase by camonagrel caused a selective release of PGI_2 and not NO (as evidenced by RIA of 6-keto-$PGF_{1\alpha}$ and c-GMP), and indeed camonagrel had thrombolytic but not hypotensive action. Low doses ($< 1\mu$g/kg) of exogenous PGI_2 or iloprost produced selective thrombolysis and not arterial hypotension. Of course, high doses of iloprost ($> 3\mu$g/kg) or NO-donors (e.g. SIN-1 $\geq 30\mu$g/kg) have produced both hypotension and thrombolysis but then it is the domain of pharmacology. Interestingly, the thrombolytic but not hypotensive action of SIN-1 was abolished after the inhibition of cyclooxygenase by aspirin as if the efficient system generating PGI_2 was required for the thrombolytic action of SIN-1. One can think about two explanations of this phenomenon, first, the "permissive" action of exogenous NO towards the thrombolytic action of pre-existing endogenous PGI_2 (5,6), and second, the stimulation of activity of cyclooxygenase by a high dose of a NO-donor (15).

However, the most unexpected finding was that streptokinase before its final thrombolytic phase induced a distinct thrombogenesis lasting for 30 -90 min. These profound changes in thromboresistance of a collagen surface which was superfused by arterial blood ranged from + 50% to -50% of the weight of thrombi. These changes in thromboresistance were not accompanied by changes in arterial blood pressure, although in some experiments the thrombotic phase was associated with shots of arrhythmias, rising ST segment in ECG and a transient decrease in dp/dt. Thrombosis by streptokinase was influenced neither by L-NNA nor by SIN-1 and nor by aspirin. It was abolished by exogenous (iloprost) or endogenous (camonagrel) PGI_2-like activities. Iloprost and camonagrel also augmented the thrombolytic phase of the streptokinase action. On the other hand ε-aminocaproic acid (as well as trasylol - not shown here) abolished both phases of the streptokinase activity. Our interpretation of these data is as follows. The streptokinase-induced thrombogenesis and thrombolysis both are mediated by plasmin. The acute thrombosis can be associated with activation of platelets by plasmin, as it has been reported to occur *in vitro* (13). and inferred to be a possibility from clinical observation on paradoxical early reocclusions of coronary arteries in patients with acute myocardial infarction who were subdued to the thrombolytic therapy (12). Our *in vivo* observations strongly support an option of combining the thrombolytic therapy with TXA_2 synthase inhibitors or PGI_2 analogues.

CONCLUSION

In vivo a coupled release of PGI_2 and NO can be induced by activation of muscarinic receptors by metacholine. The camonagrel-induced inhibition of TXA_2-synthase is followed by the uncoupled release of PGI_2. Endogenous PGI_2 is responsible for maintaining of thromboresistance while NO for controlling vascular tone, and these endogenous mediators do not interact with each other in any respect. Intravenous injections or infusions of streptokinase produce through an ε-aminocapronate-inhibitable pathway a biphasic effect on thromboresistance. The early distinct thrombogenic phase is followed by thrombolysis. Endogenous (camonagrel) or exogenous (iloprost) PGI_2-like activities are capable to abolish thrombogenesis and to enhance thrombolysis by streptokinase.

REFERENCES

1. Basista M, Grodzińska L, Święs J. The influence of molsidomine and its active metabolite SIN-1 on fibrinolysis and platelet aggregation. *Thromb Haemostas* 1985; 54:746-749.
2. Bieroń K, Grodzińska L, Kostka-Trąbka E, Gryglewski RJ. Prostacyclin and molsidomine synergise in their fibrinolytic and anti-platelet actions in patients with peripheral arterial disease. *Wien Klin Wochenschr* 1993; 105:7-11.
3. De Nucci G, Gryglewski RJ, Warner TD, Vane JR. Receptor mediated release of endothelium-derived relaxing factor and prostacyclin from bovine aortic endothelial cells is coupled. *Proc Natl Acad Sci USA* 1988; 85:2334-2338.
4. Grodzińska L, Hafner G, Darius H. Effect of molsidomine on t-PA and PAI activity in man: a double blind, placebo controlled study. *Thromb Haemostas* 1990; 64:485.
5. Gryglewski RJ. Interactions between nitric oxide and prostacyclin. Semin *Thromb Haemos* 1993; 19:158-166.
6. Gryglewski RJ, Chłopicki S, Święs J, Niezabitowski P. Prostacyclin, nitric oxide and atherosclerosis. *Ann NY Acad Sci* 1994 in press.
7. Gryglewski RJ, Korbut R, Ocetkiewicz A, Stachura J. In vivo method for quantitation of anti-platelet potency of drugs. *Naunyn-Schmiedeberg Arch Pharmacol* 1978; 302:25.
8. Gryglewski RJ, Korbut R, Trąbka-Janik E, Zembowicz A, Trybulec M. Interaction between NO donors and iloprost in human vascular smooth muscle, platelets and leukocytes. *J Cardiovasc Pharmacol* 1989; 14:S124-S128.
9. Gryglewski RJ, Moncada S, Palmer RMJ. Bioassay of prostacyclin and endothelium-derived relaxing factor (EDRF) from porcine aortic endothelial cells. *Br J Pharmacol* 1986; 87:685-694.
10. Korbut R, Lidbury PS, Vane JR. Prolongation of fibrinolytic activity of tissue plasminogen activator by nitrovasodilators. *Lancet* 1990; 335:669.
11. Musiał J, Wilczyńska M, Sładek K, Cierniewski CS, Nizankowski R, Szczeklik A. Fibrinolytic activity of prostacyclin and iloprost in patients with peripheral arterial disease. *Prostaglandins* 1986; 31:61-70.
12. Ohman EM, Topol EJ, Califf RM, et al. An analysis of the cause of early mortality after administration of thrombolytic therapy. *Coronary Artery Disease* 1993; 4:957-964.
13. Puri RN, Hu CJ, Matsueda R, Umeyama H, Colman RW. Aggregation of washed platelets by plasminogen and plasminogen activators is mediated by plasmin and is inhibited by a synthetic peptide disulfide. *Thromb Res* 1992; 65:533-547.
14. Radomski MW, Palmer RMJ, Moncada S. The anti-aggregatory properties of vascular endothelium: Interactions between prostacyclin and nitric oxide. *Br J Pharmacol* 1987; 92:639-646.
15. Salvemini D, Misko TP, Masferrer JL, Seibert K, Currie MG, Needleman P. Nitric oxide activates cyclooxygenase enzymes. *Proc Natl Acad Sci USA* 1993; 90:7240-7244.
16. Święs J, Chłopicki S, Gryglewski RJ. Kinins and thrombolysis. *J Physiol Pharmacol* 1993; 44:171-177.
17. Święs J, Radomski MW, Dembińska-Kieć A, et al. Stimulatory cholinergic effect on the release of antiaggregatory activity into the circulation of cat and man and its modification by beta-adrenergic antagonists. *Eur J Clin Invest* 1985; 15:320-326.

*Advances in Prostaglandin, Thromboxane,
and Leukotriene Research, Vol. 23,*
edited by B. Samuelsson et al.
Raven Press, Ltd., New York © 1995

Prostaglandin-Nitric Oxide Interactions in the Microcirculation

Gabor Kaley and Akos Koller

*Department of Physiology
New York Medical College
Valhalla, New York 10595*

There is a growing body of evidence to indicate that the endothelium-derived mediators, prostaglandins (PG) and nitric oxide (NO), are released in response to similar stimuli and act in concert to mediate vascular relaxation (1). The purposes of the present studies were to examine the effects of PGs and NO on the maintenance of basal tone of skeletal muscle arterioles and their interaction in the development of agonist and flow-induced changes in vessel diameter.

STUDIES IN VIVO

Basal Tone of Arterioles

The first series of studies were carried out on single cremaster muscle arterioles of 6-10 week old pentobarbital anesthetized, male Wistar rats (2). With the use of video microscopy the changes in diameter of third-order arterioles (15-22μm) to a continuous suffusion of indomethacin (28μM) and/or intra-arterial N^ω-nitro-L-arginine (L-NNA, 2.5μM), to block cyclooxygenase or NO synthase, respectively, were examined. Each of the inhibitors significantly reduced (by 15-20%) the basal diameter of arterioles. When administered in sequence, only the inhibitor administered first caused an increase in vascular tone, suggesting that PGs and NO interact and can exert similar quantitative effects in the absence of one or the other (3). These findings suggest that both endothelial prostaglandins, via causing an increase in cyclic AMP and nitric oxide, causing an increase in cyclic GMP in arteriolar vascular smooth muscle, are continuously released and thus participate in the regulation of basal microvascular tone.

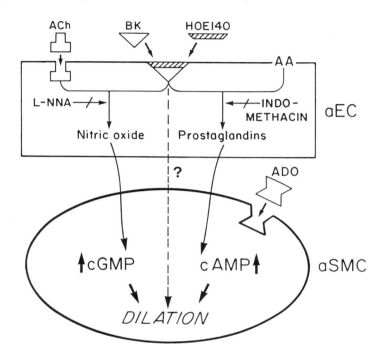

FIGURE. 1. Bradykinin (BK) stimulates arteriolar endothelial cells (aEC) to release nitric oxide and prostaglandins. These mediators, in turn, cause an increase in vascular smooth muscle cGMP and cAMP, respectively, causing arteriolar dilation. The effect of bradykinin can be inhibited by the B_2 receptor antagonist, HOE140. Acetylcholine (ACh) causes the synthesis of nitric oxide, and arachidonic acid the synthesis of prostaglandins in endothelial cells. Adenosine (ADO) affects arteriolar smooth muscle cells (aSMC) directly.

Effects of Bradykinin

In another series of experiments, using an identical in vivo experimental model, the contribution of nitric oxide and prostaglandins to the arteriolar responses of topically administered bradykinin were assessed. Bradykinin evoked dose dependent (1-100ng) dilation of arterioles that was significantly blunted in the presence of either indomethacin or L-NNA (4). Regardless of the sequence of administration their effects were additive, resulting in a practically complete elimination of the dilation to the lower doses of bradykinin. Together with our previous studies, showing that arteriolar dilations to bradykinin are completely blocked by impairment of the endothelial cell layer of the vessels, these findings strongly suggest that the vasomotor responses to bradykinin are entirely accounted for by the release of endothelial prostaglandins (PGI_2, PGE_2) and nitric oxide (Figure 1).

STUDIES IN VITRO

Effects of L-Arginine Analogs

Analogues of L-arginine, such as L-NNA, have been used extensively to study the role of nitric oxide in the mediation of vascular responses to various agonists as well as physiological stimuli (5). However, the actions of the actions of these agents may not be entirely specific and they may interfere with substances, which are believed to be unrelated to endothelial nitric oxide synthesis. Furthermore, it was recently demonstrated that NO and NO donors can stimulate cyclooxygenase with a resultant increase in PG synthesis (6). In line with the foregoing we investigated, in isolated pressurized first order arterioles (75-95μm in diameter) of rat cremaster muscle, the effects of L-NNA on dilator responses to a variety of vasoactive agents (7). At a concentration of 10^{-4}M and higher L-NNA inhibited dilations not only to acetylcholine, whose actions are in large part dependent on the release of nitric oxide from endothelium, but also those to arachidonic acid, the precursor of prostaglandins, and to PGE_2, a non-endothelium dependent dilator agent. These results suggest that L-arginine analogues, in addition to inhibiting NO synthesis, may well interfere with the endothelial synthesis and/or the vasoactivity of prostaglandins and that of other agents.

Flow Dependent Responses

Several studies have demonstrated that the increases in blood or perfusate flow cause increases in the diameter of arteries and arterioles of various sizes. There are differences, however, in the mediation of these responses, dependent upon the tissue and the size of the vessel involved. We have previously reported that in rat cremaster microvessels flow dependent dilation is mediated exclusively by endothelial prostaglandins (8). In contrast, in porcine coronary microvessels, nitric oxide is responsible for this response (9). In the present experiments, the flow (shear stress) dependent regulation of vascular resistance was studied in isolated pressurized arterioles (mean active diameter ~90μm) of rat gracilis muscle, a muscle that participates in locomotion. Step increases in perfusate flow, while pressure was maintained constant, elicited gradual increases in vessel diameter with no significant changes in shear stress. L-NNA or indomethacin reduced flow dependent dilations by ~50%, whereas combined administration of the two inhibitors or removal of the endothelium essentially eliminated the responses. In the absence of arteriolar dilation, increases in flow evoked step increases in shear stress. These studies indicate that endothelium-derived nitric oxide and prostaglandins are coreleased in response to flow, are responsible for vessel dilation and consequently for the maintenance of shear stress within normal limits.

Flow Dependent Responses After Exercise Training

Since increases in blood or perfusate flow cause release of NO and PGs from endothelial cells, the hypothesis that the intermittent increases in blood flow during a period of exercise training cause an adaptation in endothelial function resulting in an increased capacity to synthesize NO and PGs, was investigated in rat gracilis muscle arterioles. Rats underwent a mild treadmill exercise training program lasting for three weeks. Arterioles of trained rats exhibited augmented dilator responsiveness to acetylcholine and L-arginine compared to control vessels, whereas their responses to sodium nitroprusside and NaNO$_2$ remained essentially unchanged (10). These data strongly suggest that exercise training results in an upregulation of endothelial NO synthase in skeletal muscle arterioles. Enhanced flow (shear stress) dependent dilation was also observed in arterioles of exercise-trained rats. As illustrated in Figure 2, the enhanced dilator responses to step increases in perfusate flow in vessels of exercised-trained rats results in the maintenance of lower levels of shear stress compared to vessels of sedentary rats. These findings indicate that in response to exercise training, even preceding structural changes of the vessels, there is an alteration in the vasoactive function of endothelium (10,11) that may explain the increased conductance of the peripheral circulation following chronic exercise activity.

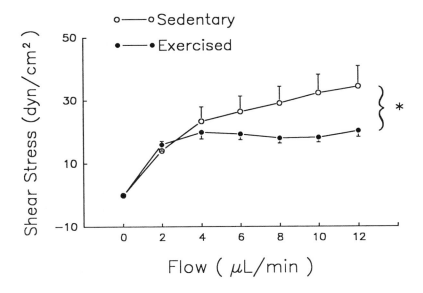

FIGURE 2. Shear stress (dynes/cm²) increases in response to step increases in perfusate flow in both groups of vessels but is maintained at a lower level in arterioles of exercised compared to sedentary rats. * indicates significant difference (p < 0.05) between the slopes of the regression lines.

The studies reviewed above reveal a close association between the synthesis and activity of NO and PGs, and strengthen the belief that these endothelium-derived dilator agents have an essential role in the regulation of peripheral resistance.

ACKNOWLEDGEMENTS

We thank Ms. Annette Ecke for her secretarial assistance. The studies were supported by NHLBI grants P01HL-43023 and HL46813.

REFERENCES

1. Furchgott RF. *Circ Res* 1983;53:557-73.
2. Koller A, Messina EJ, Wolin MS and Kaley G. *Am J Physiol* 1989;257:H1485-89.
3. Koller A, Messina EJ, Wolin MS and Kaley G. *Am J Physiol* 1989;257:H1966-70.
4. Kaley G, Koller A, Rodenburg JM, Messina EJ and Wolin MS. *Am J Physiol* 1992;262:H987-92.
5. Rees DD, Palmer RMJ, Hodson HF and Moncada S. *Brit J Pharmacol* 1989;96:418-24.
6. Salvemini D, Misko TP, Masferrer JL, Seiberg K, Currie MG and Needleman P. *Proc Natl Acad Sci* 1993;90:7240-44.
7. Koller A, Sun D, Messina EJ and Kaley G. *Am J Physiol* 1993;H1194-99.
8. Koller A, Sun D and Kaley G. *Circ Res* 1993;72:1276-84.
9. Kuo L, Davies MJ and Chilian WM. *Am J Physiol* 1991;259-H1063-70.
10. Sun D, Huang A, Koller A and Kaley G. *J Appl Physiol* 1994;(76)5:2241-47.
11. Wang J, Wolin MS and Hintze TH. *Circ Res* 1993;73:829-38.

Advances in Prostaglandin, Thromboxane, and Leukotriene Research, Vol. 23,
edited by B. Samuelsson et al.
Raven Press, Ltd., New York © 1995

Nitric oxide and the cyclooxygenase pathway. Daniela Salvemini, Karen Seibert, Jaime L. Masferrer, Steven L. Settle, Thomas P. Misko, Mark. G. Currie and Philip Needleman. G.D. Searle, Monsanto Company, 800 N. Lindbergh, St Louis, MO 63167, USA.

We have recently reported that inhibition of nitric oxide (NO) production by nitric oxide synthase (NOS) inhibitors results in inhibition of prostaglandin (PGs) formation **(1, 2)** although inhibition of PGs production by NOS inhibitors was not the consequence of direct cyclooxygenase (COX) inhibition. These findings suggested that endogenously produced NO regulates the COX pathway and that in situations in which both the NOS and COX are induced there may be a direct NO-driven production of pro-inflammatory prostaglandins which results in an exacerbated inflammatory response. We have now explored this hypothesis further by evaluating the ability of NO to alter the activity of COX *in vitro* and *in vivo.*

The inducible form of COX (COX-2) is induced approximately six fold over basal activity in fibroblasts (HFF) stimulated overnight with interleukin 1β (IL1β). Since IL1β does not induce NOS in these cells **(1)** an assessment of the action of exogenous NO on COX activity can be made. COX-2 activity in the IL1β stimulated fibroblasts was augmented at least 5 fold by NO. Pretreatment of HFF for 30 min before the addition of arachidonic acid with NO gas, sodium nitroprusside (SNP) or glyceryl trinitrate (GTN) (each at 200µM) increased prostaglandin E_2 (PGE_2) production from 166±4 to 841±28, 874±46 and 620±65 pg/µg protein/min respectively (n=7). The effects of NO, SNP or GTN were abolished by hemoglobin (Hb) which binds NO and inactivates it by oxidizing it to nitrites (NO_2^-)/nitrates (NO_3^-), but not by methylene blue, an inhibitor of the soluble guanylate cyclase.

The increase in cyclic guanosine 3'-5' monophosphate (cGMP) elicited by NO in the fibroblasts was completely abolished by these two agents indicating that COX activation is not regulated by changes in the levels of cGMP. The most likely explanation for the mechanism by which NO activates COX is a direct stimulation of the enzyme. Thus, SNP stimulates COX activity of microsomal sheep seminal vesicles as evidenced by potentiation of arachidonic acid induced PGE_2 release; removal of NO by Hb inhibits the effects of SNP consistent with a NO mediated activation of COX (from 4±0.4 for AA to 28±3 for AA+3µM SNP to 7±2 pmol/µg protein/min for AA+SNP+Hb, n=6). Similar results were obtained with murine recombinant COX-1 and COX-2 **(1)**.

These studies indicate that nitric oxide stimulates COX activity most likely in a direct manner. Does NO increase production of pro-inflammatory prostaglandins at sites of inflammation? This was tested in (A) the rabbit hydronephrotic kidney, a model of renal inflammation that is characterized by a marked increase in PGE_2 production and (B) in an *in vivo* model of endotoxin shock.

(A) The hourly stimulation of the perfused hydronephrotic kidney with bradykinin (BK) revealed a time-dependent increase in PGE_2 release (6, 7, 11 and 40 fold at 0, 1, 3 and 6h of perfusion). In the absence of BK, we observed a time-dependent release of nitrites **(2)**. The inducible forms of NOS and COX have been found to be responsible for the production of NO and PGE_2 release in the HNK **(2)**. Perfusion of the HNK with N^G-monomethyl-L-arginine (L-NMMA) a non-selective inhibitor of the constitutive and inducible forms (cNOS and iNOS) of NOS with aminoguanidine (AG, 100µM) a recently described inhibitor of iNOS (3, 4, 5) blocked NO_2^- release and attenuated BK-induced PGE_2 release by at least 50% **(Table 1)**; these effects were reversed by co-infusion with L-arginine but not D-arginine.

Perfusion of the inflamed kidney with L-arginine (1mM) increased even further the exaggerated production of PGE_2 following stimulation with BK **(Table 1)**; L-lysine (1mM), an amino acid not involved in the formation of NO had no effect **(Table 1)**.

Table 1: Effects of endogenous NO on prostaglandin production.

| | Time (h) of perfusion | | | |
Drugs	0	1	3	6
None	473±143	539±121	880±143	3079±946
L-NMMA	242±22	220±22*	418±33*	988±44*
AG	352±11	418±44	396±22*	902±77*
L-arginine	748±33	2013±143*	3982±264*	8646±162*
L-lysine	450±20	700±15	720±20	3000±70
Indomethacin	110±3*	77±22*	89±22*	87±22*

*Bradykinin was injected as a bolus (1μg) intraarterially at 0, 1, 3 and 6h of perfusion to stimulate PGE_2 release from the kidney. The venous effluent was collected for 3 min after BK injection and assayed for PGE_2 production by radioimmunoassay. Values are expressed as PGE_2 (pmol/ml/min) for 6-10 experiments. *$P<0.05$ when compared to corresponding values obtained in the absence of drug treatment.*

Inhibition of COX activity by non-steroidal anti-inflammatory drugs inhibited the exaggerated production of PGE_2 in the inflamed kidney but had no effect on the release of NO indicating that the NOS system is not directly influenced by the presence of prostaglandins (2).

(B) *In vivo* administration of E. coli lipopolysaccharide (LPS) in rats induces iNOS in a number of tissues, a phenomenon associated with the release of large amounts of nitrites in plasma (6). Furthermore, endotoxin causes marked in vivo stimulation of arachidonic acid metabolism which results in a profound increase in plasma and urinary 6-keto $PGF1\alpha$ (the stable metabolite of PGI_2) and urinary PGE_2 levels (7). We have therefore used this *in vivo* model to evaluate the contribution of NO on the increased production of PGs evoked by bolus injection of endotoxin in the conscious and restrained Sprague Dawley rat. Bolus intravenous injection of LPS (4 mg/kg) caused a time dependent increase in plasma levels of NO_2^- and 6-keto $PGF1\alpha$ (the stable metabolite of prostacyclin) and (b) urinary excretion of NO_2^-, 6-keto $PGF1\alpha$ and PGE_2. Plasma and urinary excretion of NO_2^- was completely abolished by NOS inhibitors but not by indomethacin. The NOS inhibitors also attenuated prostaglandin production by at least 50%. For instance, 5h post LPS injection, the plasma levels of 6-keto $PGF1\alpha$ increased from non-detectable values to 2.5±0.2 ng/ml (for LPS alone), 0.6±0.01 ng/ml for (LPS in the presence of LPS+LNMMA) and 1±0.01 ng/ml (in the presence of LPS+AG). Basal urinary excretion of NO_2^-, 6-keto $PGF\alpha$ and PGE_2 was 1.25±0.1 nmol/min, 177±44 pg/min and 176±23 pg/min (n=11). 5 hours post LPS injection these levels were respectively, 27, 3 and 10 fold higher. NOS inhibitors (L-NMMA and AG) inhibited the urinary excretion of NO_2^- a phenomenon associated with a marked inhibition of prostanoids release whereas indomethacin inhibited only the release of prostanoids **(Table 2)**. Dexamethasone (Dex) blocked the induction of both iNOS and COX-2 activities-pharmacological evidence that it is iNOS and COX-2 protein that are induced following the *in vivo* administration of LPS **(Table 2)**.

Our results indicate that in an inflammatory setting endogenous release of NO activates the inducible COX activity resulting in an increased release of proinflammatory prostaglandins. The enzymatic mechanisms that are involved in such activation are unknown although it has been recently reported that NO activates COX through a conformational change in the protein secondary structure rather than an interaction with the iron-heme center of the enzyme **(8)**. Other possibilities including the free radical scavenging properties of NO exists.

It is therefore conceivable that selective inhibitors of the inducible NOS may have anti-inflammatory actions as a result of their ability to remove the pro-inflammatory effects of NO and the prostaglandins.

Table 2. Effects of NOS inhibitors and indomethacin on the urinary excretion of NO_2^- and prostanoid 5 hours after a bolus administration of LPS.

	Mediators		
Drugs	NO_2^-	6-keto PGF1α	PGE_2
None	42±6	581±86	1815±81
L-NMMA	6±2	124±15	230±20
AG	4±1	188±28	76±22
Indo	40±5	78±25	127±10
Dex	6±1	165±23	70±17

Total excretion of NO_2^- (nmol/min) and prostanoids (pg/min) was calculated based on the concentration and the urine volume so as to take into account any changes in urinary output. Each point is the mean±s.e.m for n=6-10 experiments.

REFERENCES
1. Salvemini, D., Misko, T.P., Masferrer, J.L., Seibert, K., Currie, M.G. & Needleman, P. (1993). Proc. Natl. Acad. Sci. USA. 90: 7240-7244.
2. Salvemini, D., Seibert, K., Masferrer, J.L., Misko, T.P., Currie, M.G. & Needleman, P. (1994). J. Clin. Invest. 93: 1940-1947.
3. Corbett, J.A., Tilton, R.J., Chang, K., Hasan, K.S., Ido, y., Wang, J.L., Sweetland, M.A., Lancanster, J.R., Williamson, J.R. & McDaniel, M.L. (1992). Diabetes. 41: 552-556.
4. Misko, T.P., Moore, W.M., Kasten, T.P., Nickols, G.A., Tilton, R.G., McDaniel, M.L., Williamson, J.R. & Currie, M.G. (1993). Eur. J. Pharmacol. 233: 119-125.
5. Griffith, M.J.D., Messent, M., MacAllister, R.J. & Evans, T.W. (1993). Br. J. Pharmacol. 110: 963-968.
6. Moncada, S., Palmer, R.M.J. & Higgs, E.A. (1991). Pharmacol. Rev. 43: 109-141.
7. Wise, W.C., Halushka, P.V., Knapp, R.G. & Cook, J.A. (1985). Circulatory Shock. 17: 59-71.
8. Hajjar, D.P., Lander, H.M., Pearce, S.A.F. & Pomerantz, K.B. (1994). FASEB. J. A1432.

Advances in Prostaglandin, Thromboxane,
and Leukotriene Research, Vol. 23,
edited by B. Samuelsson et al.
Raven Press, Ltd., New York © 1995

NITRIC OXIDE MODULATES ANGIOGENESIS ELICITED BY PROSTAGLANDIN E1 IN RABBIT CORNEA

Marina Ziche, Lucia Morbidelli, Astrid Parenti and Fabrizio Ledda

Department of Pharmacology, University of Florence,
Viale Morgagni 65, 50134 Florence, Italy.

Angiogenesis is the process of new vessel generation which leads to neovascularization (1). In the adult tissue, angiogenesis is of importance in various physiological and pathological processes such as ovulation and corpus luteum formation, healing processes, tumour growth and metastasis, chronic arthropathies and diabetic retinopathies. The morphogenetic program of the neovascular response requires multiple steps and increase in blood flow and vasodilation of the parent venule before the emergence of the first capillary sprouts are important steps (2). Nevertheless, the relevance of vasodilation in the angiogenesis process is largely unknown.

A large number of vasoactive-vasodilating agents are reported to possess angiogenic activity (3,4), and we have previously shown that prostaglandin E_1 (PGE_1) is angiogenic in the rabbit cornea assay (5).

Endothelium-dependent vasodilation has been clearly demonstrated to be caused by the endothelium-derived relaxing factor identified as nitric oxide (NO)(6,7).

The aim of the present study was to evaluate the role played by NO in the modulation of the angiogenic process promoted by PGE_1.

MATERIALS AND METHODS

The angiogenic activity was assayed in vivo using the rabbit cornea assay (5). Slow-release pellets were prepared in sterile conditions incorporating the test substances into a casting solution of a ethynil-vinyl copolymer (Elvax-40), in 10% methylene chloride. The pellets were implanted in micropockets surgically produced into the corneal stroma. Daily observations of the implants were made with a slit lamp stereomicroscope. An angiogenic response was scored positive when budding of vessels from the limbal plexus occurred after 3-4 days and capillaries progressed to reach the implanted pellet according to the scheme previously reported (5). Angiogenic activity was expressed as the number of implants exhibiting neovascularization over the total implants studied.

RESULTS

To test the relevance of NO release in angiogenesis, two adjacent pockets were surgically produced in the same cornea, one bearing the angiogenic trigger and the other the NO-donor drug sodium nitroprusside (SNP). PGE_1 was tested at doses of 0.1 μg, which produced a weak angiogenic response (5). Pellets of Elvax alone were used as control. When SNP (1 μg) was released into the corneal stroma simultaneously with PGE_1, a sharp improvement in the efficiency of the angiogenesis response was observed (fig. 1).

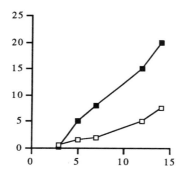

Figure 1: Effect of SNP on corneal angiogenesis promoted by PGE_1
PGE_1 (0.1 μg) was tested in the absence (□) and in the presence of SNP (■). Angiogenesis score (vertical axis) was calculated on the basis of the number of vessels and their growth rate versus time (days).

N^ω-nitro-L-arginine methyl ester (L-NAME) or the inactive enantiomer N^ω-nitro-D-arginine methyl ester (D-NAME) (7) were given to rabbits in the drinking water *ad libitum*. Drug solutions (0.5 g/l) were given for one week before surgery and 10 days following corneal implant.

Table 1: Corneal angiogenesis following systemic NO synthase inhibition

Implant (μg/pellet)	Control	Treatment L-NAME	D-NAME
Elvax	0/6	0/6	0/6
PGE_1 (0.25)	5/6	0/6	5/6

In rabbits fed with L-NAME, angiogenesis induced by 0.25 µg PGE$_1$ was drastically reduced. In control animals and in the group receiving D-NAME angiogenesis was not modified (Table 1).

DISCUSSION

The morphogenetic program of the neovascular response requires multiple steps, and increase in blood flow and vasodilation of the parent venule before the emergence of the first capillary sprouts have been observed (2,4).

We have previously reported that nitric oxide promoted DNA synthesis and cyclic GMP formation in endothelial cells isolated from postcapillary venules (8). Here we report that NO production potentiates angiogenesis elicited by PGE$_1$ in the rabbit cornea assay. Inhibition of NO production caused by chronic systemic administration of L-NAME in vivo, strongly curtailed the ability of PGE$_1$ to elicit the neovascular response.

The experimental data presented document that NO production is an essential step for angiogenesis induced by PGE$_1$ and suggest that NO production might function as an autocrine/paracrine regulator during neovascularization.

ACKNOWLEDGMENTS

This work was supported by funds from Italian Ministry for the University and for Scientific and Technological Research, Associazione Italiana per la Ricerca sul Cancro and the Italian National Research Council.

REFERENCES

1. Folkman, J. Angiogenesis: initiation and control. *Ann. N.Y. Acad. Sci.* 1982; 401: 212-227
2. Clark, E.R., and E.L. Clark. Microscopic observations on the growth of blood capillaries in the living mammal. *Am. J. Anat.* 1939; 64: 251-299 .
3. Ziche, M., L. Morbidelli, M. Pacini, P. Geppetti, G. Alessandri, and C.A. Maggi. Substance P stimulates neovascularization in vivo and proliferation of cultured endothelial cells. *Microvasc. Res.* 1990; 40: 264-278.
4. Ziada, A.M.A.R., O. Hudlicka, K.R. Tyler, and A.J.A. Wright. The effect of long-term vasodilatation on capillary growth and performance in rabbit heart and skeletal muscle. *Cardiovasc. Res.* 1984; 18: 724-732.
5. Ziche, M., J. Jones, and P.M. Gullino. Role of prostaglandin E$_1$ and copper in angiogenesis. *J. Natl. Cancer Inst.* 1982; 69: 475-482.
6. Ignarro, L.J., G.M. Buga, K.S. Wood, R.E. Byrns, and G. Chaudhuri. Endothelium-derived relaxing factor produced and released from artery and vein is nitric oxide. *Proc. Natl. Acad. Sci. USA* 1987; 84: 9265-9269.
7. Moncada, S., R.M.J. Palmer, and E.A. Higgs. Nitric oxide: physiology, pathophysiology and pharmacology. *Pharmacol. Rev.* 1991; 43: 109-142.
8. Ziche, M., L. Morbidelli, E. Masini, H.J. Granger, P. Geppetti, and F. Ledda. Nitric oxide promotes DNA synthesis and cyclic GMP formation in endothelial cells from postcapillary venules. *Biochem. Biophys. Res. Commun.* 1993; 192: 1198-1203.

Advances in Prostaglandin, Thromboxane,
and Leukotriene Research, Vol. 23,
edited by B. Samuelsson et al.
Raven Press, Ltd., New York © 1995

Human Prostanoid Receptors: Cloning and Characterization

Mark Abramovitz, Mohammed Adam, Yves Boie, Ryszard Grygorczyk, Thomas
H. Rushmore, Truyen Nguyen, Colin D. Funk*, Lison Bastien, Nicole Sawyer,
Chantal Rochette, Deborah M. Slipetz and Kathleen M. Metters

*Department of Biochemistry and Molecular Biology, Merck Frosst Centre for Therapeutic Research,
Kirkland, Quebec H9H 3L1 and Division of Clinical Pharmacology, School of Medicine, Vanderbilt
University*, Nashville, Tennessee 37232*

The naturally occurring prostanoids, derived from arachidonic acid, exert their manifold physiological and pathophysiological effects through specific interactions with a unique family of prostanoid receptors, members of the G-protein-coupled receptor (GPCR) superfamily. Until recently, characterization of these receptors has been based solely upon results from functional and radioligand-binding studies utilizing various tissues from a number of mammalian species in which a varied population of prostanoid receptors was expressed[1]. This heterogeneity together with the absence of potent and selective agonists or antagonists for these receptors has hindered our understanding of the precise role they play in normal physiology and disease states. Certainly the therapeutic potential for selective prostanoid receptor agonists and antagonists warrants their development. This requires that the prostanoid receptors be characterized at the molecular level.

The purification[2] and cloning[3] of the human thromboxane A_2 receptor (hTP), followed by the cloning of the mouse prostaglandin (PG) E_2 receptor, EP_3 subtype[4] has allowed us to devise strategies to clone these and other members of the human prostanoid receptor family. Here we summarize our results on the cloning and characterization of the human (h) EP_1[5] EP_2[6], EP_3[7], FP[8] and IP[9] prostanoid receptors.

PROSTANOID RECEPTOR CLONING

Different strategies were employed to clone the prostanoid receptors. Initially, a PCR generated mEP_3[4] cDNA probe was used to clone three isoforms of the hEP_3 prostanoid receptor from kidney and uterus cDNA libraries. The three isoforms of the hEP_3 receptor (hEP_{3-I}, hEP_{3-II} and hEP_{3-III}) code for proteins containing 390, 388 and 365 amino acids (aa) with calculated molecular masses (Mr) of 43315, 42688 and 40507, respectively[7]. The sequences diverge after the glutamine residue (aa 359) located 10 aa from the end of transmembrane domain (TMD) VII, a consequence of alternate gene splicing. This has

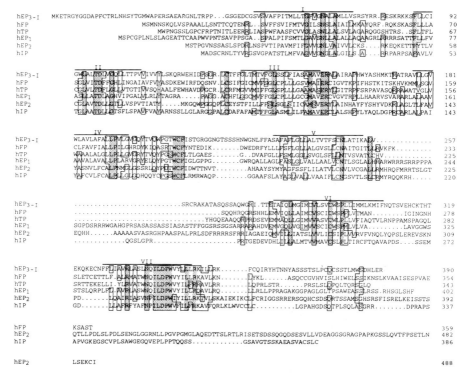

FIG. 1. A comparison of the deduced amino acid sequences of the hEP$_{3-1}$, hFP, hTP, hEP$_1$, hEP$_2$ and hIP receptors are shown. Identical aa in at least four sequences are boxed and those identical in all receptors are shaded. Dots indicate gaps introduced in the sequences for alignment purposes.

also been shown for the mouse[10,11], rat[12], rabbit[13] and bovine[14] EP$_3$ receptors. To date, nine different C-terminal tails from five different species have been described.

The hEP$_2$ receptor was cloned using a similar strategy. A partial mouse EP$_2$[15] cDNA fragment was used to clone the hEP$_2$ receptor cDNA from a lung library[6]. The cDNA encodes a 488 aa protein with a calculated Mr of 53115.

The identification of novel prostanoid receptor cDNAs required a different approach. A partial hTP cDNA was used to screen an erythroleukemia cell cDNA library, under reduced stringency conditions, from which a full length cDNA for the PGE$_2$, EP$_1$ subtype was identified[5]. The cDNA encodes a 402 aa polypeptide with a predicted Mr of 41858.

We also exploited the fact that there are nine invariant aa (NQILDPWVY) located in TMD VII of the TP[3], EP$_1$[5] and EP$_3$[4] receptors. A degenerate 27mer oligonucleotide was synthesized based on this sequence and used to probe several cDNA libraries. This resulted in the cloning of the hFP receptor cDNA from a uterus library. The FP cDNA encodes a 359 aa polypeptide with a predicted relative Mr of 40060.

We then compared the nine conserved aa in TMD VII with those from the mouse EP$_2$ receptor[15]. There were two aa differences; glutamine for proline and valine for isoleucine (N$\underline{P}$ILDPW$\underline{I}$Y). A 26mer degenerate oligonucleotide was synthesized based on these differences and used to clone the hIP receptor cDNA from a lung library[9]. The cDNA encodes a 386 aa polypeptide with a relative Mr of 40961.

Hydropathicity analysis of the human prostanoid receptor deduced aa sequences predicted the seven putative TMDs characteristic of GPCRs. Overall aa identity between prostanoid receptors ranges from 27% to 42%, mostly in the TMDs and especially in TMD VII (Fig. 1). There are 33 aa conserved in this family, 10 of which are found in almost all GPCRs and several of these have been shown to be structurally and functionally important[16]. Residues conserved only within the prostanoid receptor family may be important in their overall structure and warrant further study.

IDENTIFICATION OF THE PROSTANOID RECEPTORS

Putative prostanoid receptors were identified by functional expression in *Xenopus* oocytes and by radioligand binding assays.

Functional Expression Of Prostanoid Receptors In *Xenopus* Oocytes

Functional expression of the prostanoid receptors in *Xenopus* oocytes was assessed using three different methods; two were used for the characterization of receptors which couple to increases in intracellular Ca^{2+}, a standard voltage-clamp assay and an aequorin luminescence assay[17]. The latter assay involves injection of the Ca^{2+}-sensitive photoprotein aequorin which is used as an intracellular Ca^{2+} sensor. In this manner agonist-induced dose-dependant (10nM-1μM) increases in intracellular Ca^{2+} were demonstrated directly by light emission in aequorin-loaded oocytes, expressing either the EP$_1$[5] or FP[8] receptor.

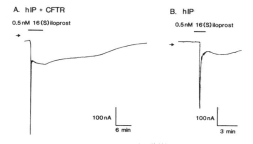

FIG. 2A. Cl⁻ current response in an oocyte co-expressing hIP and CFTR Cl⁻ channel challenged with 0.5 nM 16(S)-iloprost. **B.** Cl⁻ current response in an oocyte expressing hIP receptor alone challenged with 0.5 nM 16(S)-iloprost. Arrows indicate zero current level. See text for details and ref. 9 for method.

The third method identifies receptors which couple to increases in intracellular cAMP levels by co-expression of the receptor with the cystic fibrosis transmembrane conductance regulator (CFTR)[18], a cAMP-activated chloride channel. Oocytes co-expressing the hEP_2 or hIP receptor and CFTR, upon challenge with 0.5 to 100 nM PGE_2 or iloprost, gave prominent dose-dependent CFTR-mediated Cl^- current responses[6,9].

However, in certain batches of oocytes coupling of hIP to both Ca^{2+} and cAMP signaling pathways was detected, as shown by the characteristic Ca^{2+}-dependent Cl^- current spikes superimposed on a slower cAMP-dependent Cl^- current component (Fig. 2 A). In oocytes expressing hIP alone, only Ca^{2+}-dependent Cl^- current responses could be seen (Fig. 2B). Thus the hIP receptor can apparently signal through both increasing intracellular cAMP and Ca^{2+} as has been shown for the mouse IP receptor[19].

Radioligand Binding Studies of Prostanoid Receptors Expressed in COS Cells

Radioligand binding analyses were conducted using the plasma membrane fraction prepared from COS cells expressing the cloned putative prostanoid receptors. The rank order of affinities for prostaglandins and related analogues in competiton for specific binding to hEP_1[5], hEP_2[6], hEP_3[7], hFP[8] and hIP[9] was generally in agreement with that previously described in the literature[1] and confirmed the identity of these receptors, Table I. The metabolically stable prostacyclin and thromboxane analogues, iloprost and U46619, were used as probes for the hIP and hTP receptors, respectively. In addition, the more selective EP_1-antagonists AH6809 and SC19220, EP_2-agonist butaprost and EP_3-agonist M&B 28767 were used to discriminate between the three hEP subtypes. Suprisingly, butaprost was inactive at all three hEP receptors and was previously also shown to be inactive at the mouse EP subtypes[4,15,20]. It is probable that the methyl ester group of butaprost interferes with its binding to the EP_2 receptor, as has been reported for the binding of SM-10902, the methyl ester of SM-10906, to the IP receptor[21].

Receptor	Agonist Rank Order of Potency	K_D (nM)
EP_1	PGE_2 = iloprost > PGE_1 > $PGF_{2\alpha}$ >> U46619 > PGD_2	1.1
EP_2	PGE_2 = PGE_1 >> iloprost > $PGF_{2\alpha}$ > PGD_2 > U46619	0.63
EP_{3-I}	PGE_2 = PGE_1 >> $PGF_{2\alpha}$ = iloprost > PGD_2 >> U46619	0.64*
FP	$PGF_{2\alpha}$ = fluprostenol $\geq$ PGD_2 > PGE_2 > U46619 > iloprost	2.2
IP	iloprost >> PGE_1> carbacyclin >> PGE_2 > $PGF_{2\alpha}$ = PGD_2 = U46619	1/44**
TP	U46619 >> PGD_2 = $PGF_{2\alpha}$ = PGE_2 = iloprost	1.2

* Values for EP_{3-II} and EP_{3-III} are comparable
** Conforms to a 2-site model

TABLE I. Ligand binding properties of human prostanoid receptors

TISSUE DISTRIBUTION OF PROSTANOID RECEPTORS

Northern blot analysis has been used to assess the tissue distribution of the human prostanoid receptor family.

In general each prostanoid receptor, hEP$_1$ (Fig. 3A), hEP$_2$[6], hEP$_3$ (Fig. 3B), hFP (Fig. 3C) and hIP[9], has its own unique tissue distribution pattern. More particularly, all of them (except for FP) are well expressed in the kidney including the hEP$_1$ transcript (Fig. 3A) which is almost exclusively restricted to this tissue. Prostanoids, such as PGE$_2$ and PGI$_2$, have been shown to exert numerous effects on various aspects of kidney function[1] which are certainly mediated through the various prostanoid receptors. The expression in the kidney highlights important species differences in distribution; the FP receptor which is present in mouse kidney[22], is barely detectable in human kidney while the reverse is observed for IP, which is present in human kidney but not that of mouse[19].

Of note the EP$_2$ transcript is abundantly expressed in the thymus which is significant in light of the documented effects PGE$_2$ has on T lymphocytes[23]. The FP receptor mRNA is detected mainly in reproductive tissues such as, ovary, uterus, testis and mammary gland but also in retina (Fig. 3C). PGF$_{2\alpha}$ has a clearly defined role as a potent luteolytic agent[1] and is thought to be important in uterine contraction[1]. PGF$_{2\alpha}$ analogs have also been implicated as being intraocular pressure reducing agents[24].

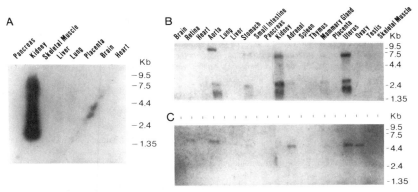

FIG. 3. Northern blot analysis of human Poly A+ RNA (2 or 3 μg) from different tissues indicated. Hybridization analysis was carried out using in **A)** a ^{32}P-labeled hEP$_1$ cDNA probe, in **B)** a ^{32}P-labeled hEP$_3$ cDNA probe, and in **C)** a ^{32}P-labeled hFP cDNA probe.

SUMMARY

Here we have summarized our work on the cloning, characterization and tissue distribution of the hEP$_1$, hEP$_2$, hEP$_3$, hFP and hIP prostanoid receptors. The availability of the prostanoid receptor cDNAs will allow for detailed localization, structure-function and binding studies to be conducted in order to understand better the physiological and pathophysiological roles these receptors play. As importantly, the development of potent and selective agonists and antagonists will allow for a rigorous assessment of their potential as suitable therapeutic targets in a number of diseases.

REFERENCES

1. Coleman RA, Kennedy I, Humphrey PPA, Bunce K, and Lumley P. Prostanoids and their Receptors. *Comprehensive Medicinal Chemistry* (Hansch C, Sammes PG, Taylor JB, and Emmett JC. eds) *Vol* 3, Pergamon Press, Oxford. 1989:643-714.
2. Ushikubi F, Nakajima M, Hirata M, Okuma M, Fujiwara M, and Narumiya S. Purification of the throm- boxane A2/prostaglandin H2 receptor from human blood platelets. *J Biol Chem* 1989;264:16496-501.
3. Hirata M, Hayashi Y, Ushikubi F, et al. Cloning and expression of cDNA for a human thromboxane A2 receptor. *Nature* 1991;349:617-20.
4. Sugimoto Y, Namba T, Honda A, et al. Cloning and expression of a cDNA for mouse prostaglandin E receptor EP3 subtype. *J Biol Chem* 1992;267:6463-6.
5. Funk CD, Furci L, FitzGerald GA, et al. Cloning and expression of a cDNA for the human prostaglandin E receptor EP1 subtype. *J Biol Chem* 1993;268:26767-72.
6. Bastien L, Sawyer N, Grygorczyk R, Metters K, and Adam M. Cloning, functional expression, and characterization of the human prostaglandin E2 receptor EP2 subtype. J Biol Chem 1994;269:11873-7.
7. Adam M, Boie Y, Rushmore TH, et al. Cloning and expression of three isoforms of the human EP3 prostanoid receptor. *FEBS Letters* 1994;338:170-4.
8. Abramovitz M, Boie Y, Nguyen T, et al. Cloning and expression of a cDNA for the human prostanoid FP receptor. *J Biol Chem* 1994;269:2632-6.
9. Boie Y, Rushmore TH, Darmon-Goodwin A, et al. Cloning and expression of a cDNA for the human prostanoid IP receptor. *J Biol Chem* 1994;269:12173-8.
10. Sugimoto Y, Negishi M, Hayashi Y, et al. Two isoforms of the EP3 receptor with different carboxyl-terminal domains. *J Biol Chem* 1993;268:2712-8.
11. Irie A, Sugimoto Y, Namba T, et al. Third isoform of the prostaglandin-E-receptor EP3 subtype with different C-terminal tail coupling to both stimulation and inhibition of adenylate cyclase. *Eur J Biochem* 1993;217:313-8.
12. Takeuchi K, Takahashi N, Abe T, and Abe K. Two isoforms of the rat kidney EP3 receptor derived by alternative RNA splicing: Intrarenal expression co-localization. *Biochem Biophys Res Commun* 1994;199:834-40.
13. Breyer RM, Emeson RB, Tarng J-L, et al. Alternative splicing generates multiple isoforms of a rabbit prostaglandin E2 receptor. *J Biol Chem* 1994;269:6163-9.
14. Namba T, Sugimoto Y, Negishi M, et al. Alternative splicing of C-terminal tail of prostaglandin E receptor subtype EP3 determines G-protein specificity. *Nature* 1993;365:166-70.
15. Honda A, Sugimoto Y, Namba T, et al Cloning and expression of a cDNA for mouse prostaglandin E receptor EP2 subtype. *J. Biol. Chem.* 1993;268:7759-62.
16. Probst WC, Snyder LA., Schuster DI, Brosius J, and Sealfon SC. Sequence alignment of the G-protein coupled receptor superfamily. [Review] *DNA Cell Biol.* 1992;11:1-20.
17. Giladi E, and Spindel ER. Simple luminometric assay to detect phosphoinositol-linked receptor expression in Xenopus oocytes. *Biotechniques* 1991;10:744-7.
18. Grygorczyk R, Abramovitz M, Boie Y, Bastien L, and Adam M. Detection of adenylate cyclase-coupled receptor expression in *Xenopus* oocytes. (Manuscript in preparation)
19. Namba T, Oida H, Sugimoto Y, et al. cDNA cloning of a mouse prostacyclin receptor. *J Biol Chem* 1994;269:9986-92.
20. Watabe A, Sugimoto Y, Honda A, et al. Cloning and Expression of cDNA for a Mouse EP1 Subtype of Prostaglandin E Receptor. *J. Biol. Chem.* 1993;268:20175-8.
21. Oka M, Negishi M, Yamamoto T, Satoh K, Hirohashi T, and Ichikawa A. Prostacyclin (PGI) Receptor Binding and Cyclic AMP Synthesis Activities of PGI1 Analogues, SM-10906 and Its Methyl Ester, SM-10902, in Mastocytoma P-815 Cells. *Biol Pharm Bull* 1994;17:74-7.
22. Sugimoto Y, Hasumoto K-Y, Namba T, et al. Cloning and expression of a cDNA for mouse prostaglandin F receptor. *J Biol Chem* 1994;269:1356-60.
23. Negishi M, Sugimoto Y, and Ichikawa A. Prostanoid receptors and their biological actions. *Prog Lipid Res* 1993;32:417-34.
24. Racz P, Ruzsonyi MR, Nagy ZT, and Bito LZ. Maintained intraocular pressure reduction with once-a-day application of a new prostaglandin F2 alpha analogue (PhXA41). An in-hospital, placebo-controlled study. *Arch Ophthalmol* 1993;111:657-61.

Advances in Prostaglandin, Thromboxane, and Leukotriene Research, Vol. 23,
edited by B. Samuelsson et al.
Raven Press, Ltd., New York © 1995

Interactions Between Prostaglandins, Muscarinic Agonists And The Adenylate Cyclase And Phospholipase C Systems In Dog Ciliary Smooth Muscle

A.A. Abdel-Latif, S.Y.K. Yousufzai and Z. Ye

Department of Biochemistry and Molecular Biology,
Medical College of Georgia, Augusta, GA 30912, USA

The physiological effects of topically administered prostaglandins (PGs) in the mammalian eye have been extensively investigated and there is now a better understanding of the relationship between prostanoid receptors and their effects in this organ (for reviews, 1-3). PGs of the E series and $PGF_{2\alpha}$ have been reported to elicit responses such as contraction and relaxation of the iris sphincter and ciliary muscles, increased permeability of the blood-aqueous barrier, and lowering of intraocular pressure (IOP). PGs exert at least part of their ocular hypotensive effect by increasing the uveoscleral pathway (1,2). While the main resistance in this pathway is constituted by the ciliary muscle (4), the mechanisms underlying the ocular hypotensive effects of PGs and the role of this smooth muscle in IOP lowering have yet to be determined. The sphincter and ciliary muscles of the iris-ciliary body are innervated by the parasympathetic nervous system and activation of muscarinic receptors (mainly M_3) in this tissue leads to: (a) Enhanced hydrolysis of phosphatidylinositol 4,5 bisphosphate (PIP_2) and the generation of the two second messengers, inositol 1,4,5-bisphosphate (IP_3) and 1,2-diacylglycerol (DAG); (b) release of arachidonic acid (AA) and its subsequent conversion into PGs; and (c) muscle contraction (for review, 5). In view of the possibility that the ciliary muscle could be the site of action of the ocular hypotensive effects of PGs, here we have investigated the relationship between PGs and muscarinic functions in the dog ciliary muscle.

METHODS

Dog eyes were obtained through the courtesy of the Richmond County Animal Control (Augusta, GA). Eyes were enucleated immediately after death and transported to the laboratory packed in ice. Ciliary muscle was dissected from the sclerae spur, lens and choroid under a binocular microscope.

Methods for incubation of ciliary muscle with myo[^{3}H] inositol and analysis of inositol phosphates by anion-exchange chromatography, assay of cAMP by means of radioimmunoassay (RIA) and measurement of agonist-induced tension responses were carried out as previously described (6,7). Briefly, in the studies on dose-response effect of PGE_2 on CCh-stimulated IP_3 production the ciliary muscles were prelabeled with ^{3}H-inositol, washed with Krebs-Ringer bicarbonate buffer containing 1 μM indomethacin and then incubated in the same buffer for 1 min with different concentrations of PGE_2 as indicated, followed by addition of 10 μM carbachol (CCh) for an additional 5 min.

In the studies on the effects of PGs on cAMP formation the dog ciliary muscle was divided into four fragments and each fragment was incubated in 1 mL of buffer containing 1 μM indomethacin for 1 hr at 37°C. The tissues were transferred to fresh buffer (1 mL/tube) containing 0.1 mM IBMX, pre-incubated first for 10 min and then incubated in absence and presence of various concentrations of PGE_2 or $PGF_{2\alpha}$ as indicated for 5 min. The reaction was killed with TCA (final conc. 2.5 %) and the cAMP extracted from the tissue and assayed by means of RIA.

For measurement of tension responses, changes in tension were recorded isometrically using a force-displacement transducer (Grass model FT.03) coupled to a polygraph (Grass model 79D).

Data presented in figures and table are means $\pm$ S.E.M.

RESULTS

Effects of PGs on CCh-induced IP_3 production and muscle contraction

To test the possibility that PGs could function in part to modulate muscle tension in the ciliary muscle we investigated their effects on CCh-induced muscle contraction and on IP_3 production. Addition of 5 μM CCh in the absence (Fig. 1A) and in the presence (Fig. 1B) of 1 μM indomethacin, which completely blocks PG synthesis in this tissue, elicited contractile responses of 11.2 and 15.6 mg tension/mg wet weight, respectively (Fig. 1). This is an increase of 39%. However, when PGE_2 (1 μM) was added to muscle precontracted with 1 μM CCh, in the presence of indomethacin, the muscle relaxed by 33% (Fig. 1C). In contrast, $PGF_{2\alpha}$ had no influence on the contractile response by the muscarinic agonist in this tissue (data not shown). Addition of PGE_2 to ciliary muscle precontracted with CCh inhibited IP_3 production in a dose-dependent manner (Fig. 2). Maximal inhibition (84%) was observed in the presence of 1 μM PGE_2. These data suggest that PGE_2-induced muscle relaxation in the ciliary muscle is mediated through cAMP.

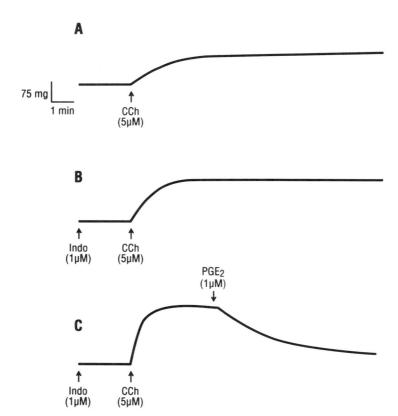

Fig. 1. Tracings showing the effects of CCh (5 μM) in absence (A) and presence (B) of indomethacin (1 μM) in dog ciliary muscle. In (C) the muscle was pre-equilibrated in Krebs-Ringer bicarbonate buffer (pH 7.2) containing 1 μM indomethacin for 90 min, then contracted by CCh (5 μM) for 3 min followed by addition of 1 μM PGE$_2$.

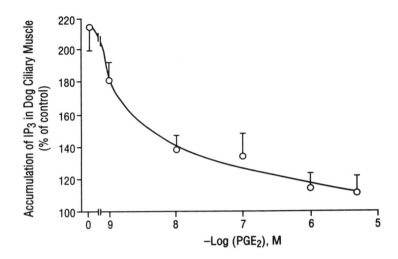

Fig. 2. Dose-response effect of PGE$_2$ on CCh-stimulated IP$_3$ production in dog ciliary muscle. The basal value for ^{3}H-IP$_3$ production was 1640 ± 171 dpm/mg of total tissue proteins. Each value represents the mean $\pm$ S.E.M. for three separate experiments each run in triplicate.

Effects of various PGs on cAMP formation

In preliminary studies we found that all PGs tested had no effect on IP$_3$ production and contraction in this tissue. This is in contrast to the sphincter muscle where both PGF$_{2\alpha}$ and PGE$_2$ increased IP$_3$ production and contraction in this tissue (6). In addition, PGs did not contract isolated ciliary muscle obtained from bovine, cat, pig, or human (data not shown). However, we found that PGE$_2$ and PGF$_{2\alpha}$ increased cAMP production in a dose-dependent manner with EC$_{50}$ values of 0.8 and 2 μM, respectively (Fig. 3). In addition, at 0.1 μM concentrations PGE$_2$, 11-deoxy PGE$_1$ and PGD$_2$ increased cAMP production by 72, 64 and 57%, respectively (Table I). 17-phenyl-ω-trinor PGE$_2$ and sulprostone had little effect on cAMP production, and PGF$_{2\alpha}$ had no effect on the cyclic nucleotide formation at this concentration. Under the same experimental conditions 0.1 μM isoproterenol increased the intracellular concentration of cAMP by 112%. These data show that PGs are involved in muscle relaxation in this tissue, via stimulation of adenylate cyclase, and furthermore demonstrate that the stimulatory effect of PGE_2 on cAMP production is mediated through the EP_2 receptor subtype.

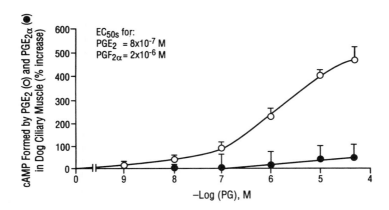

Fig. 3. Dose-response effects of PGE_2 (○) and $PGF_{2\alpha}$ (●) on intracellular cAMP formation in dog ciliary muscle. Basal cAMP formation was 8.3 pmol/mg protein. The data are averages of 3-4 experiments each run in triplicate.

TABLE I: Effects of various prostaglandins on cAMP formation in dog ciliary muscle*

Agonist and receptor subtype (0.1 μM)	cAMP (pmoles/mg protein)	% of control
None	10.0 ± 0.6	100
PGE$_2$ (EP$_2$)	17.2 ± 1.3	172
11-Deoxy PGE$_1$ (EP$_2$)	16.4 ± 1.3	164
17-Phenyl-ω-trinor PGE$_2$ (EP$_1$)	13.3 ± 1.2	133
Sulprostone (EP$_3$)	12.6 ± 0.9	126
PGD$_2$ (PD)	15.7 ± 1.1	157
PGF$_{2\alpha}$ (FP)	10.0 ± 0.7	100
Isoproterenol (β-adrenergic)	21.2 ± 1.4	212

*Tissues were incubated for 90 min, washed with buffer three times, then pretreated with 0.1 mM IBMX for 10 min, and with the agonist for an additional 5 min. Data are averages of four experiments, each run in duplicate.

DISCUSSION

The present studies on the relationship between PGs and muscarinic receptor-mediated responses in dog ciliary muscle suggest that PGE$_2$, but not PGF$_{2\alpha}$, may play an important role in regulating muscarinic functions in this parasympathetically innervated tissue. This conclusion is supported by the following findings in the present work: (a) None of the PGs we have tested had any effect on IP$_3$ production and contraction in this muscle. This was also found to be true of ciliary muscles obtained from bovine (7), pig, cat, and human (S.Y.K. Yousufzai and Abdel-Latif, unpublished observations). Instead, we observed that at lower concentrations (0.1 μM) PGE$_2$, but not PGF$_{2\alpha}$, significantly induced cAMP formation (Fig. 2, Table I). In addition, these data suggest that the stimulatory effect of PGE$_2$ on cAMP formation is mediated through the EP$_2$ receptor subtype (Table I). There are three EP receptor subtypes: EP$_1$, which is coupled to IP$_3$ production and smooth muscle contraction; EP$_2$, which is coupled to an increased intracellular cAMP; and EP$_3$, which is coupled to a decreased intracellular cAMP and inhibition of neurotransmitter release (8). The EP$_2$ receptor subtype appears to predominate in human ciliary muscle (9) and in rabbit iris-ciliary body (10). (b) Indomethacin, which blocks PG synthesis in this tissue, potentiated CCh-induced muscle contraction (Fig. 1). In the absence of indomethacin there are more PGs released, PGs in turn could inhibit, through stimulation of cAMP formation, the CCh-induced muscle contraction. Therefore, in ciliary muscle PGs released by Ca^{2+}-mobilizing agonists could be involved in the modulation of muscarinic functions. (c) Addition of PGE_2, but not $PGF_{2\alpha}$, to muscle precontracted with CCh relaxed the dog ciliary muscle (Fig. 1), and inhibited IP_3 production by 84% in the presence of 1 μM indomethacin (Fig. 2). This is in contrast to the bovine sphincter where both PGE_2 and $PGF_{2\alpha}$ contracted the muscle (6). Chen and Woodward (11) reported that PGE_2 induced relaxation of cat ciliary muscle precontracted by CCh. These data show that in ciliary muscle PGE_2 bind to EP_2 receptors, this activates adenylate cyclase and increases intracellular cAMP concentrations. Cyclic AMP in turn activates protein kinase A which phosphorylates a component of the transduction unit (receptor, G protein, or phospholipase C) and inhibits IP_3 production and Ca^{2+} mobilization. Lowering of cytosolic free Ca^{2+} concentrations results in decreased activity of myosin light chain kinase, decreased phosphorylation of myosin light chain and subsequently muscle relaxation. The modulation of muscarinic functions in ciliary muscle by PGE_2 is yet another example of a cross-talk between the cAMP and IP_3-Ca^{2+} second messenger systems in ocular tissues (3,5).

In summary, PGE_2, the major PG produced in the dog ciliary muscle, induced cAMP formation and relaxed muscle precontracted with CCh. Indomethacin, which blocks PG synthesis in this tissue, potentiated CCh-induced contraction. This suggests that PGE_2 may be involved in the regulation of muscarinic functions in this smooth muscle. $PGF_{2\alpha}$, which has been reported to lower IOP in several mammalian species, including human, had little effect on second messengers generation or muscle responses in this tissue. This could suggest either that the ciliary muscle is not the site of action of the IOP-lowering effects of $PGF_{2\alpha}$ and its analogs, or that these PGs may act at the uveoscleral pathway through a mechanism which does not involve the cAMP and IP_3-Ca^{2+} second messenger systems. Very recently, Lindsey *et al* (12) reported that exposure of human ciliary smooth muscle cells to $PGF_{2\alpha}$ induces an immediate early gene expression response that is similar to c-Fos induction in other cell systems. Thus, further studies are needed in order to delineate the mechanisms underlying the effects of PGs on uveoscleral outflow.

ACKNOWLEDGEMENTS

This study was supported by Grants R01-EY-04387 and R37-EY-04171 from the U.S. Public Health Service.

REFERENCES

1. Bito LZ and Stjernschantz J (eds). *The Ocular Effects of Prostaglandins and Other Eicosanoids*. New York:Alan R. Liss, Inc; 1989.
2. Hurvitz LM, Kaufman PL, Robin AL, Weinreb RN, Crawford K and Shaw B. New developments in the drug treatment of glaucoma. *Drugs* 1991;41:514-32.

3. Abdel-Latif AA. Release and effects of prostaglandins in ocular tissues. *Prostaglandins, Leukotrienes and Fatty Acids* 1991;44: 71-82.
4. Stjernschantz J and Resul B. Phenyl substituted prostaglandin analogs for glaucoma treatment. *Drugs of the Future* 1992;17:691-704.
5. Abdel-Latif AA. Calcium-mobilizing receptors, polyphosphoinositides, generation of second messengers and contraction in the mammalian iris smooth muscle: historical perspectives and current status. *Life Sci* 1989;45:757-86.
6. Yousufzai SYK, Chen AL and Abdel-Latif AA. Species differences in the effects of prostaglandins on inositol trisphosphate accumulation, phosphatidic acid formation, myosin light chain phosphorylation and contraction in iris sphincter of the mammalian eye: Interaction with the cAMP system. *J Pharmacol Exp Ther* 1988;247:1064-72.
7. Yousufzai SYK, Zheng P and Abdel-Latif, AA. Muscarinic stimulation of arachidonic acid release and prostaglandin synthesis in bovine ciliary muscle: Prostaglandins induce cyclic AMP formation and muscle relaxation. *Exp Eye Res* 1994;58:513-522.
8. Coleman RA, Kennedy I, Humphrey PPA, Bunce K and Lumley P. Prostaglandins and their receptors. In: Hansch C, Sammes PG, Taylor JB, Emmett JC, eds. *Comprehensive Medicinal Chemistry*, Vol. 3, Oxford: Pergamon Press; 1990;643-714.
9. Matsuo T and Cyander MS. The EP_2 receptors is the predominant prostanoid receptor in the human ciliary muscle. *Br J Ophthalmol* 1993;77:110-14.
10. Csukas S, Bhattacherjee P, Rhodes L and Paterson CA. Prostaglandin E_2 binding site distribution and subtype classification in the iris-ciliary body. *Prostaglandins* 1992;44:199-208.
11. Chen J and Woodward DF. Prostanoid-induced relaxation of precontracted cat ciliary muscle is mediated by EP_2 and DP receptors. *Invest Ophthalmol Vis Sci* 1992;33:195-201.
12. Lindsey JD, To HD, and Weinreb RN. Induction of c-Fos by prostaglandin $PGF_{2\alpha}$ in human ciliary smooth muscles cells. *Invest Ophthalmol Vis Sci* 1994;35: 242-50.

Advances in Prostaglandin, Thromboxane,
and Leukotriene Research, Vol. 23,
edited by B. Samuelsson et al.
Raven Press, Ltd., New York © 1995

Preclinical Pharmacology of Latanoprost, a Phenyl-Substituted $PGF_{2\alpha}$ Analogue

Johan Stjernschantz, Göran Selén, Birgitta Sjöquist and Bahram Resul

Glaucoma Research Laboratories, Pharmacia Ophthalmics, S-751 82, Uppsala, Sweden

Latanoprost (13,14-dihydro-17-phenyl-18,19,20-trinor-$PGF_{2\alpha}$-isopropyl ester; PhXA41) is a new prostaglandin analogue under development for glaucoma treatment. While $PGF_{2\alpha}$ and its esters are effective intraocular pressure (IOP) reducing agents they cause too many side-effects to be clinically useful. These side-effects comprise e.g. conjunctival hyperaemia, irritation, and foreign body sensation. An important property of $PGF_{2\alpha}$ is that it reduces IOP mainly by increasing the uveoscleral outflow of aqueous humour (1-3). In this outflow pathway aqueous humour by-passes the trabecular meshwork and Schlemm's canal, percolates through the ciliary muscle into the supraciliary and suprachoroidal spaces and finally leaves the eye through the sclera (4). This drainage route of aqueous humour is substantial in monkeys but may be less important in man during normal physiologic conditions (5).

Recently a group of phenyl-substituted prostaglandin analogues were described which are unique in that they exhibit a significantly improved therapeutic index in the eye with retained IOP reducing effect (6,7). The common feature of these compounds is that part of the omega chain has been substituted with a terminal ring structure (6,7). Latanoprost is one member of this group of compounds. The purpose of this paper is to give a short overview of the preclinical pharmacology of latanoprost primarily with respect to its use in the eye.

MATERIALS AND METHODS

In the *in vivo* studies to be reviewed cynomolgus monkeys, cats and albino rabbits were used as experimental animals. The experimental eye was treated with latanoprost applied topically and the other eye served as control receiving the vehicle only. For *in vitro* experiments the cat and bovine iris, guinea pig ileum, vas deferens and thrombocytes, pig cornea and bovine corpora lutea were used.

Experimental procedures in unanaesthetized animals

In unanaesthetized animals the IOP was measured with pneumatonometry. Prior to measurement local anaesthetic was applied on the cornea. The pupil diameter of cats and monkeys was measured with a ruler (in mm) under constant illumination conditions. Ocular irritation was estimated in cats on an arbitrary scale from 0 to 3, 0 corresponding to absence of irritation and 3, to marked irritation defined as complete closure of the lids. Conjunctival hyperaemia was determined in rabbits. Colour photographs were taken of the eyes at regular intervals during treatment and the photographs were evaluated to quantify hyperaemia on an arbitrary scale from 0 to 5.

Experimental procedures in anaesthetized animals

For measurement of blood flow, cardiovascular and respiratory parameters, and aqueous humour dynamics the animals were anaesthetized with ketalar and pentobarbital sodium. The aqueous humour dynamics was determined in cannulated eyes of cynomolgus monkeys. Outflow facility was determined by constant pressure infusion (9), and outflow of aqueous humour through Schlemm's canal and uveoscleral outflow by perfusing the anterior chamber with 125I- or 131I-albumin. The radioactive albumin which entered the blood represented the trabecular outflow and the radioactive albumin trapped in the uveoscleral outflow routes represented the uveoscleral outflow. Regional blood flow and cardiac output were determined with radioactively labelled microspheres injected into the left heart ventricle (9). The arterial blood pressure was measured in a femoral artery. Capillary permeability to albumin in the eye was determined by using intravenously administered 125I- and 131I-albumin and 51Cr-labelled erythrocytes. Airway resistance was estimated by determining the intrathoracic inspiration-expiration pressure difference in the oesophagus in spontaneously breathing monkeys.

In vitro and biochemical experiments

The receptor profile of latanoprost was determined in muscle bath and thrombocyte aggregation experiments. Different tissues expressing functionally homogenous prostanoid receptor populations were employed (10). EC_{50} values were used to express potency. Kd values were determined in ligand binding experiments using corpus luteum cell membranes. The permeability of the cornea to latanoprost was studied by using excised pig corneas in an *in vitro* chamber system (11). Ester hydrolysis of latanoprost in the corneal epithelium and plasma was studied using 3H-latanoprost, and metabolism of 3H-latanoprost in the eye was studied in cytosolic preparations of ocular tissues (12). Absorption, distribution, metabolism and excretion of 3H-latanoprost and its metabolites were studied in cynomolgus monkeys. Major metabolites were identified with gas chromatography-mass spectrometry.

OCULAR PHARMACOLOGY OF LATANOPROST

Latanoprost reduces IOP significantly in monkeys but has no or only a weak effect on IOP in cats. However, in the feline eye latanoprost has a marked pupillary constrictive effect, a property of the drug which is not observed in primates. Latanoprost causes no ocular irritation as determined in cats at doses as high as 10 μg applied on the eye. In rabbits latanoprost has been shown to induce significantly less conjunctival hyperaemia than equivalent doses of $PGF_{2\alpha}$-isopropyl ester ($PGF_{2\alpha}$-IE). Blood flow measurements in monkey eyes using radioactively labelled microspheres have shown that latanoprost has no significant effect on the blood flow in the iris, ciliary body, choroid or the retina. An increase in blood flow was detected only in the sclera 3 hours after topical application of 6 μg of latanoprost (Table I). This is in sharp contrast to the vascular effects of $PGF_{2\alpha}$-IE, which causes a marked increase in the blood flow of the anterior uvea of the monkey after topical application of 1 μg (13). No increase in capillary permeability to albumin was detected after topical treatment with 6 μg latanoprost. Thus, there seems to be no or only slight effects of latanoprost on the ocular microvasculature.

Table I.   Maximum effect of latanoprost on regional blood flow of the monkey eye after topical application of 6 μg (Mean ± SEM; n=6).

Tissue	Experimental Eye (mg/min)	Control Eye (mg/min)
Conjunctiva #	0.26 ± 0.05	0.18 ± 0.20
Anterior sclera	14.1 ± 3.3 *	4.4 ± 0.8
Posterior sclera	9.3 ± 2.5	2.5 ± 0.5
Iris	13.7 ± 2.3	13.9 ± 2.5
Ciliary body	57.3 ± 10.1	53.0 ± 6.2
Choroid	310.4 ± 46.2	305.0 ± 49.4
Retina	12.9 ± 1.6	16.1 ± 4.9

Blood flow given in mg/min/mg tissue. * p<0.05

The effect of topical application of latanoprost on aqueous humour dynamics has been studied in cynomolgus monkeys. Latanoprost (3 μg per day) was applied to the eye for 5 days and on the fifth day of treatment the aqueous humour dynamics and the outflow facility were determined. As shown in Table II latanoprost had a significant effect on the uveoscleral outflow but did not affect the trabecular outflow through Schlemm's canal or the outflow facility. There was a tendency towards an increase in total outflow of the experimental eye which would support the previous observation that $PGF_{2\alpha}$ may slightly increase production of aqueous humour (2).

The receptor profiles of latanoprost and $PGF_{2\alpha}$ have been studied in muscle bath and thrombocyte aggregation experiments in tissue systems expressing relatively homogenous functional receptor populations (10). From the data presented in Table III it is apparent that latanoprost is a much more selective FP receptor agonist than $PGF_{2\alpha}$. In ligand binding experiments performed on corpus luteum cell membranes the same Kd value of 2.8 nM was obtained for latanoprost and $PGF_{2\alpha}$.

Table II Effect of latanoprost on aqueous humour dynamics in monkeys after topical administration of 3 µg once daily for 5 days. (Mean ± SEM;n=6).

Variable	Experimental Eye	Control Eye
Trabecular outflow (µl/min)	0.43 ± 0.11	0.48 ± 0.07
Uveoscleral outflow (µl/min)	0.59 ± 0.14 **	0.37 ± 0.12
Total outflow (µl/min)	1.02 ± 0.16	0.86 ± 0.15
Outflow facility (µl/min/mmHg)	0.13 ± 0.02	0.12 ± 0.02

** $p < 0.01$

Table III Receptor profile of $PGF_{2\alpha}$ and latanoprost based on muscle bath and thrombocyte aggregation experiments (EC_{50} values in moles/l).

Prostanoid	FP	EP_1	EP_2	EP_3	DP/IP	TP
$PGF_{2\alpha}$	6.7×10^{-9}	3.8×10^{-7}	1.4×10^{-5}	1.1×10^{-7}	3.1×10^{-3}	2.9×10^{-5}
Latanoprost	3.6×10^{-9}	6.9×10^{-6}	3.6×10^{-4}	1.7×10^{-5}	$>1.0 \times 10^{-2}$	1.1×10^{-4}

GENERAL PHARMACOLOGY OF LATANOPROST

The cardiovascular effects of latanoprost have been studied in cynomolgus monkeys. Latanoprost administered at a dose of 0.6 µg/kg b.w. which is approximately 10 times the clinical dose on the eye (~0.05 µg/kg b.w.) had no significant effects on arterial blood pressure, cardiac output, heart rate, stroke volume or cardiac work in anaesthetized animals after intravenous injection, nor was there any effect on the coronary blood flow. Latanoprost administered intravenously had no effect on the blood flow in various parts of the brain, the stomach, small intestine or the colon, nor was there any effect on the blood flow in the liver, the kidneys, the urogenital organs or the bronchial arteries. Latanoprost had no significant effect on the respiration rate in normally breathing monkeys or on the intrathoracic inspiratory-expiratory pressure difference. Intravenous injection of latanoprost in monkeys had no effect on the blood flow in the eye.

PHARMACOKINETICS OF LATANOPROST

Latanoprost is a prodrug and as such biologically inactive. However, the prodrug is quantitatively and rapidly hydrolysed to latanoprost acid in the cornea as well as in plasma. Thus all drug that enters the aqueous humour has been hydrolysed. The permeability coefficient of latanoprost in the porcine cornea has been determined to be 6.8×10^{-6} cm x s^{-1} (12). Only a fraction of the drug applied topically penetrates into the monkey eye (about 1%), the rest being absorbed into the systemic circulation through blood vessels in the conjunctiva, and the mucous membranes of the nose, pharynx, oesophagus and gastrointestinal tract. After topical application of latanoprost in the monkey the peak concentration of latanoprost acid in the aqueous humour is reached in about one hour. The half-life of latanoprost acid in plasma is approximately 10 min in the monkey. Latanoprost acid has a small volume of distribution in the monkey (~1 l/kg).

Except for the hydrolysis of the ester moiety there is sparse metabolism of latanoprost in the ocular tissues. Latanoprost is a poor substrate for 15-PGDH (12) and its metabolism differs from that of $PGF_{2\alpha}$. Based on whole body autoradiography in monkeys it appears that very little of the drug is taken up by the lungs. Instead the main metabolism is ß-oxidation in the liver. The major metabolites in monkeys have been identified as 1,2-dinor- and 1,2,3,4-tetranor-13,14-dihydro-17-phenyl-18,19,20-trinor-$PGF_{2\alpha}$. The metabolites of latanoprost are excreted mainly into the urine but also through the biliary system into the faeces. During chronic treatment on the eye there is no accumulation of the drug or its metabolites in the monkey.

DISCUSSION AND CONCLUSIONS

Substitution of carbons 18,19 and 20 on the omega chain with a phenyl ring in combination with saturation of the 13,14 double bond resulted in a relatively selective FP receptor agonist. Analogous to $PGF_{2\alpha}$-IE, the compound penetrates well into the anterior segment of the eye when applied topically. The most remarkable property of latanoprost is that the ocular irritation, common with naturally occurring prostaglandins and their analogues, is eliminated without decrease in the IOP reducing potency. Thus, it appears that the receptors which mediate irritation, probably situated on sensory nerves in the cornea and the conjunctiva, are by-passed. The vascular effects of latanoprost are also clearly weaker than those of $PGF_{2\alpha}$.

Latanoprost reduces IOP mainly by increasing the uveoscleral outflow. The increase in uveoscleral outflow was approximately the same as that reported for $PGF_{2\alpha}$-IE in a comparable experimental model and the mechanism is probably FP receptor mediated. After treatment with latanoprost the conventional outflow of aqueous humour through Schlemm's canal is not affected, and aqueous humour is shunted into the uveoscleral outflow pathway. Latanoprost may slightly stimulate the production of aqueous humour analogous to $PGF_{2\alpha}$-IE but this effect, if true, is minimal.

No effects of latanoprost could be demonstrated in the cardiovascular and pulmonary organ systems of the anaesthetized monkey. However, it can be anticipated that high doses of latanoprost, after intravenous injection, probably cause some bronchoconstriction. This is a well-documented phenomenon with $PGF_{2\alpha}$, probably mediated by FP receptors.

Since latanoprost penetrates well into the eye but is not metabolized except for the ester hydrolysis, and since the half-life of latanoprost acid in plasma is short, latanoprost can be considered an oculoselective drug for glaucoma treatment. This is an important property since many of the drugs, such as e.g. the beta-adrenergic antagonists, adrenergic agonists and carbonic anhydrase inhibitors, currently used in glaucoma therapy cause significant systemic side-effects in many patients. Furthermore the fact that latanoprost acid is not metabolized in the eye and probably has a biochemical effect on the ciliary muscle is advantageous, as a long duration of action is achieved. Thus latanoprost can be administered once daily in patients (14).

REFERENCES

1.   Crawford K and Kaufman PL. Pilocarpine antagonizes $PGF_{2\alpha}$-induced ocular hypotension: Evidence for enhancement of uveoscleral outflow by $PGF_{2\alpha}$. *Arch Ophthalmol* 1987; 105: 1112-6.
2.   Nilsson SFE, Samuelsson M, Bill A and Stjernschantz J. Increased uveoscleral outflow as a possible mechanism of ocular hypotension caused by prostaglandin $F_{2\alpha}$-1-isopropyl ester in the cynomolgus monkey. *Exp Eye Res* 1989; 48; 707-716.
3.   True Gabelt B'A and Kaufman PL. Prostaglandin $F_{2\alpha}$ increases uveoscleral outflow in the cynomolgus monkey. *Exp Eye Res* 1989; 49: 389-402.
4.   Bill A. Conventional and uveoscleral drainage of aqueous humour in the cynomolgus monkeys (Macaca irus) at normal and high intraocular pressures. *Exp Eye Res* 1966; 5: 45-54.
5.   Bill A and Phillips CI. Uveoscleral drainage of aqueous humour in human eyes. *Exp Eye Res* 1971; 12: 275-81.
6.   Stjernschantz J and Resul B. Phenyl-substituted prostaglandin analogs for glaucoma treatment. *Drugs of the Future* 1992; 17: 691-704.
7.   Resul B, Stjernschantz J, No K, Liljebris C, Selén G, Astin M et al. Phenyl-substituted prostaglandins: Potent and selective antiglaucoma agents. *J Med Chem* 1993; 36: 243-8.
8.   Bárány EH. Simultaneous measurement of changing intraocular pressure and outflow facility in the vervet monkey by constant pressure infusion. *Invest Ophthalmol* 1964; 3: 135-43.
9.   Alm A and Bill A. The oxygen supply to the retina. II. Effects of high intraocular pressure and of increased arterial carbon dioxide tension on uveal and retinal blood flow in cats. *Acta Physiol Scand* 1972; 84: 306-9.
10. Coleman RA, Kennedy I, Humphrey PPA, Bunce K and Lumley P. Prostanoids and their receptors. In: Hansch C, Sammes PG and Taylor JB. *Comprehensive Medicinal Chemistry*. Oxford/New York; Pergamon Press: 1989; 3: 643-714.
11. Camber O. An in vitro model for determination of drug permeability through the cornea. *Acta Pharm Suec* 1985; 22: 335-42.
12. Basu S, Sjöquist, B, Stjernschantz, J and Resul B. Corneal permeability to and ocular metabolism of phehyl substituted prostaglandin esters in vitro. *Prostaglandins Leukotrienes Essent Fatty Acids* 1994; 50: 161-8.
13. Stjernschantz J, Nilsson SFE and Astin M. Vasodynamic and angiogenic effects of eicosanoids in the eye. In: Bito LZ and Stjernschantz, J. *The Ocular Effects of Prostaglandins and Ohter Eicosanoids* New York: Alan Liss, Inc.; 1989: 155-70.
14. Nagasubramanian S, Sheth GP, Hitchings RA and Stjernschantz J. Intraocular pressure-reducing effect of PhXA41 in ocular hypertension. *Ophthalmology* 1993; 100: 1305-11.

Advances in Prostaglandin, Thromboxane, and Leukotriene Research, Vol. 23, edited by B. Samuelsson et al. Raven Press, Ltd., New York © 1995

Mechanism of the Prostaglandin-Induced Reduction of Intraocular Pressure in Humans

Carl B. Camras

Department of Ophthalmology, University of Nebraska Medical Center, Omaha, Nebraska 68198

Supported in part by Grant EY 07865 from the National Eye Institute, Bethesda, Maryland; an unrestricted development grant from Research to Prevent Blindness, New York, New York; and the Gifford Laboratories, Omaha, Nebraska.
Reprint requests; Carl B. Camras, M.D., Department of Ophthalmology, University of Nebraska Medical Center, 600 South 42nd Street, Omaha, Nebraska 68198

Prostaglandin (PG) analogues show great promise as a new treatment for chronic glaucomas. They effectively reduce intraocular pressure (IOP) at least as well as beta-adrenergic antagonists, which are currently the most effective topically-applied agents used in glaucoma therapy. Once daily topical application of PG analogues produces a maintained reduction of IOP, lasting at least 24 hours after each dose. Tachyphylaxis does not develop in long term studies carried out for at least 6 months. PG analogues are well tolerated following topical application, without known systemic side effects.

Following the first study demonstrating that topically applied PGs reduce IOP in rabbits via an outflow mechanism,[1] several studies have evaluated the effects of PG analogues on aqueous humor dynamics in a variety of experimental animals, normotensive volunteers, and glaucoma patients. The purpose of this chapter is to review the clinical studies to establish a basis for the mechanism of action of PGs in humans.

PGF$_{2\alpha}$-1-ISOPROPYL ESTER

Based on the initial study in rabbits demonstrating a reduction of IOP after topical application,[1] PGF$_{2\alpha}$ tromethamine salt was found to reduce IOP in normal volunteers, but with intolerable local side effects, such as irritation, foreign body sensation, and conjunctival hyperemia.[2] Esterification of the terminal carboxylic acid group, producing the more lipophilic PGF$_{2\alpha}$-1-isopropyl

519

ester ($PGF_{2\alpha}$-IE), enhanced corneal penetration so that lower concentrations effectively reduced IOP with fewer local side effects.

$PGF_{2\alpha}$-IE 0.002% did not alter aqueous flow (F_a) in normotensive volunteers, as determined by fluorophotometric technique, either after a single dose in 20 subjects[3] or after 10 days of twice daily treatment in 10 subjects.[4]

Outflow facility (C) was not altered as determined by pneumatonography in 16 normotensive volunteers at 5 hours after receiving a single dose of $PGF_{2\alpha}$-IE 0.004%.[4] However in another study, C, as determined by electronic, Schiotz-type, indentation tonography, showed a small, but significant, increase in 13 patients with ocular hypertension or glaucoma receiving $PGF_{2\alpha}$-IE 0.002% determined at 4 hours after the last dose during the first week of treatment, but not in 11 patients receiving the 0.001% concentration.[5] This dose-dependent difference of C was noted despite the finding that both concentrations effectively reduced IOP.

Since the magnitude of the IOP reduction produced by $PGF_{2\alpha}$-IE in either normal volunteers or in patients with ocular hypertension or glaucoma cannot be explained by an effect on either F_a or C, it is concluded that $PGF_{2\alpha}$-IE reduces IOP predominantly by increasing uveoscleral outflow (F_u).[3-5] These results are consistent with assessment of F_u using invasive techniques in cynomolgus monkeys after topical application of $PGF_{2\alpha}$-IE.[6,7]

PhXA34 or PhXA41 (LATANOPROST)

Although $PGF_{2\alpha}$-IE represented an improvement in the therapeutic index compared with $PGF_{2\alpha}$ tromethamine salt, it still produced unacceptable conjunctival hyperemia and irritation. Structure-activity relationship studies found that 17-phenyl substituted $PGF_{2\alpha}$-IE analogues yielded optimal separation between ocular hypotensive efficacy and side effects.[8,9] Of these agents, PhXA34 (13,14-dihydro-15(R,S)-17-phenyl-18,19,20-trinor-$PGF_{2\alpha}$-IE) and its more active R-epimer, PhXA41 (latanoprost), have been evaluated in clinical studies.

F_a, as determined by fluorophotometry either during the day or night, was not altered by PhXA34 0.04%[10] given once daily or latanoprost 0.006%[11,12] given twice daily for 3-7 days in normotensive volunteers or in ocular hypertensive patients. PhXA34 0.04% given once daily caused a small, but significant, increase in C as determined by pneumatonography on the 7th day of treatment in 18 normotensive volunteers.[10] In one study, latanoprost 0.006% given twice daily for 5 days raised C by 25-30% as determined by electronic, Schiotz-type, indentation tonography at 4 hours after the last dose either in normotensive volunteers or in ocular hypertensive patients.[12] In another study, a similar dose of latanoprost given for 7 days did not alter C determined either by a fluorophotometric technique or by pneumatonography at 6 hours after the last dose.[11]

A fluorophotometric technique was used to calculate F_u.[11] Before and after latanoprost administration, F_a was assessed at 2 levels of IOP . IOP was altered by administration of timolol topically and acetazolamide orally to reduce IOP by decreasing F_a. The ratio of the change in F_a divided by the change in IOP reflects C as determined by this fluorophotometric technique. This non-invasive method of assessing C appears to have advantages over tonography.[11,13] F_u is calculated secondarily after determining F_a and C by fluorophotometry. This method demonstrated a 2 to 6-fold increase in F_u produced by latanoprost 0.006% given twice daily for one week. This effect of latanoprost on F_u is consistent with invasive experiments in cynomolgus monkeys demonstrating a PhXA34-induced increase in F_u by a perfusion technique with radiolabelled albumin.[14]

UF-021

UF-021 (isopropyl 20-ethyl-9a,11a-dihydroxy-15-keto-cis-Δ^5-prostanoate) is a 22-carbon chain derivative of a $PGF_{2\alpha}$ metabolite. A 0.12% concentration reduced IOP in normal volunteers by 1-2 mmHg after the first dose,   but not after one month of treatment.[15] In studies evaluating its effects on aqueous humor dynamics in normal volunteers, it did not alter F_a (determined by fluorophotometry), C (determined by an electronic computerized scanner), or episcleral venous pressure (determined by an episcleral venomanometer).[15,16] Like the other PG analogues, it is felt to reduce IOP by increasing F_u.

POSSIBLE CELLULAR MECHANISMS

With a   high degree of certainty, we can conclude that $PGF_{2\alpha}$ analogues reduce IOP in humans by increasing F_u, similar to their mechanism in non-human primates.   Although the biochemical or cellular mechanism of the increase in F_u is unknown in humans, several experiments in non-human primates suggest possible mechanisms. Since PGs do not affect F_u or reduce IOP in monkeys pre-treated with atropine[7] or pilocarpine,[7,17,18] the initial effect of PGs may be secondary to relaxation of the ciliary muscle. This ciliary muscle relaxation is not consistent with a study performed in human ciliary muscle cells in tissue culture, demonstrating PG-induced stimulation of calcium efflux across cell membranes,[19] which is usually correlated with muscle contraction.

It has been suggested that PGs cause dilated spaces between ciliary muscle bundles,[20] possibly as a result of stimulation of collagenase or other metalloproteinases, which alter the extracellular matrix. "Ripening" and "softening" of the human uterine cervix during childbirth and delivery is thought to involve a similar mechanism. In support of this mechanism is the observation

TABLE: Effect of PG Analogues on Aqueous Humor Dynamics.

PG Analogue	Subjects	n	F_a	C	F_u	Reference
$PGF_{2\alpha}$-IE	NV	20	-	NT	NT	Kerstetter et al 1989
	NV	10 or 16*	-	-	NT	Villumsen and Alm 1989
	OHT/POAG	24	-	- or ↑***	NT	Camras et al 1989
PhXA34	NV	18	-	↑	NT	Alm and Villumsen 1991
Latanoprost (PhXA41)	NV or OHT	22	-	-	↑	Toris et al 1993
	NV or OHT	40	-	↑	NT	Ziai et al 1993
UF-021	NV	10	-	-	NT	Sakurai et al 1991
	NV	8	-	-	NT	Tetsuka et al 1992

* n=10 for F_a and n=16 for C

** Higher concentration significantly increased C, but lower concentration had no effect.

Key to abbreviations: PG-Prostaglandin; n-number; F_a-Aqueous Humor Flow; C-Outflow Facility; F_u-Uveoscleral Outflow; NV-Normotensive Volunteer; OHT-Ocular Hypertensive Patients; F_u-Uveoscleral Outflow; POAG-Primary Open Angle Glaucoma Patients; - -no change; ↑-Significant Increase; NT-Not Tested.

that PGs induce c-Fos in human ciliary muscle cells in tissue culture.[21] c-Fos is the protein product of the proto-oncogene *c-fos*. *c-fos* activation may be involved in stimulation of several metalloproteinases, which may lead to extracellular matrix degradation. However, two independent studies failed to demonstrate a light or electron microscopic alteration in the ciliary muscle or other ocular tissues in PG-treated monkey eyes.[22,23] Although PGs may affect the extracellular matrix at a biochemical level to alter F_u, changes at the electron microscopic level may not be apparent.

CONCLUSIONS

Overall, based on evaluation in several studies in monkeys and humans, PGs produce either no effect or a slight increase in C, without affecting F_a (Table). In none of the studies has the magnitude of the C effect been sufficient to account for the reduction of IOP. It has been suggested that the effect on C may represent a PG-induced increase in pseudofacility or in the facility of F_u, rather than facility across the trabecular meshwork.[24,25] However, it is not unreasonable to assume that PGs may slightly increase conventional C across the trabecular meshwork.

Several $PGF_{2\alpha}$ analogues, including $PGF_{2\alpha}$-IE, PhXA34, latanoprost, and UF-021, reduce IOP primarily by increasing F_u, as determined indirectly by non-invasive measurements of F_a and C in normal volunteers and in patients with ocular hypertension or primary open angle glaucoma (Table). Since glaucoma is a disease of impaired outflow, a treatment that increases outflow has advantages over one that reduces F_a. At this time, the most commonly used agents in glaucoma therapy affect F_a. F_a suppressants may have a deleterious effect on the outflow channels by diminishing the supply of important nutrients needed to maintain health.[26] Furthermore, this outflow mechanism of action enables PG analogues to have a totally additive ocular hypotensive effect with ß-adrenergic blockers.[27-30] PG analogues will represent a welcome addition to our pharmacological armamentarium in glaucoma therapy.

REFERENCES

1. Camras CB, Bito LZ, and Eakins KE. Reduction of intraocular pressure by prostaglandins applied topically to the eyes of conscious rabbits. *Invest Ophthalmol Vis Sci* 1977;16:1125-34.

2. Giuffrè G. The effects of prostaglandin $F_{2\alpha}$ in the human eye. *Graefe's Arch Clin Exp Ophthalmol* 1985;222:139-41.

3. Kerstetter JR, Brubaker RF, Wilson SE, and Kullerstrand LJ. Prostaglandin $F_{2\alpha}$-1-isopropylester lowers intraocular pressure without decreasing aqueous humor flow. *Amer J of Ophthalmol* 1988;105:30-4.

4. Villumsen J and Alm A. Prostaglandin $F_{2\alpha}$-isopropylester eye drops: effects in normal human eyes. *British J Ophthalmol* 1989;73:419-26.

5. Camras CB, Siebold EC, Lustgarten JS, et al. Maintained reduction of intraocular pressure by prostaglandin $F_{2\alpha}$-1-isopropyl ester applied in multiple doses in ocular hypertensive and glaucoma patients. *Ophthalmol* 1989;96:1329-37.

6. Gabelt BT and Kaufman PL. Prostaglandin $F_{2\alpha}$ increases uveoscleral outflow in the cynomolgus monkey. *Exp Eye Res* 1989;49:389-402.

7. Nilsson SF, Samuelsson M, Bill A, and Stjernschantz J. Increased uveoscleral outflow as a possible mechanism of ocular hypotension caused by prostaglandin $F_{2\alpha}$-1-isopropylester in the cynomolgus monkey. *Exp Eye Res* 1989;48:707-16.

8. Stjernschantz J and Resul B. Phenyl substituted prostaglandin analogs for glaucoma treatment. *Drugs of the Future* 1992;17:691-704.

9. Bito LZ, Stjernschantz J, Resul B, Miranda OC, and Basu S. The ocular effects of prostaglandins and the therapeutic potential of a new $PGF_{2\alpha}$ analog, PhXA41 (latanoprost), for glaucoma management. *J Lipid Mediators* 1993;6:535-43.

10. Alm A and Villumsen J. PhXA34, a new potent ocular hypotensive drug. *Arch Ophthalmol* 1991;109:1564-68.

11. Toris CB, Camras CB, and Yablonski ME. Effects of PhXA41, a new prostaglandin $F_{2\alpha}$ analog, on aqueous humor dynamics in human eyes. *Ophthalmol* 1993;1297-304.

12. Ziai N, Dolan JW, Kacere RD, and Brubaker RF. The effects on aqueous dynamics of PhXA41, a new prostaglandin $F_{2\alpha}$ analogue, after topical application in normal and ocular hypertensive human eyes. *Arch Ophthalmol* 1993;111:1351-8.

13. Hayashi M, Yablonski ME, and Mindel JS. Methods for assessing the effects of pharmacologic agents on aqueous humor dynamics. In:Tasman W and Jaeger EA, eds. *Duane's Foundations of Clinical Ophthalmology, Vol. 3, Chapter 25.* Philadelphia: J.B. Lippincott Co; 1990:1-9.

14. Selén G, Karlsson M, Astin M, Stjernschantz J, and Resul B. Effects of PhXA34 and PhDH100A, two phenyl substituted prostaglandin esters, on aqueous humor dynamics and microcirculation in the monkey eye. *Invest Ophthalmol Vis Sci (Suppl)* 1991;32:869.

15. Sakurai M, Araie M, Oshika T. et al. Effects of topical application of UF-021, a novel prostaglandin derivative, on aqueous humor dynamics in normal human eyes. *Jpn J Ophthalmol* 1991;35:156-65.

16. Tetsuka H, Tsuchisaka H, Kin K, Takahashi Y, and Takase M. A mechanism for reducing intraocular pressure in normal volunteers using UF-021, a prostaglandin-related compound. *Acta Societatis Ophthalmologicae Japonicae* 1992;96:496-500.

17. Crawford K and Kaufman PL. Pilocarpine antagonizes prostaglandin $F_{2\alpha}$-induced ocular hypotension in monkeys: evidence for enhancement of uveoscleral outflow by prostaglandin $F_{2\alpha}$. *Arch Ophthalmol* 1987;105:1112-6.

18. Camras CB, Wang R-F, Podos SM. Effect of pilocarpine applied before or after prostaglandin $F_{2\alpha}$ on IOP in glaucomatous monkey eyes. *Investigative Ophthalmol Vis Sci (Suppl)* 1990;31:150.

19. Weinreb RN, Kim D-M, Lindsey JD. Propagation of ciliary smooth muscle cells in vitro and effects of prostaglandin $F_{2\alpha}$ on calcium efflux. *Invest Ophthalmol & Vis Sci* 1992;33:2679-2686.

20. Lütjen-Drecoll E and Tamm E. Morphological study of the anterior segment of cynomolgus monkey eyes following treatment with prostaglandin $F_{2\alpha}$. *Exp Eye Res* 1988;46:761-769.

21. Lindsey JD, To HD, Weinreb RN. Induction of c-Fos by prostaglandin $F_{2\alpha}$ in human ciliary smooth muscle cells. *Invest Ophthalmol & Vis Sci* 1994;35:242-50.

22. Camras CB, Friedman AH, Rodrigues MM, Tripathi BJ, Tripathi RC, and Podos SM. Multiple dosing of prostaglandin $F_{2\alpha}$ or epinephrine on cynomolgus monkey eyes: III. Histopathology. *Invest Ophthalmol & Vis Sci* 1988;29:1428-36.

23. Svedbergh B and Forsberg I. A morphological study on the effects of chronic administration of latanoprost (LP) on the ciliary muscle and trabecular meshwork in monkeys. *Invest Ophthalmol & Vis Sci (Suppl)* 1993;34:932.

24. Kaufman PL. PhXA34-induced ocular hypotension. *Arch Ophthalmol* [letter] 1992;110:1042.

25. Gabelt BT and Kaufman PL. The effect of prostaglandin $F_{2\alpha}$ on trabecular outflow facility in cynomolgus monkeys. *Exp Eye Res* 1990;51:87-91.

26. Johnson DH. Human trabecular cell survival is dependent upon perfusion rate. *Invest Ophthalmol & Vis Sci (Suppl)* 1994;35:2082.

27. Villumsen J and Alm A. The effect of adding prostaglandin $F_{2\alpha}$-isopropylester to timolol in patients with open angle glaucoma. *Arch Ophthal* 1990;108:1102-5.

28. Lee P-Y, Shao H, Camras CB, and Podos SM. Additivity of prostaglandin $F_{2\alpha}$-1-isopropyl ester to timolol in glaucoma patients. *Ophthalmol* 1991;98:1079-82.

29. Alm A, Widengård I, Kjellgren D, et al. Once daily application of latanoprost causes a maintained reduction of intraocular pressure in glaucoma patients treated with timolol. *Invest Ophthalmol & Vis Sci (Suppl)* 1993;34:932.

30. Rulo AH, Greve EL, and Hoyng PF. Additive effect of PhXA41, a prostaglandin analogue, and timolol in patients with elevated intraocular pressure. *Invest Ophthalmol & Vis Sci (Suppl)* 1993;34:933.

Advances in Prostaglandin, Thromboxane,
and Leukotriene Research, Vol. 23,
edited by B. Samuelsson et al.
Raven Press, Ltd., New York © 1995

Comparative Phase III Clinical Trial of Latanoprost and Timolol in Patients with Elevated Intraocular Pressure

Albert Alm

Department of Ophthalmology, University Hospital,
S-75185 Uppsala, Sweden

The phenyl-substituted prostaglandin analogue latanoprost (13,14-dihydro-17-phenyl-18,19,20-trinor-PGF_{2a}-isopropylester - previously PhXA41) is an effective ocular hypotensive drug in normal eyes and in eyes with elevated intraocular pressure (IOP) (1-7). Previous studies have shown that application of 0.005% latanoprost once daily causes a maximal IOP reduction. It has been established that the mechanism of action is on outflow, with little or no effect on aqueous flow (7,8). The major effect seems to be increased uveoscleral outflow (6,9). Unlike PGF_{2a}-isopropylester, latanoprost has been well tolerated and ocular irritation or conjunctival hyperaemia has not been a clinical problem. In cynomolgus monkeys an increased iris pigmentation has been observed with long-term treatment with latanoprost, but no change in iris colour was seen in Dutch belted rabbits even with 12 months treatment. In the longest human study so far there was no increased iris pigmentation observed in eyes treated with 0.006% latanoprost once or twice daily for 3 months (2). In order to collect more information on the usefulness of latanoprost as a glaucoma drug the present study was undertaken as a multi-centre, masked, long-term comparison of latanoprost and timolol in open angle glaucoma or ocular hypertensive patients. Part of the study included a comparison of morning and evening administration of latanoprost. Photographs of the iris were included in order to be able to observe any change in iris colour.

Materials and methods.

The study was designed as a randomised, double-masked comparison of timolol with two dose regimens of latanoprost over 6 months and it was performed at 13 centres in Scandinavia. (Latanoprost 1) received 0.005%

527

latanoprost each morning for 3 months and then shifted to evening application. 94 patients (Latanoprost 2) started with evening application and then shifted to morning after 3 months, and 84 patients received 0.5% timolol twice daily throughout the study. To ensure masking all patients received two identical eye drop bottles, labelled morning or evening. For patients treated with latanoprost one bottle contained only the vehicle. 267 patients with a diagnosis of unilateral or bilateral primary open angle glaucoma (POAG), capsular glaucoma, pigmentary glaucoma or ocular hypertension were included. There were 116 males and 151 females with a mean age of 66 years (range 40-85). None of the patients had received topical beta-adrenergic blockers before entering the study, and other glaucoma drugs were washed out before the start of the study.

During the study 6 scheduled visits were performed, at baseline and after 2, 6, 12, 18 and 26 weeks treatment. This report will present the effect on the intraocular pressure (IOP) after 12 and 26 weeks' treatment in the three groups and the side effects that were observed. At baseline, and after 12 and 26 weeks' treatment examinations were made at 8 AM, noon and 4 PM. The diurnal IOP is defined as the average IOP of these 3 measurements.

Results.

252 patients concluded the study. The diurnal IOP in the three treatment groups before and during treatment are presented in table I. Both drugs reduced IOP significantly with the least reduction for timolol at 6 months (26%) and the largest reduction for latanoprost group 2 (evening application) at 3 months (35%). There was no difference in diurnal IOP between latanoprost applied in the morning and timolol, but latanoprost applied in the evening reduced diurnal IOP significantly better than timolol. Thus the IOP reduction at 6 months of latanoprost in group 1 was statistically significantly ($p<0.001$) better than that of timolol at 6 months, and correspondingly the IOP reduction at 3 months for latanoprost group 2 was better than that of timolol at 3 months ($p<0.01$). The diurnal IOP reduction of timolol was 29% at 3 months and 26% at 6 months. The upward drift of 0.7 mm Hg, was statistically significant ($p<0.001$).

Table I. Diurnal IOP, mean (SD) at baseline and after 3 and 6 months' treatment.

Visit	Latanoprost 1	Latanoprost 2	Timolol
Baseline	24.8 (3.8)	24.5 (3.2)	24.6 (3.1)
3 months	17.1 (2.6)	16.4 (2.9)	17.3 (2.9)
6 months	16.2 (2.5)	17.7 (2.8)	17.9 (3.0)

Table II. Maximal grade of conjunctival hyperaemia above baseline hyperemia observed during the study. Figures represent percent of patients.

Grade	Latanoprost	Timolol
None (0)	60.8	72.6
Barely detectable (0.5)	27.1	22.6
Mild (1)	11.0	4.8
Mild to moderate (1.5)	1.1	0.0

Conjunctival hyperaemia was graded in a masked fashion by comparing external photographs with a set of standard photographs corresponding to no (0), mild (1), moderate (2) or marked (3) hyperaemia. Table II presents the maximal hyperaemia above baseline observed in the three treatment groups during the study. Mild hyperaemia was slightly more common in latanoprost-treated eyes. No aqueous flare was observed in any patient, and there was no drug-related loss of visual acuity or change in refraction.

The main ocular side effect was an increased pigmentation of the iris that was observed in 5 cases and suspected in 7 more cases, all treated with latanoprost for at least 3 months. All cases of increased iris pigmentation occurred in irides with a blue/grey-brown or green-brown colour (not including naevi or freckles). Of the 12 cases 3 were found in blue/grey-brown irides and 9 in green-brown irides.

Punctate erosions of the corneal epithelium were reported more frequently in patients treated with latanoprost (13 of 183) than in patients treated with timolol (2 of 84). Most of those punctate erosions were mild and not reported as adverse events.

Apart from a statistically significant ($p<0.005$) reduction of heart rate at 6 months in timolol-treated patients there was no obvious difference in systemic side effects between the two treatments. Blood and urine analysis before and after the study did not reveal any significant effect on the haematological, urinary or clinical chemistry parameters for either drug.

Discussion.

Latanoprost administered once daily effectively reduced diurnal IOP, and a single evening application was significantly more effective than timolol administered twice daily. When applied in the evening the day-time IOP reduction of latanoprost was superior to that of timolol with 25% ($p<0.001$). Thus, based on the results of the present study latanoprost seems to be one of the most potent ocular hypotensive drugs tested for glaucoma. It is interesting to note that application of latanoprost in the evening reduced day-time IOP more effectively that application in the morning. The cross-over design of the study permits the conclusion that this result is unlikely to be due to chance variation. The most likely explanation is that two of the three IOP measurements after the morning dose were made either before this dose had reached a maximal effect (noon, 4 hrs post-dose) or at the end of its peak effect (8 AM, 24 hrs post-dose), while those taken after the evening dose were taken during a time (12-20 hrs post-dose) when the drug has its peak effect. Latanoprost does not reach its peak effect until 8-12 hrs after its application, and part of the effect may be lost after 24 hrs.

Considering the marked ocular irritation and conjunctival hyperaemia observed with PGF_{2a}-isopropylester it is of interest to note that to a large extent these side effects have been abolished with this phenyl-substituted analogue. Thus there was no difference in incidents of reported ocular irritation between the two treatments, which is remarkable since timolol is regarded as a drug inducing minimal ocular irritation. Also the difference in conjunctival hyperaemia induced by the two drugs was surprisingly small. Once again, conjunctival hyperaemia has not been considered an ocular side effect linked with timolol eye drops. The difference in the frequency of reported corneal epithelial erosions quite possibly reflects the higher concentration of the preservative benzalkonium chloride in the latanoprost eye drops. The latanoprost eye drops contained twice as much benzalkonium chloride as timolol, and since vehicle was used as placebo eyes treated with latanoprost received twice the amount of benzalkonium chloride intended for clinical use.

The main ocular side effect observed in the present study was an increased pigmentation of the iris observed in 6-7% of eyes treated with latanoprost. Increased pigmentation of the iris has not been observed with any previous ocular drug. The iris colour is mainly determined by the melanin content of the melanocytes in the anterior stroma of the iris, and histological examination of the iris from monkeys with increased pigmentation after long-term treatment with latanoprost shows an increased melanin content in the melanocytes but no significant increase in the number of melanocytes (unpubl. obs.). This observation suggests that latanoprost is able to induce melanogenesis of the iridial melanocytes, but there seems to be no cell division involved. Further studies are obviously needed to investigate the mechanism behind this change in iris colour. It is interesting to consider that fact that all cases observed occurred in irides with a mixed blue-brown, grey-brown or green-brown colour. Therefore it may be possible to predict if a patient runs the risk of developing a change in iris colour during prolonged treatment with latanoprost. To what extent this change in colour will progress is not known since treatment was withdrawn in all patients with a clear-cut change in iris colour.

Conclusions.

The present study has demonstrated that the new prostaglandin analogue latanoprost is an ocular hypotensive drug that with once daily application in a very low concentration reduces IOP as efficiently or even more efficiently than the beta-adrenergic blocker timolol. Latanoprost has a completely different mechanisms of action to that of timolol, one increasing outflow and the other reducing inflow, and previous studies have shown that the effect on IOP of the two drugs is additive. Thus it seems clear that latanoprost may become a valuable drug for the treatment of glaucoma. However, further information on the mechanism behind the change in iris colour induced in some eyes with a mixed colour of the iris is needed before its clinical usefulness can be decided.

REFERENCES

1. Alm A, Villumsen J, Törnquist P et al. Intraocular pressure-reducing effect of PhXA41 in patients with increased eye pressure. A one-month study. *Ophthalmology* 1993;100:1312-1317.

2. Alm A, Widengård I, Kjellgren D, Söderström M, Friström B, Heijl A, Stjernschantz J. Latanoprost administered once daily causes a maintained reduction of intraocular pressure in glaucoma patients treated concomitantly with timolol. Submitted to Br J Ophthalmol

3. Friström B, Nilsson SEG. Interaction of PhXA41, a new prostaglandin analogue, with pilocarpine. A study on patients with elevated intraocular patients. *Arch Ophthalmol* 1993;111:662-665.

4. Nagasubramanian S, Sheth GP, Hitchings RA, Stjernschantz J. Intraocular pressure reducing effect of PhXA41 in ocular hypertension. Comparison of dose regimens. *Ophthalmology* 1993;100:1305-1311.

5. Rácz P, Ruzsonyi MR, Nagy ZT, Bito LZ. Maintained intraocular pressure reduction with once-a-day application of a new PGF_{2a} analogue (PhXA41). An in-hospital placebo controlled study. *Arch Ophthalmol* 1993;111:657-661.

6. Toris C, Camras CB, Yablonski M. Effects of PhXA41, a new prostaglandin F_{2a} analog, on aqueous humor dynamics in human eyes. *Ophthalmology* 1993; 100:1297-1304.

7. Ziai NZ, Dolan JW, Kacere RD, Brubaker RF. The effects on aqueous humor dynamics of PhXA41, a new prostaglandin F_{2a} analogue, after topical application in normal and ocular hypertensive human eyes . *Arch Ophthalmol* 1993;111: 1351-1358.

8. Alm A, Villumsen J. PhXA34 - a potent ocular hypotensive drug. A study on dose-response relationship and on aqueous humor dynamics in healthy volunteers. *Arch Ophthalmol* 1991;109:1564-1568.

9. Selén G, Karlsson M, Astin M, Stjernschantz J, Resul B. Effects of PhXA34 and PhDH100A, two phenyl substituted prostaglandin esters, on aqueous humor dynamics and microcirculation in the monkey eye. *Invest Ophthalmol Vis Sci* 1991;32(Suppl):869.

Advances in Prostaglandin, Thromboxane,
and Leukotriene Research, Vol. 23,
edited by B. Samuelsson et al.
Raven Press, Ltd., New York © 1995

Erectile Dysfunction - Vasomotor Actions of PGE₁, Its Metabolites and Other Prostaglandins

Karsten Schrör

Institut für Pharmakologie, Heinrich-Heine-Universität Düsseldorf, Moorenstraße 5,
D-40225 Düsseldorf, Germany

Among the numerous natural vasodilator prostaglandins, PGE_1 has found particular attention in pharmacology. One reason for this is the multitude of actions which became apparent during the more than 20 years of experimental and clinical studies on the compound. Thus, it was shown that PGE_1 combines in one molecule PGI_2-like effects on platelets and selected vascular tissues with PGE_2-like effects on polymorphonuclear granulocytes and immunocompetent white cells. Furthermore, PGE_1 appears to be the only natural prostaglandin that undergoes bioactivation in vivo, eventually resulting in generation of 13,14-dihydro-PGE_1 or PGE_o (4), a metabolic pathway which was also detected in men (23). Finally, the male reproductive system contains tremendous amounts of PGE's, including PGE_1, that are generated enzymatically (9) and are unique for men within the animal kingdom (15).

This study reviews the biological activity of PGE_1 and its primary C-20 metabolites on vascular tissue including penile smooth muscle and summarizes the pharmacological evidence for administration of the compound to treat erectile dysfunction (ED).

VASOMOTOR EFFECTS OF PGE₁ AND ITS METABOLITES

In a series of in vitro studies we have compared the action of PGE_1 and its metabolites on the tone of isolated arterial and venous tissue in different animal species and men (22). In most of the vessels studied, PGE$_1$ and PGE$_0$ acted very similar, producing a contractile response in veins in both resting state and after precontraction (Figure 1) and a relaxing response in arteries in resting state and after precontraction with norepinephrine or 5-HT. In general, the vasoconstrictor effects of PGE$_0$ were somewhat more pronounced. All contractile activity of PGE$_1$ and PGE$_0$ was antagonized by a selective thromboxane receptor antagonist (SQ 29.548) (Figure 1), suggesting that it was TP-receptor-mediated. The other enzymatic metabolites of PGE$_1$, namely the 15-keto-compounds, were inactive (22). Thus, PGE$_1$ and its active metabolite PGE$_0$ combine relaxing actions on arteries with contractile actions on veins - a useful combination in ED (14,20,21).

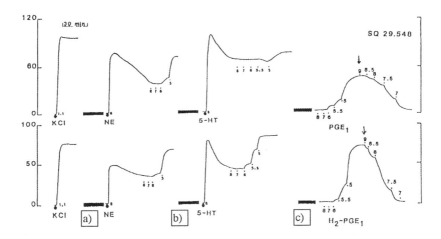

FIG. 1. Change in tension [mN] of human saphenous vein by PGE$_1$ (top) and PGE$_0$ (bottom). Vessels were precontracted by norepinephrine (a) or 5-HT (b) or remained in resting state (c). Note the dose-dependent decrease in tension by SQ 29.548. The numbers are -log M concentration. (Braun and Schrör, unpublished)

ERECTILE DYSFUNCTION (ED)

Vasoactive agents that produce erection could do so by (i) increasing the arterial flow into the penile arteries, (ii) causing sinusoidal relaxation and (iii) increasing venous outflow resistance. In 1986, Ishii and colleagues (11) reported for the first time the successful use of PGE$_1$ in patients suffering from organic impotence. Since that time the use of this compound found remarkable attention in urology. This was due to both the high success rate of this treatment (about 70%) and the low incidence of severe side effects, such as priapism, inflammatory reactions and pain as compared to other vasodilators (5,12,21,24).

SOURCE OF PROSTAGLANDINS FOR PENILE TISSUE

Since the amount of vasoactive prostaglandins, circulating in the blood, is extremely low, local generation at a site of action is necessary. Enzymatic capacity of PGE_1 biosynthesis from the respective eicosatrienoic acid precursor has been shown in homogenates of human seminal vesicles (9). In vitro studies of homogenates of human corpora cavernosa have shown the biosynthesis of PGE_2, $PGF_{2\alpha}$, PGI_2 and thromboxane (13,26) and also the capacity of the tissue to metabolize arachidonic acid-derived prostaglandins as well as PGE_1 by a 15-prostaglandin dehydrogenase (27). However, no studies appear to exist on prostaglandin generation or prostaglandin levels in penile blood in vivo.

DIRECT ACTIONS OF PGE₁ ON PENILE SMOOTH MUSCLE

In men, PGE_1 does not markedly modify the tension of corpora cavernosa (CC) or the tone of circumflex artery (CA) and vein (CV) in resting state. However, PGE_1 causes a marked, dose-dependent relaxation of both smooth muscles after precontraction by noradrenaline (Table 1) (10,17) or $PGF_{2\alpha}$ (Figure 2). Similar responses are seen with PGE_2 and PGI_2 in precontracted vessels. Interestingly, in contrast to many other tissues, PGI_2 appears not to relax precontracted CV, CC and CA as markedly as PGE_1 and in contrast to this compound rather produces contractions of CC at a resting state and concentrations of 1 µM or more (10). In the pig-tailed monkey, PGI_2 failed to increase cavernous arterial blood flow and to cause erection under conditions where PGE_1 was fully active (7).

The pharmacological investigation of prostaglandins in penile tissue is considerably hampered by species differences (18) (see below).
The effectivity of PGE_1 to relax CC appears to differ between healthy and impotent men. Knispel and collegues (19) compared the relaxing effect of PGE_1 on human CC strip preparations in vitro with that of papaverine. Papaverine caused a complete relaxation of phenylephrine-precontracted strips in all preparations. The maximum relaxant response to PGE_1 was 75% in healthy subjects (multi organ donors, n = 5), but only 45% in subjects with vascular impotence (n = 6) and 25% in diabetic impotent men (n = 5). This suggested that the physiological relaxation is not impaired in these patients but rather the PGE_1 receptor-related signal transduction. Similar differences between papaverine and PGE_1 had also been previously reported in the pig-tailed monkey (1) and may be due to a varying amount of PGE_1 receptors because the action of papaverine was unchanged. It is also possible that part of the PGE_1-induced erection in impotent patients is platelet-mediated (28).

Table 1. Actions of selected prostaglandins on human corpora cavernosa (CC), cavernous artery (CA) and circumflex vein (CV) preparations under resting conditions and after precontraction by noradrenaline in vitro

Compound	Change in tension from initial value					
	resting			precontracted		
	CC	CA	CV	CC	CA	CV
PGE_1	none	no contraction	none	↓↓	↓↓	↓↓
PGE_2	(↑)	↑	(↑)	↓	none	↓
$PGF_{2\alpha}$	↑	↑	↑	no relaxation		
PGI_2	(↑)	no contraction	none	(↓)	↓	(↓)
U 46.619	↑↑	↑↑	---	---	---	---

↑: Increase; ↓: Decrease; ---: not measured (after data from refs. 10 and 17)

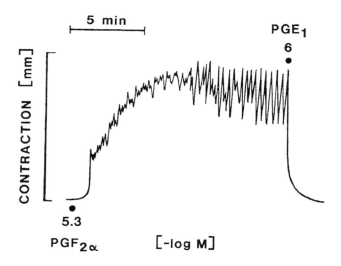

Fig. 2. Relaxation of human corpus carvernosum tissue by PGE₁; the numbers are - log M concentration (original experiment; Förster, Porst & Schrör unpublished)

INDIRECT ACTIONS OF PGE₁ ON PENILE SMOOTH MUSCLE

The stimulatory autonomic motor transmission to the smooth muscle of human corpora cavernosa is adrenergic and probably mediated by tonic norepinephrine release from adrenergic nerve terminals. The inhibitory pathways involve non-adrenergic/non-cholinergic systems, most likely nitric oxide (16) and, eventually, muscarinergic signal transduction (13). Thus, there might be a role for anti-adrenergic prostaglandins, such as PGE-type compounds. In vitro, indomethacin (3 μM) potentiated the adrenergic contractile response to electrical field stimulation of CC which was prevented by addition of PGE$_1$. This suggested that PGE$_1$ might function as an inhibitory modulator of the excitatory α-adrenergic transmission (3). A similar conclusion was reached by Porst (24) who reported an inhibition of presynaptic norepinephrine release from CC in non-impotent patients by up to 80%. It is also possible that PGE$_1$ synergizes with NO or other endogenous vasodilators, such as VIP. However, no data are available yet.

CELLULAR SIGNAL TRANSDUCTION PATHWAYS FOR PGE$_1$

Biological actions or prostaglandins are receptor-mediated. This is also valid for penile tissue where a relation appears to exist between the strength of vasomotor responses and the number of PGE$_1$-specific binding sites (2). Moreover, species with weak or no PGE$_1$ response such as rabbit (29), rhesus monkey (8) or dog (2) do not show erection subsequent to PGE$_1$ administration (2,15,29). Saturation binding studies have clearly demonstrated the existence of specific PGE$_1$ binding sites in microsomal membrane preparations from human cavernous tissue. The k$_D$ was 1 nM and the receptor density 9 fmoles/mg protein. Interestingly, the receptor density was reduced by about 80% in 3 men, suffering from ED of various causes (2). Other saturation binding studies (8) in CC penis cell fractions found about 20 pmoles PGE$_1$ specifically bound per mg cell protein. Unfortunately, the PG-receptor subtype remained unknown since no further specification was performed. Previous investigations by Bhargava et al (6) in cultured human cavernosa cells have demonstrated an increase in tissue cAMP after stimulation by PGE$_1$ and isoprenaline, however, a small increase was also seen with adrenaline and norepinephrine. Interestingly, the cAMP response to these compounds, in particular PGE$_1$, was significantly enhanced by forskolin, suggesting the existence of PG-receptors that couple to the adenylate cyclase via G-proteins. This includes IP-, EP$_2$ and the EP$_3$B and C-receptor subtypes, respectively.

There is almost no information on intracellular signal transduction by prostaglandins in human CC. One studie showed that cultured CC cells respond to PGE$_1$ (3-300 nM) with Ca^{2+}-release into the medium. These reactions were considered similar to those obtained by papaverine and phenoxybenzamine, leading to the conclusion that this Ca^{2+} exchange may indicate the relaxing response of smooth muscle (25).

REFERENCES

1. Aboseif SR, Breza J, Bosch RJLH, Benard F, Stief CG, Stacl W, Lue TF, Tanagho EA. *J Urol* 1989;142:403-8.
2. Aboseif S, Riemer RK, Stackl W, Lue T, Tanagho E. *Urol Int* 1993;50:148-52.
3. Adaikan PG, Kottegoda SR, Ratnam SS. *2nd World Meeting on Impotence*, Prague 1986, Abstr 2.6.
4. Ånggard E, Larsson C. *Eur J Pharmacol* 1971;14:66-70.
5. Bénard F, Lue TF. *Drugs* 1990;39:394-8.
6. Bhargava G, Valcic M, Melman A. *Int J Impotence Res* 1990;2 (Suppl2):35-6.
7. Bosch RJLH, Benard F, Aboseif SR et al. *Int J Impotence Res* 1989;1:211-21.
8. Gludovacz D, Virgolini I, Porst H, Friehe H, Rogatti W, Sinzinger H. *7th Intern Conf Prostaglandins Rel Compounds*, Florence, 1990. Abstr p.24.
9. Hamberg M.. *Lipids* 1976;11:249-50.
10. Hedlund H, Andersson K-E. *J Urol* 1985;134:1245-50.
11. Ishii N, Watanabe H, Irisawa C, Kikuchi Y. *Proceedings 5th Conference on vasculogenic impotence*, Prague, 1986. Abstr 11.2.
12. Ishii N, Watanabe H, Irisawa C. *J Urol* 1989;141:323-5.
13. Jeremy JY, Morgan RJ, Mikhailidis DP et al. *Prostaglandins Leukotrienes Med* 1986;23:211-6.
14. Jünemann K-P, Alken P. *Int J Impotence Res* 1989;1:71-93.
15. Kelly RW. *J Reprod Fert* 1981;62:293-304.
16. Kim N, Azadzoi KM, Goldstein I, Saenz de Tejada I. *J Clin Invest* 1991;88:112-8.
17. Kirkeby HJ, KE Andersson, A Forman. *Br J Urol* 1993;72:220-5.
18. Klinge E, Sjöstrand NO. *Acta Physiol Scand* 1977;100:354-67.
19. Knispel HH, Goessl C, Beckmann R. *Int J Impotence Res* 1992;4 (Suppl 2):A10.
20. Krane RJ, Goldstein I, Saenz de Tejada I: *N Engl J Med* 1989;321:1648-59.
21. Linet OI, Neff LL. *Clin Invest* 1994;72:139-49.
22. Ney P, Braun M, Szymanski Ch, Bruch L, Schrör K. *Eicosanoids* 1991;4:177-84.
23. Peskar BA, Hesse WH, Rogatti W, et al. *Prostaglandins* 1991;41:225-8.
24. Porst H. *Urologe [A]* 1989;28:94-8.
25. Rajfer J, Krall JF, Sikka SC. *6th Biennial Symposium on Corpus Cavernosum Revascularization*, Boston, 1988. Abstr p.46.
26. Roy AC, Tan SM, Kottegoda SR et al. *IRCS Med Sci* 1984;12:608-9.
27. Roy AC, Adaikan PG, Sen DK et al. *Br J Urol* 1989;64:180-2.
28. Sinzinger H, Stackl W, Höbarth J, Marberger M. *Thrombosis Haemostasis* 1991;65:1326.
29. Stackl W, Loupal G, Holzmann A. *Urol Res* 1988;16:455-8.

Advances in Prostaglandin, Thromboxane,
and Leukotriene Research, Vol. 23,
edited by B. Samuelsson et al.
Raven Press, Ltd., New York © 1995

The Rationale for Prostaglandin E_1 (α-Alprostadil) in the Management of Male Impotence

Harmut Porst

Urological Practice, Hamburg

Since the development and standardized use of new diagnostic procedures as doppler- and duplex-sonography of the penile vessels, pharmaco-cavernosography and measurements of the latency times of the bulbocavernous reflex a differentiated diagnosis of erectile failure has been made possible in each patient. With these recent progresses in the diagnosis of male impotence, physicians were enabled the first time to offer their patients individual therapeutic regimen which are related to the underlying etiology of erectile failure.

Both progresses in diagnosis and therapy of erectile failure were very strictly associated with the inracavernous administration of several vasoactive drugs.

Since the first reports of Virag (15) on papaverine and later on of Brindley (2) on phenoxybenzamine, as well as two years later of Zorgniotti and Lefleur (16) on the use of the mixture of papaverine and phentolamine vasoactive drugs have attained world-wide acceptance in the management of male impotence. Subsequently 1986 the first reports on PGE_1 in context with erectile failure were encountered in the literature (1,6) and especially since the reports of Stackl (12) and Porst (9) on the widespred use of this drug in patients with erectile disorders PGE_1 was going to replace the older vasoactive drugs used so far in this field.

Based on the own personal experiences on thousands of patients with erectile failure an thorough overview on the advantages and disadvantages of PGE_1 in the management of erectile failure will be presented.

Material and Method

Within the last 5 years 3362 patients with several penile disorders were referred to our andrological service. The majority of the patients was suffering from erectile dysfunction the minority from penile deviations or Peyronie´s disease (table 1).

PGE₁-Test and Etiology of Erectile and Penile Disorders

No.Pts. 3362

• Psychogenic erectile dysfunction	1082	(32,2 %)
• Mixed psych./organogenic ED	458	(13,6 %)
• Organogenic erectile dysfunction	1381	(41,1 %)
• Peyronie´s disease/penile deviation	441	(13,1 %)

Table 1

Besides a detailed sexual history all patients with erectile disorders were submitted to the following procedures : evaluation of serum hormone levels like testosterone and prolactin, intracavernous injection of Prostaglandin E_1 combined with a duplex-sonography of the penile vessels and pharmaco-cavernosography in those patients who did not respond after 20 μg PGE_1 with a complete erection sufficient for sexual intercourse. Patients with a history of neurologic disorder or trauma and therefore suspicious to show an involvement of the somatic or autonomic penile nerves (i.e. diabetes, alcoholism, multiple sclerosis, former pelvic fracture or spinal and lumbar disc lesions) underwent a thorough neurophysiologic examination with measurement of the BCR-latencies and somatosensory evoked potentials of the pudendal nerve.

In some series of patients, several vasoactive drugs like papaverine, papaverine and phentolamine, PGE_1, the NO-donor Linsidomine and the @-blocker Moxisylyte were administered in order to compare the different efficacy and side effects of the several vasoactive compounds.

Results

I Diagnostic Trials

With reference to the results of the several abovementioned diagnostic procedures in each patient a clearly definded diagnosis could be made.

Arterial insufficiency: criteria for the evidence of arterial occlusive disease of the penile vessels were duplex-sonography findings of a peak flow velocity of less than 30 cm/sec in one or two deep penile arteries.

Cavernous insufficiency: patients with maintenance flow-rates exceeding 20-25 ml/min at intracavernous pressure values of at least 90 mm Hg during pharmaco-cavernosography were diagnosed to have cavernous insufficiency.

Neurologic deficits: the diagnosis of neurologic penile disorders were depending both on the patient´s history and/or the findings of BCR-latencies and SSEP. Males with a history of relevant operation procedures like radical prostatectomy/cystectomy, rectum-amputation or those with loss of ejaculation due to diabetes a.o. were supposed to have automic neurogenic disorders of the cavernous nerves.

Males with pathologic results of the BCR-latency-time (> 42 cm/sec) and/or pathologic SSEP were diagnosed to have somatic penile neuropathy.

Endocrinologic deficits: the diagnosis of endocrinologic disorders was especially depending on the blood serum values of testosterone and prolactin.

Etiology of Erectile and Coital Disorders (table 1)

In 2280 (67,8 %) of 3362 patients one or more organogenic factors were evident contributing to the manifestation of erectile dysfunction. The distribution of the different organogenic causes was as follows:

Arterial insufficiency	903/3362	(27,0 %)
Cavernous insufficiency	933/3362	(28,0 %)
Neurologic deficits	436/3362	(13,0 %)
Endocrinologic deficits	76/3362	(2,3 %)
Penile deviation	441/3362	(13,1 %)

Results of Intracavernous Testing with Vasoactive Drugs

Responder rates (complete erection)

Papaverine (up to 50 mg)	39 % of 950 pts.
Pap./Phentolamine (up to 50 mg + 2 mg)	61 % of 249 pts.
Prostaglandin E$_1$ (up to 20 µg)	71 % of 3362 pts.
Linsidomine (up to 1 mg)	15 % of 65 pts.
Moxisylyte (up to 20 mg)	10 % of 10 pts.

Side effects

Priapism
  0,3 % after PGE$_1$, 5,3 % after Papaverine and Papaverine/Phentolamine, 0 % after Linisdomine and Moxisylyte.

Penile Pain
  8,9 % after PGE$_1$

Headache/Flush
  15 % after Linsidomine

With respect to the diagnostic use PGE$_1$ has clearly proven superiority, both in efficacy and priapism rates in comparison to the other investigated vasoactive compounds. Therefore within the last 5 years only PGE$_1$ was used for therapeutic purposes.

II   Therapeutic Trials

1. **Interval-Injection-Therapy with PGE₁:** in more than 400 patients PGE₁ was applicated in an interval-manner, that means for 6 to 10 times the patients received intracavernous injection of 10 µg to 40 µg a fortnight in the physician´s office. In 103 of these patients a comprehensive work up before and after therapy was carried out, including sexual questionnaires and duplex-sonography assessments of the penile vessels.

The results are summarized in table 2 and 3 and provide evidence of a satisfaction rate of more than 75 % of all patients. Whereas more than 50 % were unable to perform sexual intercourse at the start of the injection therapy, only 17,5 % did claim this problem after termination of therapy.

Results of Interval - Injection - Therapy with PGE₁

No. Pts.: 103	Before	After
		Therapy
• Incapable of sexual intercourse more than 6 months	51,5 %	17,5 %
• Sexual intercourse < 1 x / month	17,5 %	2,9 %
• Sexual intercourse 1 -2 x / month	23,3 %	5,8 %
• Sexual intercourse 1 -2x / week	7,8 %	73,8 %

Table 2

Results of Interval - Injection - Therapy with PGE₁

No. Pts. : 103		
※ Very satisfied	48	46,6 %
※ Satisfied	14	13,6 %
※ Fairly satisfied	16	15,5 %
※ Unsatisfied	25	24,3 %

Table 3

2. **Self - Injection Therapy with PGE₁:** in a retrospective study the results of 178 patients performing self-injection therapy with PGE₁ at home were analysed. With a mean follow up of 25 months (6-64 months) the drop-out rate was 38 % (68/178), 10 patients were lost for follow-up.

Main reasons for drop-outs were:

Recurrence of spontaneous erections	29 %
Concomittant severe diseases	25 %
Discontinuation of therapy	15 %
Partner problems	9 %
Inefficacious	7 %
Different reasons	15 %

Complications: of the 100 pts continuing self-injection therapy the following side-effects were encountered:

Penile deviation	3/100
Penile induration	5/100
Penile pain	2/100

All the patients who decided to continue self-injection therapy were satisfied with this kind of treatment.

Conclusion

Both, the own comprehensive experiences with several vasoactive drugs in erectile failure and the literature provided proof that PGE_1 represents the drug of choice in the management of male impotence. This own statement is impressively supported by the proceedings of a symposium on the role of Alprostadil in the diagnosis and treatment of erectile dysfunction, held 1993 in Kalamazoo (5).

In comparison to other vasoactive drugs like papaverine and the mixture of papaverine and phentolamine, with priapism-rates of 4 to 23 % in the literature and local complication-rates like indurations and cavernous fibrosis between 10 and 50 % in long-term follow-up (4,7,8,14) those complication-rates were significantly less encountered after the application of PGE_1 (5,10,12). Also other recently introduced new drugs like GCRP, Linsidomine and Moxisylyte seem not to be able to challenge PGE_1 in the field of impotence especially due to inferior efficacy (11,3,13). Therefore PGE_1 will furtheron represent the most frequently used drug worldwide with respect to injection therapy of cavernous bodies.

References

1. Adaikan PG, Kottegoda SR, Ratnam SS. A possible role for Prostaglandin E_1 in human penile erection. Abstract: Second World Meeting on Impotence, 1986,Prague, Abstract 2-6

2. Brindley GS. Cavernosal alpha-blockade:A new treatment for investigating and treating erectile impotence. Br. J. Psychiatry 1983; 143:332-337

3. Buvat J. Buvat-Herbaut M, Lemaire A. Marcolin G. Reduced rate of fibrotic nodules in the cavernous bodies following auto-intracavernous injections of moxisylyte compared to papaverine. Int.J.Impotence Res. (1991)3; 123-128

4. Girdley FM, Bruskewitz RC, Feyzi J, Graversen PG, Gasser TC. Intracavernous self-injection for impotence: A long-term therapeutic option? Experience in 78 patients. J.Urol 1988; 140:972-974

5. Goldstein I, Lue TF. The Role of Alprostadil in the Diagnosis and Treatment of Erectile Dysfunction. Symposium August 3-4, 1993 Brook Lodge Kalamazoo; Excerpta Medica Inc.

6. Ishii N, Watanabe H, Irisawa C, Kikuchi Y. Therapeutic trial with Prostaglandin E_1 for Organic Impotence. Abstract:Second World Meeting on Impotence , 1986, Prague,Abstract 11,2

7. Lakin MM, Montague DK, Medendorp SK. Intracavernous injection therapy: Analysis of results and complications. J Urol 1990; 143:1138-1141

8. Levine SB, Althof SE, Turner LA, et al. Side effects of self-administration of intracavernous papaverine and phentolamine for the treatment of impotence. J Urol 1989; 141:54-57.

9. Porst H. Prostaglandin E_1 bei erektiler Dysfunktion. Urologe A, (1989) 28:94-98

10. Porst H. Komplikationen vasoaktiver Substanzen in der Diagnostik und Therapie der erektilen Dysfunktion (ED). Urologe B 1993 33;13-18

11. Porst H.:Prostaglandin E_1 and the Nitric Oxide Donor Linsidomine for Erectile Failure: A Diagnostic Comparative Study of 40 Patients. J Urology 1993, 149, 1280-1283

12. Stackl W, Hasun R, Marberger M. Intracavernous injection of prostaglandin E_1 in impotent men. J Urol 1988; 140:66-68

13. Stief CG, Wetterauer U, Schaebsdau FH, Jonas U. Calcitonin-gene-related peptide: A possible role in human penile erection and its therapeutic application in impotent patients. J Urol 1991; 146:1010-1014.

14. Telöken C, Lisboa JF, Thorel E, Rössler RL, Souto CAV. Side effects of intracorporeal papaverine injection in the management of impotence: Evaluation at 30 months of follow up. JUrol 1988; 139/4(2):405A.

15. Virag R. Intracavernous injection of papaverine for erectile failure. Lancet 1982;II:938

16. Zorgniotti AW, Lefleur RS. Auto-injection of the corpus cavernosum with a vasoactive drug combination for vasculogenic-impotence. J Urol 1985;133:39.

Advances in Prostaglandin, Thromboxane,
and Leukotriene Research, Vol. 23,
edited by B. Samuelsson et al.
Raven Press, Ltd., New York © 1995

PHYSIOPATHOLOGY OF THE ERECTILE DYSFUNCTION

Franco Mantovani, Fulvio Colombo, and Edoardo Austoni

Institute of Urology, University of Milan, Italy

In the last 20 years andrology has achieved continuous and often drastic progresses, more than other branches of medical science, and there have been great advances in the fisiopathology and clinics of erectile dysfunction.

Erection is a complex event that includes a psychic trigger. At cerebral level the elaboration of fantasy and of visual, acoustic and olfactory stimulations takes place; these sensations, integrated by the memory, induce the sexual desire. This desire is transmitted through the nervous pathways of the spinal cord, to the peripheral nerves which control the miovascular system of erection. Sensorial stimulations coming from the penis are themselves important to continue that process and to promote the reflex arch which may cause erection in suitable circumstances and helping to maintain it during sexual intercourse.

Many andrological schools are nowadays active in the basic studies to understand better the deepest physiological mechanisms of erection, and above all of erectile dysfunctions to set the basis for a more correct diagnosis and the more selective therapy.

NEURO-VASCULAR ANATOMY OF ERECTIONS

The neuro-anatomical elements of erection are represented by the autonomic system, by the somatic system and by the cortical integration. The cerebral cortex, with the sub-cortical structures, takes part in the control of the erection and, generally, of the whole sexual behaviour by elaborating fantasy and visual, acoustic, olfactory stimulations. Areas destined to these control and elaboration are localised in the gyrus rectus and in the angulate gyrus, in the paraventricular nuclei, in the hypothalamus and in the mamillary bodies. Electroencephalographic studies have demonstrated that also the hippocampus place a role in the realisation of the erectile phenomenon.

In fact the hippocampus and the cingulate gyrus are the so called "cerebral emotions areas", largely connected with talamus and the hipotalamus whereas the cingulate gyrus and the mamillary bodies work in the integration of visual stimuli and the gyrus rectus in the elaboration of olfactory stimulation. These cortical elaborations are sent to the centres of autonomic innervation.

The autonomic innervation involves the sympathetic and parasympathetic system that are bases on to medullar centres:

– the lumbar center (D11-L2) (autonomic sympathetic system)
– the sacral center (S2-S4, autonomic parasympathetic system).

The sympathetic erectile centers are situated at dorsal-lumbar level (D11-L2). The fibres originated from these neuromeres reach the ganglia of the sympathetic chain where is the outcome of the sympathetic fibers, which become the nervi erigentes after having made a synapses with the efferent fibres of S2-S4. Some fibres proceeds in connection with the vessels, others enter in the mixed matrix of the pudendal nerve.

The parasympathetic erectile centres are localised in the sacral region (S2-S4). The fibres at the beginning proceed as pelvic nerves, than take part of the erigentes nerves. They run strictly connected with the rectum, in the dorso-lateral region of the prostate, passing nearby the prosthetic apex at the points 3 and 9.

Running along the bulbomembranous urethra they perforate the uro-genital diaphragm and enter in the crura penis at the points 1 and 11, in association with the artery and the deep dorsal vein, placing themselves to the erectile tissue.

Concerning the somatic innervation of the penis it is assured by the pudendal nerve. This nerve is composed by afferent fibres (gland and penile skin) and by efferent fibres coming from the metameres S2-S4.

The nerve which runs along the pudendal artery goes through the Alcock channel and then it places itself to the perineal voluntary musculature. The arterial vascularization of corpora cavernosa comes from the pudendal artery (terminal branche of the hypogastric artery) that in its internal diramation after the Alcock channel is divided in the bulbourethral artery, the cavernous artery and the penile dorsal artery. Inside the erectile tissue the cavernous artery is divided in numerous diramations: the helicine arteries.

In the 75% of cases the cavernous artery can supply on once's own the entire vascularization of corpora cavernosa; in the other cases there is blood contribution coming from the dorsal artery by perforating anastomotic branches.

The venous drainage coming from corpora cavernosa is assured by 3 systems of drainage. The principal part flows through the veins perforating the tunica albuginea. These latter flow together in the circumflex veins that flow into the deep dorsal vein and into the superficial vein which flow together into the Santorini plexus.

The second drainage system is made by the cavernous veins which come from the crura (nearby the income of the cavernous artery) and flow into the pudendal veins.

The third system is represented by the numerous shunts between corpora cavernosa and corpus spongious.

The erectile tissue is constituted by vascular sinusoides covered by epitelioid cells. The intimal structure of corpora cavernosa is made by fibromuscolar cavernula coming from the tunica albuginea. The two cavernous bodies communicate each other through the intracavernosal septum.

The numerous receptors which are present here are of great importance for the control of erection: alfaadrenergic, betaadrenergic, colinergic, vipergic, non-adrenergic/non-colinergic (NANC).

PHYSIOLOGY OF ERECTION MECHANISMS, HAEMODYNAMICS OF ERECTIONS

Erection is a complex event, controlled by a psycho neuro vascular regulation.

The neurological component is mainly under the influence of the parasympathetic system, the center of which is located in the sacral metameres S2-S4: from the efferent fibres comes the motorial component of the pelvic nerves which make possible the vasodilatation and smooth muscles relaxation of corpora cavernosa.

The sympathetic nervous system, which has its centre in the metameres D10-L12, seems to be decisive, with its postgangliar fibres of the hypogastric plexus, for the regulation of the ejaculation and the control of the psychogenic erection. Erection can therefore be reflex (parasympathetic) or psychogenic (symphatetic). In the normal subjects the two components are perfectly integrated and in presence of valid vascularisation, normal erectile tissue and absence of endocrinological disturbances, they cowork to keep a constant level of erectile stimulation in cavernous spongious district.

When the psychogenic stimulus is decresing the pudendal sensitive stimulation of the penis activates the neurogenic erectile center. The result is the perfect correlation between psychogenic and sensitive neurogenic erection, which allows to maintain a stable erection during sexual intercourse.

The target of all these factors is the erectile tissue inside corpora cavernosa. The nervous impulse allows the relaxing and the dilatation by the activation of neurotrasmitters which interfere with selective receptors located on the miovascular structures. The release of the neurotransmitters is stimulated also by the increase of the arterious influx (increase from 25 to 50 times in comparison with basic flow, that means from 5 to 250 ml/min.).

Erectile mechanism is nowadays considered as a mioneurovascular phenomenon. The endocavernous sinusoidal musculature relaxation is thought to be the central event, synchronous with the increase of the arterial flux. Recent experimental researches suggest that arteriolar relaxation is mediated by neurotransmitters non adrenergic noncolinergic (NANC). Basic research is just addressed to this particular field demonstrating that endocavernous neurotransmission is strictly connected to the dynamic endocavernous vascular mechanisms.

In fact colinergic and NANC impulses seems to be mediated by sinusoidal endothelia which produces relaxing factors for the smooth musculature, named

Endothelial Derived Relaxing Factors (EDRF), as well as contracting factors named Endotheline.

The Nitric Oxyde (NO) mediates the biological action of EDRF, as well as the vasodilatating action of the acetylcholine on the arteriolar endothelium.

On the contrary if the alfaadrenergic tone is increasing, such as in case of stress, anxiety or cold the cavernous smooth muscles contract, hindering the filling of the sinusoids and even the erection in normal subjects. In this way we can explain the psychogenic impotence due to anxiety for the sexual performance, which can involve subjects completely normal under the organic point of view.

Sinusoidal endothelium plays in fact a role of always greater importance in the realisation of erection. This must be adequatly emphasised for the clinical consequences if it is taken into account that some very frequent syndroms such as arterious hypertension, diabetes and arteriosclerosis affect the delicate endothelial functions also in early stages.

Studies on the ultrastructure of the erectile tissue have demonstrated that the degeneration of muscular smooth fibres is one of the major cause of erectile disfunction because of a complete alteration of the delicate neurovascular anatomy located just in the interstitial of the smooth muscles of erectile tissue.

The cascade of events which allows the of erection is divided in 5 phases:

1. REST: normal arterious influx, collapse of vascular sinusoides, normal venous discharge;
2. TUMESCENCE: increase of arterious influx, smooth muscles relaxation with negative pressure and sucking blood in the corpora cavernosa, normal venous deflux;
3. RIGIDITY: normalisation of arterious influx, filling of vascular sinusoides with pressure of 100 mmHg, relative decrease of venous discharge;
4. DETUMESCENCE: reduction of arterious influx, smooth muscles contraction and consequent emptying of sinusoides, probable increase of venous deflux;
5. REFRACTORY: psychic and local, both under neurological control.

The arterious inflow in tumescence increases from 8 to 60 times in comparison with the flow at rest.

In the phase of tumescence the arteriovenous shunts are closed and the arterious influx can fill in the cavernous sinusoides. On the contrary, during the stage of flaccidity most of the arterious influx is deviated from sinusoides by a capillary system. In parallel to the increase of arterious influx and the relaxing of smooth muscles a dramatic increase of venous resistences takes place, with almost a complete stop of venous discharge.

The corporo-occlusive mechanisms are identified in at least 4 different anatomical localisations of which the most known is represented by the diagonal course of the perforant veins through the tunica albuginea.

Researches with electronical microscope have found a second corporo-occlusive mechanism: the venous plexus under the tunical albuginea are compressed during tumescence by the stretching of the cavernule so reducing furthermore the venous deflux.

A third mechanism of reduction of venous discharge would be directly controlled by the neurotransmitters.

Last mechanism would be the reflex contraction of bulbo- and ischio-cavernous muscles under the influence of sexual stimulation which increases the endocavernous pressure by compressing the cavernous crura.

The phase of rigidity (with the increasing of the maximal endocavernous volume and pressure to about 160-180 mm/Hg) follows the initial phase of tumescence. This is caused by the blockage of the venous deflux and by the decrease of arterious influx to minimal values but sufficient to maintain the erection with stratching of albuginea to the limits of its compliance.

In normal subjects, the ejaculation causes, by reflex nervous mechanisms, the restoration of venous discharge, causing the end of rigidity and the beginning of a quick detumescence.

From what above we can understand how the causes of erectile dysfunction can be numerous: dynamic or functional, pure or mixed, and be the expression at local level also of pathologies which involve the entire organism.

PATHOPHYSIOLOGY OF ERECTILE DYSFUNCTIONS

During the last twenty years, the constant evolution in terms of diagnostic procedures available for the Specialist has significantly influenced the general medical opinion on the importance of the different causes of the erectile dysfunction. A good example is represented by the study of vasculogenic impotence: at the beginning of 70's, the introduction of the penile Doppler velocimetry as diagnostic tool led to a high incidence in the diagnosis of penile arterial insufficiency as cause of impotence and this was determined also by a considerable percentage of false positives.

This led to the appearance of a number of microsurgical techniques of penile revascularization, later decreased as consequence of the diagnostic evolution. Indeed in the 80's, due to the use of vasoactive drugs administered by intracavernosal injection and to the introduction of the cavernosography and carvernosometry, the so called venous leakage has been considered more and more important in the vascular impotence aetiopathogenesis. Consequently, a number of surgical procedures have been proposed in order to correct this blood escape from the corpora, such as various kind of selective venous ligations, the plication of the cavernosal crura, the corporopexy. During the 90's, the strong push of the basic research on neurophysiology and isto-anatomy of the erectile tissue reduced the role of vasculogenic impotence stressing, on the other hand, the importance of the intracavernosal smooth muscle fibres, neuromediators and receptors in the origin of the erectile disturbances. In the past, the psychogenic disturbances were thought to be the first cause of the erectile deficiency in terms of frequence, today, the organic causes (neurologic, vascular, endocrin, local and mixed) are thought to be prevalent, although the studied population are not omogeneous. Anyway, in the organic impotence of any origin a secondary psychogenic component is always present; it is due to the reduced patient's self-consideration, which worsens the primary disease and sometimes requires a concomitant psychotherapy as soon as the organic cause is removed. The natural hystory of the erectile dysfunction is not yet completely understood, especially regarding the information about the age when the disease appears, the incidence rate stratified by age, the evolution of such disease and the frequency of spontaneous recovery. Furthermore, few data are available on the concomitant morbility and the functional worsening. The available data refer mainly to the caucasian race, while the remaining races have been studied in a small number of patients, so that it is not possible to perform any sub-group analysis. The erectile dysfunction is certainly a common symptom of a number of conditions; some risk factors have been identified, and some of them could be useful in a prevention strategy. The following conditions can be regarded as risk factors: diabetes mellitus, hypogonadism in association with a number of endocrinological disorders, hypertension, vasculopathies, hypercholesterolemia, low level of HDL, drugs, neurogenic disturbances, La Peyronie's disease,   priapism, depression, alcholism, poor sexual education, scarse interpersonal relationship or their deterioration, and many chronic diseases (mainly the hepatic and the renal failure and the dialysis). The vascular surgery also represents a risck factor.

The age seems to be an indirect risk factor, since along with the age the probability of appearance of the above mentioned direct risk factors increases. Last, other conditions need further studies. Smoking has a negative effect on the erectile function, emphasizing the effects of other risk factors as vascular disease, diabetes and hypertension. We are going now into different organic causes of erectile dysfunction.

NEUROLOGICAL CAUSES

The 40% of the neurogenic erectile disturbances are consequence of a damage in the autonomic nervous system. Post-traumatic erectile dysfunctions, (for instance the trauma of the pelvis involving urethral dysrupture or the surgical consequence of radical cystoprostatectomy) represent causes of damage of the nerves erigentes; infact the symphatetic and the parasympathetic nervous systems are symultaneously destroyed togheter with pathways to the erectile tissue.

This nervous anatomic entity detailed discovered in its pathways up to the finest termination of the erigent nerves has permitted the set up of nerve-sparing operation on the pelvic viscera that is the possibility of preserving the nerves erigentes and their pathways, maintaining the oncological radicality.

Erectile disturbances deriving from abnomalities of autonomic innervation are dyagnosticable on 70% of patients suffering by meningomyelocele.

Concerning the diabetes mellitus insuline-dependent it is detectable with an incidence of 50% in erectile disturbances only five years from the appearance of the disease.

This is why the diabetes can be considered one of the most frequent and most severe cause of erectile insufficiency because it combines the cavernous microangiopathy with autonomic neuropathy.

Neurogenic erectile dysfunctions can be congenital, such as spina bifida, meningomyelocele; phlogystic: dorsal tabe, myelitis, polynevritis; degenerative:

multiple sclerosis, Parkinson's, diabetes, polyneuropathies; yatrogenic: radical pelvic surgery, vascular surgery.

In the description of neurogenic erectile dysfunctions, the level of the injury must be always carefully taken into account because, as already mentioned, in case of injury above S2 (that is upper the parasympathetic center) it is always possible a reflex erection.

In case of injury just on S2, the effect is the total impotence.

In case of trauma to the sympathetic medullar neuromeres (D10-L2) the psychogenic erection is lost.

VASCULAR CAUSES

We can distinguish two aspects of vascular impotence: arteriogenic and venogenic. When an arteriogenic damage is present the incomplete filling of the corpora cavernosa causes a reduction in erectile volume and the delay or the impossibility to obtain an effective intracavernous pressure. This condition is called insufficient inflow.

In case of venous damage, the premature emptying of corpora cavernosa causes the decrease of intracavernous pressure, normal at the beginning just beyond the critic value of 75 mmHg usefull for venous compression: it is called maintenance inability.

The two mechanisms may be associated in the same patient: it is a case of mixed insufficiency.

ARTERIOGENIC DEFICIT

Two situations can be found and can be also associated: the obstruction and the haemoderivation.

The obstruction may be present at the hypogastric level, most commonly in the situations of aorto-iliac damage and of the internal pudendal arteries and their terminal branches: dorsal and cavernous arteries.

The association of the two levels of obstruction is frequent.

In case of arterial obstruction at aorto-iliac level the phenomenon of haemoderivation (steal syndrome) is observed.

The arterial blood coming from internal pudendal artery is addressed towards the deep femoral territory for compensation of the principal branch occlusion.

The event is due to the muscular efforts during the coitus and causes a loss of erection thought to be of psychogenic origin.

Such cause of insufficiency is found on average in 40% of patients suffering with organic causes of erectile insufficiency.

As the neurogenic, also arteriogenic causes have an incidence of 40% in the population suffering from erectile organic dysfunction.

The origin of those disturbances can be congenital (vascular dysplasies or microangiopathies) or traumatic (arterial structures).

Among the causes of arterious vasculogenic impotence, arteriosclerosis plays the main role. Less frequently we can observe arterial obstructions consequent to pelvic fractures, arterial dysplasia, artero-venous fistula (located in the pelvic or perineal regions), arteriopathies in patients with collagen dystrophies and the sequelae of vascular operations for obstructive pathologies of Aorta or its branches or due to kidney transplantation.

Concerning the localisation of arterious obstructions, these can be located at various levels of aorta, up to the cavernous or dorsal arteries.

Sometimes it is possible to recognise a correlation between the site and pathogenesis of damages: this is particularly true for the obstructions of the internal pudendal artery.

The arteriosclerotic damages are more frequent in the obstructions of the first tract (ischio-rectal) of this artery, which runs from the origin of the vessel up to the ischiatic spine, and in the second tract, running from ischiatic spine to the superior border of the ischio-pubic spine throughout the Alcock channel.

The dysplasic damages, those due to diabetes mellitus and, according to some Authors, those due to a muscolar-aponevrotic compression made by the uro-genital dyaphragm are on the contrary prevalent in the obstruction of the third tract (perineal) of the artery, which runs from the ischio-pubic branch up to the terminal division.

CORPORO-OCCLUSIVE DYSFUNCTION

It seems that structural alterations of the tunica albuginea may cause an insufficient compression of perforant vein, even if largely accepted as hypotheses, it is not yet proved by ultrastructural evidencies. Disturbances of cavernous tumescence leads to an insufficient compression of the subalbugineal cavernous plexus, causing an increase of the cavernous outflow.

Recent ultrastructural evidencies on the cavernous tissue demonstrate the presence of synapsis with cavernosal endothelium and with synusoidal smooth muscle. This confirmed the theory of the terminal plurisynaptic innervation of the single muscle cells.

From that derives that a complete relaxation of erectile tissue requires a system of autonomic innervation. Therefore every injuries to those nervous fibers can only result in an insufficient relaxation of erectile smooth muscle. When the injury is severe, an alteration is produced in cavernous relaxation with secondary compressive disturbance of sub-albugineal venous system exiting in the syndrome of corporo-occlusive focal dysfunction.

OTHER CAUSES

Among the endocrine disturbances of the erection, we remind the hypogonadism (hypo- or hypergonadotropic), the hyperprolactinemia, the hypo or hyperfunctioning of thyroid or suprarenals and, according to some authors, the hyperparathyroidism.

The erectile dysfunction can also be consequence of local disturbances such as priapism and its sequelae, induratio penis plastica and mainly of the pathology related to the "ultrastructure" of the corpora cavernosa, that is the smooth muscles or the receptors; this represents the frontier of our current knowledge on this topic.

CONCLUSIONS

If the improvement of the diagnostic procedures and the progress in the comprehension of erectile neurohemodynamics has led to an evolution in the impotence pathophysiological classification, this has caused a parallel adjustment of the therapeutic approach, and the results can be judged more and more satisfying. The long-term follow up of thousands of patients treated with intracavernous medical therapy shows without any doubt that this treatment represents an efficacious therapeutic tool, with positive effects also on the anxiety components.

We can state that during the last decade the endocavernous injection of vasoactive drugs became the gold standard in patients suffering from erectile dysfunction.

The most modern drug for the intracavernous application is the PGE1 (alprostadil-alfadex) which acts through the phosphorilation of ATP and is metabolised within the lungs and partially also in the cavernous corpora, for this reason, it has surely less risk of priapism than papaverine and the combined therapy of Papaverine and Phentolamine.

In the long-term use it has been found a negligible percentage of erectile tissue fibrosis. The PGE1, which has experimentally shown to be active in relaxing the cavernous smooth muscles, has a very strong effect when administered by intracavernous route. A 50 mcg dose is sufficient to obtain a complete erectile response in 100% of cases if the neurovascular mechanisms are not compromised.

Moreover, PGE1 seems to have a residual therapeutic action more important than that of the papaverine. Some patients, completely impotent since many years, reported spontaneous erections with good rigidity rate during the days following the administration of a test-dose of PGE1. This confirm the fact that the intracavernosal injection of a drug can represent a real "medium-term therapy", playing the role of a vasoactive rehabilitating stretching of the erectile tissue. In this way, the side effects and the tolerance are reduced, maintaining the handling and the efficacy of the drug, with clear benefits for the patients.

REFERENCES

1. Austoni E., Colombo F. Trends for research and therapy in impotence studies. Int. J. Impotence Res. (1993) 5, 203-204.
2. Bush P.A. and coll. Comparison of nonadrenergic, noncholinergic-and nitric oxide- mediated relaxation of corpus cavernosum. Int. J. Impotence Res. (1992) 4, 85-93.
3. Greco E., Virag R. Impotenza. fisiopatologia e clinica. Ediz. Marrapese. Roma, 1991.
4. Krane J.R. Andrology, sexual dysfunction, infertility. Current opinion in Urol, 1992, 2: 443-445.
5. Krane J.R. Male sexual dysfunction. L.B. Company Edit. USA, 1983.
6. Lue T.F. World book of impotence. Smith Gordon Edit. Great Britain, 1992.
7. McMahon C.G. The return of spontaneous erections after self injections of Prostaglandin E1. Int. J. Impotence Res. (1992) 4, 179-186.

Subject Index

Note: Page numbers appearing in *italics* refer to illustrations; page numbers followed by t refer to tables.